# ETHICS OF MANIPULATION

# ETHICS OF MANIPULATION

*Issues in Medicine, Behavior Control and Genetics*

## Bernard Häring

*A Crossroad Book*
THE SEABURY PRESS • NEW YORK

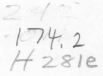
The Seabury Press
815 Second Avenue
New York, N.Y. 10017

Printed in the United States of America

Library of Congress Cataloging in Publication Data

Häring, Bernard, 1912-
   Ethics of manipulation.

   "A Crossroad book."
   Includes index.
   1. Bioethics.  2. Medical ethics.  I. Title.
[DNLM: 1. Ethics, Medical.  2. Behavior therapy.
3. Genetic intervention.  W50 H136e]
QH332.H33    174'.2    75-38960
ISBN 0-8164-0289-2

# CONTENTS

# ACKNOWLEDGMENTS

The author is greatly indebted to several institutions and to many people without whose generosity and competence this book would not have been possible.

I express my gratitude, above all, to the Joseph and Rose Kennedy Institute for the Study of Human Reproduction and Bioethics for inviting me as visiting professor and providing facilities, to the Kennedy Foundation, and especially to Mr and Mrs Sargent Shriver for continuous interest. My gratitude extends to the colleagues at the Center for Bioethics, who spent many hours discussing the subject with me, reading parts of the manuscript and offering help with the bibliography.

My special thanks go to the Director of the Institute, Professor André Hellegers, M.D., Dr LeRoy Walters, The Director of the Centre for Bioethics, Dr Roy Branson, Fr Richard McCormick, S.J., Fr James J. Doyle, C.S.C., and the always helpful and competent librarian of the Center, Mrs Doris Goldstein. My heartfelt thanks also to Mrs Alice Paroby for her most valuable and generous secretarial help.

I am grateful to the Accademia Alfonsiana (graduate school for moral theology in Rome) for freeing me from other engagements and giving time and opportunity to spend more than a year to work exclusively on this subject.

To Mrs. Josephine Ryan who again, as in various previous publications, has assisted me most generously in editing and typing the manuscript of this book, I am especially grateful. If the English is correct and the text readable, the credit is hers.

# PREFACE

Three years ago I published a book, *Medical Ethics*, on today's problems in the healing professions and in those they heal. The main perspective there is the freedom and dignity of the human person. Personal health and the health of the human society are to be measured by the criteria of freedom and of a common commitment to its growth.

In this new volume on the ethical aspects of medical, behavioural and genetic manipulation, I am applying the same lines of thought and concern to the problems of the future, while being aware that the future has already begun. It seems to me that we have to seek, above all, the ethical boundaries of manipulation, and to do this in the spirit of a dispassionate theology of liberation. We have to free ourselves and our society from all the taboos and prejudices that could block the advance of mankind, but always with extreme vigilance, in order to preserve and foster each person's dignity and freedom, and with the purpose to commit ourselves to the creation of those conditions of life that favour the growth of freedom for all people.

The content and disposition of the material of the book reflects my conviction that we can sensitize the conscience of each person and of society, regarding manipulation in the fields of medicine, behaviour modification and genetics, only to the extent that we are aware of the new opportunities to free humanity from many conditionings that are inimical to the growth of freedom, and equally aware of the manifold manipulations that threaten almost every sector of modern life.

Human freedom and health are an indivisible good. Those who receive them gratefully, as a gift from God and from those who have made efforts and sacrifices to preserve and increase them, will commit themselves not only to their own growth and integrity but also to that of their fellowmen. They will do so clear-sightedly, with convincing criteria, and will extend their joint and effective forces to the social, cultural and political spheres as well as to private life.

The problems approached here concern not only moralists, members of the medical profession and scientists. They concern all people committed to education in the Church and in the secular world, all legislators, and all mature persons who want to participate in the process of making decisions and arousing consciences about these fundamental questions that lie ahead of us and are already to be faced.

# ETHICS OF MANIPULATION

# INTRODUCTORY CHAPTER

## 1. *The relevance of this problem*

Manipulation has become a major problem in today's technical world. Outstanding scholars are focusing attention on it, and awareness is growing of the need to study all of its aspects and ramifications. There are, however, few comprehensive studies, except in the field of manipulation of the market and of public opinion.

The recent progress in biology and in the behavioural sciences has opened up totally new avenues and areas of manipulation that can be a blessing or a curse for the whole of mankind. Will the future of humanity mean a growth of liberty and of respect for everyone's freedom, or will it be shaped, managed, manipulated by the technocrats and their designs? Will the cybernetists decide what man is and what he should be? Shall we all be objects of behaviour management and of mind-changers?

The special interest of this study is manipulation in the fields of biology, medicine and psychology. Man has acquired unprecedented power to shape and reshape his biological and psychological nature. He has found new ways to liberate himself from unfavourable conditions of life. For today's citizen, respect for humanity and its world means a persistent effort to improve the conditions of life and to effect the best possible changes. Will these changes be implemented in a way that respects and

protects human dignity? Many see, in the manipulative power
we have attained, a devastating threat to the image of man
which centres on rational autonomy. We cannot avoid questions
about the ethical values that are at stake.

Humanity has now a new awareness of the many determinisms to which human life is submitted, and a growing
realization that at least some of these things can be changed in
a planned way. So we are taking nature into our hands. Matters
once decided by forces that we neither understood nor controlled
are becoming matters of human choice.[1] A full-scale planned
change includes unprecedented forms of manipulation and new
conditions to replace old ones.

The interest of this study is what manipulation means in
and for the history of freedom and liberation. What can be
manipulated? Who and what manipulates man? Who can
control the manipulators?

## 2. *The meaning of the word 'manipulation'*

'To manipulate' is of Latin origin, from *manus,* a hand, and
*pellere,* to push or *plere,* to fill. It can mean 'to get things into
one's hands' or 'to push things around with one's hands'. For
B.F. Skinner, the crucial point of departure is the hand of the
primate: what man has in common with animal. 'The primate
hand evolved *in order that* things might be more successfully
manipulated.'[2] Man 'is indeed controlled by his environment
but . . . it is an environment largely of his own making.'[3]

The word 'manipulation' was originally restricted to the
area of technology, especially in the field of mining. Only since
the end of the last century has its use been extended to other

---

[1] Cf. Amitai Etzioni, *Genetic Fix* (New York: Macmillan, 1973),
p. 188.
[2] B.F. Skinner, *Beyond Freedom and Dignity* (New York: A. Knopf
1971), p. 204.
[3] *Op. cit.,* p. 215.

fields such as psychology, psychiatry and medicine. The Oxford English Dictionary gives three senses in which the verb 'to manipulate' is used: 1. to handle, especially with dexterity, to manage, work or treat by manual and (by extension) mechanical means; 2. to operate upon with the mind or intelligence, to handle or treat (questions, artistic matter, resources etc.) with skill; 3. to manage by dexterous contrivance or influence, especially to treat unfairly or insidiously for one's own advantage.' Webster's Seventh Collegiate Dictionary also notes the unfairness of means, 'to control or play upon by artful, unfair or insidious means, especially to one's own advantage', as well as the affirmative value, 'to treat or to operate with the hands or by mechanical means, especially with skill'. So the word has various overtones according to its context. It can indicate the most beneficial achievements of man's skill and power over things; but it can also indicate the use of the most debasing and insidious means for the degradation of life and the overpowering of one's fellowmen.

With the word's gradual transferrence from its place of origin in the technical world of things to the field of life, and especially human life, there came also an attitude or outlook that to a great extent does not realize the vast qualitative difference between these fields. And therein lies our main problem. Abraham Maslow touches on the decisive point: 'I am convinced that the value-free, value-neutral, value-avoiding model of science that we inherited from physics, chemistry and astronomy . . . is quite unsuitable for the scientific study of life'.[4] Obviously he means human life, especially man 'in his inner core' and with his essential relationships.

We have to recognize the word's ambivalence and the frequent ambiguity of its use. Within the proper realm of *homo faber*, it is generally neutral or appropriate, but it acquires threatening tones and dimensions when used by those who are thoroughly shaped by a technological culture and see man only

---

[4] A.H. Maslow, *The Farther Reaches of Human Nature* (New York: Viking Press, 1973), p. 5; cf. pp. 14-15.

as a technical being, simply a manipulator. Behind the various uses of this word lies the tremendous problem of man's self-understanding in a highly developed technical civilization that must face the question to what extent methods and attitudes suitable for shaping man's environment can be applied to the shaping of human society and the realm of human life and human relationships.

It is no wonder that Skinner sees the summit of development in the total and systematic manipulation of human behaviour, since he explains man generally by comparison with animals, and especially his hand (*manus*) in the light of the hand of the higher primates. My objection is that the human hand can not only manipulate; it can and does communicate profound human relationships. To shake hands with a friend is a lie if done with intention to manipulate him, to 'push him around'. A gesture of love is as effective for and relevant to a humane world as the most skillful use of instruments and techniques to manipulate the environment. Both can contribute to human welfare and to a life in dignity and freedom.

The decisive question is whether the final orientation is given by a mainly technological view or by one of wisdom and the ability to reciprocate genuine love. The 'intelligence quotient' determined by the goals and standards of a technical culture is not man's highest endowment. 'Reason is man's faculty for grasping the world by thought, in contradistinction to intelligence, which is man's ability to manipulate the world successfully. The former is essentially human; the latter belongs also to the animal part of man.' [5]

We shall see in the course of this study that the use and

---

[5] Erich Fromm, 'Values, Psychology and Human Existence', in A.H. Maslow (ed.) *New Knowledge in Human Values* (Chicago: Henry Regnery Company, 1971), p. 160. Fromm evidently uses, in this context, the word 'intelligence' in the restricted meaning of the technocological intelligence that is measured in 'intelligence quotient' texts. The original meaning of the word, derived from the Latin *intus legere,* is to have a vision of inner meaning.

significance of the word 'manipulation' also depends greatly upon the total world view of its users. For the classical Marxist, as for the Skinnerian, everything is in final analysis a 'technology of behaviour'. [6] The manipulator, manipulated by his ideology, has his own vocabulary not only for the technical world but for the most intimate human relationships. He speaks of 'operant conditioning', 'behaviour management', 'manufacture of chimeras', of 'tailoring man', of 'inputs and outputs' in psychology, reproduction and genetic engineering.

'Manipulation' can refer also to acceptable or beneficial planned change of nature. It can mean piloting the biological or psychological nature or functions to the advantage of persons and social relationships and processes, improving behaviour through planned changes of the environment, and so on.

Even as a part of education towards liberty, mild forms of conditioning or manipulation are necessary. The question is always whether forms of conditioning and manipulation plan the use of determinisms practically to eliminate the use of freedom, or whether the manipulative tactic and practice are thoroughly subordinate to progressive education towards creative liberty and creative fidelity. In other words, certain forms of manipulation can be part of a planned change in view of greater freedom for humanity. But manipulation can also, and easily, be a means of arbitrary changes planned by a minority to exploit its fellowmen and to diminish their freedom.

## 3. *Manipulation: act, process, structures*

After exploring the various meanings of 'manipulation', one may ask who and what manipulates man? One takes it for

---

[6] Skinner, *op. cit.*, p. 25. Cf. William C. Budd, *Behaviour Modification; The Scientific Way to Self-Control* (Roslyn Heights, N.Y.: Libra Publishers, 1973), p. 49. Budd sees the essence of education and behaviour control as 'shaping technically'. The final choice is 'good riddance to man *qua* man in favour of the manipulable.' *Op. cit.*, p. 201.

granted that man's environment is in fact, and has to be, shaped and manipulated. But it is not a neutral matter how and to what purpose it is shaped and who decides about this.

We are all, by necessity, exposed to many and various influences. Human persons are interdependent, and good and bad influences interpenetrate in the world around us. But the person must never be manipulated in his inner core, never subjected to spurious or insidious influences in the use of his freedom and his search for final meaning. My attention therefore focuses mainly on those forms of manipulation that treat man as object. It will not be confined only to individual acts that intend directly to manipulate other people: that would be too narrow an approach. Each manipulative act is an investment in manipulation that takes root in human history; and there are manipulations of the environment and manipulated situations and structures in the field of technology that in many ways can threaten human freedom and dignity.

To a considerable extent we are all conditioned by our culture, and this is normal. But being conditioned can become being manipulated if we identify ourselves too uncritically with a concrete culture and fail to distinguish the liberating from the degrading elements in it. Language itself is a conditioning agent. We do share in shaping public opinion and human relationships by our use of language; but before we do, we ourselves are already conditioned by language and all the means of communication. In our spiritual, intellectual and social growth, we depend on institutions, on the structures and realities of economic life, on educational systems, social relationships, social processes. But the question is always, are these manipulating us in the pejorative sense or are they in a legitimate way influencing people for their own good?

The behavioural sciences have made us aware of the extent to which we are conditioned by all these influences. Indeed, our very freedom is conditioned by being situated in a concrete and limited world. But these sciences have also shown the actual, though sometimes limited, possibilities of growth in a common use of our freedom. To the extent of our freedom, then, it is a matter of our own responsibility if we submit passively to the manipulative structures of our environment or give ourselves over to manipulators who have no respect for human freedom.

As we become aware of the pervasiveness of manipulation and of the manipulative character of many people, it becomes easier to approach the individual phenomenon in the concrete forms of manipulation of person by person. We have to seek the causes of our vulnerability in our own personal history and in the world around us. 'Social pressure, the varied mechanisms of social control, render men manipulable.' [7]

When we face those forms of manipulation that are hostile to our freedom, we are confronted by the whole investment of humanity in oppression, coercion, deception, hypocrisy, and all the insidious means of influencing people for the selfish goals of individuals and groups. Add to this the idols and ideologies that take root in people's hearts, in traditions, customs, doctrines, and so on. The investment in inhumane manipulation operates and conditions us throughout the whole gamut of suggestions, insinuations, pressures, threats, seductive promises and unjust sanctions. And there is, besides, a powerful ally, our society's consumerism, especially when it is reinforced by widespread ideologies in a culture that confuses the distinction between the unconditioned and conditioned, between what can be marked at a price and the gratuitous gift of love. Without being aware of it, the manipulated person and the manipulators often share in a joint destructiveness. [8]

The great manipulators of the past have been the dictators, the demagogues, the exploiters, who used their ideologies and

---

[7] Heinz Otto Luthe, 'What is Manipulation?' *Concilium*, Vol. 65 (New York: Herder and Herder, 1971), p. 15.

[8] Cf. Erich Fromm, *The Anatomy of Human Destructiveness* (New York: Rinehart and Winston, 1973).

all kinds of immoral means to manipulate those whom they wanted to exploit. Today we have to add a minority of scientists, especially the behaviourists, who are convinced that they have the right and even the duty to condition and manipulate the masses.

## 4. *Conscious and unconscious manipulation*

Crucial for moral evaluation, as well as for the effectiveness of manipulation, is whether or not the subject and object of manipulation are conscious of manipulating or being manipulated. Often a part of the process is cleverly to hide the manipulative intent behind a screen of 'noble' motives, so that the manipulated person is not aware of being negatively influenced.

An uncritical mentality and a static concept of society have allowed the wealthy and powerful to preserve and even to strengthen many conditionings that are unfavourable to the development of freedom. [9] Only lately has our society acquired an ecological conscience that takes note of the interdependence between the total environment and human development or decay. The human environment can be turned into a manipulating power that can threaten not only human health but even the spirit of freedom and respect for human dignity.

The difference between pre-scientific and scientific manipulation of persons is so great that perhaps we should not even use the same word. New techniques are offered by the behavioural and other sciences for deceiving those who are to be manipulated. The skilled manipulator however, who uses these scientific tools, cannot easily conceal from his own consciousness what he is doing; yet he can somehow manipulate his moral conscience. For the technocrat, the very efficiency of his scientific methods seems to justify his manipulative plans

---

[9] Herbert Marcuse, *One-dimensional Man:* Studies in the Ideology of Advanced Industrial Society (Boston: Beacon Press, 1964).

and actions regarding people who lack his scientific knowledge. The same means by which people should be helped to overcome obstacles to freedom or to their search for truth, can be used to interfere with the normal development of their lives and their freedom. Especially in the hands of those who can summon the power of the mass media, the progress in the behavioural sciences, mass psychology and depth psychology can become dangerous tools for extending manipulative influences over the masses.

Even indirect manipulative processes are today less easily concealed from the consciences of those responsible for them. Technology assessment and similar branches of modern science are studying the indirect as well as the direct consequences of decisions about the human environment. That means that modern man can and must accept accountability for the foreseeable effects of his actions.

While the skilled manipulators are acting with increasing consciousness, this is not true of those who themselves are manipulated. The manipulator is more conscious of his manipulating action than of his own being manipulated by many conditionings. And the objects of manipulation — the masses, the poor, the underdeveloped — are only gradually becoming aware of their situation and tending to overcome their passivity.

## 5. *A new awareness and sensitivity*

While the power of systematic manipulation has grown, so also has humanity grown in awareness and sensitivity. The waves of protest, the explosions of critical minds, are protective reactions against old and new forms of manipulation which jeopardize people's freedom. The whole literature on freedom, a theology of liberation, goes hand-in-hand with the development of consciousness, the effort to make people sensitive and alert to the various forms of manipulation to which they are submitted. Strong forces are at work to help people to distinguish between those conditions and determinisms that should be changed and those which cannot yet be changed for the better. In this, we might see an analogy to psycho-analysis which brings many things from the unconscious and subconscious to full consciousness, as a necessary step towards renewed freedom, although the very tools of psycho-analysis can be, and in fact often are, abused in a dangerously manipulative way.

While one part of humanity is blinded by the ideology of technical quantitative process, others have become even more sharply aware that what is needed is a qualitative change, a change of mentality and direction that should give a new sense to all modern means and plans. Today's educated and sensitive people understand better that sin against freedom consists not only in direct and conscious manipulation of other people's minds but equally in sloth: in a failure to act against the existing conditions which oppress human freedom and block development.

There are many partial manipulations that, in the overall process of liberation and development of consciousness, can serve the history of freedom better than inactivity and sloth. A classical example exists in today's population problem. The victories of modern medicine and social planning have reduced infant mortality and enabled more people to live, to enter into marriage and to procreate. But in parts of the world, this has led to a serious population explosion and in others to grave environmental difficulties. If nothing is done to reverse the trend, people can be exposed to substantial deprivations of their freedom. In yet other parts of the world, the utilitarian technological approach has already so sharply reduced the willingness to have children, that soon the disproportion between aged people and those active in the production process will cause serious tensions. Unwarranted fear of over-population becomes, in the hands of skilled manipulators, a new tool for blinding people to basic human values such as, for instance, the life of the unborn child.

## 6. *The complexity of an ethical evaluation*

For some, manipulation is a new word for sin. However, the very ambiguity of the word forbids any generalized ethical evaluation. The fact that there are dangerous and insidious manipulations does not allow us to renounce discernment. All exaggerations and generalizations are obstacles to the serene discrimination so necessary at the present moment of new breakthroughs in biology and the behavioural sciences. [10]

Manipulation, as such, is not the great sin or a sin at all. The evil is in the transgression of the limits posed by human freedom and dignity, 'the illegitimate crossing of hierarchical boundaries', as a noted humanist (but unbeliever) expresses it. [11] Only a profound knowledge of man in his historical situation, an accurate assessment of the concrete meaning and the foreseeable and possible consequences, and the comparison of realistic choices, and of the overt and covert motives allow us to make a calm ethical evaluation of the diverse actions and processes that can be called manipulation.

To this end, I shall try to give, in a first chapter, some pictures of the various areas and forms of manipulation outside the medical and biological fields, paying particular attention to those that can interfere with people's free and full development and total health. From this basis, I shall try (in the second chapter) to find the fundamental criteria for discerning and evaluating manipulation. We should then be able to approach (in the third chapter) the main object of this study, namely, manipulation in the field of medicine, especially the medicine of the future, conditioned by the marvellous progress in biology and other sciences.

[10] Cf. Luthe, *op. cit.*, p. 17, for a typical exaggeration: 'Wherever man is manipulated, he may still persist physically (initially at least), but in the long term and without realizing it, he destroys his physical and social environment and thereby deprives himself of his basic existential principle.'

[11] Rose, Stephen, *The Conscious Brain* (New York: Alfred A. Knopf, 1973), p. 280.

## 7. *Therapy and manipulation*

Throughout this whole study, the distinction between therapy and non-therapeutic manipulation will be of paramount importance. There are unavoidably manipulative elements in education, and re-education, in the use of authority, in the whole field of the modification of behaviour, in medicine, psychotherapy and genetics (I exclude here, of course, any insidious or degrading sense of the word, any implication of an attack on people's freedom). A decisive question will be whether this or that manipulative element is an integrated part of a therapeutic process, and necessary or useful for the purpose of gradual readjustment and healing. It is not easy to determine precise limits for all imaginable cases. Almost every medical intervention manipulates or suppresses some functions in order to restore, as nearly as possible, the total health. *Again and again we are faced with the fundamental questions: What is man meant to be and to become? What is human health and wholeness? What is, then, genuine therapy?* [12]

But there is not only the problem of a holistic understanding of health and therapy. There is also the important question of whether man has a right only to such self-manipulation as is strictly necessary for therapy. Is he not also entitled to improve his historical development by conscious and direct manipulation of, for instance, his genetic heritage or the neurons of his cerebral cortex?

---

[12] Cf. my book, *Medical Ethics* (Slough: St Paul Publications, 1972), esp. pp. 42-64.

## Chapter 1

# THE MAIN AREAS OF MANIPULATION

Before we face the concrete problems of manipulation in such fields as behaviour management, brain conditioning and research, gene therapy and genetic engineering, we have to deepen and broaden our vision. Our society and its dynamics must be examined. What is sick in our society? Why does it tolerate an insidious manipulation of people in so many ways? How can we overcome the dangerous trends towards degrading manipulation in the field of medicine, and especially in the modification of behaviour and in genetic interventions?

I do not intend to give here a complete picture or a treatise on all the various forms of manipulation that pose moral problems; my choices are conditioned by a special interest in bioethics. But always it is a matter of public health — the health of the society in the broad sense of healthy or unhealthy forms of education, authority structures and so on — and a search for social remedies wherever we find degrading forms of manipulation, regardless of how acceptable they may seem to large segments of our culture.

## 1. Manipulation in the field of learning and education

If we ask why manipulation is such a complex and dangerous problem, then we must turn first to the field of learning and

13

education. These processes unavoidably contain elements which somehow can be qualified as manipulative. But the essential point is whether the process as a whole is conceived or practically carried out in the pattern of animal management, or is purposefully directed, at least in the overall of its dynamics, towards insight, motivation, goodness, a holistic vision of life, an altruistic orientation of mind, the capacity to discern values and non-values, freedom, and concern for the freedom and liberation of all people.

Education is the market-place of the various ideologies and of those who put their trust chiefly in manipulating others. In authoritarian societies and states, the whole process of education is oriented towards the submissive, manipulable citizen. Everything that could awaken a critical mind is avoided or repressed.

Learning and education lead to 'a non-inheritable, progressive and reversible change in behaviour, a change that is not attributable to maturation alone'. [1] Indeed, not all processes of learning promote a fully human maturation; some can even become serious obstacles to it. Maturation includes, above all, discernment, a sense of dignity, awareness of freedom, and motivation. There is no truly human education where there is not a constant growth in moral insights. 'The moulding of the newborn infant into an ethicizing being is not due wholly to intrinsic forces, but requires an interaction between him and his external circumstances.' [2]

Wholeness and maturation arise neither solely from nature nor solely from nurture; the process is one of interaction. 'The major ethical problems of today in the context of individual-to-individual behaviour would, I think, according to our criteria, have to be solved in those types of attitude and activity which facilitate or hinder the development of a healthy authority

---

[1] Daniel N. Robinson, *The Enlightened Machine. An Analytic Introduction to Neuro-psychology* (Encino and Belmont: Dikenson, 1973), p. 78.

[2] C.H. Waddington, *The Ethical Animal* (The Univ. of Chicago Press: Phoenix Book, 1967), p. 27.

structure'.[3] The decisive point is the use of authority in the treatment of the developing child: whether he is treated more as an object to be managed or as a partner in a process of growth, in a dialogue in which the educator as well as the young person can grow.[4]

One of the major problems in education is aggressiveness. Since the growing child wants to affirm his or her own personality, there can be aggressive reactions to aggressive methods of education. Often the educator reacts with stronger enforcements and reinforcements, and the child or adolescent is either caught in a vicious circle of aggressiveness or finally yields to passivity and easy submission. It takes a very profound education of the oppressed to make them capable of bringing about a qualitative change in their society. The beginning of liberation, the fight against oppressive and dehumanizing manipulation, begins with 'decolonizing' the child. The child must become a partner. Either learning is dialogue or it prepares the road for an oppressive and manipulative culture.

Firmness, which would include also some reinforcement or gentle punishment, cannot be lacking in the education of the child. Children cannot be spared all frustration. However, they can be motivated in such a way that conditioning does not diminish their own spontaneity and freedom. The decisive factor is always the kind of interaction that allows the child to be responsive.[5]

From the very beginning, children are extremely dependent on parental care. Gradually, however, they should be enabled to attain self-identification in growing freedom and independence. One of the educator's greatest temptations is to keep the

[3] *Op. cit.,* p. 205.

[4] Cf. Paulo Freire, *Pedagogy of the Oppressed* (New York: The Seabury Press, 1971). This is one of the major insights of Paulo Freire. There is no hope of social liberation if the educational process is thoroughly manipulative.

[5] Cf. Josef Endres, *L'uomo manipolatore* (Rome: Edizioni Paoline, 1974) pp. 100-103.

child, and then the adolescent and even the adult person, in some kind of dependence. Even affection can be a threat to liberty if it is possessive. Many researchers agree, for instance, that homosexuality is frequently due to the attitude of a mother who wants to possess the love and submission of the son for herself alone. [6]

A quite harmful feature of today's world is children's excessive exposure to television. In the United States and much of Europe, most people, at the outset of adult life, have spent more of their lifetime before television than in schools. The development of a child's capacity to interact as a partner is hampered by such constant exposure to so many strong impressions; he is, at least partially, manipulated. [7]

In a pluralistic and manipulative society, one of the most important aims of education must be to develop a critical sense; there must be education for discernment. This is possible only if the educators themselves are always open to challenge and to growth in discernment. 'Manipulation excludes the critical reasoning of the individual affected.' [8]

Luthe seems to me rather naive, however, if he thinks that our present school system and higher learning foster this critical spirit that strongly protests against manipulation. Although I do not agree with all the positions expressed by Herbert Marcuse in his book, *One-dimensional Man*, I think he has made his case and shown how much our educational system is influenced by the ideology of man-the-manufacturer, the ideologies of the market-place. [9]

Consciously or unconsciously, our public education system is to a great extent manipulated by the managers of the techno-

---

[6] Cf. my book, *Medical Ethics*, p. 184-189.
[7] Cf. Cline, V.P., et al. 'Desensitization of Children to Television', *Journal Pers. Sociology and Psychology* (Sept. 27, 1973), pp. 360-365.
[8] H.O. Luthe, 'What is Manipulation?', *Concilium* 65 (1971), p. 15.
[9] Cf. Luthe, *op. cit.*, p. 21-22.

logical culture and the consumerism typical of it. The student is 'educated' mainly for the process of production and consumption. *Homo faber* is formed to the detriment of *homo sapiens*, the discerning and loving person.

This kind of education is concerned primarily with what is directly manufacturable, manageable, marketable. The emphasis is on organization and success in the market-place. In consequence, human behaviour is largely determined by economic infrastructures and interests, by the marketable and exchangeable elements easily understood by the utilitarian, pragmatic mind. What prevails, then, in the total picture, is the kind of positivistic rationality which legitimately characterizes the restricted method of the sciences that serve technology and organization.

Nothing is to be said against this kind of rationality in its proper field. The sin is in restriction to that one dimension, an education of only the *homo faber* as member of the technological society with its rationality that practically ignores wisdom. [10] This type of rationality is at least partially blind to the scale of values, especially the higher values and the vision of wholeness. It constantly transgresses 'the hierarchical boundary lines' and invades fields that should transcend it.

The best qualified among modern scientists are aware of this danger and disturbed by it. One who has clearly discerned the phenomenon is Theodosius Dobzhansky, to whose insights this study will frequently refer. He writes, 'Dewey rightly regarded separation of science from ethics and values as "intellectual scandal".' [11] Ethics presuppose a holistic vision.

An education and educational system that care little for synthesis or a vision of wholeness shape the *homo faber*, the utilitarian man, who accepts himself as a manipulator of persons as well as of things, since he has not learned to discern. Unless

[10] Réné Simon, in *Manipolazione e futuro dell'uomo* (Bologna: Ed. Dehomiane, 1973), p. 172.

[11] Theodosius Dobzhansky, *Genetic Diversity and Human Equality* (New York: Basic Books, 1973), p. x.

he senses the flaw in the educational system and the culture that supports it, he develops no 'centre' of ordered values. Willingly or unwillingly, he becomes as easily manipulated by other people and his environment as he is inclined to manipulate others and the world around him.

The manipulative — or quasi-manipulative — elements that seem to be integral to the educational process receive, however, a totally new meaning if, in the decisive dynamics, they are oriented towards growth in insight, motivation according to a scale of values, intuition, interiorization, personal convictions and free assent to values.

## 2. *The manipulation of public opinion*

The shaping of public opinion is one of the favourite fields of the manipulator. Most human behaviour and most economic and political decisions are already conditioned by public opinion. This does not imply, however, that the conditioning is necessarily the same as manipulation in the pejorative sense; public opinion can be formed by responsible and respectful dialogue. But if many or most people refuse or neglect to participate in this fundamental dialogic task, or are unable to distinguish between insidious manipulation and genuine dialogue, then all doors are thrown open to the kind of manipulation that opposes the development of freedom and wisdom.

In today's culture, the mass media — the press, radio, television — are the most effective means of influencing public opinion. To think that manipulation is produced by the media, as such, would however, be erroneous. They can be effective means of promoting genuine and worldwide dialogue, and equally can be misused for manipulative manoeuvres.

The mass media mirror the total situation of a society, and especially its power structures. [12] Through them the 'common

---

[12] Cf. Thomas M. Garrett, 'Manipulation and Consumer Goods', *Concilium* 65 (May, 1971), p. 59.

people' have easier access to information about basic matters of culture, politics, and so on. Then there comes a moment when the masses emerge, and it is in this historical phase that manipulation can become a primary instrument for preserving the dominion and unjust privileges of the few. The very means that could allow the people to participate in a broad dialogue can become the means of manipulating them.

'Prior to the emergence of the people there is no manipulation (precisely speaking) but rather total suppression. When the oppressed are in reality almost completely submerged, it is unnecessary to manipulate them. In the anti-dialogical theory of action, manipulation is the response of the oppressor to the new concrete conditions of the historical process.' [13] Conscious and unconscious manipulation has happened and does happen in every kind of society; but the total structure of economic and political power is most decisive in the amount and forms of manipulation.

In the closed tribal societies of the past, information, education and critical capacity were kept within rather narrow limits. Tradition, custom, common religious convictions and a paternalistic style of authority almost automatically controlled the whole articulation of opinions and reflections, as well as the circulation of information. Within these limits, of course, directly intended manipulations and manipulative relationships were also possible, especially between those in power and those under them. But what typifies that kind of society is better described as uncritically accepted conditioning than as manipulation.

The tyrants of authoritarian societies could once say, 'They may hate me as long as they fear me'. Fear and the promise of 'bread and circuses' were the chief instruments of oppressive power. In modern societies, authoritarian *régimes* function somewhat differently. They take over the mass media, and

[13] Paulo Freire, *Pedagogy of the Oppressed* (New York: The Seabury Press, 9th printing 1973), p. 145.

their principal servants are the mass psychologists through whom they manipulate public opinion. This consciously contrived, and therefore more subtle and insidious kind of manipulation, becomes part and parcel of the shaping of the structures of economic, social and cultural life, of institutions and laws that condition and control information and the strictly limited participation of ordinary citizens in forming public opinion.

The dichotomy that existed in past societies between a paternalistic *élite* and the great mass of people who were taken care of was accepted as normal. If the intentions and actions of the *élite* were benevolent, the common people considered them simply as benefactors. There was less direct or conscious manipulation. Today, on the contrary, with the decline of the older cultures and traditions, a paternalistic way of telling people what they have to believe, to think and to do is usually resented; hence the powerful and overprivileged recur more to direct manipulations for preservation of the *status quo*.

In a truly democratic society there is a readiness and even an eagerness to search together for truth and truthful solutions to the problems that arise in life's new situations. Democracy functions and approaches perfection to the extent that communication is not impeded by power. Although there will always be great differences in the degree of people's intelligence, knowledge and wisdom, genuine public opinion arises only through mutual enrichment gained by listening to each other and sharing ideas. As long as a small *élite* seems to possess all the knowledge and tries only to teach or inform others about what to think and to do, there is a one-way relationship that is totally engrossed in manipulative processes.

Some neo-Marxists paint such a dark picture of the manipulative one-dimensional society, that the free democratic world seems no better off than the world under Marxist dictatorship. I want to warn against this unjust exaggeration if, in the following pages, I give a picture of the kinds and dimensions of manipulation in the competitive society.

In all times, the dominant *élite* has tried to conform the masses to its objectives and world views. The wealthy, the powerful, and those having the privilege of higher education have better access to the media of communication. The government, the military establishment, and the political parties often use these media not so much for respectful persuasion as for manipulation. On the other hand, those who want to create social unrest with slogans about freedom also capture and manipulate the public attention at times, to a point which makes impossible an open-minded dialogue with the forces that are concerned with continuity of life.

Frequently the tendency towards sensationalism, which characterizes some citizens, some journalists, and some gangsters and terrorists, can attract disproportionate public attention. Wherever the mass media prefer the chronicle of evil and sell what appeals most to passion, many people lose the capacity to see and appreciate the good and to strengthen it in our society.

Our pluralism can be a healthy challenge that invites reflection and discernment, but there is a certain myth of media pluralism that, in fact, hides a basic identicality of interests in the numerous mass media, dominated as they are more by the advertisers than by the real interests of the public. [14]

Entertainment is another and most effective means of manipulation, since people are seldom aware that a world view, or suggestions about behaviour and life style, are being communicated. 'Can one really distinguish between the mass media as instruments of information and entertainment, and as agents of manipulation and indoctrination?' [15]

The manipulative effect of mass media is by no means always the result of callous intention to manipulate, or of lust for power. Many reasons contribute to a distorted picture. Everyone bears within himself, and communicates to others, his

[14] Cf. Herbert I. Schiller, *The Mind Changers* (Boston: Beacon Press, 1973), p. 19.
[15] H. Marcuse, *One-dimensional Man,* p. 8.

own manipulated being. The necessity of communicating to a public of varied levels of education imposes a certain degree of generalization that often unwittingly becomes over-simplification. There is, besides, the necessity for almost instant reportage, which the competition within the mass media itself requires. Thus even the best and most honest journalists cannot give the full picture.

The fragmentation of modern life, the 'loss of the centre', and the decreased capacity for reflection and meditation shape the mentalities of mediators and public alike, making them both vulnerable to manipulation. [16] Journalists, readers, listeners and viewers are often so immersed in and preoccupied with the moment that they lose the sense of continuity and synthesis.

When they deliberately present messages that do not correspond to the realities of social existence, the media managers become mind-managers. 'Messages that intentionally create a false sense of reality and produce a consciousness that cannot comprehend or willfully reject the actual conditions of life, personal and social, are manipulative messages. When manipulation is successful, alternative social arrangements remain unconsidered'. [17] Not only false information, but especially the withholding or the arbitrary and intentional selection of relevant information, misleads. What is decisive is not the quantity of information but significant disclosure. [18]

Inundation of the public with all kinds of undigested information, through disputes, discussions, reflections, appeals and suggestions, easily creates a climate that perpetuates the manipulative situation. People are tempted to withdraw from commitment since, faced with such an inundation, they cannot see how to engage in debate. The result is the privatization of most of the public, which practically means submission to the mind-managers.

[16] Cf. Schiller, op. cit., p. 24.
[17] Cf. Schiller, op. cit., p. 1.
[18] Cf. Thomas McMahon, 'Manipulation and Mass Media', Concilium, Vol. 65 (1971), p. 91.

The thoroughly commercial approach of the mass media is a built-in temptation to exploit the passions and baser interests of those who buy information. Newspapers, publishing houses, radio and television stations all depend to a great extent on the good-will of advertisers who are more concerned with selling their products than with forming a mature audience. It is somehow puzzling, however, that in a society that suffers greatly from violence and terrorism, the mass media can still produce, without being strongly challenged, so much 'entertainment' and 'news' that appeal to people's inborn aggressiveness. Here again we have the vicious circle of a public already manipulated by its own aggressiveness, and perpetuating and deepening the condition.

A sense of hopelessness or helplessness on the part of the public is a potent ally of manipulation. It takes the form of silence, since a constructive and liberating dialogue cannot be carried on in the existing climate. 'If the dialoguers expect nothing to come of their efforts, their encounter will be empty and sterile, bureaucratic and tedious.' [19] A pessimistic analysis of the dimensions of manipulation could lead to this kind of hopelessness. We must therefore explore the possibilities for remedying the situation.

In all fields, manipulation of people's minds is a threat to human freedom and dignity. The question arises, 'who controls the controller?' Often, citizens want to avoid their responsibilities by calling for government controls. But the solution lies rather in the involvement of many people in the various media, on their own initiative and out of their own desire to communicate and to participate in a liberating dialogue. [20] And those who want to participate must be aware — and wary — of the deeply rooted desire to dominate others and to manipulate them. Indeed, along with a lack of respect for other persons, the deepest source of all manipulation is the lust for power.

[19] Cf. P. Freire, *op. cit.*, p. 80.
[20] Cf. Schiller, *op. cit.*, p. 186.

What we need above all is education for discernment, and a constant effort to detect manipulation and to check the mind-managers. We should all contribute to building up a widely-held, profound and loudly articulated conviction that the manipulation of persons cannot be an instrument of rehumanization. We need clear and pure motives to communicate in mutual respect and, in the process of communication, to learn from and with all those involved.

However, criticizing from the outside does not change the situation. Critical thinking is helpful to the extent that it is the expression of an indivisible solidarity between society and the individual person; but it is a virtue only to the extent that it is part of a commitment to change the world for the better. 'For the critic, the important thing is the continuing transformation of reality on behalf of the continuing humanization of man.' [21]

The role of the *élite* is of paramount importance. As long as the social and religious *élites* think in a paternalistic way and consider the general public only as objects or as inferior people to be taught and informed, they betray their proper role. Elitism is inimical to the freedom and development of all mankind. Genuine leadership in the process of liberation and humanization means dialogue, co-responsibility and education in a common process of growth towards maturity and discernment. Only they truly belong to the religious and/or social *élite* who make the best contribution to the development, maturity and discernment of all their fellowmen.

Sociology has shown that a rather small minority of one to three per cent is decisive in the formation of public opinion. It must be our concern, therefore, to form *élites* that listen as well as speak in a dialogue, and consider everyone as an equal partner from whom much can be learned.

The Church, in her preaching and teaching, should be an example of this kind of dialogue. It is true that she has received

[21] Cf. P. Freire, *op. cit.*, p. 81.

from Christ a deposit of revelation, and she is not allowed to betray it. It is very important, however, to distinguish divinely revealed doctrine from mere human opinions, regardless of how strongly they may grow into convictions. But even in the matter of the knowledge of divine revelation, nobody has a monopoly. We are all called together to grow in the knowledge of God, of Christ, and of man.

This emphasis on co-responsibility certainly does not allow the *élites* to abandon or avoid their significant function; it helps their members to understand their *rôle* better. Karl Menninger has made a strong appeal to members of the *élite*, especially the clergy, doctors and journalists, not to renounce their prophetic *rôle*. And by making his case in the best tradition of the prophets, he also shows the way of dialogue and liberating respect.[22]

## 3. *Manipulation in advertising*

The mass media are manipulated to a great extent by the powerful advertisers. Advertising itself is a privileged arena for the 'hidden persuaders'.[23] Mass-psychology is already producing the skilled manipulator in this field. To think that advertising influences only the purchase of certain things is naive. Rather, it creates a whole consumer mentality, creating new needs — especially artificial ones — and distorting in the hearts of many people their scale of values. Advertisement suggests that the person is what he buys.[24] People exposed for hours each day to such advertising gradually begin to measure everything, including their own values, in a quantitative way, as consumer

---

[22] Cf. Karl Menninger, *Whatever Became of Sin?* (New York: Haw-thorn Books, 1973) and my book, *Sin in the Secular Age* (Slough: St Paul Publications, 1974).

[23] Cf. Vance Packard, *The Hidden Persuaders* (New York: McKay, 1957).

[24] Th. McMahon, 'Manipulation and consumer goods', *Concilium* 65 (1971), p. 90.

goods are measured. They begin to measure progress and development by the quantity of goods one can buy and consume. A culture so shaped by the hidden persuaders loses insight into the hierarchy of needs. [25]

Modern advertisement has its power through the mass media but has it also from a culture of consumerism to which it then lends its own dynamics.[26] Thus the manipulating power of advertisement goes far beyond the fields of production and consumption.

Think, for instance, of the constant use of sex appeal in relation to things that, of themselves, have nothing to do with sex. Vance Packard's sardonic note is apt. 'The personal-enhancement industry has been insistently advising young females that their personal success in life is measured by their effectiveness in inspiring passes from males. And these, it is suggested, are directly related to the olfactory or visual allure a girl achieves by employing advertised products. And the boy is urged to beef up his pass-making power with girls by using the advertised scent.' [27] So sex becomes an article for the consumerist society. No wonder that, in books written by pro-abortionist doctors, the woman who seeks an abortion is spoken of — and spoken to — in marketing language simply as a 'consumer'. [28]

---

[25] Cf. Abraham Maslow, 'Psychological data and value theory', in Maslow (Ed.) *New Knowledge in Human Values* (Chicago: Henry Regnery, 1971), p. 119-136.

[26] Cf. W. Dreier, *Funktion und Ethos der Konsumwerbung* (Münster, 1965); W. Franke, *Der Manipulierte Mensch. Grundlagen der Werbung und Meinungsbildung* (Wiesbaden, 1964).

[27] Vance Packard, *The Sexual Wilderness* (New York: Simon Schuster (1970), p. 54.

[28] Howard T. Osofsky and Joy D. Osofsky (Eds.) *The Abortion Experience: Psychological and Medical Impact*. (New York: Harper and Row, 1973); Charles V. Ford comments: 'The use of marketing terminology minimizes a complex medical-emotional situation and tends to place it in the category of a hair-dressing appointment.' *JAMA* Vol. 228, No. 5 (29 April 1974), p. 634.

An equally disturbing example is the insistent advertising of psychotropic or 'mood' drugs by the drug industry. In 1973, Great Britain's drug industry spent thirty-three million pounds on advertising and only thirty million on research.[29] The United States' six billion dollar industry spends even more. John Pekkanen tells us that 'as a nation we are now purchasing, according to some estimates, more than 250,000,000 mood-drug prescriptions each year.'[30] Television viewers, deluged day by day with magic pictures of instant relief, through pills, from almost every trouble and problem of life, come to consider pills as panaceas. Those who are already partially manipulated by an ideology that promises instant happiness are especially vulnerable. They become unable to face difficulties with their normal psychic energies. 'The drug industry's wilful manipulation, done to maintain profits, has created social consequences that are only now becoming fully understood.'[31]

Again, it is not easy to define the boundaries between legitimate persuasion when useful things are offered, and spurious manipulation of millions of people when artificial and even dangerous needs are created. It is evident, however, that people need a very critical attitude and should not unnecessarily expose themselves, day by day, to the 'hidden persuaders'.

## 4. *The modern economy and manipulation*

Classical Marxism, especially in the form of Stalinism, is an elaborate system that allows, with a good conscience, the manipulation of people in the service of economic processes. The basic belief is that economic development according to dialectic materialism guarantees the best human development.

---

[29] *The New Scientist,* 18 April 1974, Vol. 66, No. 894, p. 107.

[30] John Pekkanen, *The American Connection. Profiteering and Politicking in the 'Ethical' Drug Industry,* (Chicago: Follett Publishing Company, 1973), p. 329.

[31] John Pekkanen, *op. cit.,* p. 14.

This ideology is, to a great extent, inherited from the classical liberalism of Adam Smith. The manipulation congenial to Marxism can also be violent, since the theory is that inherent growth of history makes growth in violence unavoidable. When the supreme magisterium of Marxism determines that a certain phase of economic development calls for changes in the supra-structures of cultural, political and ideological forms, then any manipulation of people seems to be justified.

I want to stress, however, that what is said against the dialectic materialism of classical Marxism is not a rejection of any and every form of socialism. Forms of socialism can be developed in the service of the maximum freedom and dignity of all persons.

Inherent in a competitive capitalistic society is the tempta-tion to manipulate economic processes and the people involved in them for the purposes or advantage of the powerful. The manipulator draws his greatest strength and justification from a widespread determinism promoted by sciences in the service of the technological society.[32] Behind many individual acts of manipulation that degrade the freedom and dignity of persons, stands the ideology that equates technological progress with human progress.

Not only Marxism but also a great many western scientists and technocrats have made a myth of technological progress, and expect from its uncontrolled growth 'the big society'. [33] But while the technological society has developed a high degree of skill in planning and futurology, it is, as a whole, irrational. 'Its productivity is destructive of the free development of human

---

[32] Cf. A. Koestler, *The Ghost in the Machine* (London: Hutchinson, 1967); Jacques Ellul, *The Technological Society* (New York: Knopf 1964; London: Jonathan Cape, 1965).

[33] Cf. Victor C. Ferkiss, *Technological Man: The Myth and the Reality* (New York and Toronto: New American Library, 1970); Alvin Toffler, *Future Shock* (New York: Random House, 19th printing, 1972).

needs and faculties.' [34] The technological culture destroys, or at least is a hindrance to man's higher capacities for contemplation and altruism. The dynamic of constant expansion, constant economic growth is, of necessity, accompanied by the creation of artificial needs while often man's most basic needs are not served because they are not seen. Whenever the positivistic sciences, including the behavioural sciences, neglect the hierarchy of values, they become the servants of power, militarism, and of wealthy minorities.

The ideology of private property in the service of uncontrolled economic growth leads to a loss of liberty for the masses. Those who regulate the tools of technology regulate also the workers, their families and their whole fate. They are manipulators in the service of a manipulated and manipulating system. 'Technological rationality has become political rationality.' [35]

Again and again, the wealthy form alliances against the weak. Yet this system of competitive, capitalistic society leads also to a continuing battle among the wealthy themselves. It is the cause of numerous wars. Stephen Rose probably hits the nail on the head when he suggests that Darwin's one-sided theory of selection and fight-for-survival reflects the ruthlessness of both capitalism and liberalism in his time. He had before his eyes daily 'nature red in tooth and claw'. [36] Darwin himself was manipulated by the fact that he and his times accepted uncontrolled capitalism as an unavoidable phase of development.

Human freedom is bound up with effective structures. Man is dependent on, or even at the mercy of the regularization of those power structures which contain manipulative processes. Interventions are not possible without a minimum of behaviour-

---

[34] Marcuse, *op. cit.*, p. ix.

[35] Marcuse, *op. cit.*, p. xiv.

[36] Rose, Stephen, *The Conscious Brain* (New York: Alfred Knopf, 1973), p. 283.

manipulation of those who are not willing to co-operate in freedom and respect. [37] So again we see that man can free himself only gradually from the tendency to manipulate not only things but also persons, since he himself is imbedded in a manipulative society and in inhuman manipulative processes. What is crucial always is the direction in which development, and especially the whole intention, is moving.

## 5. *The manipulating use of authority*

The evil of degrading manipulation originates in the lust for power, in man's desire to domineer over others, to possess and to use them. [38]

For his own protection, the human person needs healthy authority structures from the very beginning. The child owes his origin to his parents and depends upon them, but he becomes a mature person only if, from the very beginning, the parents consider the child as a person who has a right to develop towards freedom, discernment and co-responsibility.

Of necessity, parents make many decisions for the child and sometimes have to impose their reasoned will on the reluctant child. This can be called 'manipulation', but it has not the character of a degrading manipulation if it is integral to a parent-child partnership in which the child is recognized in his or her own dignity and right to develop a mature personality. A liberating education is based on dialogue which, as soon as possible, allows children to express themselves, to pose questions and to receive honest responses. Thus they develop a balanced, critical mind and gradually learn discernment. Punishment given without reasoning and without a liberating motive is always manipulation in a negative sense.

[37] Cf. K.W. Merks, 'Social Cybernetics or Social Ethics', *Concilium* 65 (1971), p. 52.

[38] Cf. K. Menninger, *Whatever Became of Sin?* (New York: Hawthorn Books, 1974), p. 108.

A marked interdependence exists between the style of authority in the family and in society at large. Where the accepted attitude in marriage and the family is authoritarian, a society is condemned to authoritarian regimes.

Dictators are always manipulators. Throughout history they have used even religious ideas and symbols — like the 'oath of allegiance' — to manipulate their subjects. In a dictatorship, everyone is manipulated. In a class society, where power and the right of decision-making are in the hands of the few, all others in the population are practically manipulated. The same is true in international relations, where powerful nations manipulate the powerless in many ways. In this context we speak of 'neo-colonialism'. While classical colonialism is outright oppression or exploitation, neo-colonialism hides the manipulative processes.

The ideal democracy is based on the equal rights of all citizens and allows for the broadest possible participation in decision-making processes. However, we have to remind ourselves that, from an authoritarian past, and especially from an authoritarian family system, a perfect democracy cannot arise at once. A long period of pedagogy is needed, beginning with the 'decolonization' of the child and of women, in order to awaken a critical mind in the whole society.

A gradual liberation from manipulative approaches calls for a loyal opposition. Where there exists no right or real opportunity to oppose, then an *élite* or a bureaucracy takes over the powers of decision-making. Either it considers itself as the holder of the truth in a kind of infallibility, or else it practically denies binding truths and norms. In either case it reserves to itself all the decisions, which are then imposed on others.

The opposition in democratic states will fulfil its function effectively only to the extent that, within the parties, there exists a readiness for dialogue, sharing and even honest disagreement. [39] When people renounce the desire to domineer

---

[39] Cf. Eugen Kogon, 'The Significance of the Opposition in the Party System of Democracy', *Concilium* 65 (1971), pp. 97-106.

over others, they can join with the conscience of all who sincerely search for truth and for truthful solutions to the problems that arise in society. [40]

Examples of arrogation of unwarranted power and of dishonest, manipulative processes by those in power are by no means lacking in our own democratic system. One of the most shocking took place when the seven judges of the Supreme Court deprived the state legislators, and therefore also the citizens of the United States, of participation in any decision about action to protect human foetuses against the arbitrary decisions of mothers and doctors to abort them. The judges' document in *Roe v. Wade*, which tries to justify the sudden change in the constitution as understood in a long tradition, is a model of manipulative language, and even more of a manipulative power structure. The point is not that the legislators' decision might be different but that it would at least be less manipulative, since it would allow the citizens their constitutional right to participate by expressing their convictions in open dialogue and by electing their candidates. [41]

The spirit of the radical manipulator is totally expressed in the prejudice that, since the foetus in her womb is not viable, a mother can arbitrarily dispose of it. In a society that considers abortion on demand as a woman's absolute right, manipulation is 'in'. There is then little hope of resolving other problems of manipulation. If the human foetus has no right whatsoever to be considered in its human dignity before birth, it can hardly be expected that the new-born child will be spontaneously accepted in its own right to development.

It is true that pro-abortionists and anti-abortionists sometimes try to manipulate public opinion and the legislators, but the situation is far more serious if citizens accept a judiciary

[40] Cf. *The pastoral constitution on the Church in the modern world* n. 16.

[41] Cf. Paul Ramsey, 'Protecting the Unborn — How Do We as People Determine the Outer Limits of Human Community?' *Commonweal*, Vol. 100 (31 May 1974), pp. 308-314.

power that does not allow for dialogue and imposes on them its lonely decisions with no ground either in the constitution or in the whole tradition of a society. Matters as grave as whether or not the human foetus is a concern of our human community, and whether or not it has a right to life, surely call for the broadest possible dialogue and the greatest care to avoid any form of manipulation. 'Dialogue does not impose, does not manipulate, does not domesticate, does not sloganize.' [42]

The authority of the state has neither the duty nor the competence to legislate in morality as such: moral convictions and decisions arise from within people's consciences. However, a society can live as a free society only when it shares common convictions and fosters a dialogue about the basic rights and values without which people cannot live together in peace and freedom.

'The principle of government by consent of the governed is the surest guarantee of individual liberty devised by man'. [43] Reinforcing just laws which reflect a society's moral convictions does not, then, at all bear the mark of unacceptable manipulation, since the law-breakers can know that the society is not imposing on them the interest of only a small minority. At times, however, a false pathos can be created in the interests of radical change, which so undermines authority that pressure groups can take over and manipulate the majority. Healthy authority structures are an absolute condition for our existence in freedom and dignity. [44]

In our advanced technological and scientific cultures, the scientist and technocrat have great power. It is normal that, within their competence, they should participate in the process of decision-making. Yet, not infrequently, scientists and technocrats are *élitists* who tend to arrogate to themselves the right

[42] Paul Freire, *Pedagogy of the Oppressed*, p. 168.
[43] Archibald Cox, *Civil Rights, the Constitution and the Courts* (Harvard University Press, Cambridge, Mass., 1967).
[44] Cf. C.H. Waddington, *The Ethical Animal*, p. 205.

to decide for the masses. Their decision can be a dangerous form of manipulation, especially when they see the whole of human life in a perspective of technology and science, and thus transgress the boundaries indicated by man's dignity and freedom. There is surely a legitimate domain for manipulation in the field of science and technology as such, but those techno-crats and scientists who do not respect persons tend to transfer manipulation into the field of human freedom and dignity. [45]

By her special vocation, the Church is expected to be an effective sign and school of liberty. Manipulations within the Church, and any attempt by her authorities to interfere in a manipulative way in the life of citizens, have therefore to be forcibly rejected. Often in the past, the Church was to a great extent manipulated by civil authorities and conditioned by the authoritarian system of society. The basic principles of the functioning of Church authority, such as subsidiarity and collegiality are, by their very nature, dialogical and anti-manipulative. However, we cannot forget that those who exercise authority and participate in dialogue within the Church bear in themselves all the manipulative input of family and society. The Church herself is only in the process of liberating herself from unacceptable forms of manipulation, and can succeed only to the extent that Christians are committed to liberation at all levels. There is need for ongoing education, dialogue and discernment.

Only in a shared effort at a development of consciousness can the Church become aware of how, in the past, political forces have manipulated her and seduced her to manipulate even the *kerygma*. She was skillfully used as a shield and pro-tector of the establishment. She has also, by identifying herself too much with Latin or other occidental cultures, sinned by her cultural invasion of people belonging to quite different cultures.

---

[45] Cf. Leslie Gould, *The Manipulators* (New York: David McKay, 1966).

## 6. *Manipulation by a permissive society*

Especially in a permissive society, a serious threat is manipulation by a certain kind of 'freedom' literature. In the name of 'freedom and liberation', a minority tries to impose its opinions, its individualism or its collective egotism on a whole society.

The permissive society lives and acts in a full-scale reaction against puritanism and rigorism. It is allergic to authority and to principles. But in turn, it tends to make permissiveness itself an absolute principle that should be adopted by all. The intolerance of this reactionary permissive society — and of certain new liberals — is often even more intense than that of an earlier rigoristic society. People who still have principles are labelled as Manicheans, outdated, passive, and so on. The manipulative slogans and the aggressive intolerance of the 'permissive' groups is a particular danger for those not educated in discernment and therefore not able to unmask and counteract this ideology.

The growing permissiveness in our society, coupled with the intolerance of the permissive subculture, causes reaction by the other side, and eventual new forms of repression.

## 7. *Manipulation of the environment and through it*

God has entrusted the earth and all that exists on it to the freedom and responsibility of humankind, created in his image and likeness. Man is free to use and to buttress the nature around him as long as he does so as that image and likeness. That means that the environment he creates has to manifest him specifically as an image of God who wants all people to grow, as persons, to their full human capacities.

In the book of Genesis, man's right to submit the earth to himself — to shape and manipulate his environment — is

related to his calling to celebrate before God, to find his repose
and peace with God and to praise him. Whoever does not adore
the true God does not recognize the message written in all
created things: that they are a gift of the one Father, entrusted
to the whole of mankind for the benefit of all. Whoever does
not adore the true God loses his inner freedom (cf. Rom
1 : 18-32).

Especially during the past few decades, a new ecological
consciousness has developed in mankind. We have become
aware of how greatly human behaviour depends upon and is
conditioned by environment. Although the crucial factor for
human growth and health is human relationships, it cannot be
denied that even those very relationships are to some degree
conditioned by the realities of the subhuman environment, the
world in which we live. It is unthinkable, therefore, that the
healing profession and the Church can fulfil their task today
without making people more sensitive to the meaning of their
environment. [48] The ecological crises have thrown new light on
the basic truth that God is the creator of all the world and that
the earth entrusted to mankind should praise him, and on the
essential dogma that Christ is the Saviour not only of individual
souls and persons but of the whole world. It makes no sense
to preach salvation to people without caring for an environment
that promotes the wholeness, health and salvation of all mankind.

Shaping the environment is one of the most important
expressions of man as a cultural being. The environment bears
the imprint of his goodness, his justice, and of his sinfulness.
It manifests somehow the scale of values, or lack of them, in
any culture.

[46] Cf. 'Manipolazione nella Chiesa', in *Manipolazione e futuro dell'uomo*
(Bologna: Ed. Dehomiane, 1972), pp. 287-290.
[47] Cf. Canial Cappon, 'Environmental Psychology and Psychiatry',
*Science, Medicine and Man*, Vol. 1 (1973), pp. 123-133; Paul R.
Ehrlich, Anne Erlich and John P. Holdren, *Human Ecology. Prob-
lems and Solutions* (San Francisco: Freeman, 1973).
[48] Cf. Karl Menninger, MD., *Whatever Became of Sin?* (New York:
Hawthorn Books 1973).

The growth mania of our technological age has already thoroughly endangered our human environment. [49] Each enterprise wants to grow, to expand, and the national economy is evaluated according to the rate of expansion. Of course consumption has to grow too. As a consequence, a depleted environment reflects little sensitiveness to the growth of the human being as person. Technology depletes the human environment and causes an enormous threat of water and air pollution, with unforeseeable consequences for the lives of persons and societies. [50]

An alarming development in our time is unbalanced urbanization: millions of people living in overcrowded cities with no space for children, where people have to cope with constant noise and unhealthy living quarters and conditions. Often this situation is the result of shameful manipulation of land and building costs, or of zoning ordinances and social pressures that successfully exclude from suburban areas the 'lower' classes and races, even when such families have given sustained evidence of responsibility for property and for the upbringing of their children. There is no longer any doubt that life in miserable urban agglomerations is a threat even to the gene pool. It engenders insecurity, promotes violence, and produces numerous forms of neurosis and psychosis, all of which contribute to the erosion of the whole society.

In the past few years, a new branch of science known as 'technology assessment' has developed rapidly. Technological initiatives are assessed in terms of their foreseeable impact on man and his environment. [51] But again, the general trend seems

---

[49] Herman Daly, in *Toward a Steady State Economy* (San Francisco: Freeman, 1973), speaks very plainly about this growth mania.

[50] Dr T. Rose (Ed.) *The Effect of Technological Advance on Environment, Life, Society* (New York-London: Gordon and Beach, Science Publishers, 1969).

[51] Cf. David Hamilton, *Technology, Man and the Environment* (New York: Scribners, 1973); Dedek Medford, *Environment Harassment or Technology Assessment?* (Amsterdam-London-New York: Else-

to be to look on the environment mainly from the point of view of technological resources and success. Human health is being taken more and more into account, but not sufficiently. Especially mental health, in a holistic vision of human health, wholeness and salvation, is not given enough attention. The 'Club of Rome' has done much to make public opinion more sensitive and to encourage a broader assessment.

Ethicists have to make a painstaking effort to see all ethical issues in their relation to the total human environment. This means a call to human freedom and responsibility about shaping our environment. The first step would seem to be a consistent application of a proper scale of values to our ecological responsibilities. A scale of values can be as high and as beautiful as possible, but it remains sterile if it is not incorporated in the human environment.

## 8.  *The manipulating power of ideologies*

Manipulators who themselves are manipulated by ideologies are often the most dangerous. To fight manipulation in a concrete case, or in a certain field such as medicine, is rather hopeless unless the manipulating power of idols and ideologies is first unmasked.

An ideology can make skillful use of ideas, moral ideals and human aspirations for the advantage of a certain group. The use, or rather misuse, of partial truth is to a certain extent unrecognized by the manipulators and even more by those who are manipulated.

To explain how an ideology operates, we need depth

---

vier Scientific Publishers, 1973); Marvin J. Cetron and Bodo Barfocha (Eds.) *Technology Assessment in a Dynamic Environment* (London-New York-Paris: Gordon and Beach Science Publishers, 1973).

psychology, psycho-analysis and mass psychology. [52] Only a deep personal conversion and a communal renewal can break the power of an ideology. Here I mention a couple of ideologies which will recur and will concern us constantly in this study.

Technological man is legitimately a manipulator. He has the right and duty to use his skills to manipulate things and conditions in his environment, for the benefit of mankind. However, he is a slave to ideology if he measures everything by criteria appropriate only to the field of technology. Often the readiness to manipulate man himself — thereby transgressing the hierarchical boundaries allowed by man's total vocation — is due to the ideology of the scientists and technocrats who consider themselves the ones most competent to determine what human life and persons should be. The ideology of the priority and supremacy of science and technology celebrates its feasts in classical Marxism but also in the western world.

The technocrats and scientists first determine that their approach is 'value free'. This could be reasonable in the sense that science itself cannot determine final moral evaluation. But often the scientists mean that their findings and the applications of them are not to be submitted to any judgment of morality or religion. Hence they make themselves the judges of the measure of all things, and even of man himself, and so come to the theory that science is 'beyond freedom and dignity'. As we have already seen, this ideology has made strong and lasting investments in our total environment, in our culture, and in our economic and political establishments.

The fight against drug addiction and the tendencies to use drugs systematically as 'mind changers' cannot be won without first unmasking the underlying ideologies that promote massive

---

[52] I do not intend to treat this important question in greater detail, since I have done so in my book, *Sin in the Secular Age* (Slough: St Paul Publications, 1974), pp. 89-96. Cf. W. Post, 'Ideology', *Sacramentum Mundi*, Vol. III (New York: Herder & Herder, 1969), pp. 94-97; Jürgen Habermas, *Knowledge and Human Interest* (Boston: Beacon Press, 1971).

manipulations in this field. There is a mixture of the utopia of 'instant happiness', the cult of efficiency, and of consumerism and utilitarianism. The patient effort to increase human freedom and preserve human dignity is disregarded. [53] Both drug abuse and the mystifying drug advertisement are culturally conditioned through ideologies and behaviour patterns. Generally speaking, the drug advertisement is not false but misleading and misled by the most dangerous ideologies of our cultures. [54]

In all fields it is difficult to obtain non-manipulated information. Dialogue is most fruitful when all those involved are aware of the need to free themselves thoroughly from any ideology: that is, from any distortion of truth that arises from the hidden or overt selfish intentions or viewpoints of individuals and groups.

Some universities have established chairs for 'the critique of ideologies'. This can be a first step towards liberation from the manipulative power of ideologies and social prejudices if it stimulates awareness and creates a concrete and systematic effort to expose them. [55] There would be little value, however, in a critique on a merely theoretical level. No substantial contribution can be made towards exposing these prejudicial slants unless the people involved in the study are existentially committed to conversion and renewal at all levels. The scientific tools of sociology, social psychology, depth psychology and philosophy would be available, but these tools can be effective only in the hands of people who are willing to free first themselves and then others from all kinds of ideologies and to dedicate themselves to the truth and to a sober scale of values.

---

[53] Cf. Skinner, *Beyond Freedom and Dignity*, p. 111. This ideology shows through quite clearly. Skinner himself is affected by this kind of ideology. He would say that everyone, including himself, is 'conditioned' by his total environment. We might say 'manipulated', wherever an ideology and its advertisers are operative.

[54] Cf. Oakley S. Ray, *Drugs, Society and Human Behaviour* (St. Louis: The C.V. Mosley Company, 1972), p. 275, cf. pp. 3-15.

[55] G.W. Allport, *The Nature of Prejudice* (Reading: Addison-Wesley, 1954).

## 9. *The vicious circle*

All the literature on liberation opposes the manipulation exercised by the oppressive establishment; yet much of this literature remains within the vicious circle when it calls for violent revolution. Those who want to carry out the revolution simply by violence do not truly liberate themselves; nor do they treat as partners in a patient dialogue those whom they want to liberate. Lacking the profound experience and conviction that liberty arises from within, and that only what is freely done with inner conviction is truly good, they are impatient. Today's myth of instant efficiency and our culture's ideology of instant happiness make their own contribution to this impatience for an instant solution through violence. [56]

Only a dialogical, non-violent action can free man from the vicious circle of manipulation and violence. This calls for humility before God, the experience of our union with God and of the unity of all mankind. Christian hope, the eschatological vision of history, does not allow a superficial trust in instant happiness and liberation. Christian freedom needs growth in endurance and perseverance.

## 10. *The manipulated ingrown group*

Certain groups exercise an enormous amount of manipulation over all those who want to be 'in'. Solidarity with the group, and unanimity, become idols. The individual renounces his own conviction in favour of the powerful team. [57]

The careerist who wants to be 'in' with the powerful group will gradually develop a very selective conscience. The classical example is the self-righteous 'pharisee' of all times, who feels

---

[56] This is well explained by James W. Douglas, *Resistance and Contemplation, The Way of Liberation* (New York: Delta Book, 1973).
[57] K. Menninger, *Whatever Became of Sin?*, p. 96.

that he is virtuous because he follows the meticulous rules of
his group. In the name of group solidarity he is ready to torture
those who challenge the group's ideology or interest. The team
player has his very specific kind of consciousness. The literature
on the Watergate scandal has given abundant documentation
on this point.

In today's society there are groupings of liberals who fear
nothing more than the label 'conservative'; it is like a social
death warrant. They would rather offend truth and justice than
risk that label. The same is true, but in reverse, of certain
conservative clubs or groups. This tribal coherence is, for
instance, behind the fanaticism of some groups in Northern
Ireland. It is characteristic also of the spirit of 'The Wanderer'
and of 'Catholics United in Faith'. Sometimes the only way to
regain one's own conscience and freedom is by having the
courage to leave the group. The one who promotes the truthful
idea of solidarity is the good Samaritan who, acting according
to his human conscience, frees himself and others from group
discrimination.

## 11. *Manipulative polls*

An unbiased study of social behaviour and public opinion
can greatly serve a growth in consciousness which increases
inner freedom. But many sociological studies and polls are
carried out in the service of the market, of politics, of ideologies,
and so on. Polls can be, and frequently are, manipulative.

In the eyes of many competent people, Kinsey's studies on
the sexual behaviour of the human male and female were, in
their very set-up, manipulative. The great publicity they received
influenced sexual behaviour not only in the United States but
in many other countries as well. When Kinsey and his associate
researchers seemed to have proved that fifty-one per cent of the
male population of the United States had some kind of homosexual experience, many more were led to seek such experience:

they wanted to be considered 'normal' according to this new standard. However, not only the poll itself but also the way the various responses were pulled together was exceedingly manipulative. [58]

These biased polls occur not only in politics, in market interests, and in connection with sex ideologies, but even in religious matters. Some years ago, a group of people who had prepared a poll on the matter of celibacy proposed to me their outline of questions. I tried to show them that the formulations of their questions were highly manipulative, since the very formulation suggested a certain response and implicitly labelled people who did not think their way. One person responded to my objections, 'But we do not want only to know about people's thinking; we want to change their attitudes. That is why we are making this investigation.'

A poll can have a final intent to change attitudes, but if it is not to be manipulative, then it first has to discover, through non-manipulative and non-suggestive questions, what people really think. Only then, in a second round, can there be a respectful effort to change attitudes by genuine persuasion. To use good arguments and to engage in dialogue for persuading people is not manipulative. It is a good thing to know first what people are really thinking, and why, before we start our dialogue and offer our own opinions, convictions and arguments.

[58] See Alfred C. Kinsey, Wardell B. Pomeroy, Clyde E. Martin, *Sexual Behaviour in the Human Male* (Philadelphia and London: W.B. Saunders, 1948), pp. 610-666; Wardell B. Pomeroy, *Dr. Kinsey and the Institute for Sex Research* (New York: Harper & Row, 1972), pp. 75-78; 126-127; 417-418; 423-427.

*Chapter 2*

# CRITERIA FOR DISCERNING THE MEANING OF MANIPULATION

In view of the tremendous power which scientific progress has given and will give to humanity to shape its world and to change even major traits in the human species, we are forced to look for criteria of judgement. We need first the virtue of a critical discernment that allows us to distinguish the proper fields of manipulation and to distinguish the boundary between the manipulation of things and of biological 'nature' and the manipulation of the human person in his inner sanctuary of freedom. For this we need, above all, mature people who excel in wisdom and goodness. But we also have to ask for objective criteria, since these grave problems must be resolved through dialogue and by sharing the search and our limited findings.

## A. OBJECTIVE CRITERIA:
## WHAT IS MAN MEANT TO BE AND TO BECOME?

We cannot expect from theology all the answers to the enormous problems that arise from a better knowledge of evolution and from new scientific insights. Humanity's growth in wisdom has not equalled its growth in scientific research. Yet we should not be pessimistic. If, in sincere conscience, we

44

all unite in searching for ultimate values and for a scale of values that allow us criteria, our situation will not be hopeless.

## 1. *The humanness of human nature*

The present chaos in such fields as behaviour modification and genetic engineering would not have developed if the first concern had been about a theory of essential human values. Lacking that, scientific research is constantly threatened by a 'conspiracy of success'. [1] Technological man, the purely empirical scientist, is always tempted to ask only whether 'it works'. Even very daring scientists are aware of this trend. 'The danger that the entire culture may become technological is obvious.' [2]

If the scientists are unable to check their own power of manipulation and to use it wisely, it is not their fault alone; rather, the technological culture that embodies the spirit of our era and the kind of education they have received incapacitates them. 'Study in the realm of philosophy and introspection is generally considered as a non-essential diversion not directly related to the preparation of future members of the industrial society, and the inference that man can succeed better in this world if he doesn't invest much time learning about his relation to it, further promotes the divergence between the technical world and that of ideas.' [3]

Theologians, philosophers and ethicists bear a good deal of responsibility for the unwillingness of many scientists to look for critical discernment and to accept objective criteria. We should try to understand their reactions against the traditionalism of moralists who so often taught as eternal principles what were only 'time-bound expressions', and whose conclusions were understandable only because of a lack of information. Philosophy

[1] Daniel N. Robinson, 'Therapies', *American Psychologist*, Feb. 1973, p. 132.
[2] J.M.R. Delgado, *Physical Control of the Mind* (New York: Harper & Row, 1971), p. 18.
[3] *Op. cit.*, p. 19.

and ethical teaching were often uninformed about the experiences, reflections and insights of the natural sciences and the behavioural sciences. They could not promote an integrated vision of life because they disregarded the facts of life known to the scientists.

On the other hand, scientific training itself tends towards such a high degree of specialization that many scientists remain, almost of necessity, imprisoned in a very partial vision of life. Sociologists sometimes tend to overlook not only creative freedom but even the contributions of empirical psychology; behaviourists see only the environmental conditionings; and geneticists sometimes explain everything by genetic determinisms. Yet we need absolutely the broadest possible interdisciplinary dialogue in order to grow in our knowledge of man and to reach convincing criteria for discernment.

But who can promote this dialogue, and what should it look like? We can agree with Delgado when he says that this can no longer be 'a purely speculative endeavour', but an exploration in a new direction already traced with scientific landmarks.' However, things are not so clear anymore if, as Delgado asserts, 'today, science is providing the means to co-ordinate the diverse fields of philosophy and biology to form a new basis of inquiry into the nature of man.' [4] The diverse sciences can, to be sure, help to co-ordinate dialogue, but it must be a dialogue that transcends the mere scientific empirical approach. A holistic approach must govern the inter-disciplinary dialogue which, by its very nature, would then give full attention to all of the results and the ongoing inquiries of the empirical sciences.

The modern concept of nature in general, and of human nature and its inborn needs and finalities, can no longer be the same as in an era when creation seemed to be a finished work and the first man was considered the model of all men. [5] In our

---

[4] *Op. cit.,* p. 19.
[5] Cf. H.J. Müller, *The Modern Concept of Nature. Essays on Theoretical Biology Evolution* (Albany: State Univ. of New York Press, 1972).

inquiry we need, surely, the modern scientists' sense of accuracy, but we also need the capacity of the prophets to see behind the phenomenon and discover ultimate meaning in a vision of wholeness. [6]

People who are experts in important scientific fields, and are also prophets or philosophers, can make a major contribution. They continue the tradition of the great physicians of the past who were philosophers; they want to know how to serve man in his quest for wholeness. There are scientists who are primarily concerned with man's ethical vocation and nature, and who try to discover God's revelation in the book of creation, just as there are theologians who try to discover it in scripture and in sacred tradition. [7] Psychologists, especially, who were or are also great therapists have made most valuable contributions to a better knowledge of man and of his ethical vocation. Among many others, I should like to mention Erich Fromm, Erik Erikson, Gordon Allport, Abraham Maslow and Viktor Frankl. [8] We can no longer speak of human nature and natural law without integrating the findings and reflections of the great scientists and therapists who are concerned about the limits of manipulation. [9]

Pessimism about man's capacity to find ultimate meaning and

[6] Cf. Abraham Heschel, *Who is Man?* (Stanford: Stanford Univ. Press, 1965).

[7] Cf. T. Dobzhansky, *Heredity and the Nature of Man* (New York: Harcourt, Brace & World, 1964); C.H. Waddington, *The Ethical Animal* (Chicago: Univ. of Chicago Press, 1960; Phoenix Book 1967); *Science and Ethics* (London: Allen and Unwin, 1942); R. Hooyass, *Religion and the Rise of Modern Science* (Edinburgh-London: Scottish Academic Press, 1972).

[8] Cf. Erich Fromm's main works: *Man for Himself; Escape from Freedom; The Art of Loving;* V. Frankl, *Man's Search for Meaning. An Introduction to Logotherapy* (London: Hodder and Stoughton, 1964). A. Maslow, *Motivation and Personality* (New York: Harper, 1954). *The Further Reaches of Human Nature* (New York: Viking Press, 1971).

[9] Cf. Carlo Caffaro, 'Legge morale naturale e manipolazione dell'uomo' in *Manipolazione e futuro dell'uomo* (Bologna: Ed. Dehomiane, 1972), pp. 253-283.

to recognize binding moral values is one of the greatest dangers for the future of man. Pessimism has ever been non-productive or counter-productive, and in this particular context it serves either to maintain the *status quo* or else to impose on others any kind of arbitrary change. For men and women to commit themselves to helping our species to attain an ever deeper knowledge and realization of our human nature, they must believe that mankind can become fully human. [10]

Joseph Fletcher, especially in his latest writings, is a shocking example of how agnosticism, combined with pragmatism, leads to the justification of any kind of manipulation. [11] His agnosticism is about the nature of man, and even about the true countenance of love; so that he can assert that a sexual reproduction by and in the artificial placenta is more 'human' than what nature provides. He also dares to say that the child is not yet human and the adult is no longer human if he is below a certain I.Q.

The great psychologist, Abraham Maslow, gives valuable indications by turning our attention to the deepest observable human experiences, which he calls 'peak experiences'. [12] He does not deny that some people can be so imprisoned in the search for material welfare and success that they are unable, or almost unable, to have such experiences. But a mature person has moments in which he or she experiences certain values — sincerity, unselfish love, gratitude, admiration, the goodness of other people — with such intensity that there can be no doubt in one's mind that this is something truly human, and that what is opposed is inhuman. [13]

[10] Cf. Leon Eisenberg, 'The Human Nature of Human Nature', *Science* 176 (1972), p. 124.

[11] Cf. Joseph Fletcher, 'Medicine and the Nature of Man', in *Science, Medicine and Man,* Vol. I (1973), pp. 93-102.

[12] A.H. Maslow, *Religions, Values and Peak Experiences* (Columbus: Ohio State Univ. Press, 1964).

[13] A.H. Maslow, 'Psychological Data and Value Theory', in A.H. Maslow (ed.) *New Knowledge in Human Values* (Chicago: Henry Regnery, 1970), pp. 119-136. This whole volume, with contributions

The heart of the best natural law traditions is the assertion that the best human qualities, like creativeness, spontaneity, caring for others, and capacity for gratitude, are not things imposed but are inborn. Similarly, Maslow insists that his study of fully humane people, and of moments in which they realize what humanness is, does not point to any kind of behaviour management but rather to the inner potentialities of mankind. 'We can certainly now assert that at least a reasonable theoretical and empirical case has been made for the presence within the human being of a tendency towards, or need for, growing in a direction that can be summarized in general as self-actualization or psychological health or maturation, and specifically as growth towards each and all of the sub-aspects of self-actualization. That is to say, the human being has within him a pressure (among other pressures) towards unity of personality, towards spontaneous expressiveness, towards full individuality and identity, towards seeing the truth rather than being blind, towards being creative, towards being good, and a lot else. That is, the human being is so constructed that he presses towards fuller and fuller being, and this means pressing towards what most people would call good values, towards serenity, kindness, courage, knowledge, honesty, love, unselfishness and goodness.' [14]

The greatest scientists emerge from the narrowness of their specific fields and show their capacity to reach out to a vision of the origin, scope and centre of human existence. 'Only when the spirit has learned to contemplate what God has made', says Johann Kepler, 'will it learn also what God has commanded. Only as one is deeply, ethically absorbed in the profound meanings of what he is doing, can he operate creatively and co-creatively'. [15] If, as responsible Christians and theologians,

---

by such scientists as Theodosius Dobzhansky, Gordon Allport, Kurt Goldstein and others, is a most encouraging example of how scientists can elaborate a holistic view in inter-disciplinary dialogue.

[14] *Op. cit.,* pp.125-126.

[15] Kenneth Vaux, *Biomedical Ethics. Morality for the New Medicine* (New York: Harper, 1974), p. 60.

we insert ourselves into the inter-disciplinary dialogue with the various sciences, we do not speak from the viewpoint of a single science but are concerned about a vision of wholeness, of ultimate meaning. We are well aware that we have constantly to learn from scientists, but we are also grateful that our faith and the tradition of believers has given us valuable insights into the meaning of our human nature. [16]

## 2. *The heart of the matter: man is a person, not a thing*

The final concern and criterion in discussing manipulation is human freedom. Man should exercise his freedom in the legitimate domain of manipulation, which is the submission of the earth to himself. But above all, he has to gain the inner freedom to be, to love, to adore. He must not allow anyone to manipulate him in his inner sanctuary, his conscience, his self-interpretation, and his reaching out for meaning and for significant personal relationships.

This is already a theme of the first chapters of the book of Genesis. God has entrusted all things to man; therefore the human person is a free steward not only of inert matter but of the plants and the animal world. He is meant to be a co-creator with God, and not just a user or consumer. Created in God's image and likeness, he is to imprint this same image and likeness on the world around him.

The fundamental condition for being truly free while acting as manipulator of the world around us is our sabbath, our repose before God. Only if man transcends himself and recognizes the gratuity of all creation and of his own call to be a co-creator, can he submit the earth to his own dignity. 'I am arguing for an understanding of human creativity which sees its mutuality with divine creativity. I prefer to think of human ingenuity as co-creativity with God'. [17]

---

[16] Cf. Paul Ramsey, *Fabricated Man. The Ethics of Genetic Control* (New Haven: Yale Univ. Press, 1970), p. 23.

[17] Kenneth Vaux, *Op. cit.*, p. 57.

Man has a creative mission not only with regard to things. Far more, he is meant to be co-creator with God in transforming human life in the direction of wholeness and fulfilment. It is absolutely necessary to see the enormous difference between the creative manipulation of things, and one's own anti-manipulative development in freedom, awareness and love, although these two different realities are inter-related.

With respect to himself, man's creativity lies primarily in his relationships with God and with his neighbour. His relations with the world around him should be effective; with God, and with individual persons and the human community (his neighbour), they should be affective. His highest creativity and dignity is in self-transcending love and genuine personal relationships. Each person discovers his own uniqueness and becomes his own artist to the extent that he recognizes the unique name of each of his fellowmen, and enhances their freedom and self-awareness.

But this does not mean that man's relations with the impersonal world and the personal world have no connection. One who finds his repose in his Creator and develops healthy relationships with his fellows will recognize something more in the created world than opportunity for consumption and management. And reciprocally, one who sees in the world around him the beauty, the splendour that invites him to adore God, will more easily develop healthy relationships with his fellow-men. If man loses the spirit of admiration and adoration, his manipulation of the world becomes depletion and alienation.

This vision, which the western world has often lost, is strongly emphasized in Mahatma Ghandi's theology of non-violent liberation. For him, the way of total liberation is through the profound consciousness of our union with God, which makes us ever more aware of our union with our fellowmen and with all of creation. Ghandi's vision is not something left over from an ancient Hinduistic vision that sees souls in all plants and animals; it is a Christian vision that recognizes all creation as a gift to mankind, a sign of God's loving presence and an invitation to reverence and respect in the use of all things. It invites to solidarity in the transformation of the world, so that all people can grow in self-awareness, inner freedom, creativity, and self-transcending human relationships.

Man becomes more and more an image and likeness of God, a co-creator and co-revealer, as he unites with his fellowmen to shape the world with a view to the freedom and co-responsibility of all mankind. Whoever approaches this transformation as a shared task in humanity's growth, experiences the world, not as 'fate' or as conditioning or as a prison of lust and greed, but as a gift of the one God and Father of all, a common heritage and a shared responsibility. Once we consider the world around us not just as 'my world' but as 'our world', then we become truly creative, and our own inner freedom and dignity develops as we make our own unique contribution to the common task.

Erich Fromm describes the free, anti-manipulative growth of the human person and community. 'Well-being I would describe as the ability to be creative, to be aware, and to respond; to be independent and fully active, and by this very fact, to be one with the world. To be concerned with *being* and not with *having*, to experience joy in the very act of living, and to consider living creatively as the only meaning of life.' [18]

Man is more than a user, consumer, manipulator of the world; he is an artist, and he grows in awareness and dignity while transforming the world, provided he sees his highest creativity in mutual respect and reverence in all his human relations. Rootedness in healthy relationships makes the world man's home. When he does not develop these diverse dimensions of his creative liberty, the will to destroy arises, and man becomes self-destructive. [19]

One who grows in his inner freedom and in self-transcendence becomes more and more aware of the yearning of

[18] E. Fromm, 'Values, Psychology and Human Existence' in Maslow (ed.) *New Knowledge in Human Values*, p. 163.

[19] Cf. E. Fromm, *Op. cit.*, p. 152-155.

the created world to have a share in the liberty of the sons and daughters of God (cf. Rom. 8:18-23). When he responds to this longing of the world by cherishing and transforming it in common freedom, he grows richer in his relationships with his neighbour and with God. Yet man must be careful never to confuse persons and things. He will try to get things into his hands, to submit them to himself; but before the other person, he should stand in awe and reverence, in respect for each person's freedom.

## 3. The one-dimensional man

As long as a person is caught in the vicious circle of 'one-dimension', he can never be more than a manipulated manipulator. The manager and organizer of the technical age is constantly tempted to consider himself only as a producer, a manufacturer, a user, organizer, consumer, and thus is caught in conflicting interests. One who knows only the single dimension of the marketable and organizable is the unredeemed person, the creator of the competitive, exploitive and violent society. Whoever lives all his life in the market-place, without any higher perspective, will always degrade his fellowman, will try to 'manufacture' him, to use, manipulate and consume him.

As he one-sidedly develops his manipulative capacities, the one-dimensional man becomes ever more dangerous. The Second Vatican Council gives a shaking description of the vicious circle of a one-dimensional world. 'Whatever is opposed to life itself, such as any type of murder, genocide, abortion, euthanasia, or wilful self-destruction; whatever violates the integrity of the human person, such as mutilation, torments inflicted on body or mind, attempts to coerce the will itself; whatever insults human dignity, such as sub-human living conditions, arbitrary imprisonment, deportation, slavery, prostitution, the selling of women and children, as well as disgraceful working conditions where men are treated as mere tools for profit rather than as free and responsible persons: all these things and others of their like are infamous indeed. They poison human society; but they do more harm to those who practise them than to those who suffer from the injury. Moreover, they are a supreme dishonour to the Creator.' [20]

Nikolai Berdyaev, whose whole life and philosophical-theological work give witness to creative liberty, sees 'objectivation' as the great enemy of liberty and liberation. [21] Berdyaev's first accusation is not against the scientists; he sees the danger of objectivation, above all, in philosophy and theology. What he rejects is an approach to ideas that looks for pure objectivity, that speaks of reality in an uncommitted way. Truth and persons become part of a 'thingified' world. They become marketable. Man becomes a number, evaluated and judged as a member of the black, white or yellow race, identified with a wealthy or powerful social class or with poverty. Practically, in a non-existential philosophy and theology, objectivation robs the person of his human dignity and freedom.

Whoever philosophizes without being existentially concerned with his own freedom and that of his fellowmen confines himself in an alienated world of objects. Cold objectivation narrows to the last degree the meagre outlook of the one-dimensional man. His fellowman is not revered or treated as an end in himself (Immanuel Kant), but only as a means. The dialectic materialism practised by Stalin and others is the bitter fruit of objectivation by one-dimensional men. Then the economic and other processes and relationships of human life are determined by the producer-consumer relationship. Any philosophy and theology that has no place, or only a secondary place, for the uniqueness of the human person, self-transcending love, and adoration produces the one-dimensional man, the manipulated manipulator.

An ethics of manipulation is concerned with any manipulation that jeopardizes human freedom and dignity. [22] We have

---

[20] *The pastoral constitution on the Church in the modern world*, n. 27.
[21] Cf. Paul Klein, *Nikolai Berdyaev und schöpferische Freiheit* (unpublished dissertation, Rome: Accademia Alfonsiana, 1974).
[22] Cf. F. Ferrero, *Manipulación* (Madrid: Perpetuo Socorro, 1973), pp. 99ff.

no reason to reject all forms of manipulation, but we must oppose any intention and practice that wants to treat a human person as if he were a thing. If we are to esteem ourselves as human persons, we have to oppose any action that endangers or practically denies anyone's humanity, his unique dignity and capacity to grow in freedom. [23] The decisive criterion in respect to psychological manipulation is concern not just for one's own freedom but for the freedom of all human beings.

I have recognized and praised the great scientists who search for ultimate meaning and warn against the danger of the one-dimensional man. The whole training of scientists, however, and the trend towards extreme specialization, create an institutionalized temptation to reductionism. Many scientists live so thoroughly in their specialization that they become increasingly unable to see the total picture of human life. They come to believe that they can decide what men should do and should become, according to their technical and scientific capacity to manipulate them, and thus they commit the sin of reduction.

Too many behaviourists, brain-changers and genetic engineers are blind with regard to human freedom. The result is that the deterministic world view of the one-dimensional man no longer sees any limits to manipulation. 'This is the combination of boundless determinism with boundless freedom.' [24]

Freedom is indivisible. It demands wholeness. The main problem for anthropology and ethics, therefore, is the overcoming of a radical objectivation that practically reduces the living person to a mere object, and limits him to a kind of knowledge and science concerned chiefly with control and utility. Where the vision of and dedication to wholeness is lost, what is identifiable becomes what can be produced. [25] In the

---

[23] Cf. Alberto Di Giovanni, 'Manipolazione e persona', *Manipolazione e futuro dell'uomo* (Bologna: Ed. Dehomiane, 1972), p. 296.

[24] P. Ramsey, *Fabricated Man*, p. 92.

[25] F. Föckle, 'Experimentation in Clinical Research', *Concilium*, Vol. 65 (May, 1971), p. 81.

technical and scientific world, the principle of isolation — the isolation of a single phenomenon — is a necessity, but in practice it leads to great dangers wherever scientists transgress the boundary lines and build their philosophy and ethical justifications on that isolated reductionism. Isolation and abstraction cause 'fade-out', and 'fade-out' is separated by no more than a hairbreadth from dilution. The human reality cannot be divided into isolated pieces. [26]

In view of the tremendous power to manipulate man in various ways, we must all be concerned with encouraging a deeper vision of wholeness. Everyone, including the scientist, needs to be made sensitive to the hierarchical boundary lines between things and persons. But only if we live fully all the dimensions of our own existence — our relationship with God in adoration, with our fellowmen in altruism and genuine respect, and with the created world in that solidarity which arises from faith — can we resist the dangers and temptations inherent in the one-dimensional approach of the individual sciences.

The vision of wholeness is particularly important in the field of medicine. Health is intimately related to wholeness, and total health can be described as the fullest possible capacity to develop relationships with God, with one's neighbour, and within the community. No one can find his true and healthy self without finding his place in the world around him, in openness to the other and to the community. [27] Those who confine themselves to a single dimension of human life tend to develop various kinds of psycho-somatic illnesses. According to Viktor Frankl, they are the most vulnerable to all forms of noogenic neuroses. Any treatment that jeopardizes the vision of human

---

[26] Dietrich von Oppen, 'Ethische Fragen um das moderne Arzneimittel', *Zeitschrift für evangelische Ethik* 9 (1963), p. 241.

[27] Cf. D. Wayne Montgomery (ed.), *Healing and Wholeness* (Richmond, Virginia: John Knox Press, 1971); David Belgum (ed.), *Religion and Medicine. Essays on Meaning, Values and Health* (Ames, Iowa: Iowa State Univ. Press, 1967); J. Bodamer, *Wege zu einem neuen Ich* (Freiburg-Wien: Herder, 2nd ed., 1968).

wholeness or the desire to reach out for wholeness is a road to unacceptable manipulation.

What I am speaking about here is a more complex concept than the traditional teaching of Catholic moral theology about the principle of totality in medical interventions. My approach includes this emphasis, but it is based on a broader concept of health as wholeness, and would define healing as aiming chiefly for wholeness.

## 4. The conditions of freedom and of its growth

'Freedom' is the key word when we seek for valid criteria to distinguish acceptable from unacceptable interferences or manipulations. So we ask ourselves first what we understand by freedom. The legalist thinks about man's obligation and capacity to obey and to abide freely within the law. The behaviourist asserts the freedom of a scientific élite to condition, to manage and to manipulate the behaviour of those who do not possess its knowledge and capacity for scientific management. The ethicist thinks, above all, about a person's inner freedom: his capacity to long for ever-growing knowledge of what is good and truthful, the capacity to love what is good and to put it into practice.

I am not, of course, dreaming of an absolute or unlimited human freedom. 'The variable overlap of the voluntary and the involuntary in human behaviour is a perennial mystery.' [28] Man has inborn drives — sex, for instance — which are to a great extent like blind forces. Their development and control depend on symbols, experience, cultural patterns, and personal and communal response. [29] Freedom is confined to each person as a germ, a talent or potentiality that cannot be preserved unless it is developed. It has to be learned and practised. It is an achievement of civilization. If we want free people, then we

[28] K. Menninger, *Whatever Became of Sin?*, p. 76.
[29] D.F. Delgado, *Physical Control of the Mind*, p. 240.

have to educate children in appreciation of freedom and in the art of growing in freedom.

Growth in freedom, and in discrimination between what is genuine liberty and what is its counterfeit, is mankind's greatest achievement. Throughout life, each person participates in the creation of this sensitiveness and openness to freedom. The process, however, is a most complex interaction of his genetic heritage with the culture, the language, the people around him: with his total environment. Ulysses says in Tennyson's poem, 'I am a part of all that I have met'. But the great difference is in whether we allow ourselves only to become a part, or, on the other hand, discern, screen, choose, and make all that we have met a part of us, in accordance with our own inner freedom and in awareness of our total vocation.

The individual freedom of each one of us is a part of the total history of the freedom of mankind. It was earned and passed on to us by all those who went before us. Gratitude for what we have received from the past, and awareness of our responsibility for the future, call us to explore the meaning and conditions of creative liberty and creative fidelity in our own era, and to seize the present opportunities to increase our own freedom and that of our fellowmen.

The freedom that I mean cannot be split into pieces. We cannot justly evaluate and foster our personal freedom without being equally concerned for the liberation of all. This concern is an essential limitation to arbitrary freedom; but it is also an essential condition for the growth of freedom and of its right understanding. It is, more than anything else, a matter of human solidarity. Our freedom can grow, thanks to all the past generations who made deposits of freedom in culture, social life and politics, in language, legislation and customs. But it cannot take root in our hearts unless it is also growing in the world around us as an on-going investment. [30]

[30] Cf. George Gurwich, *Determinismes sociaux et liberté humaine* (Paris, 1955) and *La vocation de la sociologie* (Paris, 1957). B. Häring, *Marriage in the Modern World* (Paramus, N.J.: Paulist-Newman Press, 1965), pp. 33-70.

Our genetic heritage, our environment, our culture, our life in the Church and in the secular world, are also limitations of our freedom; but they, too, are at the same time conditions for its growth for us and for all mankind. A clear understanding of the interaction between the total environment and the growth or diminishment of freedom must stimulate our interest in identifying and investigating the factors, reasons, and mechanisms of our dependence, on the one hand and, on the other, our capacity to increase liberty throughout our lifetime, both in our own inner being and in the world around us. We have to expose and eliminate the unnecessary and unjust limitations to our freedom and all oppressive manipulations in the Church and the secular world. But even more, we have to unite our energies to invest creatively in that freedom which communicates itself and inspires a growth of freedom in each individual and in the community. [31]

The battle for freedom and liberation is never over. Man is 'a creature that lives subject to natural pressures from which it frees itself by means of culture, thereby subjecting itself to new pressures which it creates and can again surmount'. [32] So the battle is an ongoing process to which all should be committed in solidarity. To win it, we need above all a sharp awareness that freedom is our most precious good, and awareness also of both the opportunities to increase it and the dangers that threaten it. Awareness is the first line of defence against degrading manipulation. However, the crucial factor is not a mere defensive attitude but our creative participation in the history of liberty and liberation.

Welfare in the affluent society has relieved much human hardship, but it has also taken away many challenges to growth in freedom. Take, for instance, the tendency of modern medicine to prescribe not only 'pain-killers' but a number of psycho-

---

[31] Cf. Karl Rahner, *Freiheit und Manipulation in Gesellschaft und Kirche* (München: Kösel, 1970).

[32] K.W. Merks, 'Social Cybernist or Social Ethics', *Concilium*, Vol. 65 (May, 1971), p. 52.

active drugs for minor difficulties which people could and should overcome by revitalizing their own inner resources. It seems that many doctors, as well as their patients, have practically forgotten that freedom and the capacity to grow in freedom are most precious elements in our own human health. So it is not only the massive manipulations which may be ahead of us but also today's actual medical practice that threatens the growth of man's freedom to cope with his minor health difficulties and his necessary adaptations. 'The greater the potential for autonomous adaptation to self and others, and to the environment, the less management of adaptation will be needed or tolerated.' [33]

## 5.  Awareness of sin

The history of each person and of all mankind is a struggle between the powers of sin and manipulation and the forces of freedom and liberating love. Any talk about freedom becomes meaningless when we forget the reality of sin. More than anything else, it is sin that threatens our freedom.

Manipulation is sin wherever it unnecessarily or unjustly jeopardizes, limits or destroys our freedom. Sin is the misuse of freedom, or equally, a refusal to use freedom to the best purpose. Each sin inscribes itself negatively in the history of freedom. It is an investment of obstruction to freedom in man himself or in his environment. But there are sins that are, in a very particular way, directed against human freedom and people's capacity to grow in it. [34] Among them must be enumerated all manipulations that diminish a person's self-interpretation, self-awareness, and his or her active insertion into the history of liberation.

We see human freedom in the light of creation: a creation that includes evolution, the gradual overcoming of chaos. I consider the freedom of mankind as the summit of all evolution

---

[33] Ivan Ilich, 'Medical Nemesis', *The Lancet* II (May, 1974), p. 921.
[34] Cf. B. Häring, 'Capital Sins Against Freedom', in *Sin in the Secular Age* (Slough:  St Paul Publications, 1974), pp. 151-154.

and of all history, if it is truly freedom for God, for our neighbour, for genuine love, justice and peace. Human history lives on hope that looks towards this final fulfilment of freedom. But in our interpretation of history and human life, awareness of the power of sin is crucial. We see our environment and our genetic heritage as 'an uneven and careless work'. [35] As Christians, we realize that there is an imperfection inherent in the created reality which calls man to be co-creator with God in bringing himself and the world to greater perfection. But there are also imperfections and real failures that are caused by man's sinfulness, by his unreadiness to do the good that he could do and to avoid the evil that he could avoid.

The history of freedom is not just a matter of development and a fight against chaotic forces. Above all, it is a battle against sin. And it has to be fought in hope. It would be easy to show that all major questions of ethics are influenced by the comparative concepts of sin and redemption. [36] The pessimistic moralist, stressing warnings, prohibitions and sanctions, emphasizes more the power of sin and the misery of sinful mankind than the liberating energy of grace and people living in grace. Pessimism leads to a kind of fatalism; it has never changed the world for the better. 'Pessimism about man serves to maintain the *status quo*. Men and women must believe that mankind can become fully human in order for our species to attain its humanity.' [37]

Those whose attention is captured more by the sinfulness of mankind than by the message of redemption and liberation react in alarm and shock to the power of modern science and technology to shape and reshape the world around us and to

---

[35] C.H. Waddington, *The Ethical Animal*, p. 203.

[36] Charles Curran, *Politics, Medicine and Christian Ethics. A Dialogue with Paul Ramsey* (Philadelphia: Fortress Press, 1973), pp. 174-176. The author exemplifies this with the diverse approaches of Paul Ramsey and Karl Rahner.

[37] Leon Eisenberg, 'The Human Nature of Human Nature', *Science* 176 (14 Apr. 1974), p. 124.

plan for profound future changes. They are unable to distinguish soberly between piloting changes and degrading manipulations; their reaction against courageous change is often wholesale condemnation. In the face of such pessimism, whether in the secular or in the religious sphere, the task of courageously promoting the good and opposing the dangerous trends becomes difficult indeed.

At the other end of the spectrum is a superficial optimism. The amazing progress of science and technique since the last century was accompanied, to a great extent, by a well-known philosophy of history that presumed that evolution and history produce, of necessity, ongoing progress and continuing humanization. This led to the conviction that scientific and technological progress was simply the summit of evolution, and that therefore, whatever science and technique could achieve was good. There was a striking lack of discernment of the difference between technological progress and progress in humanity, wisdom and unselfish love. Karl Marx adopted this philosophy of history and came to believe that progress of the economic infrastructure, including the necessary increase in tensions and class hatred, would, of necessity, lead to the highest development of the human race.

The good news of redemption tells of the basic goodness of creation and the final victory of redemption over sin. It is a message of human freedom, an appeal and a challenge to mankind to join the Redeemer and Liberator in the battle between wisdom and pride. There is no human progress without constant fight against the powers of darkness that would use the new knowledge for evil ends. Progress in science and technology is a great good if it is submitted to the discernment of wisdom.

6. *A static and a dynamic view of human nature*

In an approach to the ethical problems of manipulation, there is a fundamental choice between a static and a dynamic view of human history and nature. [38] Most of our moral principles and our teaching about natural law have traditionally been based on a rather static vision of history and human nature. But the Second Vatican Council, after exploring major cultural changes, new insights into human history, and the new powers of the various sciences, asserts: 'History itself speeds along on so rapid a course that an individual person can scarcely keep abreast of it. The destiny of the human community has become all of a piece, where once the various groups of man had a kind of private history of their own. Thus the human race has passed from a rather static concept of reality to a more dynamic, evolutionary one. In consequence, there has arisen a new series of problems, a series as important as can be, calling for new efforts of analysis and synthesis.' [39]

Moral theology has to draw its conclusion from this statement or be sincere enough to reject it. This 'effort of analysis and synthesis' concerns medical ethics and the many new ethical questions posed by the progress in biology, with particular focus on the problem of an ethics of manipulation. [40]

Our ethical reflections should not project the boring image of a God who conserves his work only by eternal repetition. 'Changelessness or eternal repetition or return is the acme of futility.' [41] It is true that profound changes disturb many people who had a false image of God as an immobile conservator, and who therefore sought security in unchanging dogmatic formulations and an equally unchanging code of morals. Yet they should have been taught better by Christ's own vision and words. 'My Father has never yet ceased his work, and I am working too' (John 5:17-18). Man the adorer is a co-creator with God in the ongoing creation.

[38] Josef Endres, *L'uomo manipolatore*, pp. 14-15.
[39] *The pastoral constitution on the Church in the modern world*, n. 5.
[40] Cf. Stacey B. Day (ed.), *Ethics and Medicine in a Changing Society* (Univ. of Minneapolis, Medical School, 1973).
[41] Theodosius Dobzhansky, *Genetic Diversity and Human Equality*, p. 111.

Creation is an unfinished work that calls for man's co-operation to bring it to greater perfection. And man himself is an unfinished work, called to become an ever better image of God. Therefore he can be faithful to himself and to his Creator only by striving for progress in a creative way. He is a cultural being. He never simply adjusts himself to nature. Rather, as co-creator and co-revealer with God, he has to take nature into his hands to transform it in accordance with his goal to grow in his capacity to reciprocate love and to discern what enhances human dignity and what blocks it.

'Wherever human life is involved, nature and culture are quite intimately connected. The word "culture", in its general sense, indicates all those factors by which man refines and unfolds his manifold spiritual and bodily qualities. It means his effort to bring the world itself under his control by his knowledge and his labour. It includes the fact that by improving customs and institutions he renders social life more human both within the family and in the civic community.' [42]

One of our great questions is, 'What is man meant to be in evolution and history? Is he a mere spectator or, perhaps, the spearhead and eventual director?' [43] He is the only being who knows about evolution. He can and must interpret it and find out his *rôle* in the continuing creation. Not only is he called to heal the wounds that sin has inflicted, but even more, to participate in the construction of the best possible world.

Since people of our era have gained a new capacity to know the course of evolution, they have also a new possibility and calling to co-operate in it creatively. If we look back on the whole of evolution, as reconstructed by scientific research and revealed by the word of God, we can say that humanity is evolution's greatest success. Humankind has gained the ability 'to adapt its environment to its genes as well as its genes to the

---

[42] *The pastoral constitution on the Church in the modern world,* n. 53.

[43] Theodosius Dobzhansky, *Op. cit.,* p. 116.

environment. This ability stems from a novel, extra-genetically transmitted complex of adaptive traits called "culture" '. [44]

We believe that the whole of evolution and history cannot be simply explained as fate, hazard or chance, nor is everything determined by iron laws. Max Planck's 'theory of quantities' and the 'uncertainty factor' as explained by Heisenberg give us some intuition about dynamism and openness in evolution. But once man has the power to interpret these dynamic forces and to open up their possibilities, then the divine mandate to submit the earth to himself includes his mission to be the spearhead of further evolution, especially of an ongoing hominization. The dogmas of creation and redemption shed their promising light on this dynamic vision of evolution and history.

Man has to be vigilant for the present opportunities to co-operate creatively with the dynamics of evolution and history. [45] But if we want to be more than manufacturers and manipulators, if we want to be co-creators with God and co-revealers of his love and wisdom, we cannot confine our attention to the scientific and technical possibilities. We have to cultivate the spirit of contemplation, the search for ultimate meaning.

The Second Vatican Council, after having affirmed the dynamic vision of evolution and history, poses the question, 'How can the vitality and growth of a new culture be fostered without a loss of living fidelity to the heritage of tradition? This question is especially urgent when a culture resulting from the enormous scientific and technological progress must be harmonized with an education nourished by classical studies as adapted to various traditions. As special branches of knowledge continue to shoot out so rapidly, how can the necessary synthesis be worked out, and how can man preserve the ability to contemplate and to wonder, from which wisdom comes?' [46] Our prin-

---

[44] Theodosius Dobzhansky, *Op. cit.*, p. 113.
[45] Cf. Herbert J. Schiller, *The Mind Changers* (Boston: Beacon Press, 1973), p. 15.
[46] *The pastoral constitution on the Church in the modern world* n. 56.

cipal concern must be to develop the whole human person harmoniously, in absolute reverence for each man's dignity and freedom, and in common striving for wisdom.

The dynamic vision of evolution, history and man's nature is not just a matter that concerns moral casework. It also makes us aware of the necessity to give people an education that enables them to grasp the meaning of the inborn dynamics of human nature. This is surely a great challenge to both the secular society and the Church. Especially the ethicist should see his task clearly in this direction. [47]

But while there are reasons to warn against a too static vision of the past, there are also reasons to warn against an extreme reaction to it. I can see the meaning of Delgado's reflection, 'We may wonder whether man's still ingrained conceptions about the uncontrollable self are not reminiscent of the ancient belief that it was completely beyond human power to alter omnipotent nature'. [48] The conclusion that Delgado draws for the new ideological and technological revolution, however, and the extent to which he would allow direct interventions in people's fate and their brains, go far beyond a balance.

## 7. Futurology and eschatology

Not only whether we have any eschatological hope, but also the kind of hope we have, determines to a great extent our understanding of responsibility, creativity, and our right and duty to shape our world and our biological and psychic nature.

The early Christians expected the second coming of the Lord and the end of this earthly history in a rather near future. This immediacy prevented them from working out a basic, constructive approach to their responsibility in cultural, economic, social and political life. Their expectation fostered detach-

---

[47] Cf. Enrico Chiavacci, 'Manipolazione politica', in *Manipolazione e futuro dell'uomo* (Bologna: Ed. Dehomiane, 1972), pp. 225-235.
[48] Delgado, *Physical Control of the Mind*, p. 246.

ment, the overcoming of greed and pride, and dedication to one's neighbour, but not any kind of planning for the future of mankind.

A hellenistic expression of Christian hope, with a one-sided emphasis on salvation of souls, is unlikely to redeem one's relationship to the bodily world and the future of this planet. Our hope is incarnate in Jesus Christ. Our expectation of the resurrection of the body, and of the world to come, our hope of the new heaven and the new earth, must be incarnate in our responsibility towards the human community and towards the created universe. 'The whole creation is groaning in all its parts, as in the pangs of childbirth' (Cf. Rom 8 : 22). Since Christ has redeemed the world and not only souls, those who have received the first fruits of the Spirit are in debt to the world around them. It should have a share of the freedom of the children of God.

Those who do not believe in 'the new heaven and the new earth', and a life in the world to come, will always be tempted to use violence to obtain that kind of earthly life that is their total hope. But those who believe in God's redeeming presence in this, our world, and in the world to come, can work with patience and endurance.

Unfortunately, we Christians do not all have the same concept of the relationship between our hope for everlasting life and our responsibility for the future of mankind on earth. Paul Ramsey is correct when he protests against desperate manipulations that arise from lack of any eschatological hope. However, I cannot agree with the vision of the impact of the eschatological hope if, in the name of it, he denies our shared responsibility for the remote future. [49] Only an apocalyptic pessimism can deny that we must care for our human environment and our genetic heritage in view not only of the next generation but of all the generations to come. I am doubtful whether my own concept of eschatological hope coincides with that of Harvey Cox, but I feel he is right if he sees sloth and lack of responsibility for

[49] Cf. Paul Ramsey, *Fabricated Man*, p. 129.

the present time and for the future as a capital sin. [50] We must never, in the name of our eschatological future, abdicate our responsibility for the near and remote future, since we are all one family of God in one history of salvation.

## 8. Man's stewardship over his own nature: how far does it extend?

The sense of history, of science, and especially of the behavioural sciences, developed best on the background of the Jewish-Christian conviction that God has entrusted to man a full stewardship over the earth. No taboo or unreasonable tradition or sacralization may limit this freedom. However, this is not the freedom of isolated individuals but the shared responsibility of mankind. Every person and every human group must absolutely respect the sacredness of each human person and contribute to the growth of freedom for all.

Man is given mastery over what we call 'nature'; but this mastery must never be exercised in a loveless attitude, in a spirit of exploitation, but with reverence for all creation as a word of the one God and Father, as a gift entrusted to us for the benefit of all humankind.

We can learn much about reverence for nature from other great cultures. The western concept of nature as an object only for utility is thoroughly alien, for instance, to the best Japanese traditions. Their concept of nature was not so much as an object of man's mastery but rather as an object of his appreciation. As his best companion, it was acknowledged in reverence and gratitude, and honoured by a sense of responsibility towards it. [51] This attitude still prevails, even in unexpected places. For example, in Japanese scientific studies about monkeys, each

---

[50] Harvey Cox, *On Not Leaving It To The Snake* (New York: MacMillan, 1967), pp. ix-xix. Cf. Charles Curran, *Politics, Medicine and Christian Ethics,* pp. 202ff.

[51] Masao Watenabe, 'The Conception of Nature in Japanese Culture', *Science,* 15 Jan. 1974, pp. 279-282.

animal has a name and is treated as an individual, not only as a number. This reminds one of the Genesis account, where 'the man gave names to all the cattle, all the birds of the air, and all the wild animals' (Gen 2:20). In exercising our stewardship over the earth and all of nature, we realize our true selves to the extent that we feel responsible before God for the fruits of the earth, for our own and our fellowmen's destiny, and for the future.

To man is submitted not only infra-human nature but also his own life. In interaction with his environment, he shapes himself regarding his own development, his own self-realization in healthy personal and communal relationships. We know more today about the interaction between self-realization and the shaping of the world we live in. We can understand that each decision to transform our environment — economic, cultural, societal and political structures — is implicitly a decision to transform also ourselves as we live within those structures. It should be a conscious decision. All our ways of submitting the earth to our use should be carefully assessed and re-assessed in view of the foreseeable influence on man's own self-realization.

With Karl Rahner, I hold that man rightly understands himself, above all, as self-creator under God and with God. All the potentialities of nature are entrusted to him. He can interpret the whole of evolution and history, and can and must shape and re-shape the material that history hands over to him. 'We can never forget that the distinctiveness of man lies in creativity and freedom, even if they are limited.' [52] God is the great artist, the Creator, and man is meant to be and to become more and more his image and likeness. We are becoming his likeness when we join him in working out his design, when we preserve our freedom, increase our capacity to love and serve one another, admire God's works, and adore him with all our heart and in all our life.

Man is entrusted to his own providence and discernment.

[52] Charles Curran, Op. cit., p. 203.

He is the only being on earth that can listen to others, can share the experience and reflections of the past and the present, and can interpret his own 'peak experiences', his inner longing for ultimate meaning, and his awareness that he is not yet fully realized.

In an ethics of manipulation, the question that interests us most is to what extent is man's own *bios* and his own psyche entrusted to him. How much, and in what ways, can he legitimately shape and re-shape them?

It is my thesis that he has to interpret his stewardship in the light of his noblest vocation. In that interpretation, he can freely interfere with and manipulate the functions of his *bios* and psyche in so far as this does not degrade him or diminish his own or his fellowmen's dignity and freedom. Not only nature around him but his own natural being — his biological, psychological reality — calls for his free stewardship, his creative co-operation with the divine artist. [53]

The person who recognizes himself as the provisional result of all previous evolution and history has a right to interfere with his physiological and psychological reality, not only for the reparation of damage, and not only for the sake of therapy in a narrow sense. Paul Ramsey, as well as most of the traditional Catholic moralists, would apply therapy as the only criterion for manipulative interference in human nature. [54] But I think that we have not only the right and duty to explore the dimensions of therapy but can go beyond that concept and acknowledge our right to plan change, to pilot evolution, even where our own physiological, biological and psychological nature is concerned. Under God, man is providence for himself. He has a right and duty to plan his future in so far as he can know and interpret his situation. He can plan his future and plan himself — always, of course, within the limits of the best possible self-interpretation and in full respect for the scale of human values.

[53] Cf. A. Portmann, *Die Natur entlässt den Menschen* (München, 1970).
[54] Cf. Paul Ramsey, *Fabricated Man*, p. 112.

Man is an unfinished experiment.[55] He is 'an experimental being in his own world.'[56] He is being in becoming, and can realize himself only in action, in response to new knowledge and insights, in self-reflection and self-interpretation, and in ongoing re-assessment of his relationship and actions. The dynamics of his growth is a part of his nature.[57]

Human progress lives from experiment, experience and constant re-assessment, and all these are of paramount importance for modern science. Scientific research is always faced with an open project. It works out theories, but in view of new verification. It is never a totally new beginning; it builds upon previous theories and their partial or complete verification.

The scientific approach to experimentation has greatly influenced all our thinking and attitudes, even in the field of ethical questions. Today's natural law concept relies heavily on shared experience and shared reflection, in openness to re-assessment of previous assumptions. But there is another side to the coin. Man has learned to be careful in experimentation with highly explosive materials. He should be equally careful in experimenting with his own biological and psychological nature, especially in matters directly concerned with his capacity as an ethical being. If he interferes with his basic biological and psychic nature, he must first carefully reflect, plan, and assess the probable results; and he must never use others as he can use infra-human material.

Our first concern should be to explore the true dimensions of freedom and never to take the risk of diminishing or losing our own freedom or jeopardizing the freedom of others. Never may we renounce a careful ethical evaluation of all interferences

[55] Cf. S.E. Luria, *Life: The Unfinished Experiment* (New York: Charles Scribner's Sons, 1973).

[56] F. Böckle, 'Experimentation in Clinical Research', *Concilium 65* (1971), p. 84.

[57] Cf. B. Häring, *Medical Ethics* (Slough: St Paul Publications, 1972), pp. 42-64 on the concept of human nature and manipulation; and pp. 208-217 on experimentation with human beings in medicine.

in manipulations of human nature. 'Whenever manipulation deprives man of his potential capacity to take up certain positions, it does not serve human progress.' [58]

### 9. The value and limits of a teleological approach to ethical evaluation

In the search for valid criteria for distinguishing constructive and valid forms of manipulation from inadmissable ones, I have drawn attention to a number of decisive values. In an ethical discussion we have to clarify in which sense these values serve the cause of discernment. I want to make clear, however, that we should not be thinking only or one-sidedly about the hoped-for outcome of manipulations; we need to give attention both to the end and to the means. If a concrete form of manipulation violates the basic values of respect for human freedom and dignity, or other equally high values, then the hoped-for consequences cannot justify the means.

In the traditional discussion about the principle that 'the end justifies the means', many disputes arose because the relationship between means and ends was not always clearly defined. Catholic theologians who asserted that the end does justify the means limited their thesis strictly to those means which are congenial to good and necessary ends. Their conviction was: 'If there is an ethical obligation to aim for a certain end, then there must be means that correspond to the quality of the end itself'. But since the end does not necessarily determine the means, we had better pronounce our conviction with the opposite formulation: 'the good end does not justify simply any kind of means that can lead to it'.

Any approach that measures the means against the background of the hoped-for ends is called 'teleological'. However, it must be realized that there are quite different forms of teleological consideration.

[58] K.W. Merks, 'Social Cybernetics or Social Ethics', *Concilium* 65 (1971), p. 52.

In a number of philosophical, ethical systems, and even more in the daily life of our utilitarian society, we find a pragmatic approach to decision-making that not only tries to justify the means by the end towards which decisions are aimed, but also betrays an individualistic, hedonistic, utilitarian, and even materialistic vision of both end and means. [59]

Since the time of Epicurus, ethicists have frequently declared that the final end of an ethical decision is man's happiness. Everyone, by an inborn dynamics (teleology), wants to be happy. The consequentialist then states that 'whatever leads to happiness is good, and whatever is an obstacle to happiness is bad'. But the understanding of happiness is open to a great diversity of even contradictory approaches. The individualist is concerned only or mainly with his own happiness, while many socialist ideologies would sacrifice the happiness and even the freedom of individuals for their concept of happiness for the masses of the future. Elitists are likely to sacrifice the happiness of the multitude to their own ideals, or dare at least to determine for the masses what kind of happiness should be allowed to them. In our efficient technological society, many would make their choices in view of 'instant happiness'. Ethicists, who are thinking about the overall happiness, have to look for further criteria.

As Christians, we believe that man is created for happiness in this life and in the life to come. God wants us to be sharers of his own blissful love. He wants us to seek and find happiness through self-purification, generosity, and that detachment that enables us to understand the true nature of love and those ways that lead to happiness by corresponding to man's vocation to be the image and likeness of God. Only by forming the best possible concept of man's vocation and acquiring an adequate knowledge of his inner dynamics can we come to an understanding of the

---

[59] Cf. Anthony Quinton, *Utilitarian Ethics* (New York: St. Martin's Press, 1973); J.J.C. Smart and Bernard Williams, *Utilitarianism: For and Against* (London: Cambridge Univ. Press, 1973); Dale Tarmovieski, *The Changing Success Ethic: an AMA Survey Report* (New York: AMACOM, 1973).

nature and quality of that happiness which can give us orientation in our ethical decisions. We believe that God, the Lord of history, has written and is constantly writing into the course of human history and into men's hearts, this longing for happiness. But since history is not completed, and is widely disturbed by sinfulness, it is not always easy to discern just what is a longing for genuine happiness and what is a craving for selfish satisfaction.

Psychology has sufficiently demonstrated that the human being has, as part of his intrinsic structure, basic needs that orient him towards self-actualization, integration, psychological health, creativity, productivity. These needs or values are related to each other in a developmental and hierarchial way. This does not mean that the highest are always the most urgent and can be experienced as the strongest. Safety is frequently more pressing than contemplation and unselfish love. The need for food is usually more strongly felt than either, but in the decisive 'peak experiences', the human person realizes that it is the higher values that make life worthwhile. [60]

The best theories about human nature and the natural law refer to this inborn need for the highest form of self-realization as a person among persons. St Paul refers to it when he says, 'When the Gentiles, who do not possess the law, carry out its precepts by the light of nature, although they have no law, they are their own law, for they display the effect of the law inscribed in their hearts. Their conscience is called as witness, and their own thoughts argue the case on either side, against them or even for them' (Rom 2: 14-15). This text seems to imply that, since we need to argue the case on either side, it is not always easy to find out what is the genuine appeal of nature. We, too, need to 'argue the case on either side' in community, sharing experience and reflection.

The whole of natural law philosophy in Europe, as well as in the great ethical religious systems of Asian cultures, is based

[60] Cf. A. Maslow, *The Farther Reaches of Human Nature* (New York: The Viking Press, third printing, 1973), pp. 41-80.

on the presupposition that there are inborn teleologies in the human being, and that by his nature, and finally by the creator of this nature, he is oriented towards the highest ethical ends.

An all too optimistic philosophy of history in the last century believed in teleology but explained it in a naive way. Each historical development was considered in an individualistic and utilitarian perspective, as the highest form of evolution. The conviction was that at the end there would be a perfect or almost perfect world.

The many disasters and the wrongdoings of mankind have led a number of people to deny teleological wisdom. One of their most outspoken representative is Monod. He suggests that evolution and human history is the result of hazard, of unpredictable coincidences, but with a kind of 'teleonomic performance'. [61] He makes his point against the over-optimistic teleology of the philosophy of history and against that deterministic world view which expected the world to develop, by inner necessity, towards the better. The latest theories of great scientists like Max Planck and Werner Heisenberg leave space for chance or relatively meaningless happenings, but the emphasis is still on a wonderful cosmic order that allows and fosters further development even through some of the unpredictable coincidences. The typical Christian vision, that speaks of a chaos that took shape only under the Spirit of God, prevents an easy sacralization of a teleology independent of God and of man's responsibility.

Creation is imperfect. Only God is absolutely holy and perfect. In the created universe there is room for more than unpredictable coincidences and meaningless hazards; sin can, at least partially, block development and human progress. However, we believe that God 'can write straight with crooked lines.'

The whole universe and man's history are an unfinished work in which there are disturbing occurrences, happenings that are neither planned nor desired. Natural catastrophes destroy the

[61] J. Monod, *Chance and Necessity* (New York: A. Knopf, 1971), p. 120.

works of man and countless human lives. But besides this we, as Christians, believe that there is the sin of man that brings an avoidable but extremely disturbing factor into human life and into the course of history. We are not only an unfinished and sometimes uneven work; we bear in our genes, in the millions of data stored in our brains and in our environment, the burden of the sins of many generations and many people.

Life is a battle between the power of the creative and redemptive spirit and the craving of incarnate selfishness. However, we believe that the totality of existence is a longing for final fulfilment, and we believe that through the presence of God, the Creator and Liberator, we can distinguish the longings of the heart for goodness, from the cravings of selfishness. Humankind is able not only to cope with unplanned and undesirable events but finally to grow in the right direction, though not without a fight against the sinfulness in the world and in each person's selfish tendencies.

An ethical system that does not take into account the hazards and the even more threatening reality of sin, the sharp conflict of values and duties in the complicated situations of an imperfect and sinful world, is worth nothing. But based on human experience, and in shared reflection, we can and must discover a hierarchy of values and needs, together with an ethics of compromise. Though we must never betray our highest vocation, in the concrete occurrence we sometimes have to be more immediately concerned with daily food and security than with the higher aesthetic values. In many conflicting situations we cannot observe and realize all the desirable values at the same time, but we can and must give preference to those that are the most valuable and most urgent for both our own self-actualization and the actualization of the human community in justice and peace.

In their declaration following Pope Paul's encyclical *Humanae Vitae* the French bishops observed that the use of mechanical or chemical means for birth regulation (which is a concrete form of manipulation) is not good in itself but can be considered as being without guilt if used in order to preserve more urgent values such as harmony and stability in a marriage. They also said this is not just an extraordinary case; rather, we know that human life is characterized by countless situations of conflicting values.

A mere teleological consideration that does not take into account the complexity of human nature, human history, and the frequent situations of conflict, is not complete. Yet we do not renounce a teleological vision of man as an ethical being, being in becoming more humane. No right and no duty is absolute when it militates against higher or equally high rights and duties to one's self or to others and to society. As creatures in an imperfect world and in a history of sin and redemption, we are not expected to make perfect decisions but only the best possible in our ongoing striving for self-realization and for building up a better world.

Having said all this, I shall now try to give a comprehensive view of the chief values that have to be considered as principal ends in a teleological vision, and as criteria in view of both the ends and the means of our decisions.

Man's noble vocation and his innermost nature include certain capacities that have constantly to be developed:

to reciprocate love, to relate to other persons and to communities, to conduct dialogue in love and to respond with discernment;

to adore, to admire, to revere, and to contemplate; to search for abiding truth and incarnate goodness, and to discover the meaning of present opportunities;

to treasure up experience and shared reflection, to foster intuition, to search for wholeness and synthesis, especially for synthesis between contemplation and action, between responsibility for one's own self-realization and love of God and one's neighbour;

to develop the sense of freedom in solidarity, out of concern for the freedom of each person and all people, and to search for a synthesis between creative freedom and creative fidelity;

to shape the world to be most expressive of and conducive
to creative freedom and fidelity, justice, love, dialogue and
mutual respect, solidarity in the search for truthfulness, sincerity
in all human relationships, readiness to act according to upright
convictions, freedom from both aggressiveness and passivity,
liberty for energetic and non-violent action in support of justice
and peace, hope and mutual trust, a sense of humour, religious
freedom and freedom of conscience, inner liberty in the experience of God's gratuitous gifts, graciousness in human relationships, and freedom to live one's own life and to die one's own
death.

These criteria are not the only ones but they are at the heart
of all the criteria in respect to manipulation, and the very remedy
against all forms of degrading manipulation.

## 10. *Ultimate theological and teleological intentionality*

Up to this point I have discussed criteria in a way that can
be shared by all the great religions and the best of humanist
tradition. The religious dimension was not left out but was
presented with concern for the broadest possible dialogue with
all believers. In dialogue with the various trends, however, we
must never forget or betray our own identity. As a Christian,
I see all human experience and reflection finally in the light of
Christ; and we Christians can enrich the dialogue with other
religions and with people of other traditions by offering our
own specific perspective.

I agree with the various teleological ethical systems which
hold that man's profound longing is for happiness, and that we
should use happiness as one of the main criteria. But we have
to seek for further criteria of true happiness, and for other
criteria besides happiness. Happiness cannot be the only
criterion.

Even those who do not believe in Christ the way we
Christians do, will not deny that he has offered a peak experience

of human freedom and dignity in the service of all others. He has come to proclaim gladdening news, to make known and to prove the way to ultimate meaning and happiness.. Christ's life and death and his teaching find a synthesis in the sermon on the mount, specifically in the beatitudes. They manifest better than anything else the dynamics of growth in freedom and in commitment to the liberation of all people and, at the same time, the dynamics of happiness.

Christ himself is the embodiment of the beatitudes. He is the peacemaker, the pure in heart, the one who hungers and thirsts for justice. He who is infinitely rich comes as a poor man, in order to free the rich from greed and lust for power, and the poor from being exploited. His inner freedom allows him to give himself to the service of his brothers and sisters. He shares with all humankind his dignity as Son of the Father, and thus communicates an ethics of open-hearted relationships, of genuine joy in mutual respect and love.

The ethics of the sermon on the mount is a call to that creative liberty which comes from inner conviction and free dedication. Christ does not impose his will; he has not come to 'control' us. He shares his life, his love and his creative freedom with us as the Emmanuel, as friend and brother, as the man for others. He looks not for servile obedience but for friends who act from personal insight and sincere conviction, with discernment, and who are motivated by love, justice and peace. 'I call you servants no longer. The servant does not know the intentions of his master. I have called you friends, since I have shared with you everything that I have received from the Father' (Jn 15:15).

In Christ's mission and work there is no talk of outside reinforcement or about control of unfree subjects. What he proclaims to his disciples is the new relationship in its very freedom, and the promise of even greater freedom and beatitude. Whoever experiences the beatitude, joy and peace of him who shares with us all that he is, knows what the loss or refusal of all this means.

The beatitudes offer a most attractive end, a clear direction for final happiness and self-realization. They also show the means and attitudes by which the end of universal beatitude may be reached in this world and in the world to come. They allow growth in patience, yet require vigilance for and response to the here-and-now opportunities. Since they neither produce nor allow any form of escapism, they free us from the dangerous 'if only', as well as from short-sighted violence and impatience in the use of present opportunities.

Christ's dedication to his mission to proclaim and bring joy and peace to the world is total. In gratitude for the gift of his sonship, he is the freest and happiest servant of all people and of all creation. His basic beatitude is that of the poor who, in the new spirit, recognize the gratuitousness of all God's gifts, of all that they are and all that they possess, and are therefore moved to share them generously with each other. The true disciples of Christ, freed from power-madness and greed, do not abuse their capacities and possessions but use them freely in the service of their brothers and sisters. Thus the liberating power and the bliss of the kingdom of God become visible. The first beatitude, which includes all the others, tells us the ultimate meaning of adoration, grace and thanksgiving. It frees us from idols and ideologies, inspires generous service to the world and the people around us. We experience then the highest, the ultimate intentionality of beatitude, which eliminates at its deepest roots any tendency towards degrading manipulation.

'Happy are the pure in heart; for they shall see God.' B.F. Skinner and others think that they could quickly make the world happy if they were allowed to manage and manipulate everyone extraneously by all kinds of reinforcement. Their ideas, ends and means of happiness differ radically from the happiness Christ proclaims and communicates.

Purity of heart means living by one's own conscience. It means morally good motives and intentions, freedom from greed and selfishness, and freedom for a life inspired by love, peace, joy and justice. These are the powers of freedom, the inner well from which liberating actions spring that show the way to abiding happiness and dignity. Skinner explicitly refuses as ineffective the teaching of Jesus on this central point. He refuses the ethics of the sermon on the mount, and looks for immediately effective means. This kind of psychology is the new secular version of the Grand Inquisitor who accuses Jesus of a misleading idealism.

Christ's way of beatitude excludes all violent means. 'Happy are those of a gentle spirit; they will gain the earth' for the gospel of love, justice and peace. Jesus teaches a liberating solidarity in non-violent action and in commitment to peace and reconciliation. By sharing with us his compassionate love, he shows us how to share in his blissful love. A theological ethics of manipulation should explore all the dimensions of gentleness, the spirit of non-violence, and discern the genuine means for a non-violent approach. Where people believe in violence because they have not discovered the liberating power of non-violent action, there is no hope of liberation from wrong manipulation.

The sermon on the mount teaches also the liberating power of repentance. Not just any kind of sorrow brings comfort and liberation, but only sorrow because God is dishonoured by sin, and his image and likeness, the human person, is degraded and offended. Man cannot free himself from the manipulative power of sin, from the contempt and abuse of others, unless he acknowledges and repents of his wrongdoing. The repentance that opens the gates to happiness is not possible without a renewed commitment to every person's dignity and freedom.

'Happy are those who hunger and thirst' for universal justice, for freedom, dignity, and true happiness for all. This beatitude includes readiness to suffer with the prophets in commitment to a healthier, happier, more fraternal world. This readiness to suffer in the way Christ suffered is an expression of inner freedom that refuses to react or counterattack by manipulative means. Suffering is not a good in itself but only in so far as it proves our willingness to bear each other's burdens and to contribute to a happier and more human world.

B. THE DISCRIMINATING PERSON

When we speak about objective criteria, we must not allow ourselves those dangerous objectivations that forget the first and basic importance of the persons involved. Objective criteria serve no purpose unless they are freely interiorized by those who have to distinguish between acceptable and unacceptable manipulations. The ethicist has not fulfilled his *rôle* if he is aiming only at objective criteria. Our main purpose is to help people to acquire the virtue of critical discernment. [62] Only when people acquire this virtue, and enough information to allow them to discriminate, can we gain from science's new knowledge without being overwhelmed by its revolutionary breakthroughs.

Both Church and society should realize that nothing is more needed than education directed towards a morality of responsibility. [63] We have to examine our whole educational system. Are we giving equal or higher place to teaching mere technical possibilities than to teaching ethical values? Are the Churches fulfilling their *rôle* as a critical conscience of society? Are we willing to listen to the prophets who want to open our eyes and show us the way to that radical conversion which develops in us the virtue of critical discernment. Everyone has to criticize himself, to discern his own life before God. Those whose fundamental option is for freedom and respect for all people attain a connatural sense of the good that helps them to interiorize the objective criteria. Their connaturality with the scale of values makes the right choices easy for them. [64]

The strongest liberating and healing power is in healthy

[62] Cf. B. Häring, *A Theology of Protest* (New York: Farrar, Strauss and Giroux, 1970).
[63] Cf. Amitai Etzioni, *Genetic Fix* (New York: Macmillan, 1973), pp. 11; 35f.
[64] A. Maslow has some beautiful reflections on this point under the heading of 'Meta-motivation'; see his book, *The Farther Reaches of Human Nature* (New York: The Viking Press, 1973), pp. 299-340.

human relationships; the most destructive power is in heartless objectivation. Wherever personal relationship gives way to an impersonal system of communication, all doors are open to manipulation, and the capacity for self-protection decreases.

In medical ethics, nothing should be emphasized more than the relationship between the doctor and patient. Therapy and all efforts to foster human growth should be directed towards an ever richer development of a person's relations with God, with his fellowmen, with the community, in self-acceptance and in a shared effort to make the environment more and more conducive to healthy inter-personal relationships.

## C. WHO CONTROLS THE MANIPULATOR?

It is in everyone's vital interest that the destructive power of atom bombs should be most strictly controlled. But the fact that the scientists did construct the bombs, and then were unable or unwilling to prevent their being exploded on heavily populated centres, leaves little hope that the scientists themselves will control the new powers of scientific manipulation acquired by the progress in biology.

It would be naive to ignore the question of whether human behaviour should be controlled in matters so decisive for the future of the human race. But it is more than a matter of control. If our society cannot develop a spirit of responsibility and the capacity to control the worst abuses, then in the end we shall all be controlled by a small *élite* of scientists who know how to manage and manipulate people. 'We should discuss what kinds of control are ethical, considering the efficiency and the mechanisms of existing procedures and the desirable degree of controls in the future.' [65]

Our first hope, however, should not be control by legislation and penal sanctions. As already emphasized, we should aim,

[65] Delgado, *Physical Control of the Mind,* p. 249.

above all, for the kind of education that prepares discriminating people. For that reason, we should speak out against an educational monopoly by the state. A pluralism in the educational system, which encourages, side by side with state schools, secular schools and schools sponsored by religious bodies, not only serves the progress of education in general but also can more easily prevent the manipulation of the educational system itself and of the people involved in the process as educators or students. The greatest attention should therefore be given to non-manipulative participation in the formation of public opinion: education towards a spirit of creative liberty, creative fidelity, and the virtue of discernment.

When public opinion is weak or misdirected, laws will be either bad or ineffective. Nevertheless, the organized society cannot function without legislation on vital matters. I agree with Daniel Robinson that 'we must protect both society and our own future with laws. Without the guidance and protection of laws, each therapist is judge, jury and ethicist. To make things worse, it is in the nature of his formal education that issues of laws and ethics have been avoided with nearly brazen assiduousness'. [66] But whether or not good laws can be passed and reasonably applied, and political power can become a non-manipulated and non-manipulative controller, depends upon our total commitment to freedom and justice in all fields, at all times, for all people. The prospect of degrading manipulation of people by *élitists* or by political power challenges everyone to work for a society that will be able to cope with the new realities. [67]

[66] Daniel Robinson, 'Therapies: A Clear and Present Danger', *American Psychologist* 28 (1973), p. 133.

[67] Cf. A. Etzioni, *The Active Society* (New York: Free Press, 1968), and *The Self-guiding Society* (New York: Free Press, 1971); Charles Wengel and Stephen E. Tinkler, 'Eugenics and Law's Obligation to Man', *South Texas Law Journal* 14 (1973), pp. 361-391.

## Chapter 3

# SPECIFIC PROBLEMS OF MANIPULATION
# IN BIOETHICS

With the scope and variety of manipulative actions in the whole of human life, and an acceptable method of formulating general principles or criteria in mind, it is now possible and necessary to look for more concrete criteria of discernment in the various fields related to medicine and biology, where manipulation is a major problem.

Though the greater part of this study is more concerned with the problems now developing or those that will be set in the future, I turn my attention first to today's problems in medicine (FIRST SECTION).

The area that seems to me most susceptible to the dangers of thoroughly unacceptable manipulations, where determination of the boundary line between therapy and insidious management is most difficult, is that of behaviour modification, especially as proposed by the Skinnerian school of behaviourism. Related to it is the picture of cybernism (SECOND SECTION).

Brain research opens new horizons for therapy but also new and very specific problems of boundary lines between therapy and manipulations that are destructive of human freedom. Enormous problems have been raised by mindchangers already present in today's life, but many new ones are in store because of the rapid progress in knowledge and techniques (THIRD SECTION).

In regard to the future of the human species, genetics is probably the field that requires the most careful attention not only by ethicists but by all those concerned for humankind's development. New knowledge has brought new powers and therefore new ethical questions in matters of genetic control, gene therapy, genetic engineering, genetic counselling and artificial reproduction (FOURTH SECTION).

*SECTION ONE*

## PROBLEMS IN TODAY'S MEDICAL PRACTICE

Unusual and exciting prospects like that of cloning must not divert our attention from the daily practice of medicine. Our attitude towards radical possibilities of manipulating mankind depends greatly on how we approach today's problems. 'Medical care will be determined less by spectacular situations than by the sum total of decisions which are far removed from the public eye. That is the medical drama of today.' [1]

We have repeatedly noted the complexity involved in discerning what is genuine therapy and what is unacceptable manipulation. It is not always easy to determine the limits. Almost every therapeutic act contains some element of manipulation, of harrassment of some biological or psychological functions or determinisms. But while suppressing some functions, therapy is always oriented towards the restoration of the more important ones. The dominant criterion is, as we have seen, the wholeness of the human person.

For an ethical evaluation of any manipulative intervention, we have to ask the decisive questions: 'what is the meaning and nature of human life?', 'what is human health?', 'what is therapy?' [2] Today we have a new understanding of the total task of the medical profession. It is no longer limited to healing the ailments of the individual person; it extends also to preventing sickness and creating the best possible conditions for the health of the whole human community. The perspectives of preventive

---

[1] Daniel Callahan, 'Medicine's "New" Ethics. A Challenge to Daily Decisions', *Prism*, Apr. 1974, Vol. 2 No. 4, p. 46.

[2] I have dedicated the major part of my book, *Medical Ethics*, to these fundamental questions.

medicine, and the social responsibility of the medical profession and of the whole society, have to be kept in mind when we discuss manipulation in medical practice.

## 1. The patient as partner

The physician has to be especially concerned about human dignity — his own and that of his patient. [3] Frequently he has to serve patients who, because of their particular illness — alcoholism or drug addiction, for instance — have partially lost the use of their freedom and the capacity to behave with dignity. But on principle, he must treat them as persons. He does so if he aims to restore the patients' sense of their personal dignity and freedom. In the process of treatment, the doctor may feel obliged to use reinforcements, but the more the patient realizes that the doctor respects him and believes in his dignity, the more he can co-operate as a partner.

Medical experimentation on human beings always has some elements of functional manipulation but is not necessarily manipulation of the person. [4] The first organ transplants in living persons, even such cases as a mother giving a kidney to save her child's life, shocked the sensitivity of many people. Some spoke of 'mutilation', and condemned the whole procedure as a scandalous manipulation. Today the judgment is quite different. Certainly to give a kidney or any other organ for the health of another person involves manipulation. However, persons who consent freely and in full knowledge of the proportionate risks exercise a high degree of freedom and promote the

[3] Cf. Thomas S. Szasz, 'Illness and Dignity', *J.A.M.A.*, Vol. 225, No. 4, 1974, pp. 543-545.

[4] Cf. J.L. Charron, *Experimentation on Humans*, unpublished dissertation (Roma, Accademia Alfonsiana, 1970); Jay Katz, *Experimentation with Human Beings* (New York: Russell Sage Foundation, 1972); Bernard Barber, John J. Kelley and others, *Research on Human Subjects: Problems of Control in Medical Experimentation* (New York: Russell Sage Foundation, 1973).

dignity of personal relationships. [5] It is not a case of manipulation of persons as persons.

Self-experimentation or co-operation in medical experimentation draws its fundamental value and justification from the social aspect of therapy. The doctors, research persons and those who co-operate have in mind the service rendered to the health of many people; but it is a question of wisdom to discern the proportion between the possible risk and the hoped-for benefit for other persons. The decisive question is whether the experimentation is agreed to in full freedom — inner and outer freedom — and with the prospect of contributing to the growth of freedom and the dignity of persons.

Whatever may be his good intention, a doctor must never use his patient as a means, or manipulate his consent. It is unethical to withhold necessary medical treatment in order to have 'control' persons. If comparison between the effectiveness of a new procedure and an old one is necessary, then a control group has to receive the standard treatment instead of being denied any treatment. The frequent use of the *placebo* for a control group poses serious problems in two instances: first, if the *placebo* is given instead of a treatment to which the person is entitled; and secondly, if there is any deception of the participants. There are, however, no ethical objections if the *placebo* is given to participants who do not need treatment, or if a delay involves no noticeable risk, and if all the participants are informed that some of them will, for a certain time, receive a *placebo*. If full agreement is given in knowledge of this practice, there is no manipulation of the person, as person. [6]

Human health and therapy are dependent on free and dignified self-realization. While healing some functions, the doctor cannot lose sight of the concept of total health and maximum autonomy as the end of therapy. Seeking this goal, the physician

[5] Cf. C. Perico, 'Trapianti', *Dizionario Encicl. di Teologia Morale* (Roma: Ed. Paoline, 1973), pp. 1889-1898 (with bibliography).
[6] Cf. F. Böckle, 'Experimentation in Clinical Research', *Concilium* 65 (1971), p. 76.

and the patient are partners in a covenant of fidelity and mutual respect. Neither should try to manipulate the other. The patient must never ask from the doctor something which he knows the doctor cannot do in accordance with his conscience. And the doctor should never make a decision for the patient that the patient can make for himself. Paternalism on the part of the doctor is not so readily accepted today as in former times. A doctor should give to his patient, and eventually to his patient's family, as much information as is necessary for co-operation as partners.

A concrete case can illustrate the problem. A man is a bearer of Huntington's disease. Should he be informed of this fact and its import: that between the ages of thirty and forty, a genetic disease will have devastating effects? An individualism and a certain paternalism on the part of the doctor may decide, 'No, the patient should not live in fear and anxiety.' A social consciousness and respect for the person, as person, suggest strongly, however, that the man has a right to be informed that he is a bearer of this disease and what the prospects are for his life. If the information is given in full sincerity, the patient and others will have no fear of being deceived, and the patient can make important decisions about his future: whether, for instance, he will or will not take the responsibility of marriage and children.[7] Yet it cannot be said that the doctor must give this information in every case, if he foresees that a certain patient is absolutely unwilling and unable to accept it and cope with it. The doctor must at least explore whether the patient is able to do so.

The physician-patient relationship is an art, and it presupposes that the physician trusts the patient's own potentialities.[8] For both doctor and patient, the process of informing the patient carefully, truthfully and respectfully is liberating.

[7] Cf. Robert S. Morison, 'Rights and Responsibilities: Redressing the Uneasy Balance', *The Hastings Centre Report*, Vol. 4, No. 2 (Apr. 1974), pp. 1-4.

[8] Cf. John H. Stone, 'The Patient as Art', *The Pharos*, Vol. 37 (Jan. 1974), No. 1, pp. 9-10.

In a technological age, we are all tempted to rely too much on manipulative means instead of seeking the kind of help that allows us to use and develop our own energies. Karl Menninger complains, 'The power of self-regulation has been seriously neglected in medicine.' But he also praises breakthroughs that have demonstrated how important active responsibility is for one's own well-being in the context of a person's total health. This is shown particularly by 'bio-feedback training for voluntary control of internal states'. [9]

Probably the greatest temptation to overstep the boundary lines of manipulation comes from the reductionism so characteristic of certain areas of medicine and science. The physician who is trained only for biochemical treatment of discrete functions will not see that limiting himself to biochemical manipulations often does violence to the person as a whole. It is not that specialization in biochemistry is wrong, but what leads to massive manipulation of human relationships is that kind of reductionism which absolutizes a particular aspect. This reductionism leads too often to a kind of anthropologic technology and biotechnic that treats the person as object. [10]

Reductionism and trends towards absolutizing one aspect of an experience expose each specialization of the healing profession to the danger of degrading manipulation. Some psycho-analysts, for instance, following their pan-sexual vision of mankind, will treat persons as if they were only sexual beings; others, following a pan-aggressive world view will focus only on aggressiveness. There can be no doubt that a doctor's one-sided approach to healing does violence to the human person and makes for a manipulative relationship with his patient. Only a holistic vision that takes into account the whole person in his or her existential relationships can allow a therapy that avoids unacceptable

[9] K. Menninger, *Whatever Became of Sin?* (New York: Hawthorn Books, 1974), p. 79. Cf. Abraham Black, 'Unlearning Visceral Learning', *New Scientist* 61, No. 883 (31 Jan. 1974), pp. 269-270.

[10] Cf. F. Böckle, *Op. cit.* 80; H. Ryffel, 'Probleme der Biotechnik in soziologischer Sicht', *Arzt und Christ* 11 (1965), pp. 193-212.

manipulations. [11] Medical progress needs specialization, but it equally needs an education that helps the specialist not to overlook the patient in his or her desire for wholeness and for personal respect. [12]

The healing profession as a whole has a co-responsibility for counteracting the various dangers of degrading manipulation. Even the doctors themselves are, to a considerable extent, exposed to manipulative information by the drug industry; and they in turn, as a professional group, can exercise a manipulative influence on public opinion. They can also act as a pressure group. Like any other social class, they are tempted to look first to their financial interest and power, and to exercise political manipulation through lobbying and manipulating public opinion.

Since the physician's healing power is practically linked to his capacity for dialogue, the medical profession must look for the best possible means of communication and dialogue with the public at large. People have to know that doctors can be trusted: that they are firmly dedicated to truthful communication and to respectful and responsible co-operation. [13]

## 2. Manipulation in contraception and population control

I have no intention of discussing all the complex questions of contraception and population problems. Catholic moral theology has, in general, spent disproportionate energy on this field while neglecting other very urgent ethical questions. However, I hope that a clear understanding and sharper discernment in respect to manipulation could help here, too, in gaining a more balanced view.

[11] Cf. John Wilkenson, M.D., 'The Christian Understanding of Health and Healing', in Claude Frazier (ed.) Faith Healing. Finger of God? Or Scientific Curiosity? (New York and Nashville: Thomas Nelson, 1973), pp. 44-55.

[12] Cf. Edmund D. Pellegrino, M.D., 'Educating the Humanist Physician', J.A.M.A., Vol. 227 (Mar. 18, 1974), pp. 1288-1294.

[13] Cf. C.M. Fletcher, Communication in Medicine (London, 1973).

An historical and sociological study of the practice of contraception and the theories about it shows that the environmental context has exercised great influence. [14] In most of past history, mankind had to give maximum emphasis to procreation, since it was a matter of survival. Today we are living under totally different conditions.

We can also see that the very different reactions to the encyclical *Humanae vitae* at all levels of the Church are conditioned to a great extent by the cultural situation of the various social classes and countries. A careful study has shown, for instance, that in North America the convictions of the various parts of the clergy are strongly related to age-group and ethnic background. [15] This does not mean that we are simply manipulated by our environment, but that we do have to face the total condition of life and the various factors that influence people's opinions, if we are to overcome, gradually and partially, the manipulative influences on our own opinions or convictions. As Catholics, we can be enlightened and helped in the fight against manipulative forces, or else we can be conditioned and partially hindered from facing the problem in all its depth and breadth, in view of the newness of humanity's situation.

Many thought that the very fact that contraception is manipulation proved its intrinsic immorality. Others objected that it is not necessarily a manipulation. It is my conviction that we cannot deny that all forms of contraception contain manipulative manoeuvres. But the decisive question is not whether it is manipulation but whether there is an illegitimate 'crossing of hierarchic boundaries'. If it is a manipulation of persons and of their free will, and degrades their dignity, then our judgment

---

[14] Cf. John T. Noonan, *Contraception: A History of Its Treatment by Catholic Theologians and Canonists* (Cambridge, Mass.: Harvard Univ. Press, 1965); L.D. Langley (ed.) *Contraception* (Dowden, Hutchin and Ross, 1973).

[15] Maurice J. Moore, *Death of a Dogma. The American Clergy's Views of Contraception* (Chicago: Community and Family Study Center, Univ. of Chicago, 1973).

cannot be anything but negative. This, however, has to be proven.

There is no doubt that all forms of contraception do manipulate physiological processes. The rhythm method is somewhat different, since there is no chemical or physical manipulation of biological functions; but the calculated use of the infertile days in order to deprive the conjugal relationship of its normal fertility contains evident elements of manipulation. This insight alone does not, however, justify a negative judgment about the method. The decisive question about all the various means of contraception is whether there is an unfavourable and unacceptable manipulation of human relationships. Each method has to be tested as to how far it manipulates the spontaneity of the marital union and endangers reciprocal love and respect. All effective means of contraception do separate the unitive end from the procreative end of the sexual act. We cannot say that the rhythm method is simultaneously effective in avoiding procreation and open to procreation. It is open to procreation only to the degree of its uncertainty and partial ineffectiveness, but this is surely not the intention of those who make a thoroughly calculated use of the method.

A completely contraceptive attitude is marked by a radical split of the unitive aspect from the procreative one. In a responsible use of contraception, there cannot be only a maximum of attention to the expression of respectful and tender love; there has to be also a fundamental intentionality to preserve and foster that unity, fidelity and vitality of conjugal love which enables the spouses to fulfil their procreative and educative vocation in the best possible manner.

Medical ethics shows generally that intervention in biological processes is never good in itself but is justified by a therapeutic end. There are even more reasons to assert specifically that contraception is not good in itself; but in a realistic ethics of compromise it can sometimes be considered as free from any subjective fault and can be, objectively, the best solution possible in painful difficulties to harmonize a responsible transmission of life with the exigencies of conjugal love. This does not, however, mean a general justification of contraception, which can in many instances be linked with a manipulative spirit in a sense that is ethically unacceptable.

Contraception can be, and, indeed, often is, a factor in the manipulation of the partner. If sex is approached in the spirit of consumerism, then unmarried and married people can dream of resolving the delicate problem of responsible parenthood either by chemical or physical means, or by a utilitarian calculation of the infertile period. Anyone who wants to resolve such personal problems automatically is on a slippery road to dangerous manipulation.

It is unethical manipulation if one spouse imposes on the other, against the other's conscience, either periodical or total abstinence or the use of contraceptive means.

The criteria which we have used thus far in the discernment of manipulation point also to the conclusion that it is sinful manipulation if a confessor or anyone else tries to impose on spouses a solution that is against their upright consciences and earnest conviction.

We can be guilty of immoral manipulation if we cause confusion in public opinion and in the consciences of many people by withholding important information and indispensable distinctions. This is surely the case if we confuse contraception and abortion, or speak of them without even a semicolon between them. Abortion is a manipulation of a totally different kind from contraception, and of a totally different ethical quality. And those who oppose both equally, or practically interchangeably, should be warned that they may be accountable for much confusion in the minds of ordinary people and of legislators who recur to abortion as a means of population regulation.

Whatever may be our personal conviction about the morality of contraception, those who have the duty to instruct people about their responsibility must clearly spell out whether or not a certain method of contraception might be abortifacient or might endanger the health of the user. Doctors have lately warned about the risk of certain birth control pills, and even more, about the use of some intra-uterine devices which can cause ectopic, hazardous pregnancies. [16] Those who recommend the rhythm method as the only acceptable method should inform spouses about the opinion of geneticists who assert that sperm from sexual intercourse that occurred several days before the ovulation of the egg they fertilize, 'are apt to produce a far greater incidence of congenital malformation than arise from sperm ejaculated closer to the time of ovulation.' [17] For those who are convinced that periodic continence is the only acceptable method of regulating conception, this means practically a strong recommendation for additional days of abstinence before the moment of ovulation. For those who feel sure about 'ensoulment' at the moment of fertilization, there is a further motive absolutely to avoid intercourse during the last six or seven days before ovulation, since fertilization of an ovule by an 'aged' sperm noticeably increases the risk of the egg's ability to survive the first critical days.

To try to make people sensitive to their responsibility in greatly overpopulated areas like India and Java (Indonesia), and to appeal for responsible limitation of the family size wherever the family is not able to provide a good education and preparation for life, is not manipulation. It may be the only way to prevent grave manipulations in the future. For if we do nothing to generate responsible co-operation, or if we fail because of inadequate approaches, then we have to fear that governments will finally use more and more pressure, coercion, and even heavy sanctions when population problems appear to be uncontainable.[18]

---

[16] Cf. M.P. Vessey, Bridget Johnson, Richard Doll, P. Peto, 'Outcome of Pregnancies in Women Using an Intra-uterine Device', *The Lancet,* 23 March 1974, pp. 495-498.

[17] P. Ramsey, *Op. cit.,* p. 98.

[18] Cf. L.H. Janssen, S.J. (ed.), *Population Problems and Catholic Responsibility* (Rotterdam–Tilburg: Tilburg University Press, 1975); B. Häring, 'Some Theological Reflections about the Population Problem', *Op. cit.,* pp. 156-163.

## 3. 'Child management'

In the child we revere humanity beyond utility and reward. Every child, and especially the handicapped, retarded or exceptional child, is a test case of respect for all humanity. Has a child, who does not meet the adult's expectation of utilitarian happiness, a right to exist and a right to humane existence? This fundamental question concerns the unborn as well as the born child, the exceptional as well as the normal one.

When the child is not truly accepted by his parents, his educators and his society, all doors are open to manipulative relationships. There is truth in the saying that 'children should be wanted children'. Transmission of life should be responsible, and each child should be welcome. But is not all this talk about 'wanted children' frequently meant to imply that parents have a free option to accept or not to accept the children they have brought to life? If we know ourselves as accepted by God and wanted by him despite our own grave faults and limitations, then we know that we have to accept our fellowmen; parents and educators especially, can and must love all their children. The way the argument of 'only wanted children' is used in favour of abortion manifests and promotes such a base approach to human life that more and more children will be rejected, not treated as wanted members of the human race.

### a. The manipulated foetus

In a society where the right to manipulate not only things but also persons is loudly asserted, it is no great wonder that the human foetus is a main object of manipulation. Even its identity is often denied; it is called 'tissue' or 'genetic material', and considered as simply a part of the mother's womb, about which she can do as she likes.

The seven judges of the United States Supreme Court have held that the pregnant woman's 'right to privacy' overrides the unborn child's right to life itself. Moreover, they have denied to the elected representatives of the states' citizens any right to protect the human foetus as such. For the manipulators, and for the pro-abortionists who accept a utilitarian calculation, abortion is no longer an ethical question. The following quotation is typical: 'The point we are making, and have made throughout this book, is that there is no right or wrong way for the unwillingly pregnant woman, only a variety of choices.' [19]

The abortionist movement is a manifestation of the consumer society where sex activity — homosexual as well as heterosexual — is considered an article of consumption, regardless of love, commitment or social responsibility. When a society holds that unborn human life can be disposed of at will, the attitude of mothers and fathers and of the wider social environment will change towards the foetus and towards newborn children — indeed towards all of us. The abortion decisions will have their impact on nursing practice, on the relationships between physician and patient, and especialy on maternal and child care. [20]

Obviously, the abortion issue is not just a legal one. It can be resolved neither by legal sanctions alone nor by legalization. But in a society that tends to be more law-oriented than conscience-oriented, people are much more easily manipulated by the managers of public opinion when official interpreters of the law declare that every mother, and every doctor with a mother's consent, may arbitrarily decide about life or death for the unborn child. The issue is a matter of social justice, and even more, a call to a necessary qualitative change in our culture. [21]

---

[19] R. Bruce Sloane, M.D., and Diana Frank Horowitz, *A General Guide to Abortion* (Chicago: Nelsontale Publ., 1973). The language in this book is characteristic of a manipulative spirit.

[20] Cf. Mary F. Liston: '*Abortion Decisions — Impact on Nursing Practice, Maternity and Child Care*', *The Jurist*, 1973; 2: *Abortion Decisions, 1973. A Response,* pp. 230-236 (other articles by D. Granfield, E. McGlynn Caffney, R.M. Nardone, Ch. Curran, J.A. Coriden, E.I. Ryle). Cf. also National Conference of Cath. Bishops and United States Cath. Conference, *Documentation on the Right to Life and Abortion* (Washington D.C.: United States Cath. Conference, 1974).

[21] Cf. Thomas W. Hilgers and Dennis I. Horan (eds.), *Abortion and Social Justice* (New York: Sheed and Ward, 1972).

Amniocentesis is a means of determining early whether the foetus is affected by genetic or other disease. This can be of great advantage for foetal therapy. A manipulative society, however, is interested also in other uses of it. Frequently we hear about the discovery, by amniocentesis, of an unborn child's sex; yet what is sometimes behind the curiosity is something else. Through the tests, the mother can know whether the foetus is male or female, and if it is not of the desired sex, she can keep on aborting until she conceives the sex she wants. In some cases, the child's father may be the manipulator of the mother, just as the mother and doctor are manipulators of the foetus.

Amitai Etzioni, who generally shows concern about new forms of manipulation, seems obsessed by the idea that mothers should have the foetus screened by amniocentesis. About twenty times in his book, *Genetic Fix*, he speaks of the necessity or duty of identifying the mongoloid foetus by this method. He feels that parents should be forced to make a declaration that they alone will take care of the mongoloid child, so that it would be no burden on society.[22] Etzioni is, however, quite critical about experimentation with foetuses, even those resulting from abortion. He is equally critical about the Supreme Court's decision, since these men have no real competence in all the fields concerned with abortion. [23]

An interesting phenomenon is the conflicting reaction of many people who accept the right of a woman to abort her unborn child without therapeutic reason, yet oppose experimentation with the aborted foetus. It shows that the deepest feelings do not really accept the thought that the foetus is 'nothing but' a

---

[22] Amitai Etzioni, *Genetic Fix* (New York-London: Collier Macmillan, 1973), pp. 179 and 188. The same position is expressed in *The Mental Health of Children: Services, Research and Manpower*. Reports of Task Force II and V, and the Report of the Committee of Clinical Issues by the Joint Commission on the Mental Health of Children (New York: Harper and Row, 1973).

[23] *Op. cit.*, p. 140. The best information about ethical questions in foetal research is to be found in P. Ramsey, *The Ethics of Foetal Research* (New Haven: Yale Univ. Press, 1975).

thing to be manipulated. People are particularly shocked if doctors view a foetus who is alive after abortion as experimental material instead of as a patient. But is there any substantial difference between destroying the foetus inside the womb and using it, outside the womb, as an object of manipulation?

I see no moral objection to using for experimentation the foetal corpse after miscarriage, if this might yield important insights for the benefit of foetology and consequently for the therapy of living foetuses. Quite different is experimentation with foetuses after an arbitrary decision to abort them. These experimentations, as well as those with foetuses who are still alive after abortion, may indeed lead to some important knowledge that can be helpful for future healing; but I am convinced that these manipulative actions, if indiscriminately approved by the public, do greater harm to humanity, to the self-understanding of men, and to reciprocal relationships. Mankind can degrade itself to such an extent that many precious medical insights cannot repair the damage.

Abortion is not the only threat to human foetuses in a manipulative, utilitarian environment where the capacity of parents to accept and love their children is diminished. An uncaring mother's recourse to excessive smoking, drinking, or drug addiction can do great harm to the foetus. There is also the danger of potentially dangerous drugs given to the mother. The thalidomide (contergan) children should be a warning to all.

b.  *Manipulation of the child after birth*

Especially defective, exceptional and retarded children are exposed to all kinds of manipulative manoeuvres. Skinnerian behaviour manipulation, as well as drugs like ritalin, are used not so much to improve the children's condition as to make them manageable. It is not therapeutic treatment but management

---

[24] Maya Pines, *The Brain Changers* (New York, 1973), p. 111. Cf. in relation to the whole problematic Joseph Goldstein, Anna Freud, Albert

that is intended to bring 'instant satisfaction for the caretaker'.[24] Yet for these children, behaviour modification processes can be therapeutic if the intention and the choice of means are directed towards helping them to become less dependent on others and at least partially self-determining.

Education is based on love and respect. The retarded child, in particular, needs a favourable environment. In ordered and tranquil surroundings and in an atmosphere of acceptance, encouragement and love, most mentally retarded children can not only make great progress in the basic human relationships of love, self-acceptance, self-respect, and the acceptance and respect of others, but often can develop their limited talents to a remarkable degree. This, however, is not possible for the child who is only 'managed', whose behaviour modification is based only on reinforcement. Nor is it possible for the child whose parents or educators reveal an attitude which makes him think that there is nothing that will improve him. Such an attitude greatly damages a mentally or physically handicapped child. For these children, we should use all the available insights of the behavioural sciences to improve their environment and their capacity for adaptation. [25]

Scientific progress is now making possible the development of preventative and therapeutic measures against mental retarda-

---

J. Solnit, *Beyond the Best Interests of the Child* (New York: The Free Press, 1973); Glenn Doman, *What to Do About Your Brain-Injured, or Your Brain-Damaged, Mentally Retarded, Mentally Deficient, Spastic, Flaccid, Rigid, Epileptic, Autistic, Atteloid, Hyperactive Child?* (Garden City: Doubleday, 1974); O. Ivar Lavaas and Bradley D. Bucher (eds.), *Perspectives in Behavior Modification with Deviant Children* (Englewood Cliffs, N.J.: Prentice Hall, 1974); Peggy Napear, *Brain Child: A Mother's Diary* (New York: Harper and Row, 1974); Sylvia Görres, *Leben mit einem behinderten Kind* (Köln: Benziger Verlag, 1974).

[25] Cf. Rudolph Schaffer, 'Behavioural Synchrony in Infancy', *The New Scientist*, Vol. 62 (4 April 1974), pp. 16-18; Roger E. Stevenson, M.D., *The Foetus and Newly Born Infant: Influences of Prenatal Environment* (St. Louis: C.V. Mosby, 1973).

tion. [26] This welcome prospect, however, poses the question of whether retarded children may be exposed to experimentation. Besides the general distinction between disproportionate and unnoticeable risk, we have to look for further criteria. There is no ethical objection to trying new therapeutic methods or new methods of behaviour modification if the hope for genuine help outweighs the risks.

I am opposed to using retarded children in mass institutions for experimentations which may benefit children generally but from which no special benefit for retarded or handicapped children can be expected. However, experimentation with no considerable risk, with a view to helping specifically retarded or handicapped children, is a different matter. I think that the social dimension of the human person and of therapy does justify well-pondered experiments that give reasonable promise of progress in therapy for exceptional children. The objection that parents and proxy-parents can never give consent to any experimentation with children seems to overlook the fact that parents have to make important decisions for their children in many other fields. Certainly, however, they may not give consent to experimentations that expose the children to any appreciable risk.

All mass institutions in which persons are housed or confined, including those for handicapped children, should be aware of the danger of massive control. Each child, and especially the mentally retarded child, needs personal relationships. There are outstanding institutions for handicapped children, with overseeing groups that act and live in a family spirit. If such institutions are not available, adoption or foster-family living is better than a totally institutionalized education. Nevertheless, the handicapped child does need, at least temporarily in his life, specialized institutions; and society should feel obliged to monitor controls and to guarantee special attention to personal relationships within these institutions.

---

[26] Cf. S.D. Elek and H. Stein, 'Development of a Vaccine Against Mental Retardation Caused by Cytomegalovirus in Utero', *The Lancet,* No. 7845, 5 Jan. 1974, pp. 1-5.

A difficult problem in the education of mentally retarded persons is sexuality. One can be able to enter marriage and experience gratifying sexual relationships without a high intelligence quotient, but not without being educated in love and respect, and helped to develop the capacity to reciprocate love. [27] In recent years the public has been made alert to the problem of sterilization's sometimes being imposed on retarded girls. Happily, measures have been taken in the United States and in other countries to prevent such imposition without proper consent by the girl and her parents or proxy-parents. Society has no right, generally speaking, to deprive them of desired happiness in a marriage. This general statement, however, leaves many questions open about how to educate the public to eugenic responsibility. [28]

## 4. The 'management of the dying'

The fundamental question 'what is death?' reproposes all the other questions of medical ethics: what is human life? what is the nature of the human person? what is health and sickness and the meaning of therapy? [29] Therefore we must probe now our criteria about acceptable and unacceptable manipulation when a patient approaches death.

[27] Cf. Felix F. de la Cruz and Gerald D. Lavek (eds.), *Human Sexuality and the Mentally Retarded* (New York: Brunner/Mazel, 1973).

[28] Cf. Jonas Robitscher (ed.), *Eugenic Sterilization* (Springfield, Illinois: Charles Thomas, 1973).

[29] Cf. my book *Medical Ethics* (Slough: St Paul Publications, 1972), pp. 120-151; Carolyn Gratton, 'Selected Subject Bibliography on Death and Dying, 1964-1973', *Humanitas, Journal of the Institute of Man* (Pittsburgh: Duquesne Univ.), Vol. 10 (1974), pp. 87-103; Edwin S. Schneidman, *Deaths of Man* (Quadrangle: New York Times, 1973); El. Kübler-Ross, *Questions and Answers on Death and Dying* (New York: Macmillan, 1974); D.P. Brooks, *Dealing with Death - A Christian View* (Nashville: Broadman Press, 1974); M.J. Krant, *Dying and Dignity: The Meaning and Control of a Personal Death* (Springfield, Illinois: Charles Thomas, 1974).

Already, expressions like 'management of the dying' warn us that not only corporal functions are managed but that the dying person himself is frequently an object of management at this decisive moment of his life. Death will reveal to each of us the value of our life, the level of our freedom and our dignity. And our attitude towards the dying person is the most revealing sign of love, respect and reverence, or lack of it, for all of our fellowmen.

a. *From therapy to caring*

Doctors and hospitals fight the battle against death. This is right and necessary. However, the moment comes when that battle is over. In many cases the doctor, or even the nurse, can determine with certainty that therapy is useless. Then there should be no simulation whatsoever of therapy. The reason is not only the injustice of imposing great expense under the name of 'therapy' when it can do no good; the chief reason is respect for the dying person and care for him. It is abhorrent manipulation if, instead of loving care and help in making this decisive moment most significant, there are all kinds of manipulation and nothing else.

Loving care for the dying is one of the supreme expressions of our respect for the human person and of truthful relationship with him. [30] Hospital chaplains, doctors and nurses should learn more about the psychology of dying persons in order to offer the most appropriate care. They should also be able to help relatives and friends to understand better what goes on in the inner life of the dying person. [31]

b. *Manipulation of the dying by stereotyped lies*

A doctor's paternalism which does not allow the patient to be a partner celebrates its triumphs of manipulation when death

---

[30] Cf. Richard Lamerton, *Care of the Dying* (St. Albans Priory Press, 1973).
[31] Cf. Ann Cartwright and others, *Life Before Death* (London: Routledge and Kegan Paul, 1973). (A description of the last moments of several hundred patients).

approaches. Then the whole system of stereotyped or studied lies, and of simulation of therapy, tries to 'manage' the person until death comes. To deceive a dying person about the most crucial personal and awesome fact of his life, his approaching death, is to treat him like an object. It can mean robbing him of the most decisive act of freedom. Not infrequently the patient is kept in unconsciousness not only by painkillers but by drugs administered with the intention of not allowing him to pose the decisive question. The treatment and care of a person when death is approaching demands a most loving and reverent way of communicating with him.

c. *The political uses of death*

A shocking manifestation of a manipulative spirit is the political use of natural death. [32] I do not refer to mass murder inspired by political interests, as most of the past wars were, or to mass killings such as Hitler's. These were not just manipulation but plain violence and annihilation. But people can easily take advantage of death, or just 'let it happen' while they wash their hands in innocence. A political decision not to help the poor and the poor countries towards better health by relieving their hunger (and all the manoeuvres and excuses to hide or rationalize it) can be an insidious form of manipulative non-action inspired by special interests of classes or nations. The same sin can be committed on the individual or group level. People can wait for the death of relatives or friends in a very selfish way. They do not kill, but they desire the death in their own interests and would make no move to prevent it by generous actions.

Here I want to raise a question for some legalistic members of the clergy. Approached by people who seek the sacraments when they are living in a healthy and stable civil marriage after the moral death of a hopeless first marriage, such a priest may tell them that their marriage can be blessed as soon as the partner

[32] Ivan Illich, 'The Political Uses of Natural Death', *Hastings Centre Studies,* Vol. 2, No. 1 (1974), pp. 3-20.

of the first marriage has died. In some cases he even suggests praying that the first spouse might die first, 'so that you, before your own death, can be reconciled'. Certainly this is not the spirit of the Church and is never done by enlightened priests; but it does happen, and manifests again a very manipulative use of natural death.

d.  *The senseless prolongation of the process of dying*

If a person has lost consciousness and there is no hope of recovering it, then the history of freedom for this person on earth has come to an end. It is one thing to heal and to prolong life; it is another to prolong only the process of dying, after a doctor realizes that healing is impossible. It is pitiful to see how persons in modern, well-equipped hospitals are manipulated by a whole system of machinery and activity, not for healing but only for prolonging the coma. [33]

The stopping of manipulative treatment that has no meaning for healing or for prolonging conscious life, but only for prolonging the death process, is sometimes called 'negative euthanasia' or 'passive euthanasia'. But this has nothing to do with the 'mercy killing' which, in modern debate, is simply called 'euthanasia'. Sometimes, however, behind the expression 'negative euthanasia' there hides a purposeful refusal of therapy which means practically the death penalty. To refuse a newborn child a minor surgery or any therapy for an accidental sickness because the child is mongoloid and not wanted, is not simply 'negative euthanasia'. The decision to refuse therapy is quite different from refusing to prolong the death process. [34]

[33] Cf. Henry Miller, 'Keeping people alive', in F.J. Ebbing (ed.), *The Future of Man* (London-New York: Academic Press, 1972), pp. 127-136; John Langone, *Vital Signs: The Way We Die in America* (Boston: Little Brown, 1974); Ernst Becker, *The Denial of Death* (New York: Free Press, 1973); D.C. Maguire, *Death by Choice* (New York: Doubleday, 1974).

[34] Cf. Joan L. Venes and Peter P. Huttenlocher, 'Management of the Infant with unmanageable Disease', *The New England Journal of Medicine*, Feb. 28, 1974, p. 518. The title might suggest that there

Re-animation is good medical practice if there is reasonable hope to restore somehow the person's health. However, if it can be foreseen that there will be only activities of the biological centre of the brain, while the higher cerebral cortex cannot be re-animated, then such a re-animation will end in nothing but manipulation of the biological functions, while the person has practically come to the end of his own personal history. Re-animation is a heroic means of therapy and should not be used where there is no reasonable hope to bring the person to consciousness and to normal mental activity.

e. *A firm 'No' to active euthanasia*

Painkillers may be given to a terminal patient in order to make the pain tolerable, even though it can be foreseen that this might somehow shorten the life expectancy. However, painkillers and narcotics may not be given with the intention and diplomatic hope of ending the patient's life sooner. Every procedure that has as end the abbreviation of life is called positive or active euthanasia. It is interesting to read the literature that glorifies euthanasia as an 'act of mercy'. One easily finds in it a utilitarian spirit and the illegitimate crossing of hierarchical boundary lines that characterize practically all the forms of hurtful manipulation of man. [35]

Representatives of a utilitarian teleology have no difficulty in justifying euthanasia. If instant happiness and avoidance of suffering is seen as the main purpose of human life, then indeed

---

the language of manipulation is used; but the authors are quite concerned for discernment. Only in the extreme cases of the anencephalic and the hydroencephalic child would they withhold life-prolonging therapy; they do not advocate positive euthanasia; cf. also Richard A. McCormick, 'To Save or Let Die', *America*, July 13, 1974, Vol. 131, No. 26, pp. 6-10.

[35] Cf. Richard Trubo, *An Act of Mercy: Euthanasia Today* (Los Angeles: Nash Publ., 1973); Marvin Kohl, *The Morality of Killing: Sanctity of Life, Abortion, Euthanasia* (London: Peter Owen, 1974); M. Kohl, 'Understanding the Case for Beneficent Euthanasia', *Science, Medicine and Man*, Vol. 1 (1973), pp. 111-121.

we shall not find any reason for prolonging the life of those who refuse the painful stage of sickness and dying.

A social and legal reasoning based on good teological orientation is against any tolerance of euthanasia. A main argument is this — if only the door is opened, the consequences are disastrous: old and ailing people will then be admonished in so many words, or without words, to ask for euthanasia. This teleological argument is fully convincing, however, only if one believes in freedom and human dignity and in the meaning of life and death. If the history of each person and all persons together is understood as a history of freedom for the sake of wisdom and growth in love, and if there is the Christian hope that life and death assimilate us to Christ and lead to resurrection, then the teleological argument is rooted in a sound foundation. Our own dignity and that of all mankind is served by the friends, the relatives, and the members. of society who give to the ailing, aging and dying person the best possible care and the highest manifestation of respect and love.

*SECTION TWO*

## BEHAVIOUR MODIFICATION: MANAGEMENT OR THERAPY?

Our attention turns now to the programme of radical manipulation proposed by behaviourism. This means that we face also the difficult determination of what is beneficial behaviour therapy, what is acceptable within certain limits, and what is insidious manipulation. A special and already burning question concerns the behaviour modification and brainwashing of political prisoners and inmates of our correctional institutions.

### 1. *The new dimension of the ethical problem*

People have always tried to manipulate others in order to submit them to either their own self-interest or their own ideas. Today, however, there is a new dimension in ethical problems. It is no longer a question of occasional manipulation; there is both a quantitative and qualitative leap towards a radical management of behaviour. It involves a scientific approach, a whole technology, and a systematic intention to modify, to manipulate and to manage the behaviour not only of individuals but of whole groups and of the masses. Highly specialized scientists have developed the techniques, often with little knowledge or interest in their possible applications. Others have developed a systematic plan of how to modify mankind by behaviour techniques. Some focus mainly on direct control of the brain, others on genetic mutations. 'It is, in fact, possible to alter behaviour by drugs, neuro-surgical intervention and systematic stimulus control.' [1]

---

[1] Gardner C. Quarton, 'Deliberate Efforts to Control Human Behavior and Modify Personality', *Daedalus* (Journal of the American Academy of Arts and Sciences, 1967), p. 837.

We face here those who consider behaviour control or behaviour manipulation to be the most effective and fastest method. One has only to look at the Index Medicus under the titles, 'Conditioning', 'Classical Conditioning' and 'Operant Conditioning' to see how much effort is being given to the study of the systematic conditioning of human behaviour.

Yet 'ethics as a discipline has so far paid little attention to the systematic problem of behaviour control, except to warn that it might be a threat to freedom.'[2] A balanced and careful assessment of the advantages and risks of various control techniques is necessary; but above all, we have to look into the world view or the ideology that is behind some of the leading schools and proposals.

By 'behaviour control' is understood the modification of other people's behaviour by means other than motivational appeal to their personal freedom. And at this point we must concentrate our attention on behaviourism and on all those forms of behaviour manipulation that stress the environmental influence, and use manipulation of the environment together with systematic conditionings and reinforcers.

A positive contribution to education and pedagogy can be made by the study of classical and operant conditionings as means of behaviour modification. They can make us alert to the limitedness of our freedom and to those conditionings that were previously unrecognized and therefore could not be changed. But we have also to know what is going on in psychology and its application. We can offer our ethical criteria only after having learned what the scientists are doing and what kind of criteria they are using.

## 2. *From Pavlov to Skinner*

Behaviour manipulation depends greatly on animal psycho-

---

[2] The Hastings Centre, *Programme in the Ethical, Social and Legal Issues of Behaviour Control*, p. 4.

logy. Pavlov's dogs have become the protagonists. [3] Pavlov paired a certain sound-tone with the process of giving food to his dogs. Food produces an 'unconditioned reflex': the dog salivates when offered food. When the same tone is repeatedly paired with feeding, the dog salivates on hearing that tone even if there is no food about. Pavlov called this phenomenon 'substitute or conditioned stimulus' or 'conditioned reflex', and built on it his psychology of the conditioned reflex. For Stalin, he wrote the textbook on 'brainwashing'.

In the English-speaking world, John B. Watson became the father of 'behaviourism'. He believed that all human behaviour can be explained in terms of conditioned reflexes. Today's behaviourism, however, relies chiefly on the research and philosophy of B.F. Skinner. [4] Skinner has experimented mostly with rats, and later with the higher primates, and has focused especially on the diverse conditionings and reinforcers of their learning process. He calls effective reinforcement 'operant conditioning'. The reinforcers can be 'adversive' (punitive) or 'non-adversive' (rewarding, remunerative).

Skinner is, in a certain sense, a humanist. He believes that the progress of science allows mankind to abandon most adversive conditionings and to concentrate instead mainly on rewarding ones. The decisive question for him is the efficiency of the conditioning: whether it is truly operant. The operant conditionings can be concealed or remain unknown to the persons who are being manipulated. The manipulator knows what kind of conditionings will be effective, and he decides alone about

[3] Cf. I.P. Pavlov, *Conditioning Reflexes and Psychiatry* (New York: International Universities Press, 1941).

[4] Burrhus Frederic Skinner, *The Behaviour of Organisms: An Experimental Analysis* (New York-London: Appleton, 1938); *Walden Two* (New York: Macmillan, 1953); *Verbal Behaviour* (New York: Appleton, 1957); *Science and Human Behaviour* (New York: Macmillan, 1953); *Contingencies of Reinforcement: A Theoretical Analysis* (New York: Appleton, Century Crofts, 1969); *Beyond Freedom and Dignity* (New York: Knopf, 1971); *About Behaviourism* (New York: Knopf, 1974).

what kind of behaviour he wants to produce and to reinforce. The justification is in humanitarian values: animals and persons are to be conditioned by reinforcers in a way that fosters their survival.

Skinner is a radical environmentalist. He believes that all human actions are nothing else than the result of the individual's environment. Since the environment does condition man, he wants to produce man as an inevitable product of an ideal environment. 'The proper application of rewards and (marginal) punishments, administered judiciously from cradle to young adulthood, will eventuate in a socialized, moral and competent character. Good and evil, by such a view, are but creations of a society, products of culture and custom which are themselves only inventions.' [5]

The underlying philosophy here is the utilitarian hedonism of Jeremy Bentham and John Stuart Mill. 'The whole fabric of behaviourism, Thorndike's law of effect, drive-reduction theories of learning, Freud's "id", Skinner's *Walden Two*, virtually all empirically-based psychological principles, spring from Bentham's twin masters, pleasure and pain.' [6]

Skinner has greatly influenced certain schools of psychology in the English-speaking world. Many share his philosophy of a utilitarian concept of happiness. Others accept his techniques and, at least partially, his philosophy. [7] On the other hand, he has been sharply criticized by psychologists of the humanist

---

[5] Daniel N. Robinson, *Psychology: A Study of Its Origins and Principles* (Encino, Cal.: Dickenson, 1972), p. 316. Robinson gives one of the most balanced judgments on Skinner's psychology. Cf. also Finley Carpenter, *The Skinner Primer: Behind Freedom and Dignity* (New York: Free Press, 1974).

[6] Daniel N. Robinson, *The Enlightened Machine. An Analytic Introduction to Neuro-psychology* (Encino, Cal.: Dickenson, 1973), p. 119.

[7] Cf. A.C. Catania (ed.), *Contemporary Research in Operant Behaviour* (60 Readings in Skinnerian Psychology) (Glenview, Ill.: Scott, Foresman, 1966); J. Wolpe, *The Practice of Behaviour Therapy* (New York: Pergamon Press, 1969); H.R. Beech, *Changing Man's*

tradition. Many consider him a threat to human freedom. Clearly, his scientific technical tools and his philosophy can be most dangerous in the hands of dictators, but they are dangerous also in psychology. One of his sharpest critics is Joseph Wood Krutch, especially in his book, *The Measure of Man*. [8]

Since the Skinnerian educator does not address himself to a conscience or to a free will, he feels entitled to manage people; and since they are manipulated anyway through their environment, he feels that they should be thoroughly and systematically manipulated for their own happiness. 'In operant conditioning, the experimenter decides on tasks, rewards and punishments, and the object of the conditioning may not even know that he is being changed. In self-education, a person learns to bring a normally unconscious process under conscious control and gains an extra measure of freedom. In B.F. Skinner's opinion, we have no choice but to use operant conditioning in one form or another to change people's behaviour. He believes this is the way to insure peace without repression.' [9]

## 3.  'Beyond freedom and dignity'

Skinner and his most ardent followers frankly confess their belief that freedom is nothing else than an illusion, and that man

*Behaviour* (Baltimore: Penguin Press, 1969); A. Robert Sherman, *Behaviour Modification: Theory and Practice* (Monterey, Cal.: Brooks, Cole Publ. Co., 1973); F.I. McGuigan and R.A. Schoonover (eds.), *The Psychology of Thinking. Studies of Covert Processes* (New York: Academic Press, 1973). Most of the 15 contributors are behaviourists. Ralph K. Schwitzgebel and David A. Kolb, *Changing Human Behaviour. Principles of Planned Intervention* (New York: McGraw Hill, 1974), p. 271: 'An ethic might ultimately be based upon both pragmatic as well as utilitarian grounds.'

[8]  Joseph Wood Krutch, *The Measure of Man: On Freedom, Human Values, Survival, and the Modern Temper* (Indianapolis: Bobbs, Merrill, 1954); *Human Nature and the Human Condition* (New York: Random House, 1959); *And Even if You Do. Essays on Man, Manners and Machines* (New York: Morrow, 1967).

[9]  Maya Pines, *The Brain Changers. Scientists and the New Mind Control* (New York: Harcourt, Brace, Javanovich, 1973), p. 83.

has to be freed from this illusion. At least, the Skinnerian scientists seem to be convinced of the emptiness of words like 'conscience', 'freedom' and 'dignity' in behaviourism. Even Skinner's hero in *Walden Two*, Dr Frazier, states, 'If man is free, then a technique of behaviour is impossible.' [10]

It is to Skinner's credit that he has lifted the curtain and made quite clear that his psychology is based on biology and technology and nothing else. 'Behaviour technology' is one of Skinnerism's most used expressions; and it is in this sense that manipulation of a person's behaviour receives a magic justification. Skinner talks plainly. What he wants is the technical controller, the *élite* of scientists who can technically shape the environment and his fellowmen's behaviour. Education and self-education is nothing but the technique to 'manipulate the variables of which his behaviour is a function.' [11] His belief in absolute determinism entitles Skinner and his students to make psychology a science of controllers. Dr Frazier says, in *Walden Two*, 'Eventually we shall have no use for planners. The manager will suffice.' 'Frazier turned to me in an open gesture of appeasement.' [12]

The managers of behaviour technology will be also the inculcators of 'wisdom'. 'The governmental design and creation of a happy people, regardless of any issue of freedom, involve some beautiful general principles.' [13] 'Where among them can you expect the inculcators of wisdom? But wait until we have developed a science of behaviour as powerful as the science of the atom, and you will see a difference quite well. What would you say to the design of personalities? There is no virtue in

[10]  B.F. Skinner, *Walden Two* (New York: Macmillan, paperback, 20th printing, 1970), p. 256. Skinner has not changed his basic philosophy over the years. In *About Behaviourism* (p. 149) he repeats: 'A self or personality is at best a repertoire of behaviour imparted by an organized set of contingencies.'

[11]  William C. Budd, *Behaviour Modification: the Scientific Way to Self-Control* (Roslyn Heights, N.Y.: Libra Publ., 1973), p. 90.

[12]  B.F. Skinner, *Walden Two*, p. 272.

[13]  *Op. cit.*, p. 281.

accident. Let us control the lives of our children and see what we can make of them.' [14] William Budd reflects his master accurately when he writes, 'Human behaviour is caused exactly as other natural events are caused. Moreover, the causes lie outside the event itself. . . We must be willing to prove a causal relationship by manipulating conditions to see if the predicted events do, in fact, occur'. [15]

Skinner radically denies freedom as well as conscience; yet he realizes that if his new 'knowledge' — that there is no freedom — is accepted, and people want to be thoroughly manipulated, the world will be radically changed. [16] According to him, only a pre-scientific and unscientific world view ascribes good behaviour to a person's merit. The scientific approach explains it through genetic endowment and, even more, through environmental circumstances. Consequently, good behaviour must be constructed through change of the gene and through technical manipulation of the behaviour. [17] With the denial of freedom, values like love are, of course, also deflated. ' "What is love", he said with a shrug, "except another name for the use of positive reinforcement?" "Or vice-versa", I said.' [18]

Those who, in freedom, do not accept Skinner's idea that there is no freedom in human life must hear his vengeful accusation, 'It is a surprising fact that those who object most violently to the manipulation of behaviour nevertheless make the most vigorous efforts to manipulate minds.' [19] This may, indeed, be true in some cases; but Skinner seems to be absolutely unable to distinguish between manipulating persons and their minds, and on the other hand, engaging in genuine, liberating dialogue. The categories of freely acquired convictions and respectful dialogue are totally absent in his technical manipulative world

[14] Op. cit., pp. 291-2.
[15] W.C. Budd, Op. cit., pp. 24-25.
[16] Cf. Skinner, Beyond Freedom and Dignity, pp. 31ff.
[17] Op. cit., p. 101.
[18] Walden Two, p. 330.
[19] Beyond Freedom and Dignity, p. 91.

view. His disbelief in freedom and unselfish motives, and his exclusive 'belief' in behaviour technology leave him no option but to be a professional manipulator and trainer of manipulators.

## 4. Typical forms of reductionism

Insofar as Professor Skinner sees his student-relationships mainly in a perspective of rigid examens, constant controls, reinforcements with benevolent rewards or (where necessary) punishments, he perfectly exemplifies the typical professor of the most conservative school. [20] It is precisely this kind of teacher who caused the student unrest of the past decade.

But Skinner not only makes a narrowing transfer from the schoolmaster to social life; he makes a far more narrowing one from *homo sapiens* to the Norway rat. His four hundred and fifty-seven page opus entitled, *The Behaviour of Organisms,* is based exclusively on the performance of rats, mostly in bar-pressing situations, in 'Skinner's box'. Because of some similitude between the associative learning of rats and human behaviour, the *rattus Norwegicus* 'soon came to be accepted as a substitute for *homo sapiens* in many psychological investigations.' [21]

It is a strange coincidence that while Adolf Hitler was trying to impose his biological racism, North American psychologists were looking to the Norway rat for an understanding of human behaviour! 'The Norway rat has been the prime favourite of psychologists working with animals. This can be understood because of the easy availability of the rats. What is more astonishing is that from 1930 to 1950, half of the published psychological studies about learning and conditioning had, as object, the Norway rat.' [22]

[20] Cf. Stephen Rose, *The Conscious Brain,* p. 281.

[21] Frank A. Beech, 'The Snark was a Boojum', in Daniel Robertson (ed.), *Heredity and Achievement. A Book of Readings* (New York: Oxford Univ. Press, 1970), p. 385.

[22] *Op. cit.,* p. 380.

Professor Skinner is a prisoner of his own world and profession. He bases most of his knowledge on experiments with animals who live in prison: in 'Skinner's box'. The rats are indeed thoroughly conditioned, but in a quite unnatural way. Ethology has abundantly demonstrated that the behaviour of an animal in prison is quite different from that in freedom. Skinner's rats are neurotic and constantly driven into deeper neuroses. The Nobel prize-winner, Konrad Lorenz, has given his attention to the social behaviour of animals who live in freedom, and has shown that it is quite different from that of domesticated animals, and much more so from that of those who are under constant control and artificial conditioning. [23]

Yet ethology has found interesting analogies between animal behaviour and human behaviour. For instance, just as animals need a certain territoriality for healthy development, so human beings need enough space. Some urban agglomerations are as bad for man as Skinner's box is for rats. [24] I consider the researches made by ethology as very enriching for the study of evolution and for all that man has somehow in common with animals. However, ethologists, too, are tempted by a constant reductionism. Stephen Rose accuses them of 'chimpomorphia'. [25]

Pavlov's dogs and Skinner's rats, and even more, the wild and free animals studied by Lorenz, can tell us wonderful things about evolution, the social behaviour of animals, and analogies

---

[23] Cf. Konrad Lorenz, *King Solomon's Ring. New Light on Animal Behaviour* (with a preface by Julian Huxley), (New York: Crowell, 1952); *Das sogenannte Böse. Zur Naturgeschichte der Agression* 15th ed., Wien: Schoeler, 1970). English version, *On Aggression,* (New York: Harcourt, Brace, 1966); *Evolution and Modification of Behaviour* (Chicago: Univ. of Chicago Press, 1965); *Studies in Animal and Human Behaviour* (Cambridge, Mass.: Harvard Univ. Press, 1970); *Civilized Man's Eight Deadly Sins* (New York: Harcourt, 1973).

[24] Cf. K. Lorenz and Paul Leyhausen, *Motivation of Human and Animal Behaviour, An Ethological View* (New York: Reinhold, 1973).

[25] Stephen Rose, *Op. cit.,* p. 381.

to human behaviour. We learn, too, that even animals are not
at their best if they are manipulated.

The main difference between man and animal is man's own
consciousness and self-determination. 'The essence of man is to
be found in precisely those behaviours which are not amenable
to manipulation and reinforcement.' [26] If human behaviour is
nothing but a function of its environment, then we are reduced
to the status of simple animals, and three million years of growth
are undone. 'The problems of the organization of the human
species are *sui generis*: very little help concerning them can be
found by looking either at evolving animal species or at developing animal individuals.' [27]

Professor Skinner probably knows more about rats and
monkeys than anyone else, but when he exposes his philosophy,
it is a futile, tiring exercise in reductionism. He explains culture
in terms of survival, and fears that if our culture would give up
concern for survival and utilitarian happiness, in favour of the
values of freedom and dignity, then other cultures might make
greater contributions to the future. [28]

For Skinnerians, thinking and self-knowledge are interesting
only in terms of reinforcement. 'Self-knowledge is valuable only
to the extent that it helps to meet the contingencies under which
it has arisen.' [29] Of course, sin and virtue can have no other
value than as successful or unsuccessful reinforcement. 'To
make a value judgment by calling something good or bad is to
classify it in terms of reinforcing effects'. [30] We have already seen
that love is nothing else than reinforcement. And so it is with
gratitude. 'To gratify is to reinforce, and gratitude refers to
reciprocal reinforcement.' [31]

[26] D. Robinson, *Psychology*, p. 315.
[27] C.H. Waddington, *The Ethical Animal* (Chicago: Univ. of Chicago
Press, 1967), p. 206.
[28] Cf. Skinner, *Beyond Freedom and Dignity*, p. 181.
[29] *Op. cit.*, p. 193.
[30] *Op. cit.*, p. 105. Cf. p. 113.
[31] *Op. cit.*, p. 108.

Imprisoned in the technological culture within the utilitarian consumer society, Skinner cannot transcend the categories of reinforcements. He exemplifies this in many ways: for instance, to him, the assertion that stealing is wrong means nothing other than that if you steal you will be punished. [32]

To be happy and manipulable, people have to forget concepts like freedom, dignity and conscience. 'If men are to think scientifically about themselves, they must step out of "selves" and manipulate their behaviour in the same way they would manipulate other natural events.' [33]

Having a sharp eye for those situations where people are manipulated and do not act according to their own conscience or in freedom, Skinnerians easily infer that all human behaviour is 'nothing else but' manipulation and being manipulated. 'Operant conditioning as an explanation of learning is based upon the assumption that much of our behaviour is controlled by its consequences.' [34] But the 'much' and 'in most of the cases' easily become 'in all of the cases'. Reductionism goes hand in hand with unjustified generalizations.

## 5. The new élitism

After having brought mankind down to the rank of highly trained rats or monkeys, behaviourists can easily arrogate to themselves the right to be leaders and manipulators of the masses who do not know their 'secrets'. Dr Frazier, in *Walden Two*, already expresses in unambiguous terms his superiority and his right to manipulate others. He feels that he makes things much better than the God of the theologians who, again and again, is disappointed by his children. [35]

Like Sigmund Freud, Professor Skinner is a pessimist about

---

[32] *Op. cit.*, p. 114.
[33] W.C. Budd, *Behaviour Modification*, p. 26.
[34] *Op. cit.*, pp. 31f, 41.
[35] *Walden Two*, p. 296.

mankind. Neither of these scientists believes that man is good by nature, and both exclude the possibility of truly altruistic motives. They could hardly be surprised by the terrifying manipulations of Hitler and his associates. Yet both are strangely optimistic about their own ability to make man happy. 'Our members are practically always doing what they want to do, what they "chose" to do, but we see to it that they want to do precisely the things that are best for themselves and the community', Dr Frazier boasts. 'Their behaviour is determined, yet they are free. . . We ask what a few men can make of mankind, and that's the all-absorbing question of the twentieth century. What kind of world can we build, those of us who understand the science of behaviour?' [36]

The pessimistic Skinnerian positivism, which vilifies all other people, is part and parcel of the arrogance of these behaviourists. Yet it is to these élitists, managers and manipulators that man becomes hopelessly a slave if he gives up his hope for freedom. 'The disciples of Skinnerism can be just as bigoted and as stubborn as the moralists and legalists who believe that everything not accidental is voluntary. The latter view makes everyone responsible for everything, while the Skinnerian position discards all responsibility as myth.' [37] Skinnerians judge as ignorant and prejudiced all those who do not 'voluntarily' renounce their faith in freedom and do not 'freely' agree to be manipulated by the new élitists.

The Skinnerian world view and the practice of total manipulation deserve a sober critique, and indeed have received it from many sides. Surely the new technology of behaviour management is the most radical and coherent denial of the whole history of the occidental, and especially of the North American emphasis on liberty and liberation. However, a criticism of this environmental determinism, and of the unambiguously proposed theory that mankind has to be thoroughly manipulated by a scientific élite through behaviour technology, deserves and needs also an

[36] *Walden Two*, pp. 296-297.
[37] K. Menninger, *Whatever Became of Sin?*, p. 79.

environmental or rather a contextual critique. Is there not possibly a dangerous *bacillus* in our present society and culture? We have to examine our whole culture and the recent development of predominant ideologies in order to understand and evaluate such a break with the best of our past history and humanistic tradition.

Skinnerian 'contingency management' experts in the field of the behavioural sciences have often expressed the following criticism: 'Single responses or a single class of behaviour have been manipulated while the syndrome or disease has been ignored'. [38] The same must also be said, however, of any critic of behaviourism who does not take into account the historical, cultural context in which it arose and grew.

Behaviour management, with no regard for freedom and dignity, is an alarming sign of the sickness of a great part of our society, and especially of our higher education. We have to face the general disease that produced such a shocking (and contagious) fever to manage people. While a great majority in our culture still believes in human freedom and dignity, and while a considerable proportion of the population believes, in theory at least, in a scale of values that is rooted in a religious tradition, practically, the majority follows a rather utilitarian approach to life in most decisions.

A criticism of Skinner's behaviourism therefore makes sense to me only in the context of a radical examination of our personal and collective conscience. His errors are a kind of mirror in which we can easily discover some of our own shortcomings, especially the loss of holistic vision and the lack of a holistic approach to our personal and social life.

We have also to acknowledge that the Skinnerian world view and technology is a reaction against an ethical or psychological

[38] I.S. Birnbrauer, 'Contingency Management Research' in Marilyn Erikson and Ben Williams (eds.), *Readings in Behaviour Modification Research with Children* (New York: MSS Information Corporation, 1973), p. 319.

approach that ignored the contextual, environmental and social factors of our behaviour. One of our greatest psychologists is ready to acknowledge the need of a broader approach that integrates some of the results of Skinner's research as well as of empirical sociology and similar sciences: 'In this respect I have learned that my earlier views seemed to neglect the variability induced by ecological, social and situational factors.' [39] I recognize, therefore, with Allport, the necessity of 'an adequate theory that will relate the inside and the outside systems more accurately.' [40]

## 6. Behaviour therapy

Critical reflections on behaviourism call for a constructive approach. We have to find out how to transcend the narrow vision of the Skinnerian school; but we also have to acknowledge that we can profit from both its positive contributions and its shocking errors. I reject the mechanistic vision of behaviour management; yet I believe thoroughly in the need for behaviour therapy as one of humanity's greatest tasks.

### a. A broader vision of therapy, responsibility and freedom

Behaviour therapy is more urgent than the therapy of any disease. It is a personal-individual and social task of enormous proportions. However, I cannot stress strongly enough that therapy is something quite different from mere management or manipulation by others, even if those 'others' are scientists.

Therapy requires, above all, great respect for persons and personal liberty: a respect which we do not find in the language and methods of behaviourism. The relationship of the behaviour therapist to his client is even more demanding than the ordinary doctor-patient relation, since the therapy of behaviour touches

[39] Gordon W. Allport, 'Traits Revisited', in Daniel N. Robinson (ed.), *Heredity and Achievement* (New York: O.U.P., 1973), p. 134.

[40] *Op. cit.,* p. 134.

a person's dignity more intimately than the healing of bodily diseases. If the doctor and patient must consider each other as partners, then even more must the behaviour therapist consider as partners both the client and the community which he is serving.

Nobody on this earth should arrogate to himself the *rôle* of therapist without being invited in freedom, or without intention to be a real partner. He should also recognize his own need for therapy: that is, for constant improvement, if not in his own behaviour, at least in his inner response to moral values.

For us Christians, a mere therapy of external behaviour is unthinkable. We do not believe that one can make good the fruits without making the tree good. If we want to heal the wounds of mankind which manifest themselves in unhealthy behaviour, we follow the vision of beatitude proclaimed by the Lord: 'Blessed are the pure in heart' (Mt 5:8). In secular language it might be expressed in this way: we believe in the reality of man's conscience, in the power of inner freedom, in the decisive value of inner convictions, and in a person's capacity to search for ultimate meaning, to search for what is truthful and good, and to act by the power of inner and freely acquired motivations.

The emphasis on this inner power of a 'pure heart' goes, however, hand in hand with our responsibility for the world in which we live. The behavioural sciences enable and oblige us to make a more conscious and systematic approach to this task. Our belief in the freedom and dignity of the human person will have its impact on our own and others' lives to the extent that we incarnate it in the whole structure of our personal life, our culture, our societal, political and international life: in effect, in our total human environment.

Psycho-analysis and behaviourism, whatever may be their errors, have made a great contribution that can no longer be ignored. They make us more fully aware of the unconscious conditionings of our lives. We can and must now, in a more realistic way, face the many conditionings of our behaviour coming from our environment, and the unconscious conditionings rooted in our psychic structure and at least partially caused by our past sins.

What specifically distinguishes us from the followers of a pessimistic psycho-analysis and behaviourism is our belief in freedom. We can freely, and with ethical motivations, change some of the conditionings. 'Notwithstanding the "evidence" of the new behaviourism, most of us favour the common sense view that by taking thought we can control, modify, restrain some of our behaviour some of the time'. [41] We know very well that we cannot change it all at once, but this does not allow us to escape into passivity or pessimism, nor does it justify the arrogance of those who want to manipulate us. We can start correcting some of our inner motivations, bring into consciousness some of the obstacles to inner freedom, and can unite with others gradually to change our environment. We can bring together the new knowledge, the new skills, and even more, our energies, in the cause of environmental medicine and behaviour therapy. [42]

b.  *An incarnate vision of freedom and of therapy*

A clear ethical vision and our belief in human freedom and dignity, far from hindering us, positively oblige us to integrate some of the insights of Pavlov, Bentham and Skinner. It is useless to warn against a total system of control in the Skinnerian manner unless we try to reconcile the scientific results of behaviour control with a humanistic conception of man. [43] Our appeal to the fullest possible use of freedom in an ethical perspective

[41] K. Menninger, *Op. cit.*, p. 185.

[42] Cf. Tee Lamont Guidotti, 'Environic Medicine: Steps in the Foundation of the Discipline', *Pharos*, Vol. 37 (Jan. 1974), pp. 17-23. Cf. Lilian Blöschl, *Grundlagen und Methoden der Verhaltenstherapie* (Bern: Hans Huber, 1974); Petra Halder, *Verhaltenstherapie* (Stuttgart: Kohlhammer, 1973).

[43] Among the authors who try to do this, I should like to mention William T. Powers, in *Behaviour. The Control of Perception* (Chicago: Aldine, 1973).

obliges us to look for genetic and environmental ameliorations, always, of course, in view of possible growth in freedom. [44]

I have already mentioned technology assessment as a more responsible approach to technical changes. We need now a new science of assessment of all the major conditionings that we introduce by our decisions into our environment and into the genetic pool. We have to assess the foreseeable consequences of our changes, using all the modern insights about conditioning. The more we know about powerful conditionings, the more we are called to examine the explicit goals of our actions and, equally, their foreseeable consequences.

In any of our decisions, we have to consider all the factors now known that allow us to assess their probable impact. For instance, if we are committed to the fundamental value of human life, we shall not only resist abortion, not only assess the new attitudes towards abortion and their foreseeable results on the whole of human relationships, but also look into all our decisions and actions in a perspective of how they influence human life. We have to examine more closely our approach to such things as population problems, birth control, food production and distribution, and our own personal and collective readiness to help any area that is plagued by malnutrition and famine.

The behavioural sciences have corrected an erroneous concept of unlimited freedom that would allow an imperative or legalistic morality. And at the same time, they have enabled us to see more clearly concrete possibilities to improve human conditions, to increase our own freedom, and to create conditions in which our freedom and that of our fellowmen can best develop.

c. *Control and motivation*

Prophets of doom like Professor Skinner predict only managers for the future. And indeed we are already in the throes of people-management by marketeers and ideologists who, through

---

[44] Cf. Th. Dobzhansky, *Genetic Diversity and Human Equality*, p. 49.

advertising, public relations campaigns, and manipulated public opinion, are trying to enforce certain ways of behaviour, not through truth and good reasoning but by constant repetition of stimuli, emotional rewards or punishments ('aversive reinforcements' such as disparaging those who are not amenable to their manipulation). These mind-managers, who appeal to the lowest level of intelligence, have to be exposed. When their tactics are brought into the open, they lose much of their power. [45]

All this presents an alarming challenge to us to bring motivation and control into proper proportion. The foundation of our own life and of our system of education must be motivational. We should not desire to change the world of people by being managers and mind-manipulators but as educators using truthful information and ethical motivation. We have not only to strengthen ideals and rational motives; we have also to educate ourselves to a keen sense of discernment and sober motivation.

In full awareness that she is called by Christ to be a spearhead of freedom and liberation, the Church has to examine her conscience radically about the place she has given to controls and sanctions. Moreover, she has to make this self-examination in the face of the new trends and dangers in our societies, and in confrontation with Skinner's total system of control.

The content and manner of evangelization must make it clearly evident that the Church's effort is not to seek power and control over people but to illumine their consciences and to promote the birth and growth of responsible freedom. [46] Law, control and sanction must be most evidently subordinated to the liberating message of the gospel and to a holistic education oriented towards inner freedom and collective commitment to liberation. This spirit must penetrate not only the life of the Church but also the education given to and through Christians.

[45] Ludwig von Bertalanffy, 'Human Values in a Changing World', in Maslow (ed.), *New Knowledge of Human Values*, pp. 71-72.
[46] Cf. B. Häring, *Evangelization Today* (Slough: St Paul Publications, 1974), pp. 115-140.

d. *The motives of reward and punishments revisited*

Skinner's plainly utilitarian and calculated distribution of reward and punishment (reinforcers) must make us all, and especially the ethicists, more alert about the proper — and improper — place of reward and punishment in a Christian presentation of ethics. It seems probable to me that Skinner may have been hurt and somehow manipulated in his youth by the frequent use of aversive reinforcers, and especially by the religious threat of divine sanctions. Preachers and educators in times past have easily resorted to God as the main reinforcer through divine threats of punishment. Even to children they spoke of mortal sin and eternal hell. This was related to a society that all too readily inflicted the death penalty and harsh treatment in prisons. In his book, *Whatever Became of Sin?*, Karl Menninger shows how casually some doctors would tell the most frightful tales about the consequences of masturbation and other kinds of behaviour. Educators in schools, too, resorted frequently to harsh punishment. Like the secular society, the Church trusted too much in non-aversive and even more in aversive reinforcers. 'This justification of the usefulness of inflicted pain (what Skinner calls aversive conditioning) has been more faintly visible in the history of even so ostensibly merciful a discipline as that of medical practice'. [47]

Skinner notes that in the religious motivation presented by the Churches lately, there has been a shift from the threat of eternal hell to emphasis on God's love. [48] But though he approves of the shift from aversive to non-aversive control, he is still convinced that the whole life of the Church and of all religions is, in the final analysis, nothing other than a system of controls and reinforcements. This massive misinterpretation is somehow understandable because of the faults committed in the past. It should, however, make us alert to the proper use and understanding of the motives of reward and punishment.

[47] K. Menninger, *Op. cit.*, p. 30.
[48] Skinner, *Beyond Freedom and Dignity*, p. 33.

Great thinkers like Immanuel Kant and Max Scheler have already criticized all forms of eudaemonism for ignoring the dignity of the good by emphasizing one-sidedly the motives of reward and punishment. We can counteract Skinnerian utilitarian eudaemonism only if we see clearly and manifest convincingly that we do not look just for self-fulfilment and reward. Goodness and truth have their own majesty that appeals to our conscience. Their own inner quality is their first attraction. We need not return to Immanuel Kant's rather arid and unattractive ethics of duty, but we should see the main point of his criticism of a mere system of reward.

What we need is to turn our attention to the immense difference between the morality of the beatitudes and any form of eudaemonistic ethics. God does not love us because he needs us. He loves us because he is love and wants sharers of his love. We find the fullness of peace, joy, graciousness to the extent that, motivated by love and gratitude, we learn to do good to those who are unable to reward or punish us. We should stop thinking about God as a superpoliceman or an embodiment of vindictive justice. He has done everything to attract us by his own love and goodness, and to teach us compassion by his own divine compassion.

The more the Skinnerian psychologists are blind to the spiritual experience — the peak experiences of so many people — and blind to the experience of goodness in itself, the sharper should be our consciousness of the difference between a simple system of reinforcers and the gospel of divine love and its ethics of the beatitudes. It is proper and just that a civilized society should defend the most basic rights also by reward and punishment. But all sanctions and all the presentations of motives of reward and sanction must be clearly subordinated to the good news of truth and goodness.

Any form of utilitarian ethics, by itself, can produce only a one-dimensional man and a one-dimensional society. Real behaviour therapy needs a qualitative change in persons according to the gospel message. Only then can mankind conquer the tremendous threats posed by the behaviour managers who have in their hands — and will have even more so in the future — a weapon more threatening to human dignity than the atom bomb.

Behaviour therapy should make use of the behavioural sciences, including some of Pavlov's and Skinner's best insights, but with great discernment. The final effectiveness and justification of genetic and environmental therapy lies in a total education towards freedom in conscience, and responsible and generous use of freedom for the common good.

## 7. *Who controls the controller?*

We come back again, now, to this basic question which arises from the threatening forms of manipulation. At this point, however, I think that we can see the threat behind the question itself when it becomes the main concern. It is that a society which, in view of grave imbalances and disorders, resorts only or mainly to controls, is already thinking and acting on the level of the Skinnerian behaviour technology and world view.

I do not deny the necessity of society's checking those who arrogate to themselves the right to become the controllers and managers of the masses; but a far more convincing approach has to be offered than the trust that someone must and can control the controllers. We have to discern and remove the social causes that give rise to this new élitism of managers and controllers. We need a qualitative therapy of our whole culture. We need an education and structures of society that give all people the greatest possible share in decision-making and in the formation of public opinion.

## 8. *Behaviour modification and the management of prisoners*

Not only typically oppressive societies but also a vindictive concept of justice has led to all kinds of manipulation of prisoners. Karl Menninger has a long list of sins of manipulation committed by police systems, by judges and courts, and especially by correctional institutions. [49] Only if and when our society sees freedom and respect for each person as one of the highest human values, will these manipulations be condemned as the serious sins they are.

War prisoners and people considered 'delinquents' have been frequently tortured or submitted to various kinds of psychological violence. The explicit intention was to force them 'to speak the truth', 'to confess'. And behaviourists have worked out increasingly effective methods of brain-washing to make the interrogations of prisoners more 'successful'. [50] A behaviourism that situates itself 'beyond freedom and dignity' has also worked out all conceivable methods of behaviour modification for delinquents, through combinations of aversive and non-aversive reinforcements. [51]

Only a utilitarian concept of teleological ethics could justify the psychological torture and the brainwashing of prisoners and of supposedly delinquent people. A civilized society should refuse to permit any tactic that destroys or degrades personalities, whether to obtain desired information or for any other purpose.

There is a heightened awareness today that many who are severely punished as delinquents are products of an unhealthy environment and of unforgivable negligence by a society that could and should have corrected harmful situations. This has led to a growing concern for the inmates of our correctional institutions. We realize that justice should be less vindictive, and punishment should yield to therapeutic treatment wherever possible. [52]

[49] K. Menninger, Op. cit., pp. 54ff.
[50] Cf. Albert D. Biderman and Herbert Zimmer (eds.), The Manipulation of Human Behaviour (New York-London: John Wiley and Sons, 1961). All the contributors to the book treat manipulation mainly in relation to interrogation.
[51] The reader will find a confrontation with and response to Skinner's ideas on this matter in Harvey Wheeler, Beyond the Punitive Society (San Francisco: W.H. Freeman and Co., 1973).
[52] Cf. Leonard Orland, Justice, Punishment, Treatment (New York: Free Press, 1973).

Of great concern to humanists is how to apply the advances in psychotherapy to delinquents, many of whom truly wish to be freed from their criminal tendencies and are ready to cooperate with therapists in the same way as anyone else who is in need of therapeutic help. [53] There is little agreement in our society about the nature of the therapy to be offered to delinquents. Many speak of 'therapy' when what they have in mind is only the application of deterrents. The first step, in any case, has to be a radical reform of the correctional institutions. [54]

The Church should take seriously her healing ministry to prisoners. We need chaplains who combine psychological expertise with great kindness and with that deep understanding of the gospel that can help to motivate prisoners to seek first their inner freedom. I have heard of fruitful efforts by members of 'houses of prayer', who have gone into jails and have succeeded in bringing prisoners together in prayer groups. In prayer, their self-discovery as sons and daughters of God can become a giant step towards self-respect, inner freedom, and right motivation. Throughout the country there are also various groups of concerned citizens whose members volunteer to become friends of prisoners in their own areas, visiting them, listening to them, caring about them on a one-to-one basis, and often helping them in their return to a decent civilian life. In our Christian mission, charity is always somehow united with conversion and renewal of the environment. No kind of therapy should be severed from help towards appropriate motivations which go far beyond the idea of mere reinforcement.

Skinnerians have developed an aversion therapy for inmates of psychiatric prisons, hospitals for the criminally insane, and for other prisoners. Electroshocks, drugs that make the patient feel miserable, and other means used as operant conditionings

---

[53] Cf. Jerome S. Stumphauser (ed.), *Behaviour Therapy with Delinquents* (Springfield, Ill.: Charles C. Thomas, 1973).
[54] Helpful proposals are offered by the United States Bishops, Nov. 1973: 'The Reform of the Correctional Institutions in the 70's,' *Catholic Mind,* June, 1974, pp. 40-51.

replace the motivational and psycho-analytic approach. But 'aversion therapy doesn't attempt to get at the psychological roots of a subject's behaviour, as psycho-analysis does. It merely conditions him not to repeat it, just as Pavlov's dogs were conditioned to salivate by the ringing of a bell.' [55]

There is sharp controversy about the legitimacy of these aversion 'therapies' which seem in some cases to be a modern version of the ancient tortures. From the press we have learned that many inmates of the correctional institutions that piloted programmes of this kind were not even told the meaning of the therapy and not asked for their consent. Indeed, there is a question whether some prisoners are at all able to give free consent to such treatment. There is, consequently, a growing conviction that legislation is necessary to control aversion therapy applied to persons confined in correctional institutions.

No person should be subjected to any aversion therapy or any attempt at behaviour modification that is devoid of genuinely humane motivation, an appeal to freedom, and respect for human dignity. Integrated into a broader and genuinely humanistic approach, however, there could be a place for the use of scientific methods of reinforcement, mostly by non-aversive but also including some aversive methods. There is nothing to be said against behaviour therapy itself. If it is truly therapy, it will never neglect education in right motivation. But techniques of behaviourism built on the conviction that there is nothing noble in man are always degrading.

Apart from other ethical considerations, we should be warned that prisoners who are submitted to the most sophisticated methods of behaviour modification are themselves becoming experts in brainwashing, and can use these techniques on others as soon as they are outside the prison walls.

I agree with Delgado in his assertion that individual freedom

[55] Stephen I. Sansweet, 'Aversion Therapy', *The Wall Street Journal*, Jan. 2, 1974, p. 1. Cf. *Newsweek*, May 20, 1974: 'Carrots and Sticks'.

should, in general, bow to community welfare, and that there is the right to limit the freedom of those who are thoroughly unable to overcome evil or who have nothing else in mind but to do evil. But manipulation by drugs or by aversion therapy must never destroy the person by treating him almost as an animal. Behaviour manipulation, especially if applied without informed consent, can never be compared with, for instance, the addition of chlorine to the water for the protection of our health, or of fluorine for better teeth. Delgado loses his sense of proportion if he compares these two forms of manipulation. [56]

Humanist therapists should offer their services to imprisoned delinquents who want to be treated for homosexuality, alcoholism, or other deviations, even if their chief reason is only to gain a more speedy release from imprisonment.

In the case of prisoners held for victimless crimes or misdemeanors, no therapist should co-operate in behaviour modification requested by the administration of the prison or the court but not by the prisoner. 'Behavioural and medical scientists have no *rôle* in arbitrating the competing claims between individuals and society in general.' [57] For delinquents who have victimized other persons and are considered too dangerous to be left in freedom, the case is different. Therapists may co-operate if compulsory therapy is determined to be an evil of lesser gravity than execution by the state. But in all cases they have to offer genuine therapy.

9. *Cybernism: a new form of total management of human life*

'Cybernetics is the theory of the relations of possible dynamic self-regulating systems'. [58] Specifically, it is (as described

---

[56] Delgado, *Physical Control of the Mind*, p. 221.

[57] Daniel Robinson, 'Harm, Offense, and Nuisance: Guides for Establishment of an Ethics of Treatment', *American Psychologist*, Vol. 29, No. 4 (April 1974), p. 238.

[58] G. Klaus, *Kybernetik in philosophischer Sicht* (Berlin, 1961), p. 27.

in Webster's Third International Dictionary) the comparative study of the automatic control system formed by the nervous system and brain and mechano-electrical communication systems and devices' such as computers, thermostats, and so on.

Technical man reached an amazing level of achievement when he produced the highly developed computer. It allows him new rationality in programming and controlling. But if he tries to make people think of their brains as computers, and tries to persuade them to allow human behaviour to be computerized, programmed and controlled, then he most illegitimately crosses the hierarchical boundaries. Stephen Rose describes as 'machineomorphs' those cybernists and behaviourists who absolutize technical rationality.

Only the most primitive functions of the human brain are computerlike. [59] The brainchangers and behaviourists who dream of programming and controlling the human brain and the whole of social life with the help of computers are true models of the one-dimensional man. They have forfeited the typically human dimensions of creativity and freedom.

Towards the end of *Walden Two*, Skinner's hero, Dr Frazier, the benevolent professor, decides to leave his university for good and settle down in Walden Two where 'there will be no planners but only managers.' Those who dream that once everything has been put into the computer it can control everything, have long ago exiled themselves from the idea of universality, of the integration of the various disciplines and dimensions of man. Cybernism has given up belief in a freely-made qualitative change in the life of persons and of society. It sacrifices higher intelligence and human wisdom in favour of cybernetic manipulation: in favour of a mere technical rationality. [60]

To confuse the difference between the unconditioned and the conditioned, between the producible and non-producible, and

[59] Stephen Rose, *The Conscious Brain*, p. 288.
[60] Cf. Italo Mancini, *Manipolazione e futuro dell'uomo*, pp. 114-115

to confine man to the mere dimension of what can be produced is the root of the most dangerous destructiveness. [61] Should man ever come to think of the computer as the only valid measurement, then he will have renounced his soul, his dignity and his freedom. 'The transfer of the natural scientific model to society is criminal in the eyes of critical theory. It represents the original sin of positivistic society.' [62]

Not only the Skinnerian school of behaviour control but also a number of advocates of genetic engineering are obviously caught in the traps of cybernism. But if man believes only in technical rationality and planning, nothing can hinder him from constructing 'cyborgs' in a strange combination of cybernetics and biology. [63]

Even for economic life and its impact on human relationships, it is catastrophic if the computer alone makes the decisions. Economic development as part of human development needs more than the design of a computer. It needs responsible persons with imagination and initiative. [64]

If cybernists are allowed to decide and plan the future of society, catastrophe for humanity will be unavoidable. With the methods of cybernetics we can comprehend only one part of the social processes. A total cybernetic planning would be one of the most violent forms of reductionism. By necessity it leads to a sterile manipulation and crippling of human society. Cybernetics must also be recognized as one of the most 'refined instruments of manipulation which guarantees the power of certain groups.' [65]

[61] Cf. Erich Fromm, *The Anatomy of Human Destructiveness* (New York: Rinehart and Winston, 1973).

[62] Heinz Otto Luthe, 'What is Manipulation?', *Concilium* 65 (1971), p. 14.

[63] Cf. Kenneth D. Eberhard, 'Genetics and Human Survival: A Christian Perspective', *Linacre Quarterly*, Aug. 1973, p. 177.

[64] Cf. Hedley Voysey, 'Computers, Conflict, and the Job', *The New Scientist*, Vol. 62 (18 April 1974), pp. 112-113.

[65] Karl Wilhelm Merks, 'Social Cybernetics or Social Ethics', *Concilium* 65 (May 1971), p. 53.

Beginning with the use of the simplest tools, and up to the invention of the highest forms of computers, mankind has manifested great rationality. But we must never forget that the human person is not a machine and not only a builder of machines. He cannot be built, manipulated, planned and controlled like a machine. [66]

Humanity can overcome the pitfalls, threats and temptations of cybernism only if we hold fast to our belief in creative freedom and creative fidelity, and find the courage to live our own life and generously to take our own share of co-responsibility for the world in which this freedom and fidelity is incarnate and has constantly to be yet more creatively incarnated.

---

[66] Cf. Mortimer Adler, *The Difference of Man and the Difference I Makes* (New York: Rinehart & Winston, 1967); Wolf Rohrer, *Is der Mensch konstruierbar?* (München: *Ars Sacra*, 1968).

SECTION THREE

# BRAIN RESEARCH AND THE MINDCHANGERS

The exploration of the deserts of the moon is surely fascinating. But what science has begun during the past few decades in exploring the human brain is of much more vital interest for mankind. [1]

The brain is the centre of life, the substratum of consciousness and of all man's spiritual activity. It would be a grave injustice to the world of scientists to think that their main goal is manipulation or control of other people's brains. Their first interest is to decipher the language of the brain. [2] Neurochemistry, neuro-biology, neuro-physiology and neuro-electricity are, in principle, seeking to aid in human transformation rather than in manipulation. [3]

A better knowledge of the functions of the brain can greatly help all branches of medicine. Here, above all, inter-disciplinary dialogue and co-operation are necessary. Such interesting and delicate research is not possible without a common effort and

---

[1] Besides the books frequently quoted in the text, I should like to mention the following for information about this most interesting field of research: S.M. Farber and R.H.L. Wilson (eds.), *Control of the Mind* (New York: McGraw Hill, 1961); Stephen Rose, *The Conscious Brain* (New York: Alfred A. Knopf, 1973); Marilyn Ferguson, *The Brain Revolution. The Frontiers of Mind Research* (New York: Toplinger, 1973). It seems that in Russia brain research is highly developed. One of the best sources of information is Alexander Romanovich Luria's *Higher Cortical Functions in Man* (authorized translation from the Russian by Basil Haigh, New York: Basic Books, 1966).

[2] Maya Pines, *The Brain Changers. Scientists and the New Mind Control* (New York, 1973), p. 31; Karl Pribram, *Languages of the Brain* (Englewood Cliffs, N.J.: Prentice Hall, 1971).

[3] Stephen Rose, *Op. cit.*, p. 295.

without special sensitiveness to philosophical and ethical problems. [4] Where inter-disciplinary dialogue is lacking, reductionism is unavoidable. 'While the respective bodies of knowledge do not rest on a theoretical substructure, their implicit hypothesis is that psychological man is *only* behaviour or a neural outcome. If we accept this assertion, then the correlated therapies constitute a veritable execution of the person being replaced.' [5]

Some researchers are interested only in mechanical processes, others in brain electricity, and so on; but in no field of research is attention to the whole more necessary than in research into the brain. Luria emphasizes especially the developmental and socio-cultural context. 'The higher mental human functions are complex reflex processes, social in origin, mediate in structure, and conscious and voluntary in mode of functions.' [6] He also turns attention to the brain as a whole. 'We therefore suggest that the material basis of the higher nervous functions is the brain as a whole, but that the brain is a highly differentiated system whose parts are responsible for different aspects of the unified whole.' [7]

While brain research opens exciting new horizons and promises results that could benefit the whole human race, it cannot be denied that the new knowledge can also be a temptation to manipulate people's brains and to control their minds. Of particular relevance for the purpose of this study of manipulation are drugs, brain surgery, brain management with electrodes, and combined methods of brainwashing. [8]

[4] Cf. J.C. Eccles, *The Neuro-physiological Basis of Mind* (Oxford: Clarendon Press, 1953); *Facing Reality* (New York: Springer, 1970).

[5] Daniel L. Robinson, 'Therapies: A Clear and Present Danger', *American Psychologist*, Feb. 1973, p. 131.

[6] A.R. Luria, *Op. cit.*, p. 32.

[7] *Op. cit.*, p. 35.

[8] Cf. E. Lausch, *Manipulation. Der Griff nach dem Gehirn* (Stuttgart, 1972); Nigel Calder, *The Mind of Man. An Investigation into Current Research on the Brain and Human Nature* (New York: Viking Press, 1973); Erwin Lausch, *Manipulation: Dangers and Benefits of Brain Research* (New York: Viking Press, 1974).

1. *Psycho-active drugs*

Neuro-chemistry is a most potent part of neuro-biology. All brain activity has a chemical component. This makes it possible to change a person's mood by chemical injections. Normally this is done by pills — psycho-active or psycho-tropic drugs — that affect the states of the neurons of certain parts of the brain. They can be tranquilizers (anti-depressant, anti-anxiety, sedative), energizers (stimulant) and hypnotics (mood elevating, hallucinogenic).

Neuro-chemistry is not related only to mood changers. Many diseases can be prevented and healed through a better knowledge of how nutrition affects the chemistry of the neurons. [9] And within a few decades, with the progress in brain research, we shall know more about how nutrition, activity, environmental variety and other factors interact to shape a baby's brain. 'The brains of millions of babies are being stunted every day as the result of poor nutrition at critical times.' [10] The more the neuronal functions of the various parts of the brain are explored, the easier it will be to influence them by chemical, electrical and other means, and thus reduce or eliminate many imbalances and sufferings.

It is known, for instance, that the hypothalamus greatly influences sexual desires and behaviour. In the study of animals' brains it has been found that 'if estrogen (a female hormone) is injected into the hypothalmus of female animals whose ovaries have been removed, they will resume mating behaviour. Injection into male animals can produce maternal behaviour (nest-building and the grooming of pups, for instance)'. [11] Male and female behaviour can be triggered by brain stimulation in either sex. However, although the study of the brains of animals gives

---

[9] Cf. John D. Fernstrom, Richard J. Wurtman, 'Nutrition and the Brain', *Scientific America*, Vol. 230 (Feb. 1974), pp. 84-91.

[10] Maya Pines, *Op. cit.*, p. 128.

[11] Daniel Robinson, *The Enlightened Machine*, p. 113.

important indications, the neurology of human beings is far more complex. [12]

A major advantage of better knowledge of neuro-chemistry and neuro-physiology will be its yield of precious results for psychiatry. [13] We are probably only at the beginning of new possibilities — and, we must be warned, also of some new dangers — in the use of drugs in psycho-therapy and psychiatry. Brainresearch has, for instance, finally found the brain receptor for opiates. This might be a great step forward towards safer use of morphine. [14]

Not only the ethical evaluation but also the effects of the use of drugs depends to a great extent upon the personal motivation. The higher the level of motivation, the less is the danger that drugs will change behaviour in an unfavourable way. 'Some drugs do have different behavioural effects depending on the type of motivation governing behaviour.' [15]

The great hopes that the development of psycho-active drugs may bring enormous progress in psychiatry and generally for medicine cannot, however, be mentioned without spelling out our concern about serious dangers, especially in view of our society's tendency to seek a drug for each and every evil. We tend to become an over-medicated society. [16] 'By now, half of the population of the United States uses mind-changing drugs

---

[12] Cf. Robinson, *Op. cit.*, p. 115; Maya Pines, *Op. cit.*, p. 131.

[13] Cf. Joseph Mendels (ed.), *Biological Psychiatry* (John Wiley Sons, 1973); W. Ruff, 'Auswirkungen der Psychopharmaka und ihre Bedeutung bei psychologischen Störungen', *Stimmen der Zeit* 92 (1967), pp. 44-51; Gerald L. Kerman, 'Psychotropic Drugs as Therapeutic Agents'. 'Controlling Behaviour through Drugs', *The Hastings Centre Studies*, Vol. 2, No. 1 (1974), pp. 81-93; R.M. Veatch, 'Drugs and Competing Drug Ethics', *Op. cit.*, p. 68-80.

[14] Cf. Roger Lewin, 'Step Towards Safer Morphine', *New Scientist*, Vol. 61, No. 880 (Jan. 10, 1974), pp. 64-65.

[15] Oakley S. Ray, *Drugs, Society and Human Behaviour* (St. Louis: Mosley, 1972), p. 48.

[16] Cf. C. Muller, 'The Over-medicated Society: Forces in the Marketplace for Medical Care', *Science* 176 (1972), pp. 488-492.

occasionally, and seventeen per cent use them frequently.' [17] About half of the almost quarter-billion prescriptions for psycho-tropic drugs brought by North Americans annually are anti-anxiety agents. [18] And the situation in Europe is not very different from that of the United States. [19]

Drug abuse is socially and culturally conditioned. Where the social pattern is to seek instant solutions for every problem, it is not too difficult for the powerful advertisers to 'extend the drug abuse into areas that call for coping, not for escape through drugs.' [20] Maya Pines echoes the opinion of many when she warns that 'the tendency to prescribe drugs for social rather than medical uses is spreading and becoming more respectable'. [21] There is an evident interaction between the strongest trends in our culture and the drug industry's wilful manipulation. It can appeal to these trends, and at the same time it strengthens them. [22]

Our society's individualistic misunderstanding of freedom, together with a utilitarian hedonism, opens wide the doors to drug abuse. [23] Dr Gerald Kernan (Harvard) sees us 'headed towards some kind of psycho-tropic hedonism in which we will be free to choose among drugs to enhance our performance, drugs to help us learn and remember better, drugs to stimulate or calm us, and a variety of drugs to increase our pleasure . . . all without fear of chemical damnation'. [24] Social reformers are alarmed.

---

[17] Maya Pines, *Op. cit.*, p. 224.

[18] Elmer Gardner, M.D., 'Implications of Psycho-active Therapy', *The New England Journal of Medicine* 290 (1974), pp. 800-801.

[19] Cf. Mitchell B. Balter, Ph.D., Jerome Levine and Dean I. Manheimer, 'Cross National Study of the Extent of Anti-anxiety, Sedative Drug Use', *The New England Journal of Medicine* 290 (1974), pp. 769-774.

[20] Maya Pines, *Op. cit.*, p. 108.

[21] *Op. cit.*, p. 224.

[22] Cf. John Pekkanen, *The American Connection: Profiteering and Politicking in the 'Ethical' Drug Industry* (Chicago: Follett, 1973), p. 14.

[23] Cf. O.S. Ray, *Op. cit.*, p. 276.

[24] Maya Pines, *Op. cit.*, p. 226.

They feel that the capitalistic establishment intentionally offers tranquilizing drugs when faced with social evils that call instead for a qualitative change of our lives and our society.

There is great concern about the vast use of psycho-active drugs for children while medicine cannot yet establish the long-term effect on their mental and bodily health. 'Right now, doctors are free to give any young child powerful mindchanging drugs simply because his teachers or parents find him hyperactive.' [25] In this case the most used drug is ritalin. Used by adults, this is a powerful stimulant, but for children it functions as a sedative. 'Ritalin enjoys more than a third of the amphitamine market. It is prescribed in large quantities for hyperkinesis, the childhood malady which still escapes a precise medical definition. The use of stimulants for hyper-kinetic children is under stronger and stronger criticism.' [26]

Even among those who seem the most competent persons in the field, there is considerable disagreement about what prospects and hopes the psycho-active drugs might offer in the future. Some are extremely optimistic. 'When more is known about the mosaic of differential maturation in various regions of the brain, it may be possible to shape the brains of infants, or even foetuses, quite effectively, much as Huxley foresaw in Brave New World.' [27] Many others are cautioning us not to expect too much. There is not much hope that drugs will improve bad memory, and even less that they will give strength to our will. Indeed, there is a danger that a great part of the population seek tranquilizing pills so easily that they will gradually lose the energy of the free will that can cope with normal situations. [28]

Stimulation of the brains of rats by growth hormones led to

[25] Op. cit., p. 212.
[26] John Pekkannen, Op. cit., p. 326. Cf. D. Safer, R. Allen, E. Barr, 'Depression of Growth in Hyper-active Children on Stimulant Drugs', New England Journal of Medicine 287 (1972), pp. 217-220; Stephen Rose, Op. cit., p. 300.
[27] Maya Pines, Op. cit., p. 130.
[28] Cf. Stephen Rose, Op. cit., p. 298f.

growth of the brain and could somehow stop the process of aging. But there is doubt whether this will occur with stimulation of the human brain, and nobody can yet indicate the risks inherent in such experimentations. [29]

There seems to be no doubt that progress in neuro-chemistry and neuro-biology does open new horizons for therapy, but it also brings new dangers of manipulation. [30] Controlling behaviour through drugs means always a manipulation of the human brain and therefore risks more manipulation of freedom than does the manipulation of any other biological function of the human body. [31] Even optimistic doctors warn that psycho-active drugs can be a dangerous manipulative weapon. Anti-anxiety sedative drugs, for instance, may be used not only to alleviate the loneliness of an elderly person or to decrease the anxiety of unhappy people; they may be used mainly to decrease the caretakers' trouble. 'In the future, as drugs become available to modify aggression or sexual desire, to enhance memory and to accelerate learning, the rôle of the physician in the prescription of psycho-active drugs will require even more public scrutiny, definition and sanction.' [32]

The medical use of drugs that alter mood, enhance performance and provide' a variety of pleasurable sensations can lead to social abuse and drug addiction. Doctors may not always realize that they do manipulate beyond therapy. The criteria should always be freedom, enhancement of inner freedom, and

---

[29] Cf. P. Overhage, 'Manipulation am menschlichen Gehirn', *Stimmen der Zeit* 184 (1969), p. 54.

[30] H.L. Lennard, L.I. Epstein, A. Bernstein and others, 'Hazards Implicit in Prescribing Psycho-active Drugs', *Science* 169 (1970), pp. 438-441.

[31] Cf. R. Neville, R.M. Veatch, G.L. Kerman, P.H. Wender, L.J. West, 'Controlling Behaviour Through Drugs', *The Hastings Centre Studies* 2 (1974), No. 1, pp. 65-112; Kenneth Vaux, *Biomedical Ethics* (New York: Harper and Row, 1974), pp. 85-95.

[32] Elmer A. Gardner, M.D., 'Implications of Psycho-active Drug Therapy', *New England Journal of Medicine* 290 (April 4, 1974), p. 801.

respect for the consent of the patient. 'In neo-psychiatric medical practice the boundaries between voluntary and involuntary treatment, informed and uninformed consent, and social and medical treatment with psycho-active agents are, if anything, more easily unrecognized or ignored.' [33]

## 2. Psycho-surgery

Brain surgery is always a serious intervention and requires extraordinary skill. In the past thirty years brain surgery has frequently been used for intentional destruction of some part of the brain in order to modify behaviour. It is still used in many hundreds of cases each year throughout the world.

Psycho-surgery is adopted when the behaviour of a person departs radically from the standards of social acceptability. But the hazards are formidable. It changes the behaviour and the character of the person. Even now, despite growing knowledge of the structure of the brain, it cannot be predicted what the consequences will be. Daniel Robinson notes that it 'is performed in the absence of any collection of ideas warranting the name theory.' [34] And he warns forcibly that psycho-surgery, drugs, electrodes, and carefully administered reinforcers can lead to harmful changes of personality. 'Only this or that is changed while the "person" survives. But who is this person or who was he?... Unlike the traditional approaches, we are not in a position to specify the range of consequences, nor can we offer the possibility of reversion of the unnatural state once the treatment is discontinued.' [35]

Psycho-surgery introduces profound lesions and partial destructions. Whenever possible it should be avoided, especially in view of the present imperfection of our knowledge about the

[33] Op. cit., p. 801.
[34] Daniel N. Robinson, 'Therapies: A Clear and Present Danger', American Psychologist, Feb. 1973, p. 131.
[35] Op. cit., p. 132.

development of the brain. 'The character of the cortical inter-central relationships does not remain the same at different stages of development of a function, and the effect of a lesion of a particular part of the brain will differ at different states of functional development.' [36]

Ethicists have, however, generally justified this risky intervention whenever the overall situation of the patient will probably be improved.

## 3. Brain management with electrodes

One of the keenest forms of brain research is into the stimulation of various parts of the brain by electricity. Electrodes are introduced into the most sensitive centres of the brain, and the emotional behaviour reactions are observed. This experimentation yielded astounding results with animals — rats, monkeys, steer, and so on. The transition from the animal world to the human brain is not at all easy, but it has been made. The researchers are well aware that this is a most risky experimentation and manipulation, and is therefore to be done with great prudence. Indeed, some express confidence that it may yield good results for even better understanding and promotion of human freedom.

We have already become aware of the many genetic and environmental influences that condition, promote or hinder the development of human freedom. Why, then, should we not also study the functioning of the neurons: the way the different parts of the brain interact with the heritage and environment in human activity? 'The element most essential to the achievement of maximal freedom is awareness of the many factors influencing our actions, in order to assure us that our responses will not be automatic but deliberate and personal.' [37] Awareness of all

[36] A.R. Luria, Op. cit., p. 37.
[37] José M.R. Delgado, M.D., Physical Control of the Mind. Towards a Psycho-civilized Society (New York: Harper and Row, 1971), p. 8.

the factors influencing us can appeal to greater individual and social responsibility. 'If we were cognizant of the factors influencing our behaviour, we would accept or reject many of them and minimize their effects upon us.' [38] Better knowledge of psychology and sociology, and of other behavioural sciences, have surely hit hard at a number of illusions about freedom, but at the same time they help us to find the real doors through which freedom can enter and be encouraged.

Delgado describes his research and that of his friends in the following way: 'In my discussion of the physical exploration of the mind, I proposed to examine the problem not in general but in some detail, asking questions and presenting experimental data about modifications of pleasure sensations, behavioural responses and other manifestations of mental activities obtained by direct manipulation of the brain.' [39] The scientist frequently uses the word 'manipulation' and he is well aware of what it means. 'The ability to influence mental activity by direct manipulation of cerebral structures is certainly novel in history, and present objectives are not only to increase our understanding of the neuro-physiological basis of mind but also to influence cerebral mechanisms by means of instrumental manifestion.' [40]

Delgado is interested not only in localizing the various functions but also in exploring the interaction between brains, heredity and environment. When he stimulates the brain electrically, he touches the control centres in order to discover how they react to what he calls 'input' from the outside world. His main interest is, however, the relation between mind and brain. 'The master control for the whole body resides in the brain, and the new methodology of implanted electrodes has provided direct access to the centres which regulate most of the body's activity. The brain also constitutes the material substratum of mental functions, and by exploring its working

[38] Op. cit., p. 10.
[39] Op. cit., p. 35.
[40] Op. cit., p. 67.

neurons, we have the possibility of investigating experimentally some of the classical problems of mind-brain relationships.' [41]

From this arises the most radical question about man's possibility to manipulate others or himself in the most delicate sphere. The new problem is: 'Could drives, desires and thoughts be placed under the artificial command of electronics? Can personality be influenced by electrical stimulation of the brain? Can the mind be physically controlled?' [42]

The working hypothesis of Delgado's brain research is based on the four following propositions. First, there are basic mechanisms in the brain that are somehow responsible for all mental activities, social relations, creative art, and so on; secondly, these mechanisms can be detected, analyzed, influenced, and sometimes replaced by means of physical and chemical technology. Of course this does not mean that love and thought are nothing else than a neuro-physiological phenomenon, but the evident fact is that the nervous system is indispensable for any behavioural manifestation. The third proposition is that predictable behavioural and mental responses may be induced by direct manipulation of the brain. The fourth is the most puzzling: 'we can substitute intelligent and purposeful determination of neuronal functions for blind, automatic responses.' [43]

Like Luria, the great Russian brain researcher, Delgado stresses again and again the interaction of the brain with the total environment and the genetic heritage. The total making of the brain depends on its inherited potentiality, and on the influence of the world around the child and adult, and on the person's own responses. It seems to me, however, that while Delgado emphasizes 'the need for a continuous flowing in of sensory input' and 'a maximum input of information' by impulse, language and so on, he does not see the need for discernment

[41] Op. cit., p. 97.
[42] Op. cit., p. 97.
[43] Op. cit., p. 68.

about the desirable amount and quality of information. However, when he quotes Tennyson's line, 'I am a part of all that I have met', I do not think that he means it in a passive way. [44] He would probably accept the other version: man, in one way or another, chooses to make a part of himself whatever he meets. In relation to the genetic heritage, Delgado agrees with Dobzhansky that 'genes determine not characters or traits but reactions and response.' [45]

In his reflections on brain research, Delgado comes to conclusions that favour the influence of the environment more than that of the genetic heritage. Man is an unfinished task but, through his genetic heritage and through the environment, he has the endowment that allows him to develop his mind. Like language, freedom too must be taught and created. The brain has the capacity to respond to the total wealth of thought, freedom and information gathered in the environment. 'The major differences between a cave man and a modern scientist are not genetic but environmental and cultural.' [46]

Delgado is convinced that brain research must insert itself into the inter-disciplinary dialogue if it is to have beneficial results. 'Both neuro-physiological and environmental factors must be evaluated, and today methodology is available for their combined study... Experimental investigation of the cerebral structures responsible for aggressive behaviour is an essential counterpart of social studies, and this should be recognized by sociologists as well as biologists.' [47]

It is not Delgado's intention to supplant patient education, dialogue and self-control by electronic controls. He does not at all believe in permissiveness. 'I would like to point out the fallacy in the theory that permissiveness develops the "true" and "free" personality of the child... We should understand that a

[44] *Op. cit.*, pp. 236-237.
[45] *Op. cit.*, p. 63.
[46] *Op. cit.*, p. 64.
[47] *Op. cit.*, p. 123.

permissively-structured child is as much the product of his parents' manipulation as a child of the most authoritarian mother.' [48] Freedom must be learned. It is an achievement of civilization and of the effort of each individual person. If we want to have free people, we must educate our children to responsible freedom. [49]

About the immediate medical therapeutic use of brain research with electrodes, Delgado expresses himself quite optimistically. 'Experience has confirmed the safety and usefulness of long-term implantation of electrodes in man, and the procedure has been used in specialized medical centres around the world to help thousands of patients suffering from epilepsy, involuntary movements, intractable pain, anxiety neuroses and other cerebral disturbances.' [50] He and his colleagues have developed very small and sensitive instruments for radio-missions called 'stimo-receivers', but he is probably too optimistic when he says, 'stimo-receivers offer great promise in the investigation, diagnosis and therapy of cerebral disturbances in man... It is reasonable to hope that in the near future the stimo-receiver may provide the essential link from man to computer, with reciprocal feedback.' [51] His optimism is tempered with respect to the capacity to decipher the electrical codes of transmitted signals in the brain. Even the most developed methodology 'would only be able to detect the carrier and not the meaning.' [52]

Elliot S. Valenstein, who admires the research of Delgado and others, is less optimistic, at least for the time being. He takes a position severely critical of the presidential address of K.B. Clark, who said at the American Psychological Association Convention, 'We might be on the threshold of that type of scientific biochemical interventions which could stabilize and make dominant the moral and ethical propensities of man, and

[48] *Op. cit.*, pp. 239-240.
[49] *Op. cit.*, pp. 240-242.
[50] *Op. cit.*, pp. 87-88.
[51] *Op. cit.*, p. 91.
[52] *Op. cit.*, p. 227.

subordinate, if not eliminate, his negative and primitive behavioural tendencies.' Valenstein insists that there is not the slightest probability of reaching this goal either with electrical stimulation or with chemical intervention. We do not possess any technique 'for suppressing socially undesirable behaviour by people with normal brains. It has yet to be demonstrated that electrical or chemical stimulation of any region of the brain can modify one, and only one, specific behaviour tendency. Interfering with a transmitter system must necessarily affect very many behaviours.' [53] Although Delgado's views are somewhat different, he does underline the fact that personal identity and reactivity depend on a large number of factors of experience interacting with genetic trends within the complexity of the neuronal networks. However, he is convinced that a limited modification of a determined aspect of personal reactions is possible through electronic stimulation of the brain. [54]

Delgado is not blind to the risks and ethical problems involved in experimentations in such a delicate field; but he overstresses the necessity of experimentation in medicine as well as in the whole of human life. He realizes that it is not at all easy to close the gap between animal and human biology, but he feels that it is the task of the researcher to seek 'a compromise between reasonable precautions and possible risks'. [55] Although he has expressed great optimism on other occasions, he warns his colleagues that 'therapeutic use of electrodes in cases of mental illness has been more doubtful and must still be considered in an experimental phase.' [56]

A highly qualified researcher feels himself particularly committed to the common good of all men, those now living and those who will come after us. At the same time, in all his

---

[53] Elliot S. Valenstein (ed.), *Brain-stimulation and Motivation. Research and Commentary* (Glenview: Scott, Foresman and Co., 1973), p. 32.
[54] Delgado, *Op. cit.*, p. 193.
[55] *Op. cit.*, p. 208.
[56] *Op. cit.*, p. 209.

research, he must respect the most precious heritage of mankind, the liberty and dignity of every person. Research in this most delicate field of brain stimulation therefore requires the greatest care for informed and free consent. In this regard, Delgado adds rightly, 'Procedures which represent risk or discomfort should be ruled out.' [57]

The absolute boundaries that must never be transgressed are determined by the dignity and inner freedom of the human person. The new neurological technologies have developed a refined efficiency, greater even than the tortures of past times. 'The individual is defenceless against direct manipulation of the brain because he is deprived of his most intimate mechanisms of biological reactivity.' [58] During the experimentation, the electrical stimulation of the brain is more powerful than the free will. This imposes sharp limits, and demands a high measure of responsibility on the part of the experimentator. However, I do not think that the conclusion must necessarily be that any attempt to modify individual behaviour by electrical stimulation is unethical. If both partners, therapist and patient, agree about the behaviour to be modified and about the means, and if the end is better behaviour, there can be no substantial objections.

4. *Brainwashing with combined methods*

All the various methods of brain research, if combined, can contribute greatly to mankind's healing power. They can also be abused in a combined effort. Neuro-biology can become a tool in the hands of those who wish to manipulate or reduce man's freedom. Neuro-chemistry can produce nerve cases; personality changing drugs, neuro-physiology, and the use of electrodes can control the brain and the mind; and mathematical biology can anticipate a future dominated by computers. [59] If the secrets of

[57] *Op. cit.*, p. 212.
[58] *Op. cit.*, p. 214.
[59] Cf. Stephen Rose, *Op. cit.*, p. 293.

the brain and its functions are deciphered, 'people will become powerful and vulnerable as never before. The issue of brain control will loom over them as ominously as atomic power hovers over us.' [60]

Our future will depend greatly on whether we keep a close watch on what the brain-changers are doing today and what they are prepared to do tomorrow.

The various methods of psycho-analysis can make a precious contribution to therapy. Yet they too can become a dangerous technique in the hands of the manipulator. There is an uneasiness about certain trends and methods of psycho-analysis. 'And since some of the champions of "growth" are frauds whose main motives are money-making, or feeling powerful by manipulating people's feelings, the suspicion has some foundation.' [61]

One of the chief complaints against the behaviour modifiers — including some trends in psycho-analysis — in the past decade was that 'they were mechanistic, dehumanizing and impersonal.' [62] It cannot be made too clear that I do not want to generalize. There is today, as in the past, an effort in psycho-therapy at looking for the meaning of life, and at doing so in full respect for man's freedom.

Psycho-analysts seem sometimes to be only listeners when actually they use a transference to make the patient dependent upon them and to modify his world view and behaviour according to their own ideology. Karl Menninger rightly insists that the patient should know clearly what the psycho-analyst stands for. Then he can be a partner in the dialogue, and the psycho-

[60] M. Pines, Op. cit., p. 236. Cf. K. Thomas, Die künstlich gesteuerte Seele (Stuttgart, 1970); F.A.M. Meerlo, The Rape of the Mind (London, 1957); Elliot S. Valenstein, Brain Control. A Critical Examination of Brain Stimulation and Psycho-surgery (New York: John Wiley, 1973).

[61] Perry London, 'The Future of Psycho-therapy', The Hastings Centre Report, Vol. 3, No. 6, Dec. 1973, p. 11.

[62] Op. cit., p. 11.

therapist will be able to offer advice in such a way that the patient's freedom is not jeopardized. With his whole profession, Menninger condemns most severely the analyst who abuses his patient sexually. He warns that the analyst should know that, in the long run, this can only do grave damage to his patient and to himself. [63]

The criterion for the best use of the transference which, in psycho-analysis, is unavoidable, is whether it enables the patient 'to find freedom from re-enacting the infantile dependencies and distortions of attitude to the analyst as parent... Obviously a lot of medical practices do not permit this goal, that is, freeing the individual from his infantile dependency on an all-giving or withholding parent.' [64]

If we want to avoid future threats of brainwashing with all the combined means provided by better knowledge of the unconscious and of the brain, then we have to fight on the whole front against a technical concept and a materialistic view of medicine. Ivan Illich warns: 'By transforming pain, illness and death from a personal challenge into a technical problem, medical practice expropriates the potential of people to deal with their human condition in an autonomous way, and becomes the source of a new kind of unhealth.' [65]

## 5. The main issue: freedom

The better knowledge of the brain and its functioning forces us to rethink and reformulate a number of traditional themes such as that of the soul, the mind, and freedom. Scientists who approach their research with traditional concepts of these fundamental realities will unavoidably be troubled. This is especially the case if one was taught a platonic idea of soul as a disincarnate spirit.

[63] K. Menninger, *Whatever Became of Sin?*, pp. 214-216.
[64] Lee H. Beecher, in Claude A. Frazier (ed.), *Faith Healing* (New York-Nashville: Thomas Nelson, 1973), p. 59.
[65] Ivan Illich, 'Medical Nemesis', *The Lancet* 11, May 1974, p. 918.

It seems that Delgado has received this concept. In many places in his publications he manifests his disarray. 'The dilemma of the soul is this: if we accept mental activities as manifestations of the soul, then the modification of these functions by physical means, such as electrical stimulation of the brain, would signify the manipulation of the soul by electricity, which is illogical because the soul is incorporeal by definition.' [66] If, on the other hand, we deny that the soul exercises mental functions which are conditioned by brain physiology, what then, he wonders, remains of the soul if not a mere abstraction? Then the soul would be not only incorporeal but with a minor symbolic relation to reality.

Our response can be given only in view of the biblical concept of the human person: man is an embodied soul, or better, an embodied spirit; and equally we have to say that human freedom is an embodied freedom. It is a spiritual reality that is, however, incarnate. For a Christian thinker there should be no substantial difficulty if we see more concretely how memory, understanding and will 'are now known to be activities subject to experimental investigation and related to the chemistry of ribo-nucleic acids, electric activity of the hippocampus, and anatomical integrity of the frontal lobes.' [67]

It is a basic human experience that the human spirit can transcend the dimensions of the material world, reaching out for values and truth with a passionate love for truth and goodness. This, however, does not hinder us from seeing how it is related to the marvellous organization of the human brain. If we accept both the spiritual transcendent dimension and the bodily aspect, then we have no less profound admiration for the mystery, and at the same time we accept our own human limitedness.

One may doubt whether scientists like Delgado have expressed this finitude in the best way, but we should take their consideration seriously. 'The brain is not able to produce

[66] Delgado, Op. cit., p. 30.
[67] Op. cit., p. 30.

absolute thoughts, to create absolute values, or to unveil intrinsic principles of ethics. . . . In rejecting the immutability of values, we also reject the fatal determination of destiny, and instead of accepting natural fate, we may gain a new personal freedom by using intelligence, considering that the systems of ideology and behaviour re-activity are only relative human creations which can be modified by feedback of reason.' [68]

I do believe that man, with the finitude of his being, can unveil intrinsic principles of ethics. He cannot create absolute values but he can discover binding values. However, we should realize that the way in which his values are expressed and manifested is finite and imperfect, and can and must be modified by feedback of new experience and shared reasoning.

Human development and all human activity is responsive to the heritage and to the environment, and therefore open to plastic effect. Today's generation is aware not only of 'the continuity of evolution and the specificity of genetics, but of the potential for change within the brain.' [69] It also knows that the concept of human freedom and responsibility can be expressed significantly only when 'associated with social interaction'. [70]

Freedom is an embodied reality with a most marvellous interplay between the genetic endowment, the total environment and personal responsiveness, which cannot be thought about without the function of neurons. We should surely be on the wrong track if we would like to seek and to prove freedom in some specific actions and functions of our human brains. Rather, it is the all-pervading reality that gives meaning to this wonderful interaction between heritage, environment and the embodied spirit of man.

I do not think that Stephen Rose speaks successfully on human freedom in distinguishing the 'explanatory power of

[68] *Op. cit.*, p. 234.
[69] Stephen Rose, *Op. cit.*, p. 294.
[70] *Op. cit.*, p. 291.

neuro-biology' from 'any predictive power'.[71] The fullness of human freedom cannot be explained by the mere fact that neuro-biology has no predictive power. Neuro-biology tells us wonderful things, but the total human reality is infinitely greater. There is danger in scientists' thinking and speaking as if the human person were nothing else than what the chemistry and electricity of human brains can capture.

Some scientists rooted in Christian tradition have felt that Heisenberg's theory of indeterminacy could somehow be helpful in gaining an intuition of the mystery of freedom. But, freedom and awareness, which surely cannot take place without corresponding cerebral change, transcend the categories of Heisenberg's indeterminacy. 'It is suggested that the invocation of Heisenberg's indeterminacy, though potentially relevant to our picture of spontaneous human activity, is logically unnecessary in order to make room for the kind of freedom that goes with responsible choice, and that objections *a priori* to a closed loop model of the conscious human control of action are without foundation.'[72]

It is one thing to conceptualize human freedom in a metaphysical perspective and in a language that takes into account the new world view conditioned by the behavioural sciences and by brain research. It is quite another thing to believe in freedom or to deny it. Freedom is a reality much greater than our capacity to conceptualize; but we can no longer overlook the fact that freedom exists only as an embodied reality. The consequence is that the main objective cannot be to explain freedom; we cannot even approach this miraculous reality in an abstract language remote from reality. We have to accept the finitude of human freedom. But I believe that, in its greatness and its

---

[71] *Op. cit.*, p. 292.

[72] D.M. McKay, 'Cerebral Organization and the Conscious Control of Action', in John Eccles (ed.), *The Brain and Conscious Experience* (Texts of the Study Week, Sept. 28 - Oct. 4, 1964, of the Pontificia Academia Scientiarum), (New York: Springer, 1966), p. 440. Cf. John Eccles, *The Understanding of Brain* (New York-London: McGraw Hill, 1973).

limitedness, it points to the mystery of God's infinite freedom. However, even that freedom of God cannot be thought of by human beings without the experience of our embodied freedom. God reveals the freedom of his love in the reality of history.

Realizing in a more concrete way how much freedom depends on the interaction between heritage and environment, we can speak about it significantly only if we accept it as a creative freedom in creative fidelity, and are ready to incarnate it in all of human life and human conditions of life. If we are ready to do this, our incapacity to explain freedom in terms of scientific language will not disturb us. On the contrary, it corroborates in us the conviction that the total reality is greater than the object of the empirical sciences. We all live by the profound intuition and experience that without freedom and commitment to it, all scientific and technical progress would be meaningless. The conclusion cannot be other than a firm purpose to protect and encourage freedom, whatever may be the price.

The healing profession, therefore, has to reject any kind of brainwashing, all forms of psycho-active drugs, brain surgery, and electric stimulation of the brain wherever the main intention or a secondary intention is to change people's ideas with no respect for their freedom. We should realize the immense danger that people whose ideas and behaviour are socially disliked could be submitted to brain-manipulation in a way that has nothing to do with healing. Nevertheless, this is no reason 'for not seeking to learn how to control murderous behaviour in those individuals who have demonstrable brain disease.' [73]

The new insights of the behavioural sciences and brain research, and the progress that can be reasonably hoped for in these fields, give to man an ever greater power to shape his own being and the world around him. He can intuit both his finitude and the real possibilities of improving the quality of life: his heritage, his environment, and even the development of his

[73] Maya Pines, *Op. cit.,* p. 207.

brain. Man is the only being known to us that is conscious of evolution and can take an active part in it. His decision to do so is not necessarily *hubris*. [74] For instance he will never totally prevent aging, but he can postpone it and increase the number of years to be lived in full health and energy. Why, we ask, should he not try similarly to increase intelligence and consciousness, and the total conditions of life that allow him to live his freedom more fully?

---

[74] Cf. Charles E. Curran, *Politics, Medicine and Christian Ethics: A Dialogue with Paul Ramsey* (Philadelphia: Fortress Press, 1973), p. 177. Cf. C. Feinberg, *The Prometheus Project* (Garden City, N.Y.: Doubleday, 1968).

SECTION FOUR

# MANIPULATION IN THE FIELD OF GENETICS

My first reaction to the astonishing beginnings and development of brain research was not a warning against manipulation but an expression of awe and admiration for man's capacity to decipher gradually the language of the brain, the code of the neurons, and their message. Admiration is my first response also to the findings of science in the field of genetics, where scientists have been able to decipher the language of the genes.

The gene communicates a marvellous and rich message in a coded language that can be translated into our language. It consists of sixty-four characters in which the DNA articulates our genetic heritage. The gene of the fertilized egg spells out the biological uniqueness of each individual except identical twins. It also spells out a most admirable rootedness of this individual in the whole of human history and evolution. The language of human genes has something in common with the DNA of all that is living, and at the same time it manifests the differentiation of man from all subhuman life. [1]

The more we understand the language and message of the genes of human beings and of all other living beings, the more we come to realize man's historicity, our rootedness in the total evolution of the world and in the past history of mankind. We can then understand what the great ethologist, Konrad Lorenz, means when he says that a break in tradition is one of the deadly sins. [2] Genetics, by uncovering the marvels of evolution and

[1] Cf. Leon Kass, 'New beginnings of Life', in Michael Hamilton (ed.), *The New Genetics and the Future of Man* (Grand Rapids, Mich.: Eerdmans, 1973), pp. 15-63.

[2] Konrad Lorenz, *Civilized Man's Eight Deadly Sins* (New York: Harcourt, 1974).

man's unique position in the midst of all other beings, lets us understand better that humanity is, biologically, an extraordinary success. 'It has gained the ability to adapt its environment to its genes as well as its genes to the environment.' [3]

Having uncovered new aspects of the evolution of all that is on earth, and the evolutive character of the human gene, man has now opened new avenues for a better understanding of human life and of the possibilities of eventually controlling it in response to the givenness and adaptability of the genetic endowment. Our growing knowledge about the language and message of the genes not only enriches our general knowledge, and not only makes possible genetic therapy and all kinds of genetic manipulation; it also, and above all, sharpens our sense of life-long responsibility for the world around us — which means, implicitly, also our responsibility for the human gene pool.

We are concerned here with the problem of manipulation in this field. To assess its value and to elaborate criteria, we have to face at least the main ethical problems arising from the growing knowledge and consequent power in the fields of genetics and eugenics. I shall treat the general questions of our growing awareness first in eugenics, then in gene therapy (manipulations of the gene with a clear therapeutic end), and then in genetic engineering (manipulation with a constructive end of changing traits of genes, regardless of therapy). I shall then face some problems of genetic screening which imply gross manipulative manoeuvres, and give some attention to questions about the artificial placenta in conjunction with genetic or non-genetic manipulations. Finally, we cannot avoid asking what kind of ethical problems would arise if scientists should one day succeed in cloning a human being: that is, in producing a boring repetition of the genetic message of one individual.

[3] Theodore Dobzhansky, *Genetic Diversity and Human Equality* (New York: Basic Books, 1953), p. 113.

## 1. Man's responsibility for the genetic heritage

From the moment man knows the trends, laws and dynamics of genetic development or decay, he cannot avoid the ethical issues of responsibility. During thirty years, Russian scientists were forbidden to study Mendelian genetics, since the Marxist ideology held that the transformation of the environment is the only decisive factor of human history. Consequently, Russia was thirty years behind the genetic biology of the western world. But finally the conviction broke through that human genetics is a necessary subject for inquiry: that man should know and be fully aware of what his capacities and responsibilities are in this field. [4] For Christians, the theological themes of creation and procreation bring genetics into the field of ethics. The divine mandate to submit the earth and to fill it includes man's mission to transform life according to his finest vision of humankind's future. [5]

The progress already made in genetic knowledge and technical capacity, and the foreseeable progress still in store, require all responsible people to give serious attention to this field. It becomes a fundamental question of conscience to foster the right kind of research, to guarantee the best possible information for those involved in it and for the public at large. We have to face the facts and the problems without bias, without exaggeration and without hiding any of the problems before us. [6]

### a. The specifically human nature of human genetics

Genetics has been greatly enhanced by the study of plants and by research and experimentation with animals. There is a

[4] Cf. C.P. Snow, 'Human Care', *Journal of the American Medical Association* 225 (5 Aug. 1973), pp. 817-821.

[5] Kenneth Vaux, *Biomedical Ethics*, p. 54.

[6] Cf. Martti Lindquist, *The Biological Manipulation of Man and the Quality of Life*, Publication No. 6 of the Research Institute of the Lutheran Church in Finland, pp. 190-192, where a good catalogue of ethical problems to be studied is clearly indicated.

link between all of life and human life. But reflection and solid scientific research abundantly demonstrate the tremendous difference. Only technological narrowness and unacceptable reductionism have made it possible for some scientists to overlook the hierarchical boundaries. Great men in the field, like Theodore Dobzhansky, have warned repeatedly against the danger of overlooking the uniqueness of human life and of each human person. 'Individuality, uniqueness, is not outside the competence of science. It may, in fact it must, be understood scientifically. The individuality of the human self becomes comprehensible in the light of genetics.' [7]

As in many other fields, in genetics too, there is danger of the kind of reductionism and transgression of the borderline that we have seen in those who studied the behaviour of the white rat and, naively or purposefully, allowed themselves an inductive leap that hurdles over successive species in order to establish a uniformity hypothesis. [8] Ethologists as well as biologists could assert genetic determinism only in consequence of various manoeuvres of extrapolation. [9]

The dangers of extrapolation and reductionism lurk everywhere in the field of genetics. Scientists who are unaware even of the type of society and culture that has given them their education and the funding for their research are not likely to be aware of how many of their assessments and evaluations are conditioned by that culture of the 'technical man'. One example concerns 'the genetic aspects of intelligence and performance. They are not only at best socially irrelevant; they are scientifically spurious.' [10]

No one, whether scientist, philosopher or ordinary citizen, can face the new responsibilities laid upon us by the increased

---

[7] Th. Dobzhansky, 'Of Flies and Man', in Daniel N. Robinson (ed.), *Heredity and Achievement* (New York, 1970), pp. 425-441 (429).
[8] Daniel N. Robinson, *Heredity and Achievement*, p. 352.
[9] Stephen Rose, *Op. cit.*, p. 279.
[10] Stephen Rose, *Op. cit.*, p. 295

knowledge of genetics unless he or she is keenly aware of the equality and dignity of human persons, the uniqueness of human history in all its diversities, and the plasticity of the human genes and brain to both transient and long-term changes, in their interaction with the whole social environment and with individual experience.

Brain research and psychology have demonstrated that all our perception operates selectively. We become easily protective and selective in important aspects of the problems we face. The besetting problem in all the questions that surround genetics is a one-sided technological thinking which either cannot or will not face ethical values and standards. [11]

In the theories that guide research, in explanation, and above all, in the ethical questions asked, there must be the greatest concern for holistic vision. A number of outstanding scientists and ethicists have emphasized this and have given it appropriate attention. [12] 'Only by constantly renewing our sense of what it is to be radically and simply human, will we retain the vision — and the humility — necessary to avoid becoming victims of our theory of what we ought to be.' [13] Survival, as well as any other biological concept, is a poor value without the freedom, dignity and beauty that give life its abiding meaning.

O.B. Hardison, who has chosen to entitle his book, *Toward Freedom and Dignity,* as a sharp criticism of Skinner's *Beyond*

[11] Leon R. Kass, 'New Beginnings in Life', in M. Hamilton (ed.), *The New Genetics and the Future of Man*, p. 16.

[12] Cf. C.H. Waddington, *Science and Ethics* (London: Allen and Unwin, 1942); *The Strategy of Genes* (London: Allen and Unwin, 1957); *The Nature of Life* (London, 1961); *The Ethical Animal* (Chicago: Univ. of Chicago Press, 1960, Phoenix Book, 1967); R. Kaufmann, *Die Menschenmacher. Die Zukunft der Menschen in einer biologisch gesteuerten Welt* (Hamburg, 1964); F. Wagner (ed.), *Das Problem der genetischen Manipulierung des Menschen* (München, 1969).

[13] O.B. Hardison, Jr., *Toward Freedom and Dignity. The Humanities and the Idea of Humanity* (Baltimore-London: The John Hopkins Univ. Press, 1972), p. xxi.

*Freedom and Dignity*, sees the optimistic prospect of man's overcoming 'future shock' if we are able to integrate the technical aspect into a better understanding of what is specifically human. 'I assume that there will be, in fact, a future society. I assume that it will be highly technical, but I am willing to believe that it will be a society for human beings rather than the technocratic nightmare described in *1984* or *A Clockwork Orange*.' [14]

What Abraham Maslow wrote on the health of individual persons can be applied also to the health of mankind as a whole in the matter of genetic responsibility. Health includes 'the ability to master the environment, to be capable, adequate, effective in relation to it . . . to be in good relations to it.' [15] Without this effort to regain, deepen and act upon a holistic vision, all casuistry and casework in the field of genetics, and all education towards responsibility, will be in vain.

Inter-disciplinary dialogue is surely not easy. The ethicist often is not sensitive enough to new avenues of science and, on the other hand, the scientists and the public are shaped by the world view and the particular language of the technical man. A careful language analysis of the publications in the field of genetics gives plenty of evidence for the 'Sapir-Whorf hypothesis which embodies the notion that world views are as much shaped by language as they are shapers of language itself.' [16] Everyone, and especially every scientist who is a leader in the field of genetics, should be aware of the limitations of the technical language when he faces ethical questions. 'The only choice he must make is whether to bring his assertions to consciousness (and hence expose them, to criticism) or leave them buried in his scientific language and thought.' [17]

---

[14] *Op. cit.*, p. 121.

[15] Abraham Maslow, *Toward a Psychology of Being* (New York-Cincinnati: D. Van Nostrand, 1968), p. 179.

[16] Marc Lappé, 'Allegiances of Human Genetics: a Preliminary Typology', *Hastings Centre Studies*, Vol. 1, No. 2 (1974), p. 64.

[17] Kenneth Eberhard, 'Genetics and Human Survival', *Linacre Quarterly*, Vol. 40, No. 2 (1973), p. 175.

b.  *Interaction between freedom, gene and environment*

Skinnerians do not believe in man's inborn goodness or in his freedom; and since they undervalue the genetic heritage, they put all their trust in manipulation through conditioning and the shaping of the environment. Geneticists, or rather genetic engineers, frequently overlook both man's freedom and the importance of the environment. Yet development of consciousness and education towards an ethical approach of shared responsibility for our world presuppose not only full awareness of our freedom but also a basic knowledge about the interplay of genes and the cultural heritage. In other words, we have to recognize the interaction between our genetic shape and the shaping power of the environment in order to discover the possibilities and our corresponding responsibility freely to shape our environment.

That man is a cultural being means, among other things, that even in his genetic heritage he is conditioned by his culture. 'Life in a culture changes man's biological nature.' [18] The biological nature, and especially the genetic heritage, is a part of the cultural project that affects, conditions and changes various aspects of human nature. From this arises the question of how far we can consciously and intentionally condition and thus change our genetic heritage, and even directly interfere with and modify the genes. The response can be sought and found only through the most conscientious use of our present knowledge and of our hoped-for future knowledge about the interplay between genetic endowment and cultural evolution.

It seems to me that Theodosius Dobzhansky achieves one of the most balanced approaches. 'That the cultural evolution is conditioned by the genetic endowment of our species is evident enough.' [19] But this obvious truth does not allow us to forget

[18] Daniel Callahan, 'New Beginnings in Life: A Philosopher's Response', in Michael Hamilton, *The New Genetics and the Future of Man* (Grand Rapids, Mich.: Eerdmans, 1973), p. 100.

[19] Theodosius Dobzhansky, 'Human Nature as Product of Evolution', in A. Maslow (ed.), *New Knowledge in Human Values*, p. 80.

for one moment the importance and finality of human responsibility for the cultural environment. 'The diversity we observe is a joint product of genetic and environmental differences. The observed diversity is, in principle, controllable by genetic as well as environmental means.' [20]

Throughout the history of evolution and culture, man has influenced his genetic heritage indirectly by exercising his total responsibility for the conditions of life. And even today, while we have new knowledge and new technical capacities, it is still true that 'eugenic amelioration can only be successful, given antecedent environmental and sociological improvement.' [21]

The progress of ecology in our own time is a case in point. Recognition of the connection between environmental pollution and public health has led to intensive studies about health hazards caused by mutagenicity. 'The first evidence that environmental pollutants may influence the genetic constitution of future population came some four decades ago from the discovery that high energy radiation induces mutations. The likelihood that some highly mutagenic chemicals may come into wide use, or indeed may already be in wide use, is now causing serious concern.' [22]

A change in the genetic material may be simply a chemical transformation of one individual gene that alters its function; or it may involve a whole group of genes or even a gain or loss of parts of chromosomes. Since every part of the body and every metabolic process is influenced by genetic control, the mutagenic effects are of a great diversity. 'There are numerous known inherited diseases, and probably many more that are unknown, all of which owe their ultimate cause to mutation. While these are individually rare, collectively they are a cause for serious

[20] Th. Dobzhansky, *Genetic Diversity and Human Equality* (New York: Basic Books, 1973), p. 49.

[21] *Op. cit.*, p. 49.

[22] Samuel S. Epstein, 'Pollution and Health', in M. Hamilton (ed.) *The New Genetics and the Future of Man*, p. 194.

public health concern. Mutations can produce a wide diversity of deleterious effects, many of them similar to those produced by non-genetic causes.' [23]

It would be an error, however, to think about the environment only as a threat or a cause of harmful mutations. The environment can also be, and often has been, a decisive factor in evolution. 'In any case, genetic conditioning, no matter how strong, does not preclude improvement by manipulation of the environment.' [24]

In the past years, alarming voices have been heard lamenting that the progress in medicine allows many genetically defective people to reach the reproductive age and thereby become a threat to the hereditary health of mankind. The most competent researchers seem less pessimistic. The gene pool of mankind is of tremendous dynamism and richness. Even without direct human intervention there is a high capacity for adaptive mutation. 'This vastness suggests that it is difficult to dirty the pool by human intervention.' [25]

Everything seems to indicate that mankind best fulfils its responsibility towards genetic heritage by a maximum of responsibility for good behaviour and for the shape of the total environment. This does not, of course, exclude the necessity to explore, in multi-disciplinary analyses ranging from biochemistry through evolution, all the various possibilities to improve mankind's condition, including the gene pool. 'The provision of an optimum environment for the optimum development of the various aspects of human behaviour should follow such increased understanding.' [26]

The findings of genetics do not at all indicate a genetic

[23] Op. cit., p. 185.
[24] Th. Dobzhansky, Genetic Diversity and Human Equality, p. 10.
[25] A. Etzioni, Genetic Fix, p. 83. Cf., however, pp. 24ff., where the same author expresses an extremely pessimistic view.
[26] Irving I. Gottesman, 'Heritability and Personality', in D.N. Robinson (ed.), Heredity and Achievement, p. 217.

determinism. 'What actually develops is conditioned by the interplay of genes with the environment. . . What the genes really determine are the reaction ranges exhibited by individuals with more or less similar genes over the entire gamut of possible environments.' [27] 'The genotype determines not rigid traits of the organism (the phenotype) but rather its norm of reaction to the environment.' [28] Both outstanding psychologists and outstanding geneticists are recognizing more and more the importance of the ecological factors. They acknowledge frankly that they have had to correct an earlier neglect of the variabilities induced by ecological, social and situational factors and by man's spontaneous and/or free response to them. [29]

There have been, in the past decades, efforts to trace the influence of the genetic heritage on the intelligence quotient (I.Q.) and other human traits, by comparing the achievements of various races. Many of these studies were biased either by racial prejudice or by a lamentable lack of awareness of the environmental influence. 'The controversial question of the race differences arise from failure to understand the genetics of the individual and population differences, and the rationale of their statistical analysis.' [30] Unprejudiced studies seem to yield a more balanced view. 'The degree to which differences in I.Q. arrays between races are genetically conditioned is at present an unsolved problem.' [31] Human development is 'a result of a complex, little understood interaction between heredity and environmental factors. To construct questions about complex behaviour in terms

[27] Theodosius Dobzhansky, *Genetic Diversity and Human Equality*, p. 8. Cf. also his *The Biological Basis of Human Freedom* (New York: Columbia Univ. Press, 1956).

[28] Paul Ramsey, *Fabricated Man*, p. 6.

[29] Cf. Gordon Allport, 'Traits Revisited', in Daniel N. Robinson (ed.) *Heredity and Achievement* (New York: Oxford Univ. Press, 1970) p. 134.

[30] Jerry Hirsch, 'Behaviour, Genetics and Individuality Understood' in D.N. Robinson, *Op. cit.*, p. 372.

[31] Th. Dobzhansky, *Op. cit.*, p. 90. Cf. R.J. Herrnstein, *I.Q. in th Meritocracy* (Boston: Little, Brown, 1973).

of heredity *versus* environment is to over-simplify the essence and nature of human development and behaviour.' [32]

A number of careful studies comparing white and negro children of the same social and economic background and exposed to the same cultural influences show a minimal difference regarding intellectual performance. It seems to be more and more proved that the I.Q. differences in the United States are due mostly to socio-economic and cultural factors. [33] Often, studies about differences in the I.Q. suffer from an almost complete unawareness that the means of the measurement itself, and its particular evaluation, are tied to the specific culture of the one-dimensional, technical man.

This is, however, only one example of a wrong emphasis. The alarmists about genetic deterioration are frequently 'worried about the wrong genes.' I agree with Leon Kass who asserts that today's world suffers more from the morally and spiritually defective than from the genetically defective. [34] If mankind would overcome water and air pollution, the depletion of the environment, the abuse of alcohol and drugs, and numerous other vices, there would be much more achieved for the genetic pool and the future of mankind than by genetic crusaders who approach the complicated problems as one-dimensional biological beings.

Those who are emphasizing one-sidedly man's responsibilty for direct genetic interventions must be asked whether they can give us a proper evaluation of the genes they want to change or to foster. The intelligence quotient alone cannot be the decisive criterion; there are too many people with a relatively high I.Q.

[32] Council of the Society for the Psychological Study of Social Issues Statement, *Harvard Educational Review* 39 (1969), pp. 625-627.

[33] Cf. Paul L. Nichols and V.E. Anderson, 'Intellectual Performance, Race and Socio-Economic Status', *Social Biology* 20 (Dec. 1973), pp. 367-374; David Layzer, 'Heritability Analysis of I.Q. Scores: Science or Numerology?', *Science,* Vol. 183, No. 4, 413 (March 29, 1974), pp. 1259-1266.

[34] Leon Kass, *Op. cit.,* pp.18-19.

but with a vicious character. Others may have inherited or developed a lower I.Q. but are distinguished by kindness, gentleness, altruism, and by the capacity for careful and hard work. [35] The great scientists are far from denying that intelligence does have a genetic background, but they do not stress as the critical factor only the interaction of genes and environment when the quality of the intelligence resides in human liberty and responsibility.

The final question is, again and again, what kind of man we desire: the highly qualified technical and perhaps emotionally and morally underdeveloped man, or the human person with, perhaps a less developed I.Q. when measured for technical capacities, but more human, more able to grow in love and to discern with wisdom what is truly love, inner freedom, generosity, and so on.

c.   *Some examples of genetic responsibilities and social control*

It is highly desirable that genetic information should become a part of general education. Before young people prepare themselves to choose their future partners, they should know about the general risks of genetically conditioned diseases and their transmission. I consider the premarital genetic test to be highly advisable. Indeed, as our genetic information and our responsibilities grow, I think that the premarital exchange of a genetic testimony may be considered a basic moral duty. A different question, however, is whether, or to what extent, a society should use pressure or make compulsory this type of premarital test. Some people are proposing that society should 'keep on record the genetic pedigree of each citizen.' [36]

Paul Ramsey is quite outspoken in favour of the test, to

---

[35] Cf. Th. Dobzhansky, *Op. cit.*, p. 11.
[36] Hermann Muller, 'What Genetic Course Will Man Steer?', in James F. Crow and James V. Need (eds.), *Proceedings of the Third International Congress of Human Genetics* (Baltimore: John Hopkins Press, 1967), pp. 532f.

protect the ignorant and avoid 'complicity in a tragic birth'. He would approve the use of the state's marriage-licensing power to help prevent the transmission of highly negative genes. I agree with him that, from a moral point of view, nobody has 'an unqualified right to have children', and that 'children are not simply for one's own fruition'. [37] However, I am hesitant to recommend or simply approve law enforcement that would keep people from marrying when they are able to enter into marriage and to conduct mature relationships. I agree, rather, with Amitai Etzioni, who says, 'I oppose genetic intervention, not the setting and promotion of genetic codes.' [38]

For a state to refuse to contribute to the care of genetically defective children would be, practically, one of the strongest reinforcements, but it would be simply unjust to the children. On the other hand, those who are opposed to governmental intervention should do more to make consciences sensitive to genetic responsibility, because in the long run we can surely expect reinforcement by law if institutions like the Church and the educational system neglect their duty to inform people's consciences and appeal to their sense of responsibility. [39]

To avoid irresponsible transmission of life, the proper means for unmarried people is abstention from intercourse. It is not easy, however, to decide the moral question for married people who feel obliged in conscience not to transmit defective genes.

[37] P. Ramsey, *Fabricated Man*, p. 97. Of the same opinion is J. Endres, *L'uomo Manipolatore*, p. 71.

[38] A. Etzioni, *Genetic Fix*, p. 108. However, the author practically takes back what he said by asserting, 'the societies can try to persuade people to have fewer children or to abort severely defective ones, but they cannot force the choices. However, the individuals' rights do not include the liberty to charge the upbringing of their children to the public.'

[39] Cf. Gordon Rattray Taylor, *The Biological Time Bomb* (New York: World Publishing Company, 1968); Dwight J. Ingle, *Who Should Have Children? An Environmental and Genetic Approach* (Indianapolis: Bobbs and Merrill, 1973); Summer B. Twiss Jr., 'Parental Responsibility for Genetic Health', *The Hastings Centre Report*, Vol. 4, No. 1 (Feb. 1974), pp. 9-14.

Total continence can jeopardize the very existence of the marriage. Periodical continence often does not offer the necessary degree of certainty, and this may be true also of other contraceptive means. Preventive sterilization could, in some cases, tempt to sexual licence, even when there was no such original intention. But pregnancy in these cases could present a strong temptation to resort to abortion. In comparison with abortion, the preventive sterilization might be the minor evil. If spouses have come to the firm conviction of conscience that, for them, transmission of life must be now and forever excluded, sterilization may sometimes be the proper means to resolve the problem. It has then the character of a preventive therapy.

Worries about defective genes can, however, be exaggerated. I disagree with Paul Ramsey who strongly recommends sterilization, or at least abstension from procreation, for spouses who would transmit diabetes as genetic disease. [40] To my mind, diabetes is no reason for such action, when the spouses know quite well that they transmit also a most precious heritage of strong faith, the capacity to love, harmony of character, and a number of other qualities that outbalance minor defects. I also would not dare recommend generally to women, as Ramsey does, that they abstain from childbearing after the age of thirty-five. [41] It is true that with a woman's increasing age, the risk of having a mongoloid child does increase; but at the age of thirty-five the probability of having such a child is still far below one per cent. I am afraid that the fear of having defective children could easily become psychotic in our society. Genetic education and the development of consciousness must be aware of the danger that when a society is unwilling to bear the burden of handicapped children, it manipulates people through unnecessary fear, and is increasing the already widespread anti-baby attitude.

---

[40] P. Ramsey, *Fabricated Man*, p. 118.
[41] Cf. *Op. cit.*, p. 98.

## 2. Gene therapy

Medicine achieved a great breakthrough when antibiotics made possible a direct attack on the many diseases caused by bacteria. Now it is hoping for a similar breakthrough in the treatment of the numerous diseases caused by errors in the human genetic code. Success in this direction would be one of the greatest benefits to mankind, since 'fifteen out of every one hundred newborn infants have hereditary disorders of greater or lesser severity. More than two thousand genetically distinct inherited defects have been classified. Many are mild, but a large number are not. Forty per cent of all non-traumatic deaths in children's hospitals can be attributed to diseases that are partly or wholly genetic in nature.' [42] Biology is still far from being able to determine accurately all the kinds of defects in the expression of genetic information in DNA. The pace of progress, however, is astonishing.

Gene therapy is a part of a broader field of genetic medicine which involves the diagnosis, prevention and treatment of hereditary diseases. It is a whole new approach — often called 'eugenetic engineering' — based on the assumption that man may attain the power directly to manipulate his genes for his own improvement. It can be called 'gene surgery' when parts are removed or replaced, and 'eugenic engineering' when modification or alteration of genes or gene actions is undertaken to eliminate genetic disorders. Gene therapy differs from 'eugenics', which makes no direct attempt to change the gene itself but tries to improve the quality of the human gene pool by improving the environment and the total human condition. It differs from positive genetic engineering, whose 'patient' is the whole human species, while gene therapy treats the individual living patient at the beginning of his existence.

[42] W. French Anderson, 'Genetic Therapy', in Michael P. Hamilton (ed.), *The New Genetics and the Future of Man* (Grand Rapids, Mich.: Eerdmans, 1972), p. 110. Cf. Harmon Smith, 'Genetics and Ethics: Reaffirming the Tragic Vision', *Linacre Quarterly* 40 (Aug. 1973), p. 160.

The term 'genetic engineering' can be 'considered as covering anything having to do with manipulation of the gametes or the foetus, for whatever purpose, from conception by other than sexual union, or the treatment of disease *in utero*, to the ultimate manufacture of a human being to exact specifications.' [43] Obviously, then, gene therapy is but a modest part of this whole field of biologic engineering. It differs from traditional eugenics which has developed various methods of treating genetically-caused disorders, for instance, treating foetal Rh anemia by replacement of the blood of the foetus, and PKU (phenylketonuria) by a special diet for the newborn.

The new type of gene therapy that interests us here attacks deleterious genes surgically, by chemical means or radiation, to reverse a mutation or eliminate wrong information in the DNA. The chances and the prospective techniques of gene therapy differ according to the main forms of genetic disorder. There are diseases caused by: (1) aberration in the number of chromosomes and the quality of the gross structures (for example, mongoloidism is caused by an additional disturbing forty-seventh half-chromosome and there are gross chromosomal errors, especially in sex abnormalities) [44]; (2) mutations affecting only a single gene (for instance, hemophilia); (3) interaction of several genes (here, the problem of identification is extremely difficult if not impossible); (4) materno-foetal blood incompatibility (for instance, Rh diseases of the newborn).

Some writers speak very optimistically about the future of

[43] *Journal of the American Medical Association*, Vol. 220 (1972), p. 1356.

[44] Cf. R. Walbaum et al., '48 XXX Syndrome in an Infant', *Journal of Genetics and Humanity*, Vol. 21 (March 1973), pp. 43-65. Al. Christensen et al., 'Psychological Studies of Ten Patients with the YYY Syndrome', *British Journal of Psychiatry*, Vol. 123 (Aug. 1973), pp. 219-221. Kenneth Burke, 'The XYY Syndrome: Genetic Behaviour and the Law', *Denver Law Journal*, Vol. 46 (1969), pp. 261-284. Marg. A. Telfer, David Baker, Gerald Clark and Claude Richardson, 'Incidence of Gross Chromosomal Errors Among Tall Criminal American Males', *Science* 159 (March 15, 1968), pp. 1249-1250.

gene therapy.[45] Other experts in the field of biology make sharp distinctions between genetic disorders that might be reasonably accessible to gene mutations, and those more complicated disorders for which the present state of biology can offer no reasonable hope of healing, at least in the foreseeable future. Motulsky gives quite a clear picture of this situation. The less accessible to direct therapy are chromosome aberrrations. In Down's syndrome (mongoloidism) an additional small chromosome (called † 21) is present, and the condition may be compatible with a fairly long life. Gene therapy would require the removal of the additional chromosome very early in embryonic life, at least before the formation of the brain, where the major damage occurs. Such micro-surgery of individual cells is not feasible now nor in the foreseeable future. A similarly unfavourable prospect holds for other chromosome disorders.

Gene therapy also appears to be impossible for diseases where multiple genes are involved. It is highly unlikely that it would be possible to reach, by direct manipulation, a group of genes located on different chromosomes.[46] In those genetic disorders that affect structural protein (DNA), genetic therapy is theoretically conceivable but practically not yet available. Disorders caused by deficiency of protein or enzymes are most accessible to genetic manipulations. The therapy involves administration of normal DNA in various ways. The cure for these diseases is, in theory, to correct a wrong message or to replace it by accurate code words in the DNA and message molecules.

Although progress in research is enormous, and is being carried on by numerous groups of highly qualified scientists, it has to be said that at the present moment there is still a

[45] Cf., for instance, Joseph Fletcher and Joshua Lederberg. See J. Fletcher, *The Ethics of Genetic Control. Ending Reproductive Roulette* (Garden City, N.Y.: Anchor Press/Doubleday, 1974). A more balanced optimism is expressed by outstanding scientists like Anderson, 'Genetic Therapy', in Hamilton, *Op. cit.*, pp. 109-124.

[46] Arno G. Motulsky, 'Genetic Therapy', in Hamilton, *Op. cit.*, p. 127.

great lack not only in knowledge but especially in techniques necessary to manipulate genes and chromosomes in a reasonable way.[47] Researchers believe they now have the necessary knowledge to decipher the language of the cell. Actually (in 1970) a complete gene has been synthesized in the test tube.[48] Cytogenetists have made great progress in animal experimentation.[49] But the step from the animal world to the world of the human species is particularly difficult in this field.

Before we try to evaluate direct genetic manipulation as a new form of therapy, it may be well to look at the alternatives. Anderson, dramatizing the danger of the increasing number of defective genes in the total population, evaluates the various alternatives proposed by modern scientists and/or ethicists, journalists and politicians. The most radical proposal is to stop treating serious genetic diseases and thus allow natural selection to take control again. But this is no real alternative for Christians or for anyone who takes seriously the individual person. 'To refuse to treat a child who has a treatable disease is inhumane, reprehensible, and totally against the ethics of the medical profession.'[50]

A second proposal is to treat individuals but to block the further pollution of the gene pool by means of contraception, sterilization and restrictive marriage licenses for carriers of gravely defective genes. I have already expressed my own opinion on this view. Anderson speaks out sharply against mandatory restrictions. 'Who would make the final decision as

---

[47] Cf. Paul Overhage, 'Die Evolution zum Menschen hin', in Johannes Hüttenbügel, *Gott, Mensch, Universum* (Graz/Köln: Styria, 1974), p. 404.

[48] Cf. Anderson, *Op. cit.*, p. 112.

[49] Cf. Monitor, 'Cell Fusion to Repair Genetic Defects', *New Scientist,* Vol. 61 (3 Jan. 1974), p. 3. Graham Chedd, 'How to Repress an Operator', *New Scientist,* Vol. 61 (3 Jan. 1974), pp. 7-9. Monitor, 'Shooting Genes in the Dark', *New Scientist,* Vol. 61 (24 Jan. 1974), p. 18.

[50] Anderson, *Op. cit.*, p. 123.

to which defective genes are "bad" and which are simply less than "good"?' [51]

A third alternative is already widely practised. It allows those individuals who, because of medicine's tremendous advances, have reached the reproductive age, to marry and to have children, but would determine by amniocentesis during each pregnancy whether a defective foetus was conceived, and if so, would abort it. This is an especially frightening prospect, since it will be very difficult to convince people of the unacceptability of such an approach in a society which tolerates and legalizes abortion of the normal foetus.

The last alternative is to continue the present research efforts to treat genetic diseases in every way other than by direct gene therapy. There already exist many techniques for the treatment, and partially even for the prevention of genetic diseases. The best known are the following.

1) Diets: in mental retardation caused by PKU (an anomaly in protein metabolism), dietary phenylalanine restriction from birth may allow normal mental development.

2) Supply of missing factors: pernicious anemia can be treated by vitamin $B^{12}$ injection; hemophilia can be treated by injection of the missing protein substance, anti-hemophilic globulin, factor VIII.

3) Immunologic prevention: for instance, injection of Rh globulin destroys Rh positive cells of foetal origin in mothers with Rh positive babies, and prevents build-up of Rh antibodies which cause hemolytic diseases of the newborn in the next foetus.

4) Enzyme inducements: certain enzymes can be induced by drugs; for instance, some types of hereditary jaundice can be treated by phenobarbital which stimulates production of the missing enzyme; Motulsky completes the list by mentioning removal of excess toxic substances, surgery and transplantation. [52]

*(margin handwritten note: what's most commonly helped by gene therapy)*

[51] Op. cit., p. 124.
[52] Motulsky, Op. cit., p. 128.

There is no doubt that research in this more traditional direction can still bear considerable fruit. However, it is evident that direct therapy of the genes could bring tremendous progress, over and beyond all the other methods. Not only would future generations profit greatly, but also the individual person thus healed would be free from the fear of transmitting defective life.

We can say that genetic surgery, *if* done effectively and with no disproportionate risks, would be the most moral and potentially the most promising of genetic alternatives. [53] The same criteria apply to gene therapy as to therapy in general. Hopes and risks have to be carefully weighed, one against the other. It is true that human life is, at its very source and beginning, a most delicate object of therapeutic manipulation. However, in many genetic disorders, if nothing is done, the risks are enormous. In many cases, gene therapy would be the only hope to save life or to save human life from mental decay.

Some ethicists, like Paul Ramsey, reject gene therapy radically whenever it means gametic manipulation (manipulation of the sperm and eggs). His main argument is that 'it is not a proper goal of medicine to enable women to have children and marriages to be fertile by any means necessary, even one which imposes an additional hazard upon the child not yet conceived.' [54] I think he under-evaluates the legitimate desire of spouses to have children. We have already seen that he would not allow potential parents to transmit life even when there is no greater risk than diabetes. I agree with him if he stresses that not all means necessary to this end can be approved, but he goes beyond traditional moral theology in both the Catholic and the Protestant tradition if he demands that there should be no risk whatsoever in this matter. Transmission of life always includes risk. 'In cases involving both genetic therapy and gametic manipulation, the unknown and unforeseen risks to future generations may

[53] Cf. Kenneth D. Eberhard, 'Genetics and Human Survival: A Christian Perspective', *Linacre Quarterly* (Aug. 1973), p. 178.

[54] P. Ramsey, 'Genetic Therapy', in Hamilton (ed.), *Op. cit.*, p. 160.

outweigh any benefit that might be secured for the individual patient; in a matter of such great importance, "no discernible risk" is not an adequate protection. We need to know that there are no risks — a requirement which inheritable gene therapy is not apt to meet'. [55] However, in cases where there is no gametic manipulation involved, but healing of a conceptus, Ramsey would be less severe about the dangers of methods to eliminate an extremely grave genetic defect. He would approve genetic surgery even with a discernible risk whenever it is the only way to save life or to save it from total decay. [56]

One of the methods of gene therapy is a process called 'transduction', which has already been thoroughly tested *in vitro,* at least with animals. The desired gene is attached to a non-pathogenic virus particle which then carries the gene into the cell where it is incorporated into the cell's gene pool. 'Theoretically, the carrier virus should have no effect on all the other genes in the gene pool; but therein, of course, lies the problem. It is not known, nor can it be clearly tested, what effect any virus, believed to be non-pathogenic, will have on the gene pool. In other words, we may have the ability to manipulate genes long before we know whether it is safe to do so. The same argument can be made against almost any new agent or procedure.' [57]

The first attempts at this method have already been made in cases where there would otherwise be no hope whatsoever of saving life or of guaranteeing the most basic capacity of human consciousness and freedom. There seems to be little doubt about moral justification in such extreme cases. Then, gradual progress may be hoped for that can justify application to less drastic cases.

[55] P. Ramsey, *Op. cit.,* p. 169
[56] Cf. Ramsey, *Fabricated Man,* p. 119; Ch. Curran, *Politics, Medicine and Christian Ethics,* pp. 167f.
[57] Anderson, *Op. cit.,* p. 117.

## 3. Genetic engineering

The term 'genetic engineering' can be used in a broad and in a strict sense. Here I intend to use it in the strict sense, as direct attempt to change the genes of the embryo, not only to eliminate gene disorders but with the intent to add new traits and to construct a more desirable or more desired human being. Some scientists think that it is possible to reconstruct genetically a more perfect human being than the one that has resulted from millions of years of evolution. 'Perhaps the great breakthrough of the future will be in changing the species through genetic manipulation.' [58]

I do not take into consideration the dreams and proposals of extremists like Joseph Fletcher who hope that genetic engineers can and will construct cyborgs (combining human bodies and technical electrical adjuncts) and a totally new species through hybridization between, for instance, *homo sapiens* and high primates. For those who believe that all surprising new scientific possibilities automatically mean human progress, it is usual to disparage those who do not greet all this with enthusiasm. Fletcher writes, 'Bizarre certainly, repellant to some, but it spells out the radical character of the new frontier.' [59] Not only for the serious ethicist but also for almost all scientists, it is evident that here the boundary lines demanded by the uniqueness of humankind are grossly overstepped.

Until about ten years ago, scientists and theologians used the term 'genetic manipulation' or similar expressions almost exclusively in reference to selection of sperm and ova for artificial insemination or fertilization. They spoke mainly or only about the baby to be produced *in vitro*. Karl Rahner's oft-quoted

---

[58] *The Mental Health of Children: Services, Research and Manpower.* Reports of Joint Commission on Mental Health of Children (New York: Harper and Row, 1973), p. 259.

[59] J. Fletcher, *The Ethics of Genetic Control*, pp. 4-5. Cf. pp. 43-45

article of 1967 is typical. [60] Now, most of the abundant literature under the heading 'genetic engineering' treats of all kinds of manipulation in the field of the transmission of life. It discusses not only those manoeuvres now possible but almost everything conceivable between what is already possible and utopia. In the foreground are the technical questions and the foreseeable impact of genetic manipulation on the whole of society and culture. [61]

Direct engineering, or reconstruction of the genes, is conceivable in regard to the gametes (sperm and ova) or the fertilized egg in its successive phases of development. It could be practised by changing, more or less radically, the genetic information of the DNA which guides the whole development from fertilization to the formation of the adult organism, and is operative even in the future transmission of life.

Also discussed is the possibility of adding or subtracting chromosomes. In the opinion of some serious scientists, a *homo novus*, belonging to the species of *homo sapiens*, will be not

[60] K. Rahner, 'Zum Problem der genetischen Manipulation', in *Schriften zur Theologie* (Benziger: Zürich, 1967), pp. 286-321. English version: 'The Problem of Genetic Manipulation', in *Theological Investigations* (New York: Herder and Herder, 1972), Vol. IX.

[61] Cf. Aldous Huxley, *Brave New World* and *Brave New World Revisited* (New York: Harper and Row, 1965). Fred Warshofsky, *The Control of Life in the 21st Century* (New York: Viking Press, 1967). Gerald Feinberg, *Prometheus Project* (New York: Doubleday, 1968). Gordon Rattray Taylor, *The Biological Time Bomb* (New York: World Publishing Company, 1968). David Paterson (ed.), *Genetic Engineering* (London: British Broadcasting Corporation, 1969). Albert Rosenfeld, *The Second Genesis: The Coming Control of Life* (Englewood Cliffs, N.J.: Prentice Hall, 1969). Philip Handler (ed.), *Biology and the Future of Man* (New York: O.U.P., 1970). Robert T. Francoeur, *Utopian Motherhood: New Trends in Human Reproduction* (Garden City, N.Y.: Doubleday, 1970). Henry Still, *Man-made Man* (New York: Hawthorn Books, 1973). H.J. Muller, *Man's Future Birthright: Essays on Science and Humanity* (New York: State Univ. of New York Press, 1973). Carl Heintze, *Genetic Engineering* (Nashville: Th. Nelson, 1974). Darrel S. English, *Genetic and Reproductive Engineering* (New York: MSS Information Corporation, 1974).

only thinkable but also constructable in the near future: this would be achieved by directed and enforced evolution of the chromosomes with diploid of only forty-four chromosomes. [62] Even more discussed is a plan to insert one gene or a number of gene informations into human cells — for instance, the brain cells — at decisive moments of development.

The difficulties in all these proposals are colossal. Any important change could possibly be effected only by multiple gene mutations. Important traits such as intelligence, strength of will and, creativity, do not depend on a single gene but are the result of a considerable number of genes and multiple interdependencies. 'It is possible to produce defective intelligence (mental retardation) by any one of many different single gene mutations, in the same sense that one can obtain a defective automobile by any one of many different manufacturing errors. But to improve intelligence genetically, it would be necessary to make precise changes in such a way that all interrelated components would work with increased efficiency... Our present understanding of brain function, however, is still extremely rudimentary. Nonetheless, even after saying all of this, it is possible that efforts to "improve" intelligence might be attempted some day.' [63]

Other interventions which do not attempt direct gene mutation might be more promising. There is, for instance, a reasonable prospect of obtaining a multiplication of the neurons, and thus a higher intelligence quotient, through the use of human growth hormones (HGH) before and immediately after the birth of the child. [64]

In the effort to come to a moral evaluation of directly intended gene mutations, we can distinguish three questions.

---

[62] P. Overhage, Op. cit., p. 403. Cf. P. Eberle, 'Spontane und induzierte Gen-Anderungen beim Menschen', Arzt und Christ 11 (1935), pp. 129-146.

[63] Anderson, Op. cit., p. 119.

[64] P. Overhage, Op. cit., p. 406.

(1) Is mankind allowed to try, by direct gene manipulation, to improve the human species beyond the indications of therapy? (2) If so, can we offer criteria? (3) Can we have any trust that the technical man of today will approach such a daring enterprise in the right spirit? Or should we discourage or hinder any movement in the direction of constructing a better biological substrate for man's existence? Could the necessities of survival or any other reason justify any attempt to change the human species?

I think that, on principle, we cannot simply condemn man's desire to improve directly, and even by constructive manipulation of the genes, the genetic basis of human existence. Karl Rahner notes that, in so far as self-realization as a person is concerned, most people have a rather poor biological heritage. [65] Since man's biological nature is entrusted to his freedom and wisdom, he is, by his very historical nature, the steward of his genetic heritage. The real question is not whether we should or should not influence genetic evolution. Consciously or unconsciously, willingly or not, man does constantly influence genetic history by how he shapes his own behaviour and his total environment. 'Our fundamental decision, then, is whether or not we should intervene in our own evolution deliberately, rather than continue to do so haphazardly.' [66]

We know now that, throughout history, man has manipulated himself and, in many ways, has caused the present condition of his biological genetic heritage. We also realize that, through negligence, sloth and ignorance, he has caused not only certain ailments and genetic disorders but also insufficient development. From this awareness, it is only a step to a serious consideration of the prospect of using all modern knowledge and available technique to improve humankind's genetic heritage, wherever

[65] K. Rahner, 'Zum Problem der genetischen Manipulation', *Op. cit.*, p. 297.

[66] Bernard D. Davis, 'Threat and Promise in Genetic Engineering', in R.H. Williams (ed.), *Ethical Issues in Biology and Medicine* (Cambridge, Mass.: Schenkman, 1973), p. 18.

and whenever this may be reasonably possible. [67] Self-manipulation, which heretofore was almost totally unplanned, can in the future become a planned and systematic piloting of biological nature.

Christians and other representatives of the humanist tradition concur in the view that the meaning of history is an increasing hominization. That means not only a continuing growth in the intelligence quotient but also the gradual overcoming of unreasonable aggressive tendencies and a greater adaptability to co-operation. [68]

The conclusion might well be that we are not only allowed to use gene therapy — that is, to eliminate an additional chromosome or a wrong genetic information that causes decay and disrupture of human relationships — but may also be entitled to accelerate hominization by direct improvement of the genetic heritage if this is possible. The careful planning of constructive changes that work in the direction of that common task of hominization cannot be rejected a priori as being against man's nature or vocation. [69]

Here, the point has to be stressed that I am not speaking of arbitrary genetic changes but only of the general principle of whether, if there should be the necessary knowledge, techniques, and especially the necessary criteria, mankind might be entitled to pilot its genetic development. Regarding genetic manipulation that does not take into account man's total vocation, I agree wholeheartedly with C.S. Lewis, that 'if any one age really attains, by eugenics and scientific manipulation, the power to make the descendants what it pleases, all men who live after it are patients of that power. They are weaker, not stronger.' [70]

In such a sensitive field, all people and all disciplines have

---

[67] Cf. K. Rahner, Op. cit., p. 263.
[68] Cf. Bernard D. Davis, Op. cit., p. 30.
[69] Cf. K. Rahner, Op. cit., p. 295.
[70] C.S. Lewis, The Abolition of Man (New York: Collier-McMillan, 1965), pp. 70-71.

to co-operate in finding criteria and in creating that firm conviction that makes unrealistic and irresponsible interventions impossible. 'We are not fated to do everything genetically which we now have or will have the power to do. Nor are we utterly free to manipulate our human future. Genetic manipulation can either be responsible or irresponsible.' [71]

If we look for criteria for realistic attitudes and interventions in this most delicate matter, we have to be aware of the total situation in our highly technical society, and especially of those who are leading in genetic research and technique. We have not only to try to become immune to the fascination of the new and astonishing possibilities but also to be critically aware of the major trends.

Many scientists, honest and good men, are thoroughly shaped by the educational system in which they have developed their extraordinary capacities. They have in mind the development of the *homo faber*. What they want to develop through genetic improvement is, to a great extent, that intelligence quotient which is measured by the criteria of this technical man. Along with many others, Karl Rahner puts the question whether the intelligence that can be genetically influenced is really the kind of intelligence we need most, namely, that of wisdom, moral responsibility and altruism. The purely technical intelligence can already be increased though computers and cybernetics. [72]

We have substantial reasons to fear that genetic engineering could fall under the heartless rules of the market. Studies have already been published on the interdependence between market profits as a main incentive and the actual possibilities of biomedical engineering. [73] Will such an important matter finally be regulated by the rules of the market? LeRoy Walters touches

[71] James B. Nelson, *Op. cit.*, p. 121.
[72] K. Rahner, *Op. cit.*, p. 317.
[73] Typical is the following publication: Committee on the Interplay of Engineering with Biology and Medicine, *An Assessment of Industrial Activity in the Field of Biomedical Engineering* (National Academy of Engineering, Washington, 1971).

a sensitive point: 'Because of its intellectual rootage in utilitarianism, the TA (technology assessment) movement tends to focus primary attention on man the maker' [74] — by which he means man the producer, not man the poet, man the artist.

The present situation is one of abundant technical knowledge faced with a great lack of wisdom for guiding the evolutionary process. To discuss such a grave matter in the abstract is thoroughly unreasonable. We shall have to deal with genetic engineers who are products of the technical culture, and with scientists for whom the genetic sources of human behaviour are particularly useful for exoneration. Where human behaviour and misbehaviour are explained chiefly by the genes, there will be a tendency to claim that the only reasonable use of freedom lies in a calculated change of the genes; technical progress, and the satisfaction gained from calculated manipulation of man's future, will count much more than man's dignity and freedom. [75] All too easily forgotten or denied will be the normative value of human wisdom. [76]

Under such circumstances, even if ethical problems are seen, they will be easily discounted. The task forces and committees that published the book *The Mental Health of Children* acknowledge that they are aware of social, juridical and moral questions but are convinced that technical progress cannot and must not be stopped. 'Theoretically, some day — and not in some impossibly remote future but within decades — it might become possible to add specific traits or to delete given genes from a particular pair of gametes by some combination of microsurgery and biochemical effect.' And for them it would be the great breakthrough 'to change the human species' through genetic manipulations. Their practical conclusion is that research

---

[74] LeRoy Walters, 'Technology Assessment and Genetics', *Theological Studies* 33, (1972), p. 683.

[75] Cf. B.F. Skinner, *Beyond Freedom and Dignity,* pp. 77-78.

[76] Cf. James M. Gustafson, 'Genetic Engineering and the Normative View of the Human', in R.H. Williams (ed.), *Ethical Issues in Biology and Medicine* (Cambridge, Mass.: Schenkman, 1973), pp. 46-58.

should be continued 'by all means'. [77] It is one thing to improve the genetic heritage, with maximum care for continuity; it is another is to 'change the human species'.

Even the expressions 'genetic engineering' or 'genetic technology' indicate how great is the danger that the methods of the natural sciences — 'experimentation, error, risk' — will be applied uncritically to the field of man's biological substratum and even to the transmission of life (typically called 'reproduction'). 'Biology will take this risk and carry on the genetic manipulation, whatever may be the price. However, man should not forget how precious the unique substance of man is, and that it is the result of millions of centuries of evolution until he became what he is in the breadths of variations and in his adaptability.' [78]

One of the most worrying aspects of all the new initiatives is the danger of coldly eliminating mishaps or, as scientists might say, 'disposing' of them. It is true that 'genetic and reproductive engineering do not necessarily involve the intention to discard human mishaps'. [79] But as long as society legalizes, without any therapeutic indication, the killing of healthy foetuses, there is little hope that scientists will respect the human life of the 'mishaps' of their own engineering.

The minimum that we should ask is that experimentation should go slowly, step by step, and never further than the present knowledge allows. The risks should be carefully evaluated in comparison with the risks in spontaneous evolution with no direct interference by man. [80] Yet it seems to me too rigoristic to demand that direct interventions in the evolution of the gene should exclude any noticeable risk whatsoever. Of course, I

---

[77] *The Mental Health of Children: Services, Research and Manpower* (New York: Harper and Row, 1973), p. 259.

[78] Paul Overhage, *Op. cit.*, p. 423. Cf. Paul Overhage, *Experiment Menschheit, Die Steuerung der menschlichen Evolution* (Frankfurt: Knecht, 3rd ed., 1969).

[79] Charles Curran, *Op. cit.*, p. 211.

[80] Cf. Ch. Curran, *Op. cit.*, p. 212.

speak only about interventions that respect the dignity of the human person, and are inserted into the history of liberty in a positive way.

An over-emphasis on direct genetic manipulation, or unrealistic hopes for it, can have a negative impact on man's primary responsibility to promote genuinely human evolution and development through better attitudes, better behaviour and a wiser ordering of the world in which he lives. Genetic engineering which intends to change the human species could become a great threat if it were launched on a broad level in the service of economic or political power. There is also danger that a manipulated public opinion could facilitate unreasonable experimentations, even where there is no political pressure. 'Presently, not enough is known about either genetics or psychology for a social experiment to be launched with enthusiasm. Even if the mental and behavioural dispositions of man prove to be genetically manipulable, it is by no means clear what the desirable types should be.' [81]

I shall try, now, to synthesize my conclusions: Man has a limited right of self-modification. However, he has to carry it out with wisdom and responsibility for future generations. It seems to me that man's right of intervention goes beyond therapy in the strict sense; but, as Paul Ramsey warns, 'the practice of medicine in the service of life is one thing; man's unlimited self-modification of the genetic conditions of life would be quite another matter.' [82] I agree with him that there is not an unlimited right; but in my opinion, there is a limited one. However, it is no easy matter to determine accurately the legitimate limits of such a new venture. There are extreme forms of genetic manipulation envisaged which manifest a clear immorality. This is so wherever they deny man's essential vocation or radically jeopardize it. 'It could, for instance, be said that a genetic manipulation is to be condemned if it destroys or damages

[81] D.N. Robinson, *Psychology*, p. 311.
[82] P. Ramsey, *Fabricated Man*, p. 95.

the vital substrate for genuine human intercommunication.' [83] Increase in technical intelligence can in no way justify an intervention which probably jeopardizes or decreases the growth in wisdom.

## 4. Genetic counselling and prenatal diagnosis

Interest in eugenics and in the new knowledge and techniques is proved by hundreds of counselling units which operate mostly with a negative eugenic policy, that is with the only goal of preventing genetically undesirable marriages and/or pregnancies. Until a few years ago, genetic counselling was confined almost exclusively to premarital situations. Its concern was whether a marriage might be advisable or whether, in a given marriage,' transmission of life would bring a disproportionate risk. To facilitate this counselling, a genetic screening of the population for the most wide-spread genetic diseases was strongly advertised. [84]

Recent years have brought a great shift in genetic counselling, owing to new methods of prenatal diagnosis and the strong trend towards abortion. Since 1966, the method of the photographing and systematic cataloguing of chromosomes has developed. A process called 'amniocentesis' (tests of amniotic fluid taken from the mother's womb between the twelfth and fifteenth weeks of pregnancy) now allows detection of genetic disorders with approximate accuracy. [85] Much of genetic coun-

[83] K. Rahner, Op. cit., p. 296.
[84] Cf. Marc Lappé, 'Ethical Issues in Screening for Genetic Diseases', New England Journal of Medicine, Vol. 286 (25 May, 1973), pp. 1129-1132. Harry Harris and Kurt Hirschborn (eds.), Advances in Genetic Screening (New York: Plenum Press, 1973).
[85] Cf. Daniel Bergsma et al. (eds.), Intra-uterine Diagnosis: Birth Defects. Original Article Series, Vol. VII, No. 5 (Baltimore: Williams and Wilkins, 1971). A.E.H. Emery, Prenatal Diagnosis of Genetic Disease (Baltimore: Williams and Wilkins, 1973). Aubry Milunsky, The Prenatal Diagnosis of Hereditary Disorders (Springfield, Ill.: Charles C. Thomas, 1973). Arno G. Motulsky et al., The Role of Genetic Counselling (New York: MSS Information, 1974).

selling has therefore become associated with amniocentesis. In some cases it is used in view of foetal therapy; for instance, for rhesus iso-immunization. But when amniocentesis is used in the context of genetic counselling, the usual purpose (at least in the United States) is to find out whether the foetus has any grave genetic disorder, with implicit or explicit intention to abort it if such is the case.

What especially motives this is the fear of Down's syndrome and similar disorders that cause mental retardation. [86] The present confusion in vision and language becomes evident when we hear even serious scientists speak easily of 'therapeutic abortion' in these cases where the mother's unspecified 'disease' is the fear of having a defective child. [87] Even some people who are worried about the overall effects of genetic engineering become fanatic apostles of amniocentesis and abortion in all cases where serious genetic disorder can be found. [88]

For serious ethicists, genetic counselling in these new situations has become one of the major fields of concern and reflection. [89] It should be noted that there is often not even a reasonable proportion between the hope of detecting the genetic disorder or the probability of the givenness of a serious genetic disease on the one hand and, on the other, the risks involved in this procedure. Amniocentesis still represents a one to two per

---

[86] Cf. I.M. Berg (ed.), *Genetic Counselling in Relation to Mental Retardation* (New York: Pergamon Press, 1971).

[87] Cf. W.F. Anderson, in Hamilton, *Op. cit.*, p. 116.

[88] For instance, A. Etzioni, in his book *Genetic Fix*, stresses this point at least fifteen times in various contexts in which one would not expect this problem. No wonder that J. Fletcher is one who sees in amniocentesis and in the follow-up of abortion one of the greatest successes of modern science, since his thesis is, 'abortion is far safer than pregnancy.' (*The Ethics of Genetic Control*, p. 58).

[89] Cf. Roger Shinn, 'Genetic Decisions: A Case Study in Ethical Method', *Soundings* 52 (1969), pp. 299-310. Alexander Morgan Capron, 'Informed Decision-making in Genetic Counselling: A Dissent to the "Wrongful Life" Debate', *Indiana Law Journal*, Vol. 48 (1973), pp. 581-604.

cent risk of hurting the foetus and provoking irreparable damage or miscarriage through infection or trauma. From the viewpoint of Catholic moral doctrine, it is never licit to terminate a pregnancy because of genetic defects in the foetus. 'Hence, it is difficult to see the justification for performing amniocentesis for the prenatal diagnosis of hereditary diseases unless it is done with a view to real therapy.' [90]

The rush to amniocentesis, with abortion in mind, is a sign of a manipulated public opinion; and a genetic counselling unit that performs routine amniocentesis under these circumstances can only increase this manipulative process. Daniel Callahan warns, 'Society has taken many centuries to develop sensitive, receptive response to the defective person. That gain should not be jeopardized by new-found powers to ameliorate defectiveness'.[91]

Many think that the genetic counsellor's *rôle* is only to provide strictly neutral information. I agree with James Nelson who feels that this impersonal attitude treats the counselees as medical cases rather than truly as persons. [92] This very appearance of neutrality by the one who provides information, where such a grave decision is at stake (whether or not to terminate a pregnancy), is a kind of manipulation. It suggests that, after all, an abortion to avoid the risk of a defective child is as neutral as the information. I agree with those counsellors who insist that they do not want to intrude on the consciences of their clients, since the clients should make their own decision. However, the way in which they give information should make it clear that they do not consider the decision as a neutral one but as one of grave consequences, involving the highest human values.

In some cases, counselling with the prospect of abortion is

---

[90] George V. Lobo, S.J., *Current Problems in Medical Ethics* (Allahabad: St Paul Publications, 1974), p. 155.

[91] D. Callahan, 'Ethics, Law and Genetic Counselling', *Science* 176 (1972), p. 199.

[92] James Nelson, *Human Medicine,* p. 101.

linked with a desired sex: someone absolutely wants a boy, and therefore each female foetus is aborted. In a few cases, sex selection is linked with genetic disease: a man who has a recessive gene of hemophilia can pass it on only to daughters, who then do not have the disease, since it is sex-linked, but become carriers and pass it on their children. Joseph Fletcher says, 'By controlling his reproduction through sex selection or pre-emptive abortion, keeping only male embryos, this man would stop, once for all, the scourge of his family line. That is his moral responsibility.' [93] This is an example of the manipulative power of a permissive society and its prophets.

## 5.  *Artificial human reproduction*

An early capitalism which considered even the transmission of life under the 'iron law' of interdependence with the problems of production, coined the chilling phrase, 'human reproduction'. It implied the same mechanistic spirit now at work in the type of genetic technology that is producing test-tube babies and planning many more technical inventions for the manufacture of human beings.

While the possibility and feasibility of direct gene manipulation is still in the discussion stage, eugenetic engineering is already being practised in many ways. Man can be thoroughly manipulated in his ontogenesis before and after conception, until his birth. Various forms of engineering are possible: the exchange of the nucleus in sperm or ovule, the fusion of human cells including ovules, the development of unfertilized ovules (parthenogenesis), artificial insemination and egg grafts, fertilization *in vitro* (in the test tube), the growth of early embryos in the laboratory (in a glass womb or steel womb with an artificial placenta), with selective destruction of those who cannot pass genetic muster. All these forms of breeding human beings are

---

[93]  J. Fletcher, *Op. cit.*, p. 157.

already practised or are at least in an advanced phase of preparation. [94]

These experimentations have various goals: for instance, the improvement of the gene pool, the battle against sterility, the selection of the sex of children. [95] The main purposes, as expressed by pioneers in this work, are research and progress in medicine and, finally service to life. 'We are all aware that this work presents challenges to a number of established social and ethical concepts. In our opinion, the emphasis should be on rewards that may be promised in fundamental knowledge and in medicine.' [96]

The scientific world was not surprised when, in June 1974, the two English scientists, Steptoe and Edwards, could announce that three test-tube babies had been born and were thriving. Already, twelve years before, the world had been surprised by the news that Petrucci, a professor at the University of Bologna, had succeeded in artificial fertilization in the test-tube, and had kept one of the foetuses alive until the twenty-ninth day. Later, it was heard that he succeeded even to the fifty-ninth day. In

---

[94] Cf. F. Wagner (ed.), *Menschenzüchtung: Das Problem der genetischen Manipulierung des Menschen* (München, 1969). David M. Rorvik, 'Taking Life Into Our Hands: The Test Tube Baby is Coming', *Look*, May 18, 1971, pp. 83-88. P.C. Steptoe, R.G. Edwards and I.M. Purdy, 'Human Blastocysts Grow in Culture', *Nature* 229 (1971), pp. 132-133. R.G. Edwards, 'Problems of Artificial Fertilization', *Nature* 233 (1971), pp. 23-25. Dr. Kratzer et al., 'Transfer of Human Zygotes', *Lancet* (Sept. 29, 1973), pp. 728-729. Mark Lipkin Jr. and Peter T. Rowley (eds.), *Genetic Responsibility: On Choosing Our Children's Genes* (New York: Plenum Press, 1974).

[95] With his usual enthusiasm for the new and the unusual, J. Fletcher (*The Ethics of Genetic Control*, p. 62) writes, 'individual fertilization . . . invaluable means to select the sex of children.' The suggested method is to induce super-ovulation and then to fertilize *in vitro* the one zygote of the desired sex while 'discarding the surplus' (*Op. cit.*, p. 63). For a serious treatment of the present possibilities of sex choice, see Leon R. Kass, 'New Beginnings in Life', in Hamilton, *Op. cit.*, pp. 24-25.

[96] R.G. Edwards and R.F. Fowler, 'Human Embryos in the Laboratory', *Scientific American* 233 (Dec. 1970), p. 54.

1966, medical magazines published the news that a team of Russian researchers had been able to keep about two hundred and fifty foetuses alive for as long as two months. One was kept alive for six months and had reached the weight of half a kilo. [97]

It is no wonder that some scientists are fascinated by their new power, and go ahead with their experimentations whatever the cost may be. An anonymous scientist is quoted as saying, 'If I can carry a baby all the way through to birth *in vitro*, I certainly plan to do it, though obviously I am not going to succeed on the first attempt or even on the twentieth.' [98] Artificial fertilization *in vitro*, and subsequent implantation even after hibernation, is already successful in breeding animals. The first implantation of human blastocysts, after about five days' growth *in vitro*, was tried in 1971.

Those who follow an older, static natural law concept that virtually sacralizes the biological processes can only look with horror on all these phenomena. Most of us react, or reacted, with negative feelings when we first heard about these interventions into processes concerning the beginning of human life. However, a moral evaluation based on a personalistic view and concerned mainly with the dignity and freedom of man, must look at each phenomenon individually.

a.   *AIH — homologous insemination*

Tens of thousands of persons now living owe their existence to artificial insemination either with the husband's sperm (AIH), or with the sperm of an anonymous donor (AID). Pius XII declared both illicit, although his emphasis was on the rejection of artificial insemination with the sperm from a donor, leaving seemingly open an unspecified kind of 'assisted insemination' with the sperm of the husband. [99]

[97] P. Overhage, *Op. cit.,* p. 408.
[98] Albert Rosenberg, *The Second Genesis: The Coming Control of Life* (Englewood Cliffs, N.J.: Prentice Hall, 1969), p. 117.
[99] Address to Catholic Doctors, Sept. 29, 1949, *AAS* 41 (1949), p. 560.

The two cases must be thoroughly distinguished. Today, outside the Catholic Church very few ethicists reject AIH in cases where spouses, with good reason, desire to have their own child. Even Paul Ramsey, a moralist who is generally extremely severe in the whole field of genetic engineering, gives approval to AIH in certain circumstances, including even the hibernization of the husband's sperm in the case of an unavoidable vasectomy.[100] In the Catholic Church the question is very much under discussion. Before the papal intervention of 1949, a number of balanced and rather conservative moralists — for instance, A. Vermeersh and G. Kelly — approved AIH, at least when the sperm was obtained in a licit way.[101] George Lobo expresses today's more common opinion: 'It seems that in the present state of the question, a couple, eagerly desiring a child, and sincerely finding the procedure of assisted insemination unsatisfactory, would not be doing wrong by having recourse to AIH'.[102]

Moral questions are not decided by majorities. However, ethicists do well to take seriously into consideration the moral convictions of good people. According to a poll taken in the United States, ninety per cent of the women who were interrogated would be ready for AIH, but only fourteen per cent for AID; sixty-six per cent would be ready to resort to fertilization *in vitro* with the sperm of the husband, if this would be the only way to have children, while only eleven per cent would do so with the sperm of a donor.[103]

---

[100] Paul Ramsey, *Fabricated Man*, pp. 110-112. Cf. Ch. Curran, *Politics, Medicine and Christian Ethics*, p. 192. Herein, Curran is substantially in agreement with Ramsey.

[101] G. Kelly, 'The morality of Artificial Insemination', *American Ecclesiastical Review* 101 (1939), p. 113.

[102] George V. Lobo, *Current Problems in Medical Ethics*, p. 132. Cf. R. Van Allen, 'Artificial Insemination (AIH): A Contemporary Re-analysis', *Homiletic and Pastoral Review* 70 (1970), pp. 363-372.

[103] W.B. Miller, 'Reproduction, Technology and the Behavioural Sciences', *Science* 183 (18 Jan. 1974), p. 4121.

b.  *AID — Sperm shopping*

The great majority of people consider artificial insemination with the sperm of an anonymous donor appalling. However, some genetic engineers and their prophets do everything in their power to make it not only acceptable but even dutiful. The same Joseph Fletcher who thought Truman's decision to drop atom bombs was a classical case of his concept of *agape* and pragmatic love, and a 'moment of truth',[104] thinks that 'our notion of avarice may have to be broadened to condemn the selfishness of keeping our sperm and ova to ourselves exclusively.'[105] Of course he also considers as avarice and selfishness the attitude of a husband who regards the marital rapports with his wife as his exclusive right. Sperm banking, in this enthusiast's opinion, would provide a wonderful possibility for women to conceive a child from their lover long after he is dead.[106]

Etzioni considers as 'an ignoble sentiment' the objection against AID that the child would not be of the husband's blood.[107] In view of sperm shopping he recommends consumer education but sees 'no reason to protect individuals from sperm salesmen or to stigmatize such a procedure.'[108] However, because of the dramatic evidence that the risk of abormality is great among offspring of incestuous unions, he recommends that society should somehow control the physician who wants to act as the sperm donor for a number of women without revealing the fact to his clients.[109]

Hermann Muller is not so much concerned for an individual couple who desires a child which cannot be obtained with the husband's sperm, as for the general improvement of the genetic

---

[104] J. Fletcher, *Situation Ethics* (Philadelphia: Westminster Press, 1966), p. 168.
[105] J. Fletcher, *The Ethics of Genetic Control*, p. xiv.
[106] J. Fletcher, *Op. cit.*, p. 69.
[107] A. Etzioni, *Genetic Fix*, p. 80.
[108] *Op. cit.*, p. 122.
[109] *Op. cit.*, pp. 159-160.

pool. He recommends sperm banks with frozen sperm from outstanding men and ovum banks from outstanding women. AID, in cases where the husband is a carrier of genetic disorder, or implantation of another woman's fertilized ovule in the wife who does not possess the desired genetic quality, would, he feels, lead to ideal 'love children'. [110]

Paul Ramsey considers AID as immoral not only because of the 'anonymous parentage' and the danger of inbreeding but, above all, because it bypasses the fundamental oneness of the unitive and the procreative vocation of spouses. [111] Catholic moral theology argues the same way; and Karl Rahner adds a number of other arguments. He feels that the sperm donor refuses his responsibility and his name as father: he does not want to offer his sperm to a mother known by name, but hides from the prospective mother and child in his anonymity. The relationship of the child to his physical father is only as to a sperm salesman. If this kind of genetic manipulation should become ingrained in the public consciousness, then we should have two quite different human races: the one, a technically manipulated 'chosen race' and the other a non-selected 'lower' race reproduced in the old-fashioned way. [112]

It can be foreseen that the practice of AID would, in many cases, weaken the relationship between husband and wife. When a woman, after this procedure, 'becomes conscious of the new life waxing within her, she will realize that she is bearing a child that has no relation to the love that binds her to her partner who, in turn, will feel that he is a stranger to the new

---

[110] Hermann Muller, 'What Genetic Course Will Man Steer?', in James F. Crow and James V. Need (ed.), *Proceedings of the Third International Congress of Human Genetics* (Baltimore: Johns Hopkins Press, 1967), pp. 532f. H.J. Muller, 'Genetic Progress by Voluntarily Conducted Germinal Choice', in Paul T. Jersild and Dale A. Johnson (eds.), *Moral Issues and Christian Response* (New York: Holt, Rinehart and Winston, 1971), pp. 422ff.

[111] P. Ramsey, *Fabricated Man*, p. 128.

[112] K. Rahner, 'Zum Problem der genetischen Manipulation', *Op. cit.*, pp. 313-315.

life developing in his home.' [113] The relationship with an adopted child is much better, since both spouses equally chose this relationship in an act of responsibility to a human person already born and known.

Robert Francoeur, as in many other questions, easily abandons the traditional doctrine of the Church and favours AID under certain conditions. Since he is convinced that extramarital rapports cannot be absolutely immoral for married people, he has an *a fortiori* argument in favour of AID. [114]

c. *Fertilization* in vitro

Fertilization *in vitro* was first done simply for research, to gain greater knowledge about the beginning of life, evidently in the hope that this would yield valuable help for foetal therapy and for the whole plan of genetic engineering. Since it is experimentation with human life, it poses serious moral questions. Most researchers recognize this honestly. However, here again, there is no problem for extremists like Joseph Fletcher, because for them, the product of this fertilization is nothing else than 'laboratory reproduction of human tissue', or nothing more than 'fallopian and uterine material'. [115]

All who are convinced that fertilization coincides with the givenness of a human person must sharply condemn these experimentations. Others recognize that there is a serious doubt about whether we are faced with a human person or, let us say, a human being with the absolute right to life. But the very probability that we may be faced with a human person in the full sense constitutes in my opinion, an absolute veto against this kind of

[113] G. Lobo, *Op. cit.*, p. 150.

[114] Cf. Robert Francoeur, *Adam's New Rib* (New York: Harcourt Brace, Javanovich, 1972). Cf. J.K. Sherman, 'Synopsis of the Use o Frozen Human Sperm Since 1964: State of Art of Semen Banking' *Fertility and Sterility* 24 (1973), pp. 397-412.

[115] J. Fletcher, *Op. cit.*, pp. 78 and 88.

experimentation. [116] On this point, Karl Rahner, who is strongly opposed to genetic engineering by AID and by implantation of artificially fertilized ovules, does not feel so sure. In view of the doubt about whether 'immediately with the fertilization a human person is already substantially given', he does not want to assert that there could be no justification whatsoever for some experiments; the overall good might even outbalance this doubt. [117]

A number of ethicists and moralists feel almost or fully convinced that, in the early stage between fertilization and implantation, there is not yet given a human person. However, they would stress the point that we are still faced with human life that deserves great respect. The consequence of this deliberation is well expressed by Nelson: 'One could say that these disposed eggs do have human value and hence there is moral ambiguity surrounding their death; nevertheless, their value, even to life's creator, may be far outweighed by the value of the personhood in the potential child of a hitherto childless couple.' [118]

In view of the fact that some of the pioneers of in vitro fertilization are thoroughly dedicated to serve life, some moralists incline to a mild judgment of it when it is done with the sperm of the husband and the ovule of the wife, and in order to fulfil the desire of the spouses to have a child of their own. Although it can be foreseen that several oozytes will perish after fertilization, they feel that 'considering the little possibility of "hominization" until about the time of implantation, the moral

---

[116] Cf. Gonzalo Higueira, in Hans-Ruedi Weber and Gonzalo Higueira, 'Experimentos con el hombre' (Santamder: Ed. Sal Terrae, 1973), p. 188. Angelo Perego, La Fecondazione in vitro e sua problematica morale e teologica (Brescia: Paideia, 1964), pp. 16-18.

[117] K. Rahner, Op. cit., p. 301. In the same sense, E. Chiavacci, 'Problemi morali della manipolazione dell'uomo con particolare riguardo alla sperimentazione in embriologia', in Morale e Medicina (Rome, 1970), pp. 409-421. Cf. J. Ferin, 'Fertilization in vitro et transfert d'oeufs', in Ch. Robert (ed.), L'homme manipulé. Pouvoir de l'homme sur l'homme, ses chances et ses limites (Strasbourg: Cerdic, 1974), pp. 25-34.

[118] James Nelson, Human Medicine, p. 117.

difficulty on this score does not seem to be insurmountable, provided the risk is kept within reasonable limits.' [119]

After having considered the *pro* and *contra*, I would not, at least for the time being, dare to approve *in vitro* fertilization and implantation even with the gametes of the spouses. As for AID, in agreement with the strong convictions of many open-minded moralists and ethicists against it, [120] I see no justification for this kind of genetic engineering with sperm and ovule shopping.

The chief reason for the negative evaluation of *in vitro* fertilization is not the fact that it is artificial but that it is manipulation not only of sperm but of the embryo itself, with no safety and with numerous hazards imposed on another being, the child-to-be. [121]

d. *The foster womb*

A woman in whom the fertilized egg (other than her own) is implanted is a 'host mother'. She offers her womb as a 'foster womb'. In doing so, she may be acting as a mercenary or be motivated by generosity. A great variety of situations and motivations can be imagined: a healthy woman might not want to jeopardize or interrupt her career by the inconveniences of a pregnancy; another might desire a child but be anguished by the prospect of pregnancy and childbirth; the health of still

---

[119] George V. Lobo, *Op. cit.,* p. 153. In a similar sense B. Webb, OSB, cautions against a radical condemnation *Catholic Medical Quarterly* 24 (Oct. 1972), pp. 69-75.

[120] Cf. Helmut Thielicke, *The Ethics of Sex* (New York: Harper and Row, 1964), pp. 252-258. Harmon L. Smith, *Ethics and the New Medicine* (Nashville and New York: Abingdon Press, 1970), pp. 70-74.

[121] Leon R. Kass, 'New Beginnings in Human Life', in Hamilton, *Op. cit.,* p. 27. Cf. Leon R. Kass, "Making Babies - the New Biology and the "Old" Morality', *The Public Interest* 26 (Winter 1972), pp. 18-56. Cf. P. Ramsey, 'Shall We Reproduce? The Medical Ethics of in vitro Fertilization', *Journal of the American Medical Association* 220 (June 5, 1972), pp. 1364-1380.

another might not allow a pregnancy although she wanted a child. These might seek a foster-mother in whom would be implanted the blastocyst gained through *in vitro* fertilization of the sperm and ovule of the couple who desired the child. It is also thinkable that the egg could be fertilized through normal intercourse of the couple and then, at the most favourable moment, transplanted into the womb of the hired woman who, after pregnancy and childbirth, would give back the child to those who had hired her.

A first objection comes from the health risk — for instance, chromosomal damage to the embryo. But the psychological objections are even stronger. 'What of the host mother (whether mercenary or unpaid volunteer) who becomes psychologically attached to that which is physically attached to her? What of the genetic mother who has good intentions at the start of the procedure but who, months later, finds herself psychologically unable to accept the child who has been carried by another and born of another?... These difficult questions make the host-mother procedure greatly suspect as a morally humanizing option.' [122] I generally agree with this judgment. However, if some day it will be possible to transplant safely an embryo from the uterus of a woman who is in imminent danger of death, or who cannot be saved without interruption of the pregnancy, I would have no substantial moral objections. A different opinion is expressed by the Ethical Committee of the British Guild of Catholic Doctors, which declares such a procedure always unethical. [123]

e.   *The artificial placenta*

When medically indicated, a foetus can be removed from the womb as early as twenty-five weeks after conception, and safely raised in an incubator. Hopeful attempts are now being

[122] James B. Nelson, *Human Medicine*, p. 115.
[123] Cf. *Catholic Medical Quarterly*, 24 (1972), p. 242. Of the same opinion is George Lobo, *Op. cit.*, pp. 153-154.

made to keep alive human foetuses expelled by miscarriages as early as ten weeks after conception. [124] The efforts to construct a placenta-lined incubator are not made just for scientific curiosity or unmotivated manipulation. When successful, an interruption of the pregnancy due to grave therapeutic indications would no longer be an abortion but a transplant of the foetus into the glass womb. Of course this would be a case of manipulating the embryo or the foetus, but one motivated by the sole intention to save life.

Quite different is the ethical evaluation of ecto-genesis, the 'pregnancy' in the laboratory from artificial fertilization to birth. Leon Kass calls this laboratory production of human beings 'the complete dehumanization of procreation'. [125] Not less severe is the judgment of Paul Ramsey who calls the procedure an 'unethical experimentation' with human beings, not for their own good but exclusively for the future shape of the species. [126] For the time being, regardless of any other consideration, our response must be a firm 'no' because the risks to human life would be much greater than the risks entailed in ordinary procreation. But even if, in the future, the biological risk could be reduced to normal proportions, the procedure would still be unacceptable, because there is at least 'grave psychological danger for a foetus bred outside the human *milieu* without the essential symbiotic mother-child relationship. Here there would be complete separation of human generation from conjugal love.' [127]

f. *Asexual reproduction*

A climax of genetic engineering, and a total separation of the beginning of life not only from marriage but from all sexual

---

[124] Cf. E. Fuller Torrey, *Ethical Issues in Medicine: The Future* (Boston: Little Brown and Company, 1968), pp. 380f.

[125] Leon R. Kass, 'New Beginnings in Life', in M. Hamilton, *The New Genetics and the Future of Man*, p. 53.

[126] P. Ramsey, *Fabricated Man*, p. 113.

[127] G.V. Lobo, *Op. cit.*, p. 153.

relationships, is or will be possible in the not too remote future, through parthenogenesis and through cloning.

Mono-genesis, called also parthenogenesis or virgin birth, can happen as a natural event. It seems to be proven in frogs, rabbits and turkeys, and is probably not excluded in human-kind. We are concerned here, however, with induced mono-genesis, which can be done by chemical, electrical or other processes. Boston's famous scientist, Pincus, succeeded some time ago in obtaining well-developed and fertile rabbits by starting off by cooling the eggs and other manoeuvres of stimulation. Gynogenesis can also happen as a natural event in the rare case that the sperm activates the egg but fails to fuse with its nucleus. The development of embryonic life can then possibly succeed if diploidation occurs: that is, if one haploid set of twenty-three chromosomes, with the genes they contain, duplicates to the normal set of forty-six. [128]

A different procedure, but still parthenogenesis, involves the infusion of a nucleus with diploid genome; that is, with the normal forty-six chromosomes of good genetic quality. This is a conceptually simple but technically complicated form of cloning. The nucleus of an unfertilized egg is removed and replaced by the nucleus of an asexual cell of a male or female adult organism. It can be taken, if desired, from an intestinal or skin cell of the woman whose egg is enucleated. For reasons not yet known, the egg with its transplanted nucleus develops as if it had been fertilized by a sperm.

The gene, in these cases, is determined only by the donor of the nucleus. [129] If the nucleus is taken from a cell of the woman whose egg is activated, then her child will be her identical twin. If the nucleus is from a cell of the husband or of a donor, then the child will be a twin or 'double' of the husband or of the donor whose cell-nucleus activates the egg. In this kind of reproduction, one person could become the parent of the nume-

[128] Cf. Paul Overhage, *Op. cit.*, pp. 408f.
[129] Cf. James B. Nelson, *Op. cit.*, pp. 110-113.

rous duplications of himself or herself. This also makes possible the choice of the child's sex. [130] A fatherless society of only women could be produced, or one almost exclusively of men. The male children produced by cloning would have nothing in common with the genetic heritage of the mother.

Scientists have all the clues for cloning. It has been successful with frogs, but a large number of grossly deformed frogs resulted from the experiments. Can we hope at least that scientists will not try cloning human beings until the hazards are eliminated by sufficient experience in cloning animals, including the most highly developed mammals?

But the risk of producing and then discarding mishaps is surely not the only objection. The total bypassing of the sexual relationship, the total severance of the unitive and procreative purposes of sexuality, would have profound repercussions on all human relationships. What would be its effect on the new generations' need for identity, for belonging, for continuity, and on their willingness to accept interpersonal responsibility and commitment, all of which are somehow implicit in the fusion of the procreative and unitive ends of human sexuality? 'The conquest of evolution by setting sexual love and procreation radically asunder entails depersonalization in the extreme. The entire rationalization of procreation — its replacement by replication — can only mean the abolition of man's embodied personhood.' [131] This procedure would pave the way to a more thoroughly manipulated fatherless society.[132] By abolishing the normal biological relationship, the 'irreversible commitment of specific adults to specific children would be massively endangered.' [133] If cloning were to become a widespread practice, it

[130] Cf. Marc Lappé and Peter Steinfels, 'Choosing the Sex of Our Children', *The Hastings Centre Report*, Vol. 4, No. 1 (Feb. 1974), p. 14.

[131] P. Ramsey, *Op. cit.*, p. 89.

[132] Cf. A. Mitscherlich, *Die vaterlose Gesellschaft* (München, 1963).

[133] Daniel Callahan, 'New Beginnings in Human Life', in M. Hamilton, *Op. cit.*, p. 102.

would thoroughly undermine the stability of marriage and family, with unthinkable consequences for the whole culture. Man is an embodied person who needs to belong, to trust, to be accepted. He cannot separate the biological belonging from the rootedness in irreversible human responsibility.

Besides weakening marriage and family, and consequently all social relationships and the stability of society, cloning poses 'the most obvious kind of problems concerning the social and ethical acceptability of one group of people manufacturing another group with pre-established genetic characteristics.'[134] As for the individual products of cloning, there would be new hazards even beyond birth. What, for instance, would be the parent-child relationship and its psychic and social effect on a child, where the parent has deliberately chosen to produce, not a person with a unique identity, but one who is the duplicate of himself or herself?

I think that Leon Kass draws the right conclusion: 'Among sensible men there would be no human cloning.'[135] In a world in which the transmission of life is transformed into manufacture in the laboratory, the scientists' skill increases but the sense of mystery in mankind decreases. 'To the extent that we view as knowable only those aspects of nature which are reducible to material for population, to that extent we shall surrender our human and humanizing ability to perceive and sense the mysteries of nature.'[136]

Genetic engineering alone will surely not resolve all the genetic problems of mankind. Ever and again, a decaying culture produces new disorders. For example, some think that homosexual tendencies are to some extent genetically determined; but the paradox is that although homosexuals produce fewer children than normal people, the incidence of homosexuality is

[134] Daniel Callahan, 'Human Rights: Biogenetic Frontier and Beyond', *Hospital Progress* 54 (1973), p. 83.
[135] Leon Kass, *Op. cit.*, p. 44.
[136] Leon Kass, *Op. cit.*, p. 59.

not diminished. Rather, the 'unculture' of the consumer society produces an ever greater number of homosexuals.[137]

The new knowledge and new techniques of genetic engineering, if wisely used and wisely limited, can be a great blessing to mankind. But where the sociality of mankind is jeopardized, even the most sophisticated technology cannot improve that human health which depends upon healthy relationships in healthy self-acceptance, with God, with our fellow-men, and with the world around us.

[137] Cf. Kenneth Eberhard, 'Genetics and Human Survival', *Linacre Quarterly* 40 (1973), p. 172.

# CONCLUSION

The dedication and courage of our scientists awakens in us a sense of admiration and gratitude. Their capacity is awe-inspiring. What they discover and plan is a part of man's 'future shock'. The researchers who are working to decipher the language of the neurons and the geography of the human cerebral cortex, the message of the DNA, the many conditionings of human behaviour, and the depths of the unconscious and subconscious, are no less the 'spacemen' of our age than the astronauts who set foot on the moon and prepare even greater ventures. Our horizons are broadened no less by the amazing progress in biology and medicine than by the new knowledge about the world's past evolution and the dimensions of the cosmos.

Man has reached a new crossroad. 'We have come to the point in biological history where we now are responsible for our own evolution. We have become self-evolvers. Evolution means selecting and therefore choosing and deciding, and this means valuing.' [1]

Our humanist tradition surely does not favour a rush towards all kinds of controls. Rather, just as good pedagogy trusts a child's own impulses towards growth and self-realization, and good psychology helps a person to discover the healing energies of his own inner core, so do we hope that the new knowledge will further mankind's progress towards greater consciousness and

[1] A.H. Maslow, *The Farther Reaches of Human Nature,* pp. 11-12.

freedom. In our concept of human progress and health, a person's inner freedom has high priority. I agree with Maslow who writes, 'I can certainly say that descriptively healthy human beings do not like to be controlled. They prefer to feel free and to be free.' [2]

Working through an immense literature, I frequently had great difficulty in understanding the language and sometimes even the mentality of some scientists. But as a citizen of this new world, and as an ethicist, I feel great respect and gratitude for those eminent scientists who — along with incredibly detailed information — convey a message of scientific consciousness, awareness of the limits of their results and working hypotheses, and above all, a passionate concern for human wholeness and health. They are not only our partners but frequently our masters in the ethical dialogue. If a certain proportion of scientists remain imprisoned in a technical world view, this is not the case with many others. They perceive the appeal, arising from the new discoveries and addressing itself to all, to grow in the spirit of co-responsibility and wisdom. They realize that technology alone must not be allowed to determine behaviour, structures of human society, or the uses to which the new knowledge in biology, and especially in genetics, is put.

But any substantial optimism in this matter would be an irresponsible evasion if we failed to summon the energies of all people of good will to face the new situation and to guard its progress. More than half a century ago, Max Scheler, in a sharp analysis of our culture, distinguished 'control knowledge' (*Herrschaftswissen*), 'essential knowledge', (*Wesenwissen*), and 'salvific knowledge' (*Heilswissen*). [3] We need each of these kinds

---

[2] *Op. cit.*, p. 14.
[3] Cf. M. Scheler, *Vom Umsturz der Werte* (Leipzig, 1919); *Vom Ewigen im Menschen* (Leipzig, 1921); *Schriften zur Soziologie und Weltanschauungslehre* (Leipzig, 1926). Cf. my book, *Das Heilige und das Gute* (Krailling vor München: Erich Wewel Verlag, 1950); Alfons Deeken, *Process and Permanence in Ethics: Max Scheler's Moral Philosophy* (New York: Paulist Press, 1974).

of knowledge but, above all, a clear scale of values and an education conducive to living in accord with it.

Not only the Christian Churches and other religions, but every community and every individual person must look for balance through renewed emphasis on salvific knowledge. What is at stake is the integration of all our knowledge and research, and indeed of all our life, in that knowledge which leads to radical commitment to the wholeness, health and salvation of all mankind. [4]

There can be no doubt that the wholeness of the human person is in jeopardy today. Neither the individual nor organized society can remain indifferent to the new powers that can manipulate man in his very substance, or to the mentality that is willing, even anxious, to proceed with such manipulation. So the questions press as to who should decide, what ends to select and by what methods they are to be achieved and who should control the controller. [5]

In matters that touch the foundations of life, the whole of society is concerned, as well as the lawgiver. [6] We have to recognize that both the content and the efficacy of all laws depend greatly on the quality of public opinion and on the broadest possible participation in forming, strengthening and purifying it. A special responsibility for the quality of this participation rests on those involved in education and those who have

---

[4] Cf. my book, *Prayer: the integration of faith and life* (Slough: St Paul Publications, 1975).

[5] George A. Hudock, 'Gene Therapy and Genetic Engineering: Frankenstein is still a myth, but it should be re-read periodically', *Indiana Law Journal* 48 (Summer, 1973), pp. 533-558; cf. Marc Lappé, 'Allegiances of Human Geneticist: A Preliminary Typology', *Hastings Centre Studies*, Vol. 1, No. 2 (1973), pp. 63-78.

[6] Cf. Charles L. Weigel and Stephen E. Tinkler, 'Eugenics and Law's Obligation to Man', *South Texas Law Journal* 48 (1973), pp. 361-391. Harold P. Green, 'Genetic Technology: Law and Policy for the Brave New World', *Indiana Law Journal* 48 (1973), pp. 581-604. Michael H. Shapiro, 'Legislate the Control of Behaviour Control: Autonomy and the Coercive Use of Organic Therapy', *Southern California Law Review* 47 (2) (February, 1974), pp. 237-338.

ready access to the public mind: teachers, counsellors, authors, newsmen, lecturers, broadcasters. They cannot neglect the constant and deep study of trends which can gravely affect the future of all mankind. Nor can any individual person abdicate his personal share of responsibility in the matter.

What is at stake is more than an increase of consciousness in order to obtain proper laws and a public opinion favouring them; it is quite simply a matter of conscience that unites all men in the search for what is true and good, and for truthful solutions to problems that concern the future of all humankind.

History should have taught us that we cannot entrust our present and our future to governments or to scientific *élites*. In his shocking novel, *Die Sintflut: Das Tier aus der Tiefe* [7] (The Flood: The Animal Rising from the Abyss), Stefen Andres treats of the tyranny of Hitler. A main figure, representing the 'Propagandaminister' Göbbels, is simply called 'the controller' (*der Normierer*), the man who imposes his norms on all by powerful controls and conditioning. It all can happen again. If all people do not unite in a sincere and passionate search for ethical norms, we shall inevitably suffer under highly inappropriate juridical norms and unjust controls.

Particularly now, in such new areas as behaviour control, mind manipulation, genetic control and genetic engineering, we have to pool our energies and our wisdom. 'The criteria of genetic good set up by persons and societies are culturally conditioned and far from certain. Particular societies and powerful cliques within them claim for their particular prejudices the status of norms for all human life for all time.' [8]

I have not ignored in this study the grave question of

[7] Stefan Andres, *Die Sintflut: Das Tier aus der Tiefe* (München: Pieper, 1949).

[8] Roger L. Shinn, 'Ethical Issues in Genetic Choices', in Mark Lipkin Jr. and Peter T. Rowley (eds.), *Genetic Responsibility. On Choosing Our Children's Genes* (New York and London: Plenum Press, 1974), p. 115.

legislation on dangerous forms of manipulation; but the emphasis is on moral insight and ethical norms. I hope the reader will recognize that the great moral questions of today are not chiefly of a private nature, and that our problem is not just a matter of solving some cases of casuistry. The main task for all of us is to acquire that broad and profound vision of life, that spirit of contemplation, that synthesis of 'control knowledge' and 'salvific knowledge', and that kind of dialogue and shared responsibility that can enable us to face the new situation with courage and with hope.

The new and constantly increasing knowledge about the various conditionings of behaviour and the techniques of behaviour modification, the growing capacity to decipher the language of the brain, the various forms of mind-moulding and brain-changing, and last but not least, the new knowledge and technology in the field of genetics that can be foreseen for the next decades, constitute a tremendous appeal to make good use of all this new knowledge. To that end we shall have to learn to discern better what genuine therapy and human progress mean in a perspective of human dignity and freedom. Those who belittle, ignore or plainly deny these basic values of dignity and freedom have, willingly or unwilllingly, called for the animal arising from the abyss. It is urgent, therefore, that we confront him now, before he is fully aroused. Once aroused, as history has shown, he will demand the holocaust.

Man's true humanity has constantly to be guarded and defended. He is a creature of many dimensions; and only by a radical commmitment to the basic value of salvific knowledge, altruism, respect for every persons's dignity, and concern for life conditions that favour the growth of genuine freedom, can we assure his gradual progress in hominization. We need, above all, to hold fast to our sense of mystery, our capacity for admiration, for celebration, for contemplation, and for a wholehearted common search for ultimate values.

# INDEX

214

218

W9-ASJ-376

# Judicial Proces in Americ

Robert A. Ca
Ronald Stidl

# Judicial Process in America

# Judicial Process in America

Robert A. Carp
University of Houston

Ronald Stidham
Lamar University

PRESS

A Division of Congressional Quarterly Inc.
1414 22nd Street, N.W., Washington, D.C. 20037

Grateful acknowledgment is made to the following publishers for granting permission to reprint from copyrighted material: Princeton University Press, from J. Woodford Howard, Jr., *Courts of Appeals in the Federal Judicial System: A Study of the Second, Fifth, and District of Columbia Circuits*, copyright © 1981; Simon & Schuster, from Bob Woodward and Scott Armstrong, *The Brethren*, copyright © 1979; University of Chicago Press, from Walter F. Murphy, *Elements of Judicial Strategy*, copyright © 1964; University of Tennessee Press, from Robert A. Carp and C. K. Rowland, *Policymaking and Politics in the Federal District Courts*, copyright © 1983.

Cover design by Dmitri Lipczenko.

Library of Congress Cataloging-in-Publication Data

Carp, Robert A., 1943-
    Judicial process in America / Robert A. Carp, Ronald Stidham.
    p. cm.
    Bibliography: p.
    Includes index.
    ISBN 0-87187-485-7
    1. Courts--United States. 2. Judges--United States. 3. Judicial process--United States. I. Stidham, Ronald, 1940- . II. Title.
KF8700.C37 1990
347.73' 1--dc20
[347.3071]
                                                                89-34955

*To my father and friend, Samuel M. Carp*

R.A.C.

*To my daughter, Heather Elizabeth*

R.S.

# Contents

# Preface

Our goal has been to prepare a comprehensive and highly readable textbook about the judicial process in the United States. The primary emphasis is on the federal courts, but we offer full coverage of state judicial systems, the role of the lawyer in American society, the nature of crime, and public policy concerns that color the entire judicial fabric. The book is designed as a primary text for courses in judicial process and behavior; it will also be useful as a supplement in political science classes in constitutional law, American government, and law and society. Likewise it may serve as interesting reading in law-related courses in sociology, history, psychology, and criminology.

In preparing this text we have been careful to minimize the use of jargon and the theoretical vocabulary of political science and the law, without condescending to the student. We believe it is possible to provide a keen and fundamental understanding of our court systems and their impact on our daily lives without assuming that all readers are budding political scientists or lawyers. At times, of course, it is necessary and useful to employ technical terms and evoke theoretical concepts; still, we address the basic questions on a level that is meaningful to an educated layperson. For students who may desire more specialized explanations or who wish to explore more deeply some of the issues we touch on, the footnotes and selected bibliography contain ample resources.

We have also tried to avoid stressing any one theoretical framework for the study of courts and legal questions, such as a systems model approach or a judicial realist perspective. Instructors partial to the tenets of modern behavioralism will find much here to gladden their hearts, but we have also tried to include the insights that more traditional scholarship has provided over the years. The book reflects the contributions not only of political scientists and legal scholars but also of historians, psychologists, court administrators, and journalists.

Throughout the text we are constantly mindful of the interrelation between the courts and public policy. We have worked with the premise that significant portions of our lives—as individuals and as a nation—are affected by what our state and federal judges choose to do and refrain from doing. We reject the common assumption that only liberals make public policy while conservatives practice restraint; rather, we believe that to some degree all judges engage in the inevitable activity of making policy. The question, as we see it, is not whether American judges make policy but rather which direction the policy decisions will take. In the chapters that follow we shall explain why this has come to be, how it happens, and what the consequences are for the United States today.

In Chapter 1 we set the theoretical stage. While noting Americans' great respect for the law, we also document the traditional willingness of Americans to violate the law when it is morally, economically, or politically expedient to do so. We also examine sources of law in the United States and several of the major philosophies of the role and function of law.

Chapter 2 provides a brief sketch of the organizational structure of the federal and state judiciaries, placed in historical perspective. As we shall see, the state and federal judicial systems are the product of two centuries of evolution, trial and error, and a pinch of serendipity. The distinction between routine norm enforcement and policy making by judges is first addressed in this chapter.

The third chapter underscores the theme that "judging" is more and more a team effort. This chapter describes the duties and contributions of the staff and administrative agencies that support the federal and state courts today, including law clerks, state judicial councils, magistrates, the Federal Judicial Center, and the Administrative Office of the U.S. Courts.

Chapter 4 discusses the role of the lawyers in American society—their training, their values and attitudes, and the public policy goals of their professional associations. In this chapter we also explore the impact of interest groups in the judicial process and the importance of judicial lobbying.

Chapter 5 outlines the jurisdiction of the several levels of U.S. courts and provides current data about the workload of state and federal tribunals. We believe that a full understanding of how judges affect our daily lives also requires us to outline those many substantive areas into which state and federal jurists may not roam.

In Chapter 6 we focus on the criminal court process at both the state and federal levels. We begin with a discussion of the nature and substance of crime; we then examine, step by step, the key stages of the criminal court process. Chapter 7 examines the civil court process. We begin with a discussion of the various types of civil cases and the options available to the complainant and the respondent. Then we proceed through the pretrial hearing and jury selection. After a look at the trial and judgment we turn to the alternative methods available to resolve civil disputes, such as mediation and arbitration.

In Chapter 8 we take a close look at the men and women who wear the black robe in the United States. What are their background characteristics and qualifications for office? How are they chosen? What are their values, and how do these values manifest themselves in their behavior as judges and justices? In a key segment on the federal courts we find a discernible policy link among the values of a majority of voters in a presidential election, the values of the appointing president, and the subsequent policy content of decisions made by judges nominated by the chief executive.

Chapter 9 is the first of two on judicial decision making. Here we outline those aspects of the decision-making process that are characteristic of all judges, in the context of the "legal subculture"—the traditional legal reasoning model for explaining judges' decisions—and the "democratic subculture"—a number of extralegal factors that appear to be associated with judges' policy decisions. Chapter 10 examines the special case of decision making in collegial appellate courts. We explore the assumptions and contributions of small-group theory, attitude and bloc analysis, and the fact pattern approach to understanding the behavior of multijudge tribunals.

Chapter 11 explores the policy impact of decisions made by federal and state courts and discusses the process by which judicial rulings are implemented—and why some are not implemented.

The last chapter has two general goals: to outline the primary factors that impel judges to engage in policy making and then to suggest the variables that determine the ideological direction of such policy making.

Many people contributed to the writing of this book, and to all of them we offer sincere thanks. Russell R. Wheeler of the Federal Judicial Center read the entire manuscript and provided us with many useful criticisms and additions. Houston police officer Robert Nelson read our chapter, "The Criminal Court Process," and suggested numerous ways to improve the accuracy of our discussion of police procedures and the law. Thomas G. Walker, Emory University, and Wayne V. McIntosh, University of Maryland, provided detailed suggestions that added greatly to the scope and precision of the text. For any errors that remain, we assume responsibility.

Our relationship with CQ Press has been a most pleasant one. Joanne Daniels, director of CQ Press, offered encouragement, sound advice, and helpful suggestions at crucial stages of the project. We also appreciate the fine work of our copy editor, Nola Lynch.

We owe a special debt of thanks to John McElroy, a former undergraduate research assistant at Lamar University. He provided valuable help in preparing tables and checking citations in the library.

Stidham would like to express a deep debt of gratitude to his personal support group: Laquita, Sam, and Heather. Their constant love, encouragement, and understanding during the long periods when "Dad was working on the book" made the project much easier.

# 1  Foundations of Law in the United States

Law is an appropriate subject to begin this text with because without law there would be no courts and no judges; there would be no political or judicial system through which disputes could be settled and rendered. In this chapter we examine the sources of law in the United States, that is, the institutions and traditions that establish the rules of the legal game. We discuss the particular types of law that are used and define some of the basic legal terms. Likewise we shall explore the functions of law for society—what it enables us to avoid and accomplish as individuals and as a people that would be impossible without the existence of some commonly accepted rules. Finally we examine America's ambivalent tradition vis-à-vis the law, that is, how a nation founded on an *illegal* revolution and nurtured with a healthy tradition of civil disobedience can pride itself on being a land where respect for the law is ideally taught at every mother's knee. We also take note of the degree to which American society has become highly litigious and why this is significant for the study of the American judicial system.

## Sources of Law in the United States

Where does law come from in the United States? At first the question seems a bit simpleminded. A typical response might be: "We get it from legislatures; that's what Congress and the state legislatures do." This answer is not wrong, but it is far from adequate—in fact, law comes from a large variety of sources in this country.

### Constitutions

The U.S. Constitution is the primary source of law in the United States, as indeed it claims to be in Article VI: "This Constitution . . . shall be the supreme Law of the Land; and the Judges in every State shall be bound thereby, any Thing in the Constitution or Laws of any State to the Contrary notwithstanding." Thus none of the other types of law that we shall subsequently mention may stand if it is in conflict with the Constitution of the United States. Similarly, each state has its own separate constitution and all local laws must yield to its supremacy.

1

## Acts of Legislative Bodies

Laws passed by Congress and by the various state legislatures constitute a sizable bulk of law in the United States. Statutes requiring us to pay income tax to Uncle Sam and state laws forbidding us from robbing a bank are both examples of this. But there are many other types of legislative bodies that also enact statutes and ordinances that regulate our lives as citizens. Country commissioners (also known as county judges or boards of selectmen) act as legislative bodies for the various counties within the states. Likewise city councils serve in a legislative capacity when they pass ordinances, fix property tax rates, establish building codes, and so on, at the municipal level. Then there are the thousands upon thousands of "special districts" throughout the country, each of which is headed by an elected or appointed body that acts in a legislative capacity. Examples of these would be school districts, fire prevention districts, water districts, and municipal utility districts.

## Decisions of Quasi-Legislative and Quasi-Judicial Bodies

Sprinkled vertically and horizontally throughout the U.S. governmental structure are thousands of boards, agencies, commissions, departments, and so on, whose primary function is not to legislate or to adjudicate but which still may be called on to make rules or to render decisions that are semilegislative or semijudicial in character. The job of the U.S. Postal Service is obviously to deliver the mail, but sometimes it may be called on to act in a quasi-judicial capacity. For example, a local postmaster may refuse to deliver a piece of mail because he or she believes it to be pornographic in nature, for Congress has mandated that pornography may not be sent through the mails. The postmaster is acting in a semi- or quasi-judicial capacity in determining that a particular item is pornographic and hence not protected by the First Amendment.

The Securities and Exchange Commission is not basically a lawmaking body either, but when it determines that a particular company has run afoul of the securities laws or when it rules on a firm's qualification to be listed on the New York Stock Exchange, it becomes a source of law in the United States. That is, it makes rules and decisions that affect a person's or a company's behavior and for which there are penalties for noncompliance. Although decisions of agencies such as this may be appealed to or reviewed by the courts, they are binding unless and until they are overturned by a judicial entity.

A university's board of regents may also be a very real source of law for the students, faculty, and staff members covered by its jurisdiction. Such boards may set rules on such matters as which persons may lawfully enter the campus grounds, procedures to be followed before a staff member may be fired, or definitions of plagiarism. Violations of these rules or procedures carry with them penalties backed by the full force of the law, for such boards are themselves a source of law.

## Orders and Rulings of Political Executives

We learn in our school history classes that legislatures make the law and executives enforce the law. That is essentially true, but it is also a fact that political executives have some lawmaking capacity. This occurs whenever presidents, governors, mayors, or others are called upon to fill in the details of legislation passed by legislative bodies, and sometimes when they promulgate orders purely in their executive capacity.

When Congress passes reciprocal trade agreement legislation, the goal is to encourage other countries to lower trade and tariff barriers to U.S.-produced goods, in exchange for which the United States will do the same. But there are so many thousands of goods, hundreds of countries, and countless degrees of setting up or lowering trade barriers. What to do? The customary practice is for Congress to set basic guidelines for the reciprocal lowering of trade barriers but also to allow the president to make the actual decisions about how much to regulate a given tariff on any given commodity for a particular country. These "executive orders" of the president are published regularly in the *Federal Register* and carry the full force of law. Likewise at the state level, when a legislature delegates to the governor the right to "fill in the details of legislation," the state executive uses what is termed "ordinance making power," which also has lawmaking capacity.

Political executives may promulgate orders which within certain narrow but important realms constitute the law of the land. For example, in the wake of a natural disaster such as a flood or tornado, a mayor may declare an official state of emergency that empowers him or her to issue binding rules of behavior for a limited period of time. A curfew ordering persons to be off the streets at a given hour is an example of a "law" made by a municipal chief executive. Though limited and usually temporary, such orders are indeed law and violations invoke penalties.

## Judicial Decisions

When we learned in school that legislatures make the law and executives enforce the law we were told that judges are supposed to *interpret* the law. So they do, but as we shall see again and again throughout this text, judges in fact make law as they interpret it. And we must note that judicial decisions themselves constitute a body of law in the United States. All the thousands upon thousands of court decisions that have been handed down by federal and state judges for the past two centuries are part of the *corpus juris*—the body of law—of the United States.

Judicial decisions may be grounded in or surround a variety of entities: any of the above-mentiond sources of law, past decisions of other judges, or legal principles that have evolved over the centuries. (For example, one cannot bring a lawsuit on behalf of another person unless that person is one's minor child or ward.) Judicial decisions may also be grounded in what is called "the common law," that is, those written (and sometimes unwritten) legal traditions and principles that have served as the basis of court decisions and accepted human behavior for many centuries. For instance, if a couple lives together as husband and wife for a specified period of years, the common law may be invoked to have their union recognized as a legal marriage.

## Types of Law in the United States

Now that we have examined the wellsprings of American law, it is appropriate to take a brief look at the vessels wherein such laws are contained, that is, to examine the formal types of categories of law in the United States. What follows are definitions or explanations of the primary kinds of law that we shall make reference to subsequently in this text. (Note that types of law are not necessarily mutually exclusive.)

### Statutory Law

Whereas the common law has dealt traditionally with matters of a private character (such as the relations between individuals), statutory law is concerned more frequently with society as a whole. It is law that originates with specifically designated, authoritative lawmaking bodies such as legislatures, but it may also take in executive-administrative decrees, ordinances, treaties, and protocols, all of which are committed to paper. Statutes outlawing murder or burglary would be examples of statutory law.

### Civil Law and Criminal Law

We shall have much more to say about these terms in Chapters 6 and 7, but suffice it to say here that the former deals with relations between individuals, such as ownership of private property. It also deals with corporations, admiralty matters, and contracts. Criminal law, on the other hand, pertains to offenses against the state itself—actions that may be directed against a person but that are deemed to be offensive to society as a whole. Crimes, such as drunken driving, armed robbery, and so on, are punishable by fines or imprisonment.

## Equity

Equity is best understood when contrasted with law; the primary difference between the two terms is, as we shall see, in the remedy involved. Equity begins where the law ends. It takes the form of a judicial decree— not of an ordinary yes or no judgment. Equity leaves the judge reasonably free to order *preventive* measures—and under some circumstances even *remedial* ones. Such measures are in the form of special writs, such as injunctions or restraining orders, that are designed to afford a remedy not otherwise obtainable. For example, let's say you were the owner of an old cabin located in the center of town and that this structure was the first built in the community. You wish to preserve it because of its historic value, but the city decides to expand the adjacent street and thereby destroy the cabin. Your remedy at law is to ask the city for monetary compensation, but to you this is totally inadequate. The cabin has little intrinsic value, although as a historic object it is priceless. Thus you may wish to ask a judge to issue a writ in equity which might order the city to move the cabin to another site or perhaps even to order the city to reconsider its plan to widen the street.

## Private Law

Private law governs the relationship between private citizens or persons, that is, it regulates the relations of individuals with each other. Much civil law is obviously in this category, for it deals with subjects such as contracts between individuals and corporations and statutes pertaining to marriage and divorce.

## Public Law

In contrast to private law, public law is a branch or department of law very much concerned with the state in its political or sovereign capacities— including the important two subheadings of administrative law and constitutional law. Public law deals with the regulation and enforcement of rights in those cases where the state is viewed as the subject of the right or the object of the duty, including criminal law and procedures. Public law applies and affects the entire people of a nation that adopts it. Thus the vast majority of legislation enacted by Congress is in the category of public law; indeed, when it is codified, it is preceded by the term "Public Law" and a number. Social welfare legislation, defense appropriations, aid to farmers, and the control of subversive activities are all illustrations of the vast and diversified content of public law.

## Administrative Law

Administrative law consists of those rules and regulations that are promulgated by the various administrative agencies that have been empowered to deal with the operation of government under the delegated rule-making authority of a legislative body. This branch of law prescribes in detail the activities of the agencies involved, such as those concerned with the collection of revenue, regulation of competitive practices, public health, and the armed forces.

## Constitutional Law

Basically, constitutional law prescribes the plan and method under which the public business of the political organ, known as the state, is conducted. In the United States, with its written constitution, constitutional law consists of the application of fundamental principles of law based on that document, as finally interpreted by the Supreme Court. For example, in 1952 the Supreme Court ruled that nothing inherent in Article II of the Constitution gave the president the right to seize and run the steel mills— even in time of emergency—without specific congressional authorization.[1]

## Functions of Law

What is the function of law in the United States (or in any country, for that matter, because the function of law is more or less universal)? That is, what dire things would occur in this land were there no law or, conversely, what positive things can we do as a people through law that would be impossible without it?

Some persons in history have believed that there should be no government (and hence no laws) at all. Such individuals, called anarchists, have argued that governments by nature make rules and laws and that such restrictions impinge on personal freedom. In the past anarchists have used violence to overthrow governments and have assassinated heads of state. Such attempts to abolish law and authority have resulted in much destruction of life and property and temporary reigns of terror, but they have never brought about the elimination of law or government. Instead of increasing personal freedom, a state of anarchy virtually destroys personal freedom for all but the most powerful and savage of individuals. Few would deny that in today's world if people are to live together amicably, law must be an essential part of life. As our population expands and modern transportation and communication link us all together, every action that each of us takes affects another either directly or indirectly and may even cause harm. When the inevitable conflict results, it must be resolved peaceably using a rule of law. Otherwise there is just disorder, death, and chaos. We must have some common set of rules that we agree to live by—a rule of law and order.

But what kind of law and order? There is truth to the anarchist's argument that laws restrict personal freedom. If there are too many rules, laws, and restrictions, totalitarianism results. That may be just about as bad as a state of anarchy. The trick is to strike a balance so that the positive things that law can do for us are not strangulated by the tyranny of the "law and order" offered by the totalitarian state.

Assuming, then, that we reject both anarchy and totalitarianism, what are the positive functions of law when it exists in a reasonable degree? Legal theorists tell us that there are several.

## Resolving Disputes

No matter how benign and loving people can be at times, altercations and disagreements are inevitable. How disputes are resolved between quarreling individuals, corporations, or governmental entities tells us much about the level and quality of the rule of law in a society. Without an orderly, peaceful process for dispute resolution there is either chaos or a climate in which those with the strongest fists or the largest gang of thugs prevail.

Let us say that big, rugged New England fisherman Cabot Quincy suspects that his frail neighbor, Angus Shortfellow, has been tampering with the lobster pots that lie in the waters along Cabot's jetty. Cabot has the strong desire and the physical capacity to "thrash that little wimp within an inch of his life." But what will happen to Shortfellow's wife and children if their breadwinner and father is beaten near to death? And indeed what might happen twenty years hence when Cabot is ailing and elderly and Shortfellow's now grown son decides to take revenge on the once powerful man who pummeled his father? Better that the original matter be taken before a justice of the peace and settled quietly by rules of law on which all agree.

## Providing Order and Predictability in Society

We live in a chaotic and uncertain world. People win lotteries while stock markets collapse; more and more persons are living to the age of a hundred while babies die of AIDS; some ranchers manage to enlarge their herds just at the time of a beef shortage while corn farmers suffer from the worst drought in decades. Laws cannot avert most natural disasters, nor can they prevent random episodes of ill fortune, but they can create an environment in which people can work and invest and pursue pleasure with a reasonable expectation that their activity is worth the effort. Without an orderly environment based on and backed by law the normal activities of life would be lacerated with chaos.

When we drive a car, for example, there must be rules to tell us which side of the road to drive on, how fast we can safely go, and when to slow down and stop. Without rules of the road there would be horrible traffic jams and terrible accidents because no driver would know what to expect from the others. Or, for example, without a climate of law and order no parent would have the incentive to save for a child's college education. The knowledge that the bank will not simply close and that one's saving account will not be arbitrarily confiscated by the government or by some powerful party gives the parent an environment in which to save. Law and the predictability it provides cannot guarantee us a totally safe and predictable world, but it can create a climate in which people believe it is worthwhile to produce, to venture forth, and to live for the morrow.

## Protecting Individuals and Property

Even libertarians, who take a very narrow view of the role of government, will readily acknowledge that the state must protect citizens from the outlaw who would inflict bodily harm or who would steal or destroy their worldly goods. Because of the importance to us of the safety of our persons and our property, many laws on the books deal with protection and security. Not only are laws in the criminal code intended to punish those who steal and do bodily harm, but civil statutes permit many crime victims to sue for monetary damages. The law has created police and sheriffs' departments, district attorneys' offices, courts, jails, and death chambers to deter and punish the criminal and to help people feel secure. This is not to say that there is no crime; everyone knows differently. But without a system of laws, crime would be much more prevalent and the fear of it would be much more paralyzing. Unless we could afford to hire our own bodyguards and security teams we would be in constant anxiety of loss of life and limb and property. However imperfect our system of law prevention and enforcement may be, it is certainly better than none.

## Providing for the General Welfare

Laws and the institutions and programs they establish enable us to do corporately what would be impossible, or at least prohibitive, to do as individuals. Providing for the common defense, educating young people, putting out forest fires, controlling pollution, and caring for the sick and aged are all examples of activities that we could do only feebly, if at all, acting alone but that we can do efficiently and effectively as a society. As citizens we may disagree about which endeavors should be undertaken through the government by law. Some may believe, for example, that the aged should be cared for by family members or by private charity; others see such care as a corporate responsibility. But while we can disagree about the precise activities that the law should require of government, few would deny that there are many significant and beneficial results that are achieved through corporate endeavors. After all, the foundation of our legal system, the U.S. Constitution, was ordained to "establish Justice, insure domestic

Tranquility, provide for the common defence, promote the general Welfare, and secure the Blessings of Liberty to ourselves and our Posterity. . . . "

## The United States and the Rule of Law

We Americans pride ourselves on being a law-abiding people, and to the casual observer so we are. Few of us would question Abraham Lincoln's admonition that respect for the law should be taught the child at every mother's knee, and most of us are glad to proclaim that ours is a government of *law*, not of individuals. The fact that over a half million of our fellow citizens reside in jail or prison on any given day is seen not as evidence that our society is lawless but rather as proof that in the United States respect for the law is paramount and disobedience to the law is punished. A careful analysis of our history and traditions would reveal, however, that our view of the law has in reality been ambivalent. A few examples from our history will illustrate our love-hate relationship with the rule of law.

An appropriate place to begin is the American Revolution. Few Americans can look back on that seven-year struggle and feel anything but pride from the images that come to mind: the bold act of defiance of the Boston Tea Party, the shot fired at Concord that was "heard 'round the world," George Washington's daring attack on the Hessian troops at Trenton. But in all the goosebumps raised in this patriotic reverie, we lose sight of one bothersome little fact—the Revolution was illegal! The wanton destruction of private property that comprised the Boston Tea Party and the killing of British troops sent to this land for the colonists' protection were illegal in every sense of the word. Indeed, the Founders were so keenly aware of this that they prepared a Declaration of Independence to justify to the rest of the world why a bloody and illegal revolt against the lawful government is sometimes permissible:

> When in the Course of human events, it becomes necessary for one people to dissolve the political bands which have connected them with another, . . . a decent respect to the opinions of mankind requires that they should declare the causes which impel them to the separation. . . .
> [W]hen a long train of abuses and usurpations . . . evinces a design to reduce them under absolute Despotism, it is their right, it is their duty, to throw off such Government, and to provide new Guards for their future security.

The irony of our nation's birth is often overlooked: this citadel of law and order was born under the star of illegality and revolution.

Let us stroll a little further along our historical path and view John Brown's famous raid on the U.S. arsenal at Harpers Ferry in the fall of 1859. With thirteen white men and five black men this militant opponent of slavery began his plan to lead a mass insurrection among the slaves and to create an Abolitionist republic on the ruins of the plantation South. After a small but bloody battle that lasted several days, Brown was captured, given a public trial, and duly hanged for murder and other assorted crimes. But were Brown's flagrantly violent and illegal actions justifiable, given the nobility of his vision? Many in the North believed so. Its moral and cultural elite took the line that Brown might have been insane, but his acts and intentions should be excused on the grounds that the compelling motive was divine. Horace Greeley wrote that the Harpers Ferry raid was "the work of a madman," but he had not "one reproachful word." Ralph Waldo Emerson described Brown as a "saint." Henry Thoreau, Theodore Parker, Henry Longfellow, William Cullen Bryant, and James Lowell—the whole Northern pantheon—took the position that Brown was an "angel of light," and not Brown but the society that hanged him was mad. It was also reported that "on the day Brown died, church bells tolled from New England to Chicago; Albany fired off one hundred guns in salute, and a governor of a large Northern state wrote in his diary that men were ready to march to Virginia." [2] Again the ambivalence: one ought always to obey the law—unless, of course, one hears a divine call that transcends the law.

Skipping over dozens of other keen illustrations of this truth, let us look at a couple of events from the middle part of this century. The civil rights movement that began in the 1950s caused many Americans to be torn between their natural desire to obey the law of the land and their call to change the system. As the Reverend Martin Luther King, Jr., sat in a Birmingham jail, he wrote a now famous letter to supporters who were disturbed by his having disobeyed the law during his civil rights protests:

> You express a great deal of anxiety over our willingness to break laws. This is certainly a legitimate concern. Since we would diligently urge people to obey the Supreme Court's decision in 1954 outlawing segregation in the public schools, at first glance it may seem rather paradoxical for us consciously to break laws. One may well ask: "How can you advocate breaking some laws and obeying others?" The answer lies in the fact that there are two types of laws: just and unjust. I would be first to advocate obeying just laws. One has not only a legal but a moral responsibility to obey just laws. Conversely, one has a moral responsibility to disobey unjust laws. . . . Thus it is that I can urge men to obey the 1954 decision of the Supreme Court, for it is morally right; and I can urge them to disobey segregation ordinances, for they are morally wrong. [3]

Even a member of the Supreme Court of the United States sanctioned civil disobedience during the heady days of the civil rights movement. Justice Abe Fortas said:

If I had been a Negro living in Birmingham or Little Rock or Plaquemines Parish, Louisiana, I hope I would have disobeyed the state laws that said that I might not enter the public waiting room in the bus station reserved for "Whites." I hope I would have insisted upon going into parks and swimming pools and schools which state or city law reserved for "Whites." I hope I would have had the courage to disobey, although the segregation ordinances were presumably law until they were declared unconstitutional.[4]

Those who opposed the civil rights movement and the Supreme Court decisions and congressional statutes that supported it likewise believed that their form of civil disobedience was in response to a higher calling. Quoting scripture as support of their belief that God created the white race separately from the colored races, segregationists argued that it was the divine will to keep the races apart. Thus defiance of integration orders was seen by many traditionalists as keeping in touch with the natural order of the universe as God had established it. That black and white should not mix with one another was believed to be "a self-evident truth," not to be overturned by the courts' desegregation orders.

The recent "pro-life offensive" being conducted by opponents of abortion is a final example of how basically law-abiding persons may be ready and willing to break the law in furtherance of their response to what they believe is a higher calling. For example, in dozens of "rescue actions" at abortion clinics, protesters all across the country have blocked access to these facilities, harassed doctors and nurses, and tried to persuade pregnant woman that "Abortion is murder.... Don't kill your baby." As of November 1988, over 3,000 protestors have been arrested. Many have refused to give their names to the police, thus making it legally impossible to set bail. Some have spent as long as forty days in jail.[5]

Civil disobedience does not need a divine call. There are ample illustrations of the wholesale avoidance of laws that were thought to be economically harmful and unfair or that were seen as beyond the rightful authority of the state to enact.

American farmers are probably as law abiding a segment of the population as any, but they, too, can thwart the law when their economic livelihood is at stake. As early as George Washington's administration, state militias were activated and sent out to quash what has come to be known as the Whiskey Rebellion, a series of lawless acts by the tillers of the soil who objected to the federal tax on their homemade elixirs. And during the terrible Depression days of the 1930s, when, for example, one-third of the state of Iowa was being sold into bankruptcy, farmers often revolted. Thousands with shotguns held at bay local sheriffs who tried to serve papers on fellow farmers about to be dispossessed.

During the Prohibition era, from 1919 to 1933, many Americans refused to obey a law they thought to be unfair and in excess of the legitimate bounds of state authority. Not only did the laws prohibiting the production and sale of alcohol prove to be ineffective and unenforceable, but Americans actually seemed to relish flouting the law. The statistics of prohibition enforcement reveal how the laws were honored in the breach: in 1921 the government seized a total of 95,933 illicit distilleries, stills, still worms, and fermenters; this number went to 172,537 by 1925 and jumped to some 282,122 by 1930.[6] By 1932 President Herbert Hoover, who had originally supported Prohibition, now talked about "the futility of the whole business."

One last example. In the vast majority of the states it is against the law to engage in a whole host of forbidden sexual activities—fornication, sodomy, adultery, homosexuality. The legislatures in most of the states have gone to great trouble to spell out for us which parts of our bodies may be touched by the parts of other people's bodies. That these laws are seldom obeyed or enforced is a secret to no one. Although most Americans still approve of forbidding sexual practices and acts that they find personally distasteful, few have much enthusiasm for putting police officers in every bedroom or for strictly enforcing laws that touch on very personal issues.

So, are we a law-abiding people or are we not? Is our respect for the law only superficial and our belief that everyone ought to obey the law mere cant? The truth, it would appear, is that Americans do honestly have great respect for the law and that our abhorrence of lawbreakers is genuine. But it is also fair to say that mixed with this tradition and orientation is a longstanding belief that sometimes people are called to respond to values higher than the ordinary law and thereby to illegal behavior. Of course, one person's command to disobey the law and follow the dictates of conscience will appear to another as mere foolishness. Furthermore, Americans possess a hefty pragmatic tradition vis-à-vis the law. Laws that drive us to the wall economically (such as farm foreclosures during the 1930s) and laws that are seen to needlessly impinge upon our personal pleasures (such as Prohibition and laws forbidding fornication) are just not taken as seriously as those that forbid bank robbery and rape.

Like the law, judges are viewed ambivalently by Americans. In general, judges are held in inordinately high esteem in the United States, and most Americans would be proud if a son or daughter grew up to become one. Yet Americans can be very quick to condemn judges whose rulings go against deeply held values or whose decisions are not in the best interests of their pocketbooks.[7] Whether this is hypocrisy or merely the complex and ambivalent nature of humankind is perhaps all in the eye of the beholder.

## A Litigious Society

The raw statistics reveal that we Americans readily look to the courts to redress our grievances. The quarter of a million cases that are filed in the federal courts each year are dwarfed by the 80 to 100 million cases filed in the courts of the fifty states and the District of Columbia. That's about one for every two people in the United States; although many of these deal with relatively minor matters, still about 12 million are filed in the *major* state and federal trial courts.[8] As one contemporary expert has noted:

> Ours is a law-drenched age. Because we are constantly inventing new and better ways of bumping into one another, we seek an orderly means of dulling the blows and repairing the damage. Of all the known methods of redressing grievances and settling disputes—pitched battle, rioting, dueling, mediating, flipping a coin, suing—only the latter has steadily won the day in these United States.
>
> Though litigation has not routed all other forms of fight, it is gaining public favor as the legitimate and most effective means of seeking and winning one's just deserts.
>
> So widespread is the impulse to sue that "litigation has become the nation's secular religion," and a growing array of procedural rules and substantive provisions is daily gaining its adherents.[9]

This virtual explosion of primarily civil litigation in the United States has led the courts to enter realms that in years past were settled privately among citizens or which often went unresolved. Some obviously deal with momentous subjects, such as the right of the states to curtail abortion and efforts by the Environmental Protection Agency to enjoin polluters of the environment. But many suits stagger the imagination by their audacity or triviality:

1. In Boulder, Colorado, a man sued his parents for $350,000, alleging that they had provided him with inadequate home life and psychological support and were thus guilty of "malpractice of parenting."
2. A woman in the state of Washington was dismissed from the Gonzaga University School of Law because of a poor grade point average. She promptly initiated a suit asking either for a law degree or the sum of $110,000. Her argument was that given her mediocre college grades and aptitude test scores, the law school admissions board should have advised her that her chances of graduating from law school were slim.
3. A long-time employee of the Los Alamos Scientific Laboratory sued for occupational disability benefits, claiming that although he had never suffered any physical injury, he had become mentally disabled "by a neurotic fear that radiation would kill him."[10]

True, many suits of this nature are frivolous, but they do require the time and efforts of the jurists who must at least consider their merits from within the 17,000 courthouses that dot the landscape. For example, a federal judge in West Virginia took several printed pages of the *Federal Supplement* to explain why the punishment of a state prisoner for his refusal to bury a dead skunk was not a violation of the prisoner's civil rights. A federal judge in Pennsylvania agonized at length in print as to whether the First Amendment protected from a tort action *Time* magazine, which had published a photograph of a man whose fly had become unzipped.[11]

While there has in fact been a burst of litigation in the United States during the past several decades, we must not lose sight of the fact that Americans have always been litigious people. As early as 1835 the highly perceptive French observer Alexis de Tocqueville acutely noted that "there is hardly a political question in the United States which does not sooner or later turn into a judicial one."[12] Indeed, as one contemporary scholar has said: "To express amazement at American litigiousness is akin to professing astonishment at learning that the roots of most Americans lie in other lands. We have been a litigious nation as we have been an immigrant one. Indeed, the two are related."[13] This scholar goes on to argue that our history was made by diverse groups who wanted to live according to their own customs but found themselves drawn haphazardly into a larger political community. As these groups bumped into one another and the edges became frayed, disputes resulted. But given a fairly strong common law legal tradition, such disputes were for the most part channeled into the courtroom rather than onto the battlefield. There are, of course, many reasons why Americans have been and continue to be a highly litigious people, and it is beyond the scope of this chapter to examine them all systematically. Suffice it to say that in the United States the courthouse has been and is the anvil on which a significant portion of our personal, societal, and political problems are hammered out.

America's judicial caseload is so enormous and far ranging that to understand fully how our nation is governed and how its resources are allocated, we must study the courts that are such a vital part of this process. Given the significance of courts in formulating and implementing public policy in the United States, it is important that we know who the judges are, what their values are, and what powers and prerogatives they possess. And it is essential that we study how decisions are made and how they are implemented if we are to follow the judicial game.

## Summary

In this chapter we looked briefly at law in the United States—the wells from which it springs, its basic types, and its functions in society. We also examined the ambivalent attitude that Americans have about the rule of law; this is a nation birthed in an illegal revolution, yet proud of our respect for law and order. Finally, we noted that our contentiousness as a people has been channeled largely through our legal and court systems. As a consequence, the high priests of our judicial temples, the judges, play a very significant role in our personal lives and in our evolution as a society and political entity.

## Notes

1. *Youngstown Sheet & Tube Co. v. Sawyer*, 343 U.S. 579.
2. T. R. Fehrenbach, *Lone Star: A History of Texas and the Texans* (New York: American Legacy Press, 1968), 336.
3. Martin Luther King, Jr., "Letter from Birmingham Jail, April 16, 1963." The full text of the letter may be found in Martin Luther King, Jr., *Why We Can't Wait* (New York: Harper & Row, 1963).
4. Abe Fortas, *Concerning Dissent and Civil Disobedience* (New York: Signet, 1970), 18.
5. "The New Pro-Life Offensive," *Newsweek*, September 12, 1988, 25, and "Abortion Protests Sweep Nation; 2200 Are Jailed," *Houston Chronicle*, October 30, 1988, A1.
6. Andrew Sinclair, "Prohibition: The Era of Excess," in Lawrence M. Friedman and Stewart Macaulay, eds., *Law and the Behavioral Sciences* (New York: Bobbs-Merrill, 1977), 353.
7. See, for example, Jack W. Peltason, *Fifty-Eight Lonely Men* (New York: Harcourt, Brace & World, 1961), and Jack Bass, *Unlikely Heroes* (New York: Simon & Schuster, 1981).
8. Jethro K. Lieberman, *The Litigious Society* (New York: Basic Books, 1983), ix.
9. Ibid., viii.
10. Ibid., 4.
11. Robert A. Carp and C. K. Rowland, *Policymaking and Politics in the Federal District Courts* (Knoxville: University of Tennessee Press, 1983), 18.
12. Alexis de Tocqueville, *Democracy in America*, ed. J. P. Mayer and Max Lerner, trans. George Lawrence (New York: Harper & Row, 1966), 248.
13. Lieberman, *The Litigious Society*, 13.

# 2 History, Function, and Organization of the Federal and State Judicial Systems

One of the most important, most interesting, and most confusing features of the judiciary in the United States is what is known as the *dual court system*. This term simply means that each level of government (state and national) has its own set of courts. Thus, there are fifty-one separate court systems in the United States, one for each state and one for the federal government. As we shall see more clearly in Chapter 5, some legal problems are resolved entirely in the state courts, while others are handled entirely in the federal courts. Still others may get attention from both groups of courts. To simplify matters as much as possible, our approach in this chapter will be to discuss the federal and state courts separately.

Because a knowledge of the historical events that helped shape the national and state court systems can shed light on the present judicial structures, our study of the federal and state judiciaries begins with a description of the court systems as they have evolved over two centuries. We will first examine the three levels of the federal court system in the order in which they were established: the Supreme Court, the courts of appeals, and the district courts. The emphasis in our discussion of each level will be on historical development, policy-making roles, and decision-making procedures.

In a brief look at other federal courts we will focus on the distinction between constitutional and legislative courts, using the example of bankruptcy courts to illustrate a major difference in the two types. Our overview discussion will conclude with an examination of the role of the federal courts in the American political system. We will be particularly interested in comparing the courts' role in public policy making with that of the president and the Congress.

Following our examination of the federal judiciary we will turn our attention to the state court systems. Their development will be traced from the colonial period to the present in terms of organization, functions, and procedures.

## The Historical Context

Prior to the adoption of the Constitution, the country was governed by the Articles of Confederation. Under the Articles, practically all functions of government were vested in a single-chamber legislature called a Congress. There was no separation of executive and legislative powers.

The absence of a national judiciary was considered a major weakness of the Articles of Confederation. Both James Madison and Alexander Hamilton, for example, saw a need for a separate judicial branch. Consequently, the delegates gathered at the Constitutional Convention in Philadelphia in 1787 expressed widespread agreement that a national judiciary should be established. There was a good deal of disagreement, however, on the specific form that the judicial branch should take.

## The Constitutional Convention and Article III

The first proposal presented to the Constitutional Convention was the Randolph, or Virginia, Plan, which would have set up both a Supreme Court and inferior federal courts. Opponents of the Virginia Plan responded with the Paterson, or New Jersey, Plan, which called for the creation of a single federal supreme tribunal. Supporters of the New Jersey Plan were especially disturbed by the idea of lower federal courts. They argued that the state courts could hear all cases in the first instance and that a right of appeal to the Supreme Court would be sufficient to protect national rights and provide uniform judgments throughout the country.

The conflict between the states' rights advocates and the nationalists was resolved by one of the many compromises that characterized the Constitutional Convention. The compromise is found in Article III of the Constitution, which begins, "The judicial Power of the United States, shall be vested in one supreme Court, and in such inferior Courts as the Congress may from time to time ordain and establish." Thus the conflict would be postponed until the new government was in operation.

## The Judiciary Act of 1789

Once the Constitution was ratified, action on the federal judiciary came quickly. When the new Congress convened in 1789, its first major concern was judicial organization. Discussions of Senate Bill 1 involved many of the same participants and arguments as were involved in the Constitutional Convention's debates on the judiciary. Once again, the question was whether lower federal courts should be created at all or whether federal claims should first be heard in state courts. Attempts to resolve this controversy split Congress into two distinct groups.

One group, which believed that federal law should be adjudicated in the state courts first and by the United States Supreme Court only on appeal, expressed the fear that the new government would destroy the rights of the states. Other legislators, suspicious of the parochial prejudice of state courts, feared that litigants from other states and other countries would be dealt with unjustly. This latter group naturally favored a judicial system that included lower federal courts. The law that emerged from this debate, the Judiciary Act of 1789, set up a judicial system composed of a Supreme Court, consisting of a chief justice and five associate justices; three circuit courts, each comprising two justices of the Supreme Court and a district judge; and thirteen district courts, each presided over by one district judge. The power to create inferior federal courts, then, was immediately exercised. In fact, Congress created not one but two sets of lower courts.

## The U.S. Supreme Court

### A First Look

A famous jurist once said, "The Supreme Court of the United States is distinctly American in conception and function, and owes little to prior judicial institutions." [1] To understand what the framers of the Constitution envisioned for the Court, we must consider another American concept: the federal form of government. The Founders provided for both a national government and state governments; the courts of the states were to be bound by federal laws. However, final interpretation of federal laws simply could not be left to a state court, and certainly not to several state tribunals, whose judgments might disagree. Thus, the Supreme Court must interpret federal legislation. Another of the Founders' intentions was for the federal government to act directly upon individual citizens as well as upon the states. The Supreme Court's function in the federal system may be summarized as follows:

> In the most natural way, as the result of the creation of Federal law under a written constitution conferring limited powers, the Supreme Court of the United States came into being with its unique function. That court maintains the balance between State and Nation through the maintenance of the rights and duties of individuals. [2]

Given the High Court's importance to our system of government, it was perhaps inevitable that the Court would evoke great controversy. A leading student of the Supreme Court says:

> Nothing in the Court's history is more striking than the fact that, while its significant and necessary place in the Federal form of Government has always been recognized by thoughtful and patriotic men, nevertheless, no branch of the Government and no institution under the Constitution has sustained more continuous attack or reached its present position after more vigorous opposition. [3]

### The Court's First Decade

George Washington, in appointing the first Supreme Court justices, established two important traditions. First, he began the practice of naming to the Court those with whom he was politically compatible.

Washington, the only president ever to have an opportunity to appoint the entire federal judiciary, did a good job of filling federal judgeships with party bedfellows. Without exception, the federal judgeships went to faithful Federalists.

The second tradition established by Washington was that of roughly equal geographic representation on the federal courts. His first six appointees to the Supreme Court included three northerners and three southerners. On the basis of ability and legal reputation, only three or four of Washington's original appointees actually merited their justiceships. Many able men were either passed over or declined to serve.

The chief justiceship was the most important appointment Washington made. The president felt that the man to head the first Supreme Court should be an eminent lawyer, statesman, executive, and leader. Many names were presented to Washington, and at least one person, James Wilson, formally applied for the position. Ultimately, Washington settled upon John Jay of New York. Although only forty-four years old, Jay had experience as a lawyer, a judge, and a diplomat. In addition, he was the main drafter of his state's first constitution. Concerning the selection of Jay as chief justice, it has been said:

> That Washington picked Jay over his top two rivals for the post, James Wilson and John Rutledge, was either fortuitous or inspired—for it would scarcely have added to the fledgling Supreme Court's popular prestige to have its Chief Justice go insane, as Rutledge later did, or spend his last days jumping from one state to another to avoid being arrested for a debt, as did Wilson.[4]

Washington did, however, appoint both Wilson and Rutledge to the Court as associate justices. Neither man contributed significantly to the Court as a government institution; thus Washington became the first of many presidents to misjudge an appointee to the Court.

The remaining three associate justices who served on the original Supreme Court were William Cushing, John Blair, and James Iredell. Cushing remained on the Court for twenty years, more than twice as long as any of the other original justices, although senility affected his competency in later years. Blair was a close personal friend of Washington's, and Iredell was a strong Federalist from North Carolina who was instrumental in getting that state to join the Union. The appointment of Blair and Iredell, then, has been seen as sheer political reward. Despite the generally mediocre quality of the original six appointees, they were held in somewhat higher esteem by their contemporaries, according to studies of early letters and correspondence.[5]

The Supreme Court met for the first time on Monday, February 1, 1790, in the Royal Exchange, a building located in the Wall Street section of New York City. Compared with today's Supreme Court, that first session was certainly unimpressive. Tongue in cheek, one Court historian noted: "The first President immediately on taking office settled down to the pressing business of being President. The first Congress enacted the first laws. The first Supreme Court adjourned." [6]

Only Jay, Wilson, and Cushing, the three northern justices, were present on opening day. Justice Blair arrived from Virginia for the second day, while Rutledge and Iredell, the other southerners, did not appear at all during the opening session.

The Supreme Court's first session lasted just ten days. During this period the Court selected a clerk, chose a seal, and admitted several lawyers to practice before it in the future. There were, of course, no cases to be decided. In fact, the Court did not rule on a single case during its first three years. In spite of this insignificant and abbreviated beginning,

> the New York and the Philadelphia newspapers described the proceedings of this first session of the Court more fully than any other event connected with the new Government; and their accounts were reproduced in the leading papers of all the States. [7]

The minor role the Supreme Court played continued throughout its first decade of existence. The 1790-1799 period saw several individuals decline their nomination to the Court and one, Robert H. Harrison, chose to accept a *state* position rather than a Supreme Court justiceship.

During its first decade the Court decided only about fifty cases. However, one of these, *Chisholm v. Georgia,* involved the Court in considerable controversy. [8] In *Chisholm* the justices held that a citizen of one state could sue another state in a federal court. That decision was vigorously attacked by states' rights forces and was ultimately overturned by ratification of the Eleventh Amendment in 1798.

Given the scarcity of Supreme Court business in the early days, Chief Justice Jay's contributions may be traced primarily to his circuit court decisions and his judicial conduct. In one circuit court opinion Jay and his colleagues, Justice Cushing and district judge Henry Marchant, unanimously held that Rhode Island could not permit a debtor to extend his obligations for three years and grant him immunity from arrest and penalties during that time. [9] Jay viewed such an action as a violation of the contract clause contained in Article I, Section 10. His view, a clear affirmation of national supremacy and federal judicial authority, may well have set the stage for John Marshall's later opinions along these lines.

In another circuit court case, Jay held that Congress had no authority to assign nonjudicial functions to the courts. [10] Congress had attempted to give the courts the duty of approving applications for military pensions, subject to suspension by the secretary of war and revision by Congress.

Perhaps the most important of Jay's contributions, however, was his insistence that the Supreme Court could not provide legal advice for the

executive branch in the form of an advisory opinion. Jay was asked by
treasury secretary Alexander Hamilton to issue an opinion on the constitutionality of a resolution passed by the Virginia House of Representatives
which declared that a congressional bill for the assumption of the state
debts was unconstitutional. President Washington also asked Jay for advice
on questions relating to Washington's Neutrality Proclamation. In both
instances, Jay's response was a firm no. On balance, "despite his lack of
judicial craftsmanship and the brief time in which he might display his
personal talents, Jay was successful in establishing the dignity of the office
and the independence of the Supreme Court." [11]

## The Impact of Chief Justice Marshall

John Marshall served as chief justice from 1801 to 1835 and dominated
the Court to a degree unmatched by any other justice. In effect, Marshall
*was* the Court—perhaps because, in the words of one scholar, he "brought
a first-class mind and a thoroughly engaging personality into second-class
company." [12]

Marshall's dominance of the Court enabled him to initiate some major
changes in the way opinions were presented. Prior to his tenure, the
justices ordinarily wrote separate opinions (called *seriatim* opinions) in
major cases. Under Marshall's stewardship, the Court adopted the practice
of handing down a single opinion. As one might expect, the evidence
shows that from 1801 to 1835 Marshall himself wrote almost half the
opinions. [13]

It was Marshall's goal to keep dissension to a minimum. Arguing that
dissent undermined the Court's authority, he tried to persuade the justices
to settle their differences privately and then present a united front to the
public. No doubt his first-class mind and engaging personality aided him
in this endeavor. As strange as it may sound, so did the cozy living
arrangements of the time. The justices lived in the same Washington, D.C.,
boardinghouse while the Court was in session. Thus, they were together
before, during, and after work in a pleasant, comfortable routine that
discouraged deep disagreements. Can you imagine having breakfast,
lunch, and dinner every day with a fellow justice whom you have sharply
criticized in a public opinion? Human nature, it would seem, was on
Marshall's side in keeping dissension to a low level.

In addition to bringing about changes in opinion-writing practices,
Marshall used his powers to involve the Court in the policy-making
process. Early in his tenure as chief justice, the Court asserted its power to
declare an act of Congress unconstitutional, in *Marbury v. Madison*
(1803). [14]

This case had its beginnings in the presidential election of 1800, when
Thomas Jefferson defeated John Adams in his bid for reelection. Before

leaving office in March 1801, however, Adams and the lame-duck Federalist Congress combined efforts to create several new federal judgeships. To fill these new positions Adams nominated, and the Senate confirmed, loyal Federalists. In addition, Adams named his outgoing secretary of state, John Marshall, to be the new chief justice of the Supreme Court.

As secretary of state it had been Marshall's job to deliver the commissions of the newly appointed judges. Time ran out, however, and seventeen of the commissions were not delivered before Jefferson's inauguration. The new president ordered *his* secretary of state, James Madison, not to deliver the remaining commissions.

One of the disappointed nominees was William Marbury. He and three of his colleagues, all confirmed as justices of the peace for the District of Columbia, decided to ask the Supreme Court to force Madison to deliver their commissions. They relied upon Section 13 of the Judiciary Act of 1789, which granted the Supreme Court the authority to issue *writs of mandamus*—court orders commanding a public official to perform an official, nondiscretionary duty.

The case placed Marshall in an uncomfortable predicament. Some suggested that he disqualify himself because of his earlier involvement as secretary of state. There was also the question of the court's power. If Marshall were to grant the writ, Madison (under Jefferson's orders) would be almost certain to refuse to deliver the commissions. The Supreme Court would then be powerless to enforce its order. On the other hand, if Marshall refused to grant the writ, Jefferson would win by default.

The decision Marshall fashioned from this seemingly impossible predicament was sheer genius. He declared Section 13 of the Judiciary Act of 1789 unconstitutional because it granted original jurisdiction to the Supreme Court in excess of that specified in Article III of the Constitution. Thus the Court's power to review and determine the constitutionality of acts of Congress was established. This decision is rightly seen as one of the single most important decisions the Supreme Court has ever handed down. A few years later the court also claimed the right of judicial review over actions of state legislatures; during Marshall's tenure it overturned more than a dozen state laws on constitutional grounds.[15]

## The Changing Issue Emphasis of the Supreme Court

We complete our brief historical review of the Supreme Court by looking at the major issue areas that have occupied the Court's attention. Until approximately 1865 the legal relationship between the national and state governments, or cases of federalism, dominated the Court's docket. John Marshall believed in a strong national government and was not hesitant to restrict state policies that interfered with its activities. A case in point is *Gibbons v. Ogden* (1824), in which the Court overturned a state monopoly over steamboat transportation on the ground that it interfered with national control over interstate commerce.[16] Another good example of Marshall's use of the Court to expand the federal government's powers came in *McCulloch v. Maryland* (1819), in which the chief justice held that the necessary-and-proper clause of the Constitution permitted Congress to establish a national bank.[17] The Court also ruled that the state could not tax a nationally chartered bank. The Court's insistence on a strong government in Washington did not significantly diminish after Marshall's death. Roger Taney, who succeeded Marshall as chief justice, served from 1836 to 1864. Although the Court's position during this period was not as uniformly favorable to the federal government, the Taney Court did not reverse the Marshall Court's direction.

During the 1865-1937 period issues of economic regulation dominated the Court's docket. The shift in emphasis from federalism to economic regulation was brought on by a growing number of national and state laws aimed at monitoring business activities. As such laws increased, so did the number of cases challenging their constitutionality. Early in this period the Court's position on regulation was mixed, but by the 1920s the bench had become quite hostile toward government regulatory policy. Federal regulations were generally overturned on the ground that they were unsupported by constitutional grants of power to Congress, while state laws were thrown out mainly as violations of economic rights protected by the Fourteenth Amendment.

Matters came to a head in the mid-1930s as a result of the Court's conflict with President Franklin D. Roosevelt, whose New Deal program to combat the effects of the Depression included broad measures to control the economy. However, "in the 16 months starting in January 1935, the Supreme Court heard cases involving ten major New Deal measures or actions; eight of them were declared unconstitutional by the Court." [18] Following his overwhelming reelection in 1936, Roosevelt fought back against the Court. On February 5, 1937, he proposed a plan whereby an additional justice could be added to the Court for each sitting justice over the age of seventy. The result of FDR's "Court-packing" plan would have been to increase the Court's size temporarily to fifteen justices.

While Roosevelt's proposal was being debated in Congress, the Court made an about-face and began to uphold New Deal legislation and similar state legislation.[19] This "switch in time that saved nine," as it has been called, came about because Chief Justice Charles Evans Hughes and Justice Owen Roberts changed their votes to establish majority support for the New Deal legislation. As a result, the Court-packing plan became a moot issue and quietly died in Congress.

Since 1937 the Supreme Court has focused on civil liberties concerns—in particular, the constitutional guarantees of freedom of expression and freedom of religion. In addition, an increasing number of cases have dealt with procedural rights of criminal defendants. Finally, the Court has decided a great number of cases involving equal treatment by the government of racial minorities and other disadvantaged groups.

The Supreme Court's position on civil liberties and civil rights has varied a good deal over the years. Without doubt, it gave its strongest and most active support for civil liberties and civil rights during the 1953-1969 period, when Earl Warren served as chief justice. Perhaps the best known decision of the period was *Brown v. Board of Education* (1954), which ordered desegregation of the public schools.[20] Other notable decisions guaranteed the right to counsel in state trials, limited police search and seizure practices, required that police inform suspects of their rights, mandated legislatures to be apportioned according to population, and prohibited state-written and state-required prayer in public schools.[21] These and many other controversial decisions led to heavy criticism of the Warren Court.

During his 1968 presidential campaign Richard Nixon pledged that, if elected, he would appoint more conservative individuals to the Court. In 1969 he took the first step toward making good on that promise by naming Warren Burger to replace the retiring Earl Warren as chief justice. Over the next two years Nixon appointed three other justices and did indeed produce a Court whose aggregate viewpoint was more conservative. The conservative trend of the Supreme Court was continued with President Ronald Reagan's appointees. In addition to elevating William Rehnquist to the chief justiceship, he also named Sandra Day O'Connor, Antonin Scalia, and Anthony Kennedy to the High Court.

We next turn our attention to the various roles played by the Supreme Court, in particular, its policy-making function and its role as court of final appeal.

## The Supreme Court as a Policy Maker

The Supreme Court's role as a policy maker derives from the fact that it interprets the law. Public policy issues come before the Court in the form of legal disputes that must be resolved.

> Courts in any political system participate to some degree in the policymaking process because it is their job. Any judge faced with a choice between two or more interpretations and applications of a legislative act, executive order, or constitutional provision must choose among them because the controversy must be decided. And when the judge chooses, his or her interpretation becomes policy for the specific litigants. If the interpretation is accepted by the other judges, the judge has made policy for all jurisdictions in which that view prevails.[22]

An excellent example may be found in the area of racial equality. In the late 1880s many states enacted laws requiring the separation of blacks and whites in public facilities. In 1890, for instance, Louisiana enacted a law requiring separate but equal railroad accommodations for blacks and whites. A challenge came two years later. Homer Plessy, who was one-eighth black, protested against the Louisiana law by refusing to move from a seat in the white car of a train traveling from New Orleans to Covington, Louisiana. Arrested and charged with violating the statute, Plessy contended that the law was unconstitutional. The U.S. Supreme Court, in *Plessy v. Ferguson* (1896), upheld the Louisiana statute.[23] Thus the court established the *separate-but-equal* policy that was to reign for about sixty years. During this period many states required that the races sit in different areas of buses, trains, terminals, and theaters; to use different restrooms; and to drink from different water fountains. Blacks were sometimes excluded from restaurants and public libraries. Perhaps most important, black students often had to attend inferior schools.

Separation of the races in public schools was contested in the famous *Brown v. Board of Education* case. Parents of black schoolchildren claimed that state laws requiring or permitting segregation deprived them of equal protection of the laws under the Fourteenth Amendment. The Supreme Court ruled that separate educational facilities are inherently unequal and, therefore, segregation constitutes a denial of equal protection. In the *Brown* decision the Court laid to rest the separate-but-equal doctrine and established a policy of desegregated public schools.

In an average year the Court decides, with full opinions, only about 150 cases. Thousands of other cases are disposed of with less than the full treatment. Thus the Court deals at length with a very select set of policy issues that, as noted, have varied throughout the Court's history.

In a democracy broad matters of public policy are, in theory at least, presumed to be left to the elected representatives of the people—not to judicial appointees with life terms. Thus, in principle, U.S. judges are not supposed to make policy. However, as we shall demonstrate when we discuss decision making in Chapters 9 and 10, in practice judges cannot help but make policy to some extent.

It should be noted that the Supreme Court differs from legislative and executive policy makers. Especially important is the fact that the Court had no self-starting device. The justices must wait for problems to be brought to them; there can be no judicial policy making if there is no litigation. The president and members of Congress have no such constraints. Moeover, even the most assertive Supreme Court is limited to some extent by the actions of other policy makers, such as lower-court judges, Congress, and the president. The Court depends upon others to implement or carry out its decisions. This process of implementation will be discussed in detail in Chapter 11.

## The Supreme Court as Final Arbiter

The Supreme Court has both original and appellate jurisdiction. The two types of jurisdiction will be discussed in detail in Chapter 5, but a brief definition of each will be helpful at this point. In *original jurisdiction* a court has the power to hear a case for the first time. In *appellate jurisdiction*, on the other hand, a higher court has the authority to review cases originally decided by a lower court.

The Supreme Court is overwhelmingly an appellate court since most of its time is devoted to reviewing decisions of lower courts. Regardless of whether its decisions are seen as correct, it is the highest appellate tribunal in the country. As such, it has the final word in the interpretation of the Constitution, acts of legislative bodies, and treaties—unless the Court's decision is altered by a constitutional amendment or, in some instances, by an act of Congress.

Since 1925 a device known as *certiorari* has allowed the High Court to exercise discretion in deciding which cases it should review. Under this method a person may *request* Supreme Court review of a lower-court decision; it is then up to the justices to determine whether the request should be granted. If review is granted, the Court issues a *writ of certiorari*, which is an order to the lower court to send up a complete record of the case. When certiorari is denied, the decision of the lower court stands.

## The Supreme Court at Work

The formal session of the Supreme Court lasts from the first Monday in October until the business of the term is completed, usually in late June or July. Since 1935 the Supreme Court has had its own building in Washington. The imposing five-story marble building has the words "Equal Justice Under Law" carved above the entrance. It stands across from the Capitol. Formal sessions of the Court are held in a large courtroom that seats 300 people. At the front of the courtroom is the bench where the justices are seated. When the Court is in session, the chief justice, followed by the eight associate justices in order of seniority (length of continuous service on the Court), enters through the purple draperies behind the bench and takes a seat. Seats are arranged according to seniority, with the chief justice in the center, the senior associate justice on the chief justice's right, the second-ranking associate justice on the left, and continuing alternately in declining order of seniority. Near the courtroom are the conference room, where the justices decide cases, and the chambers that contain offices for the justices and their staff.

The Court's term is divided into *sittings*, of approximately two weeks each, during which it meets in open session and holds internal conferences, and *recesses*, during which the justices work behind closed doors as they consider cases and write opinions. The 150 or so cases per term that receive the Court's full treatment follow a fairly routine pattern, which is described below.

*Oral Argument.* Oral arguments are generally scheduled on Monday through Wednesday during the sittings. The sessions run from 10:00 a.m. until noon and from 1:00 until 3:00 p.m. Since the procedure is not a trial or the original hearing of a case, no jury is assembled and no witnesses are called. Instead, the two opposing attorneys present their arguments to the justices. The general practice is to allow thirty minutes for each side, although the Court may decide that additional time is necessary. The Court can normally hear four cases in one day. Attorneys presenting oral arguments are frequently interrupted with probing questions from the justices. The oral argument is considered very important by both attorneys and justices because it is the only stage in the process that allows such personal exchanges.

*The Conference.* On Fridays preceding the two-week sittings the Court holds a conference; during sittings it holds conferences on Wednesday afternoon and all day Friday. At the Wednesday meeting the justices discuss the cases argued on Monday. At the longer conference on Friday they discuss the cases that were argued on Tuesday and Wednesday, plus any other matters that need to be considered. The most important of these other matters are the certiorari petitions.

Prior to the Friday conference each justice is given a list of the cases that will be discussed. The conference begins about 9:30 or 10:00 a.m. and runs until 5:30 or 6:00 p.m. As the justices enter the conference room they shake hands with each other and take their seats around a rectangular table. They meet in secret behind locked doors, and no official record is kept of the discussions. The chief justice presides over the conference and offers an opinion first in each case. The other justices follow in descending order of seniority. At one time a formal vote was then taken in reverse order (with the junior justice voting first); however, today the justices usually indicate their view during the discussion, making a formal vote unnecessary.[24]

A quorum for a decision on a case is six members, but there is seldom any difficulty in obtaining a quorum. Cases are sometimes decided by less than nine justices because of vacancies, illnesses, or nonparticipation because of possible conflicts of interest. Supreme Court decisions are made by a majority vote. In case of a tie the lower-court decision is upheld.

*Opinion Writing.* After a tentative decision has been reached in conference, the next step is to assign the Court's opinion to an individual justice. Chief justices in the majority assign the opinion, either to themselves or to another justice who voted with the majority. When the chief justice votes with the minority, then the most senior justice in the majority makes the assignment.

After the conference the justice who will write the Court's opinion begins work on an initial draft. Other justices may work on the case by writing alternative opinions. The completed opinion is circulated to justices in both the majority and the minority groups. The writer seeks to persuade justices originally in the minority to change their votes, and to keep his or her majority group intact. A bargaining process occurs and the working of the opinion may be changed in order to satisfy other justices or obtain their support. A deep division in the Court makes it difficult to achieve a clear, coherent opinion and may even result in a shift in votes or in another justice's opinion becoming the Court's official ruling.

In most cases a single opinion does obtain majority support, although only a few rulings are unanimous. Those who disagree with the opinion of the Court are said to *dissent*. A dissent does not have to be accompanied by an opinion; in recent years, however, it usually is. Whenever more than one justice dissents, each may write an opinion or they may join in a single opinion.

On occasion a justice will agree with the court's decision but differ in his or her reason for reaching that conclusion. Such a justice may write what is called a *concurring opinion*. A good example may be found in Justice Potter Stewart's concurring opinion in *Stanley v. Georgia* (1969).[25] In that case an investigation of Stanley's alleged bookmaking activities led to the issuance of a search warrant for his home. Federal and state agents conducting the search found three reels of film, a projector, and a screen. After viewing the films, the state officers seized them as pornographic. Stanley was convicted of "knowingly having possession of obscene matter" in violation of Georgia law. The Supreme Court overturned the Georgia trial court's decision on the ground that mere private possession of lewd material could not constitutionally be made a crime. Justice Stewart agreed that the lower court decision should be overturned, but he did so for quite a different reason; he felt that the films had been seized unlawfully in violation of the Fourth and Fourteenth Amendments.

An opinion labeled *concurring and dissenting* agrees with part of a Court ruling but disagrees with other parts. Finally, the Court occasionally issues a *per curiam opinion*—an unsigned opinion that is usually quite brief. Such opinions are often used when the Court accepts the case for review but gives it less than full treatment. For example, it may decide the case without benefit of oral argument and issue a *per curiam* opinion to explain the disposition of the case. Table 2-1 shows the types of opinions written by the individual justices for the 1985, 1986, and 1987 terms of the Supreme Court.

**Table 2-1**  Types of Opinions Written by Supreme Court Justices, 1985, 1986, and 1987 Terms

| Justice | Opinions of the Court | | | Concurring opinions | | | Dissenting opinions | | | Total | | |
|---|---|---|---|---|---|---|---|---|---|---|---|---|
| | 1985 | 1986 | 1987 | 1985 | 1986 | 1987 | 1985 | 1986 | 1987 | 1985 | 1986 | 1987 |
| Blackmun | 14 | 13 | 14 | 10 | 13 | 4 | 16 | 16 | 10 | 40 | 42 | 28 |
| Brennan | 13 | 16 | 15 | 7 | 8 | 11 | 28 | 24 | 13 | 48 | 48 | 39 |
| Burger | 14 | — | — | 15 | — | — | 5 | — | — | 34 | — | — |
| Kennedy | — | — | 7 | — | — | 4 | — | — | 3 | — | — | 14 |
| Marshall | 15 | 16 | 15 | 6 | 1 | 1 | 31 | 20 | 13 | 52 | 37 | 29 |
| O'Connor | 17 | 18 | 16 | 12 | 11 | 8 | 7 | 13 | 12 | 36 | 42 | 36 |
| Powell | 18 | 20 | — | 10 | 7 | — | 11 | 11 | — | 39 | 38 | — |
| Rehnquist | 19 | 17 | 15 | 3 | — | 2 | 15 | 9 | 7 | 37 | 26 | 24 |
| Scalia | — | 12 | 16 | — | 17 | 15 | — | 13 | 11 | — | 42 | 42 |
| Stevens | 17 | 16 | 19 | 15 | 14 | 6 | 36 | 32 | 17 | 68 | 62 | 42 |
| White | 19 | 17 | 20 | 11 | 5 | 13 | 12 | 16 | 11 | 42 | 38 | 44 |
| Per curiam | 13 | 7 | 5 | — | — | — | — | — | — | 13 | 7 | 5 |
| Total | 159 | 152 | 142 | 89 | 76 | 64 | 161 | 154 | 97 | 409 | 382 | 303 |

*Sources*: "The Supreme Court, 1985 Term," *Harvard Law Review* 100 (November 1986): 304; "The Supreme Court, 1986 Term," *Harvard Law Review* 101 (November 1987): 362, and; "The Supreme Court, 1987 Term," *Harvard Law Review* 102 (November 1988): 350. Copyright 1986, 1987, 1988, by the Harvard Law Review Association. Reprinted by permission.

## The U.S. Courts of Appeals

The courts of appeals have been described as "perhaps the least noticed of the regular constitutional courts." [26] They receive less media coverage than the Supreme Court, in part because their activities are simply not as dramatic. However, one should not assume that the courts of appeals are unimportant to the judicial system. As we shall see, their role has increased significantly over the years.

### Circuit Courts: 1789-1801

As noted earlier, the Judiciary Act of 1789 created three circuit courts—the southern, middle, and eastern circuits—each composed of two justices of the Supreme Court and a district judge. The circuit court was to hold two sessions each year in each district within the circuit.

It was the district judge who became primarily responsible for establishing the circuit court's workload. The two Supreme Court justices then came into the local area and participated in the cases. This practice tended to give a local rather than national focus to the circuit courts.

The circuit court system was regarded from the beginning as unsatisfactory, especially by Supreme Court justices, who objected to the traveling imposed upon them. As early as September 1790, Chief Justice Jay wrote to the president urging changes in the circuit-riding duties prescribed by the Judiciary Act of 1789. Justice Iredell, who resided in North Carolina, was particulary hard pressed; in addition to some 2,000 miles of travel between his home and Philadelphia (where Supreme Court sessions were held), he was required to tour the states of Georgia, North Carolina, and South Carolina twice annually. It is no wonder Iredell referred to his life as that of a "travelling postboy." [27]

Supreme Court justices were not the only ones who objected to the circuit-riding duties. Attorney General Edmund Randolph and President Washington also urged relief for the Supreme Court justices. Congress made a slight change in 1793 by altering the circuit court organization to include only one Supreme Court justice and one district judge. The Randolph proposal for separate circuit court judgeships to replace Supreme Court participation was not implemented, however. The circuit courts had become the center of a political controversy, with the Federalists urging passage of Randolph's proposal for separate circuit judges, while the Anti-Federalist leaders saw the Randolph proposal as an attempt to enlarge the federal judiciary and remove it from state surveillance.

### Circuit Courts: 1801-1891

In the closing days of President Adam's administration in 1801, Congress passed the "midnight judges" act, which eliminated circuit riding by the

Supreme Court justices, authorized the appointment of sixteen new circuit judges, and greatly extended the jurisdiction of the lower courts.

Some saw the Judiciary Act of 1801 as the Federalists' last-ditch effort to prolong their domination of government, while others viewed it as an extension of federal jurisdiction to suits that previously had been tried only in state courts. Certainly the Federalists were interested in federal judgeships, and they wanted to protect the judiciary from Anti-Federalists. The act of 1801, however, was not a last-minute effort. As we have seen, efforts to change the circuit courts had been going on for more than ten years.

The new administration of Thomas Jefferson strongly opposed the "midnight judges" act, and Congress wasted little time in repealing it. The Circuit Court Act of 1802 restored circuit riding by Supreme Court justices and expanded the number of circuits. However, the 1802 legislation allowed the circuit court to be held by a single district judge. At first glance, such a change may seem slight, but it proved to be of great importance. Increasingly, the district judges began to assume responsibility for both district and circuit courts. In practice, then, original and appellate jurisdiction were both in the hands of the district judges.

The next major step in the development of the courts of appeals did not come until 1869, although there had been a growing recognition that some form of judicial reorganization was necessary. The pro-state and pronationalist interests disagreed on the exact form of judicial relief that should be enacted. The pronationalists did not want a plan that would transfer power from the national government to the states. They favored shifting many conflicts to the lower federal courts under the supervision of the Supreme Court. Thus, "reorganization of the circuit courts continued to be the key to the nationalists' strategy." [28]

Expansion of the circuit courts with greater control over appeals would free the Supreme Court to concentrate on the key cases as well as to formulate policy. The pro-state interests also wanted to lessen the High Court's burden, but by reducing its power. Unable to do so, they were willing to accept only minor changes in the basic judicial structure established in 1789.

The political stalemate prevented any major reorganization between 1802 and 1869. Consequently, the courts simply were unable to handle the flood of litigation. Then, in 1869, Congress approved a measure that authorized the appointment of nine new circuit judges and reduced the Supreme Court justices' circuit court duty to one term every two years. Still, the High Court was flooded with cases because there were no limitations on the right of appeal to the Supreme Court. Six years later Congress broadened the jurisdiction of the circuit courts. The workload of the Supreme Court was not significantly decreased, however, since there was still an automatic right of appeal to the High Court. A more drastic revision of the federal judicial system was to come in 1891.

## The Courts of Appeals: 1891 to the Present

On March 3, 1891, the Evarts Act was signed into law, creating new courts known as circuit courts of appeals. These new tribunals were to hear most of the appeals from district courts. The old circuit courts, which had existed since 1789, also remained—a situation surely confusing to all but the most serious students of the judicial system. The new circuit court of appeals was to consist of one circuit judge, one circuit court of appeals judge, one district judge, and a Supreme Court justice. Two judges constituted a quorum in these new courts.

Following passage of the Evarts Act, there were two trial tribunals in the federal judiciary: district courts and circuit courts. There were also two appellate tribunals: circuit courts of appeals and the Supreme Court. Most appeals of trial decisions were to go to the circuit court of appeals, although the act also allowed direct review in some instances by the Supreme Court. In short, creation of the circuit courts of appeals released the Supreme Court from many petty types of cases. There would still be appeals, but the High Court would now have much greater control over its own workload. Much of its former caseload was thus shifted to the two lower levels of the federal judiciary.

The next step in the evolution of the courts of appeals came in 1911. In that year Congress passed legislation abolishing the old circuit courts, which had no appellate jurisdiction and frequently duplicated the functions of district courts.

Today, as a result of a name change implemented in the 1948 Judicial Code, the intermediate tribunals are officially known as courts of appeals. Despite their official name, they continue to be referred to colloquially as circuit courts. Nine regional courts of appeals, covering several states, were created in 1891. Another, covering the District of Columbia, was absorbed into the system after 1893. The Court of Appeals for the Tenth Circuit was carved from the Eighth Circuit in 1929, and the Court of Appeals for the Eleventh Circuit was carved from the Fifth in 1981. Figure 2-1 shows the boundaries of each circuit and indicates the states contained in each.

On April 2, 1982, President Reagan signed the Federal Courts Improvement Act, which created a thirteenth circuit court. The act, which took effect on October 1, 1982, created the United States Court of Appeals for the Federal Circuit. This newest appellate court consolidated the Court of Claims and the Court of Customs and Patent Appeals (types of courts which will be described later in this chapter).

**Figure 2-1** District and Appellate Court Boundaries

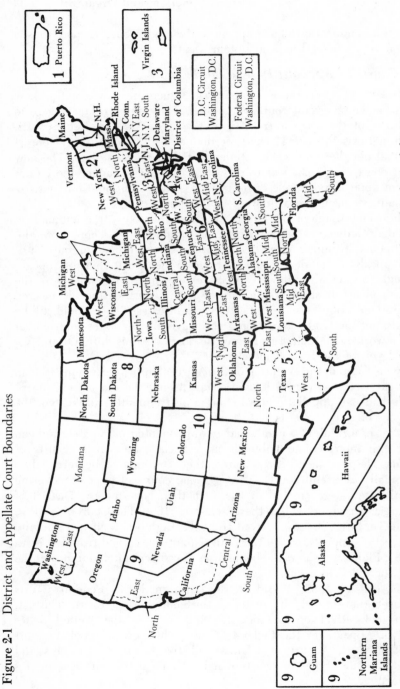

*Note:* The large numerals indicate the Courts of Appeals, and the broken lines represent jurisdiction boundaries of district courts.

*Source:* Administrative Office of the U.S. Courts.

## The Review Function of the Courts of Appeals

As one modern-day student of our judiciary has noted:

> The distribution of labor among the Supreme Court and the Courts of
> Appeals, implicit in the Judiciary Act of 1925, has matured into fully
> differentiated functions for federal appellate courts. Substantively, the
> Supreme Court has become more and more a constitutional tribunal.
> Courts of Appeals concentrate on statutory interpretation, adminis-
> trative review, and error correction in masses of routine adjudi-
> cations.[29]

Although the Supreme Court has had discretionary control of its
docket since 1925, the Courts of Appeals still have no such luxury.
Instead, their docket depends on how many and what types of cases are
appealed to them.

Most of the cases reviewed by the courts of appeals originate in the
federal district courts. Litigants disappointed with the lower court
decision may appeal the case to the court of appeals of the circuit in
which the federal district court is located. The appellate courts have also
been given authority to review the decisions of certain administrative
agencies. This type of case enters the federal judicial system at the court
of appeals level rather than at the federal district court level.

Since the courts of appeals have no control over which cases are
brought to them, they deal with both highly important and routine
matters. Scholars identify five general types of appeals that the circuit
judges consider:

1. *Ritualistic appeals*—petitions that are expected or demanded even
   though the odds of winning are very low. Such appeals were quite
   common following the school desegregation decision (*Brown v.
   Board of Education*) in 1954. Those favoring the continuance of
   segregated schools routinely appealed their cases from the federal
   district courts to the Court of Appeals for the southern-oriented
   Fourth or Fifth Circuit. Although they were almost certain to lose,
   they were able to shift the burden for defeat outside the local area
   and, at the same time, convince their supporters they had done
   everything possible under the law to defend segregationist interests.
2. *Frivolous appeals*—cases and claims that have no substance and
   little or no chance for success. Many of these appeals come from
   prisoners who have everything to gain and nothing to lose. Such
   appeals are no doubt encouraged by the fact that the Supreme
   Court has ruled that assistance of counsel for first appeals should be
   granted to all indigents who have been convicted of a crime.[30]
   Occasionally a claim is successful, however, and then other prisoners become motivated to appeal.

3. *Bureaucratic appeals*—challenges of federal agencies and commissions. Outright reversal of agency decisions is rare, but modification of administrative orders is not uncommon.

4. *Consensual appeals*—cases in which there is substantial agreement on how the issue should be resolved. Petitioners who have lost, however, hope to change the original verdict. In other words, the litigants seek modifications of the lower-court monetary awards. Such appeals, called the "bread and butter" issues of the appellate docket, include income tax, corporate activity, and eminent domain cases.

5. *Nonconsensual appeals*—cases that raise major questions of public policy and evoke strong disagreement. Decisions by the courts of appeals are likely to establish policy for society as a whole, not just for the specific litigants. Civil liberties, reapportionment, religion, and education cases provide good examples of the kinds of disputes that may affect us all.

There are several purposes of review in the courts of appeals. The first is *error correction*. Judges in the various circuits are called upon to monitor the performance of federal district courts and federal agencies and to supervise their application and interpretation of national and state laws. In doing so, the courts of appeals do not seek out new factual evidence, but instead examine the record of the lower court for errors. In the process of correcting errors the courts of appeals also settle disputes and enforce national law. Since the Supreme Court intervenes so infrequently, the courts of appeals become the last resort in the overwhelming majority of cases.

The courts of appeals perform a second function: sorting out and developing those few cases worthy of Supreme Court review. The circuit judges tackle the legal issues earlier than the Supreme Court justices and may help shape what they consider review-worthy claims. Judicial scholars have found that appealed cases often differ in their second hearing from their first. An analysis of cases that raised civil liberties issues when taken from district courts to Court of Appeals for the Third, Fifth, and Eighth Circuits during the 1956-1961 period revealed that only about one-third had had a civil liberties content in the trial court. [31] In other words, the substance of the case shifted on appeal, and routine cases were given greater political significance. More recently, however, a study of Courts of Appeals in the Second, Fifth, and District of Columbia Circuits showed that in only 7 percent of the opinions had circuit judges reformulated the issues. [32]

## The Courts of Appeals as Policy Makers

We noted earlier that the Supreme Court's role as a policy maker derives from the fact that it interprets the law; the same holds true for the court of appeals. The scope of the courts of appeals' policy-making role takes on added importance when we recall that they are the courts of last resort in the vast majority of cases. A couple of examples illustrate the far-reaching impact of the circuit judges.

In 1966 the Court of Appeals for the District of Columbia Circuit decided a case involving an application for a license renewal by television station WLBT in Jackson, Mississippi.[33] Complaints against WLBT included charges of racial and religious discrimination and excessive use of commercials. The first major complaint dated back to 1955, when it was alleged that WLBT had deliberately cut off a network program about race relations on which the general counsel of the National Association for the Advancement of Colored People was appearing; according to the complaint, the station flashed on the screen a sign reading "Sorry, Cable Trouble."

In 1957 WLBT was accused of presenting a program that urged the maintenance of racial segregation and then refusing requests for time to offer an opposing viewpoint. When WLBT applied for its license renewal in the mid-1960s, the Office of Communications of the United Church of Christ asked the Federal Communications Commission (FCC) for permission to present arguments and evidence in opposition to the renewal application. The FCC dismissed the Church of Christ's petition and took the unusual step of granting a conditional license to WLBT for one year instead of the usual three. Speaking for the court of appeals, Judge Warren Burger (later chief justice of the United States) held that the granting of WLBT's license was erroneous and ordered the FCC to hold hearings allowing opponents of the license renewal to present their arguments.

The second example involves a case that began in the Cleveland, Ohio, suburb of Parma. In April 1973 the U.S. Department of Justice, in a suit filed in the district court for the Northern District of Ohio, alleged that the city of Parma had violated the Fair Housing Act. The suit contended that Parma's conduct and practices had the effect of making equal housing opportunity unavailable. On June 5, 1980, Chief Judge Frank Battisti held that Parma had intentionally engaged in discrimination in violation of the Fair Housing Act. Parma appealed the district court's ruling, however, and on October 14, 1981, the Sixth Circuit Court of Appeals affirmed Judge Battisti's decision.[34] The city of Parma continued its fight by seeking review by the U.S. Supreme Court, which early in 1982 denied certiorari. Thus, a major decision affecting equal housing opportunities for hundreds of people was rendered by the Sixth Circuit Court of Appeals.

A major difference in policy making by the Supreme Court and by the courts of appeals should be noted. While there is one High Court for the entire country, each court of appeals covers only a specific region. Thus, the courts of appeals are more likely to make policy on a regional basis. Still, they are a part of the federal judicial system and "participate in both national and local policy networks, their decisions becoming regional law unless intolerable to the Justices." [35]

## The Courts of Appeals at Work

As we noted earlier, the courts of appeals do not have the same degree of discretion as the Supreme Court to decide whether to accept a case for review. Still, as we shall see, circuit judges have developed methods for using their time as efficiently as possible.

*Screening.*   During the screening stage the judges decide whether to give an appeal a full review or to dispose of it in some other way. The docket may be reduced to some extent by consolidating similar claims into single cases, a process that also results in a uniform decision. In deciding which cases can be disposed of without oral argument, the courts of appeals increasingly rely on law clerks or staff attorneys. These court personnel (discussed in greater detail in Chapter 3) read petitions and briefs and then submit recommendations to the judges. In 1975 the Second Circuit Court of Appeals instituted a Civil Appeals Management Plan (CAMP). The plan is aimed at promoting settlements and reducing the proportion of appeals that require oral argument. An evaluation of CAMP conducted in 1983 concluded that the plan does produce the benefits expected of it: settlement or withdrawal of a significant number of appeals and an improvement in the quality of briefs and oral arguments.[36] Several other circuits have adopted their own variations of CAMP. The screening process is very effective. According to Chief Judge Charles Clark of the Fifth Circuit, in fact, it results in a decision without oral argument in over half of the circuit's cases.[37]

*Three-Judge Panels.*   Those cases given the full treatment are normally considered by panels of three judges rather than by all the judges in the circuit. This means that several cases can be heard at the same time by different three-judge panels, often sitting in different cities throughout the circuit.

As one might guess, there has been some past criticism of panel assignments, especially those made by a chief judge. An excellent example is offered by the Fifth Circuit in the early 1960s. Judge Ben F. Cameron claimed that Chief Judge Elbert F. Tuttle stacked the panels hearing civil rights cases so that they would be decided favorably to black claimants.[38]

Today panel assignments are typically made by the circuit executive or someone else and then a clerk assigns cases blindly to the panels. In the Eleventh Circuit, for example, a committee of judges that does not include the chief judge uses a computer-generated random matrix to set the composition of every panel a year in advance.[39] Since all the circuits now contain more than three judges, the panels change frequently so that the same three judges do not sit together permanently. Regardless of the method used to determine panel assignments, one fact remains clear: a decision reached by a majority of a three-judge panel does not necessarily reflect the views of a majority of the judges in the circuit.

*En Banc Proceedings.*    Occasionally, different three-judge panels within the same circuit may reach conflicting decisions in similar cases. To resolve such conflicts and to promote circuit unanimity, federal statutes provide for an *en banc* procedure, in which all the circuit's judges sit together on a panel and decide a case. The en banc procedure may also be used when the case involves an issue of extraordinary importance, as in the famous *Tinker* decision.[40] That case raised the question of whether high school students wearing black armbands in the classroom to protest the Vietnam War should be protected by the First Amendment. When the Court of Appeals for the Eighth Circuit heard that case in 1967, the en banc procedure was used.

The en banc procedure may be requested by the litigants or by the judges of the court. The circuits themselves have discretion to decide if and how the procedure will be used. Clearly, its use is the exception rather than the rule. For example, the Administrative Office of United States Courts reports that of the 18,502 appeals terminated on the merits during the twelve-month period that ended on June 30, 1987, only 99 were handled by en banc panels.[41] Recently, however, it had been argued that appeals court judges placed on the bench by President Reagan are, where they are in the majority, using en banc panels to overturn precedents they do not like. A recent study found that in the last four years the number of en banc decisions increased by 33 percent. By contrast, from 1976 through 1983 the number of en banc hearings grew only 5 percent.[42]

*Oral Argument.*    Cases that have survived the screening process and have not been settled by the litigants are scheduled for oral argument. Attorneys for each side are given a short amount of time (in some cases no more than ten minutes) to discuss the points made in their written briefs and to answer questions from the judges.

*The Decision.*    Following the oral argument the judges may confer briefly and, if they are in agreement, may announce their decision immediately. Otherwise, a decision will be announced only after the judges confer at greater length. Following the conference some decisions will be announced with a brief order or per curiam opinion of the court. A small portion of decisions will be accompanied by a longer, signed opinion and perhaps even dissenting and concurring opinions. Recent years have seen a general decrease in the number of published opinions, although circuits vary in their practices.

## U.S. District Courts

The U.S. district courts represent the basic point of input for the federal judicial system. While some cases are later taken to a court of appeals or perhaps even to the Supreme Court, most federal cases never move beyond the U.S. trial courts. In terms of sheer numbers of cases handled, the district courts are the workhorses of the federal judiciary. As we shall see, however, their importance extends beyond simply disposing of a large number of cases.

### The First District Courts

Congress made the decision to create a national network of federal trial courts when it passed the Judiciary Act of 1789. Section 2 of the act established thirteen district courts by (1) making each of the eleven states then in the union a district, and (2) making the parts of Massachusetts and Virginia that were to become Maine and Kentucky into separate districts. That organizational scheme established the practice, which still exists, of honoring state boundary lines in drawing districts. Thus, from the very beginning "the federal judiciary was state-contained, with the administrative and political structure of the states becoming the organizational structure of the federal courts." [43]

### The First District Judges

Each federal district court was to be presided over by a single judge who resided in the district. As soon as this became known, President Washington began receiving letters from individuals desiring appointment to the various judgeships. Many asked members of Congress or Vice President Adams to recommend them to President Washington. Personal applications were not necessarily successful and were not the only way in which names came to the president's attention. Harry Innes, for example, was not an applicant for the Kentucky judgeship but received it after being recommended by a member of Congress from his state.[44]

Not everyone nominated was willing to serve as a district judge, however, and three of the thirteen whose names were originally submitted to the Senate for confirmation declined the appointment—perhaps because the nominating process "did not permit consultation either with the individuals concerned or representatives of the 'neighborhood' who might know if the office would be accepted." [45] The rejections were somewhat embarrassing, and we are told that Washington resorted to careful preliminary screening of future appointments and relied more heavily on his secretary of state for recommendations.

In our discussion of early Supreme Court nominations we noted that many prospective nominees preferred state level appointments. The same held true for district court appointments. Some declined judgeships in order to pursue other positions. Still others simply held both a district judgeship and a state office simultaneously.[46] Eventually, states began to pass laws prohibiting state officeholders from accepting federal positions.

As new states came into the Union, additional district courts were created. The additions, along with resignations, gave Washington an opportunity to offer judgeships to thirty-three people, twenty-eight of whom accepted. A student of the early courts offers a profile of the twenty-eight judges Washington appointed. Their average age at appointment was forty-six. All but three were born in the United States, and sixteen had received college educations. All were members of the bar, and all but seven had state or local legal experience as judges, prosecutors, or attorneys general.[47] As we shall see in Chapter 8, presidents have continued to appoint lawyers with public service backgrounds to the federal bench.

## Present Organization of the District Courts

The practice of respecting state boundaries in establishing district court jurisdictions began in 1789 and has been periodically reaffirmed by statutes ever since. As the country grew, new district courts were created. Eventually, Congress began to divide some states into more than one district. California, New York, and Texas have the most, with four each. Figure 2-1 shows the number of districts and their boundaries in each state. Other than consistently honoring state lines, the organization of district constituencies appears to follow no rational plan. Size and population vary widely from district to district. Over the years, a court was added for the District of Columbia, and several territories have been served by district courts. There are now U.S. district courts serving the fifty states, the District of Columbia, Guam, Puerto Rico, the Virgin Islands, and the Northern Mariana Islands.

Congress often provides further organizational detail by creating divisions within a district. In doing this, the national legislature precisely lists the counties included in a particular division as well as the cities in which court will be held.

As indicated, the original district courts were each assigned one judge. With the growth in population and litigation, Congress has periodically had to add judges to most of the districts. In 1978, for example, it passed the Omnibus Judgeship Act, which created 177 new federal district judgeships and 35 new court of appeals judgeships—the largest number of judgeships ever created by a single act of Congress. The net effect of the legislation was to increase the number of federal district judges from 398 to 515. Legislation passed in 1984 added 61 new federal district judges, bringing the total to the current 576. Today all districts have more than one judge; the Southern District of New York, which includes Manhattan and the Bronx, currently has 27 judges and is thus the largest. Since each federal district court is normally presided over by a single judge, several trials may be in session at various cities within the district at any given time. The judges fulfill several functions, which we examine next.

### The District Courts as Trial Courts

Congress established the district courts as the trial courts of the federal judicial system and gave them original jurisdiction over virtually all cases. They are the only federal courts in which attorneys examine and cross-examine witnesses. The factual record is thus established at this level; subsequent appeals of the trial court decision will focus on correcting errors rather than on reconstructing the facts. The task of determining the facts in a case often falls to a jury, a group of citizens from the community who serve as impartial arbiters of the facts and apply the law to the facts.

The Constitution guarantees the right to a jury trial in criminal cases in the Sixth Amendment and the same right in civil cases in the Seventh Amendment. The right can be waived, however, in which case the judge becomes the arbiter both of questions of fact and of matters of law. Such trials are referred to as *bench trials*. Two types of juries are associated with federal district courts. The *grand jury* is a group of men and women convened to determine whether there is probable cause to believe that a person has committed the federal crime of which he or she has been accused. Grand jurors meet periodically to hear charges brought by the U.S. attorney. *Petit jurors* are chosen at random from the community to hear evidence and determine whether a defendant in a civil trial has liability, or whether a defendant in a criminal trial is guilty or not guilty. Federal rules call for twelve jurors in criminal cases but permit fewer in civil cases. The federal district courts generally use six-person juries in civil cases.

### Norm Enforcement by the District Courts

Some students of the judiciary make a distinction between norm enforcement and policy making by the courts.[48] Trial courts are viewed as engaging primarily in norm enforcement, while appellate courts are seen as having greater opportunity to make policy.

Norm enforcement is closely tied to the administration of justice, since all nations develop standards considered essential to a just and orderly society. Societal norms are embodied in statutes, administrative regulations, prior court decisions, and community traditions. Criminal statutes, for example, incorporate concepts of acceptable and unacceptable behavior into law. A judge deciding a case involving an alleged violation of that law is basically practicing norm enforcement. Because cases of this type rarely allow the judge to escape the strict restraints of legal and procedural requirements, he or she has little chance to make new law or develop new policy. In civil cases, too, judges are often confined to norm enforcement; opportunities for policy making are infrequent. Rather, such litigation generally involves a private dispute whose outcome is of interest only to the parties in the suit.

## Policy Making by the District Courts

The district courts also play a policy-making role. One leading judicial scholar explains how this function differs from norm enforcement:

> When they make policy, the courts do not exercise more discretion than when they enforce community norms. The difference lies in the intended impact of the decision. Policy decisions are intended to be guideposts for future actions; norm-enforcement decisions are aimed at the particular case at hand.[49]

The discretion that a federal trial judge exercises should not be overlooked, however. As Americans have become more litigation-conscious, disputes that were once resolved informally are now more likely to be decided in a court of law. The courts find themselves increasingly involved in domains once considered private. What does this mean for the federal district courts? According to a recent study, "These new areas of judicial involvement tend to be relatively free of clear, precise appellate court and legislative guidelines; and as a consequence the opportunity for trial court jurists to write on a clean slate, that is, to make policy, is formidable."[50] In other words, when the guidelines are not well established, district judges have a great deal of discretion to set policy. Some district judges, in fact, have gained considerable notoriety because of their policy-making activities. Two good examples are Judge Frank M. Johnson of the Middle District of Alabama (now a judge on the Eleventh Circuit Court of Appeals) and Judge William Wayne Justice of the Eastern District of Texas.

In the early 1970s Judge Johnson sent shockwaves throughout Alabama when he ruled that conditions in one of that state's mental hospitals prevented patients from receiving adequate treatment and thus deprived them of due process guaranteed by the Constitution.[51] Johnson mandated more than fifty specific changes that he felt were necessary to bring the state's mental facilities up to minimum constitutional standards. His guidelines required changes in state budgetary and personnel policies as well. In short, Judge Johnson translated constitutional standards into policies affecting every mental patient in a state facility and, indirectly, every taxpayer in Alabama.

Judge Justice has become familiar to public officials in Texas. It was said that "while he will never win a popularity contest among Texas lawmakers, no one can dispute the fact that his bold and aggressive rulings are changing the face of Texas politics." Justice is perhaps best known in the state for rulings in three particular areas: public education, criminal justice, and legislative redistricting. For example, he has ruled that bilingual educational programs must be extended through the twelfth grade. In another case he required the state to provide one-prisoner cells or at least sixty square feet of space for each inmate.[52] Like Johnson's rulings in Alabama, Justice's decisions in Texas have had an impact upon the state budget and, ultimately, on all taxpayers.

Texas legislators have not been reluctant to express their dissatisfaction with Judge Justice's policy-making activities. For example, following a court-ordered reform of the state's juvenile justice system in 1977, the Texas House of Representatives retaliated by amending an appropriations bill to require construction of a new juvenile halfway house next door to Justice's home in Tyler.[53]

## Three-Judge District Courts

In 1903, Congress passed legislation providing for the use of special three-judge district courts in certain types of cases. Such courts are created on an ad hoc basis, with the panels being disbanded when a case has been decided. Each panel must include at least one judge from the federal district court and at least one judge from the court of appeals. Normally, two district judges and one appellate judge comprise the panel. Appeals of decisions of three-judge district courts go directly to the Supreme Court.

The earliest types of cases to be heard by three-judge district courts involved suits filed by the attorney general under the Sherman Antitrust Act or the Interstate Commerce Act. Congress later provided that these special courts could decide suits brought by private citizens challenging the constitutionality of state or federal statutes and seeking injunctions to prevent enforcement of the challenged statutes.

An example of the use of a three-judge district court is provided by the abortion case of *Roe v. Wade*.[54] Jane Roe (a pseudonym), a single, pregnant woman, challenged the constitutionality of the Texas antiabortion statute and sought an injunction to prohibit further enforcement of the law. The case was initially heard by a three-judge court consisting of district judges Sarah T. Hughes and W. N. Taylor and Fifth Circuit Court of Appeals judge Irving L. Goldberg. The three-judge district court held the Texas abortion statute invalid but declined to issue an injunction against its enforcement on the ground that a federal intrusion into the state's affairs was not warranted. Roe then appealed the denial of the injunction directly to the Supreme Court.

Over the years congressional statutes, such as the Civil Rights Act of 1964, the Voting Rights Act of 1965, and the Presidential Election Campaign Fund Act of 1974, have specified the use of three-judge district courts. However, increases in the number of cases decided by such courts led to complaints about caseload problems, since appeals from the three-judge panels go directly to the Supreme Court. To relieve some of the caseload pressure, Congress passed legislation in 1976 restricting the use of three-judge district courts.

## Constitutional Courts and Legislative Courts

The Judiciary Act of 1789 established the three levels of the federal court system in existence today. Periodically, however, Congress has exercised its power, based on Article III and Article I of the Constitution, to create other federal courts. Courts established under Article III are known as *constitutional courts,* and those created under Article I are called *legislative courts.* The former handle the bulk of litigation in our system and, for this reason, will remain our focus. The Supreme Court, courts of appeals, and federal district courts are, of course, constitutional courts. The U.S. Court of Military Appeals is one example of a legislative court. It was created in 1950 under authority found in Article I, Section 8 of the Constitution, "To constitute Tribunals inferior to the supreme Court," and "To make Rules for the Government and Regulation of the land and naval Forces." Another important legislative court currently in existence is the United States Tax Court (formerly an administrative agency called the Tax Court of the United States until its name was changed by a 1969 statute).

The newest Article I court is the Court of Veterans Appeals, which was established by legislation signed by President Reagan on November 18, 1988. This court has exclusive jurisdiction to review decisions of the Board of Veterans Appeals. Judges on this newest court will serve fifteen-year terms of office. The two types of courts may be further distinguished by their functions. Legislative courts, unlike their constitutional counterparts, often possess administrative and quasi-legislative as well as judicial duties. Another difference is that legislative courts are often created for the express purpose of helping to administer a specific congressional statute. Constitutional courts, on the other hand, are tribunals established to handle litigation.

Finally, the constitutional and legislative courts vary in their degree of independence from the other two branches of government. Article III (constitutional court) judges serve during a period of good behavior, or what amounts to life tenure. Since Article I (legislative court) judges have no constitutional guarantee to "good behavior" tenure, Congress may set specific terms of office for them. Judges of Article III courts are also constitutionally protected against salary reductions while in office. Those who serve as judges of legislative courts have no such protection. In sum, the constitutional courts have a greater degree of independence from the other two branches of government than the legislative courts. How important is such independence? Recent events surrounding the fate of federal bankruptcy courts reveal independence to be a major consideration.

On November 6, 1978, President Jimmy Carter signed into law the Bankruptcy Reform Act. That legislation (1) required that bankruptcy cases be filed in bankruptcy courts rather than in district courts; (2) extended the terms of current bankruptcy judges through March 1984; (3) provided that after March 3, 1984, bankruptcy judges were to be appointed by the president, with Senate confirmation, for fourteen-year terms; (4) simplified existing bankruptcy law; and (5) expanded the jurisdiction of bankruptcy judges. A system of bankruptcy courts was seemingly in place.

Trouble began, however, less than three years later. In a brief order issued on April 23, 1981, and a supplemental memorandum issued on July 24, 1981, U.S. District Judge Miles W. Lord of Minnesota held that the Bankruptcy Reform Act's delegation of Article III authority to bankruptcy judges was unconstitutional.[55] Judge Lord argued that Congress had exceeded its constitutional power when it authorized bankruptcy judges to exercise the jurisdiction and duties of district judges without at the same time vesting them with the tenure and salary protections given Article III judges. The independence question was at the heart of Judge Lord's decision.

The case was appealed to the Supreme Court, which, in a June 1982 decision, agreed that portions of the Bankruptcy Reform Act were unconstitutional. The Court held that certain powers granted by the act to bankruptcy judges could be exercised only by Article III judges, who are insulated from political pressures by life tenure and protection from pay cuts.[56] The Supreme Court asked Congress to pass remedial legislation aimed at handling the bankruptcy problem. After several failures on Congress's part, the federal district courts put into operation a contingency plan recommended by the Judicial Conference of the United States in September 1982.[57] Among other things, the Judicial Conference's emergency rule removed contested matters from bankruptcy judges to district court judges.

After several unsuccessful attempts Congress passed a law in July 1984 to correct the problem. The new legislation provided for the creation of bankruptcy courts as units of the district courts. Bankruptcy judges are now appointed for fourteen-year terms by the court of appeals for the circuit in which the district is located. Most bankruptcy cases can be handled entirely by the bankruptcy judge. However, in certain types of cases, such as those involving personal injury or wrongful death, the bankruptcy judge may only submit proposed findings of act and the district judge then enters the final order or judgment.

## The Federal Courts in the American Political System

The role of the federal courts in the American political system generally, and in the policy-making process specifically, has long been debated by students of the judiciary. There is widespread agreement that all three levels of federal courts engage in policy making to some extent. How the courts handle this function has been subject to a good deal of controversy, however.

In a 1957 article focusing on the Supreme Court's power of judicial review, political scientist Robert A. Dahl concluded that "the policy views dominant on the Court are never for long out of line with the policy views dominant among the lawmaking majorities of the United States." In other words, according to Dahl the Supreme Court justices generally hold policy views that are similar to those espoused by a majority of the Congress. Obviously, the Court does not always agree completely with the policies developed by Congress. He argued, however, that the Supreme Court's weaker position in relation to Congress and the president means that "it would be most unrealistic to suppose that the Court would, for more than a few years at most, stand against any major alternatives sought by a lawmaking majority." Only during a period of political upheaval or transition from one electoral coalition to another might we expect to find the Court in a position to block a particular policy. In short, this approach sees the Court not so much a protector of fundamental minority rights as a legitimator of the policies of the majority.[58]

This view of the Supreme Court and its role in the American political system has been widely debated by judicial scholars.[59] A 1973 study by David Adamany, for example, focused on the historical periods of party realignment and found that there was intense conflict between the High Court and the lawmaking majority after each realigning election. Perhaps even more important is Adamany's conclusion that the historical evidence simply does not support the earlier assertion that the Supreme Court serves to legitimize the policies of the new coalition.[60] Two years later, however, political scientist Richard Funston, also analyzing Supreme Court activity during periods of electoral realignment, concluded that earlier studies "have been correct in emphasizing the Court's function as a legitimating agency." [61]

Jonathan D. Casper entered the debate by pointing out two serious limitations of Dahl's 1957 study: (1) that its time frame did not include the entire Warren Court period and (2) that it did not include judicial review over actions of the states. Extending the analysis to cover the 1958-1974 period and including state cases presented a different picture of the Supreme Court's policy-making role. Casper noted several areas in which the Court was influential in developing policy; he pointed out that "the Court can and does get its way a good deal more frequently than [the 1957] analysis implies." [62]

The debate over the Supreme Court's role in the American political system has been a lively one. Depending upon the scope of the study and the particular method of analysis, scholars have reached different conclusions. Whatever their conclusions, however, there can be no doubt that the Supreme Court is involved in the policy-making process. The following statement aptly summarizes current thinking in the debate: "The Court may be a legitmator . . . but it is also a significant wielder of power." [63]

The lower federal courts, as we have noted, also operate within the context of the larger political system and thus are participants in the policy-making process. Not only has increasing litigation opened up new areas of district court decision making but, like the appeals courts, the bottom rung of the federal judiciary is the tribunal of last resort in the vast majority of cases it hears. In the late 1960s, for example, one judicial scholar stated:

> Trial Judges, because of the multitude of cases they hear which remain unheard or unchanged by appellate courts, as well as because of their fact- and issue-shaping powers, appear to play an independent and formidable part in the policy impact of the federal court system upon the larger political system. [64]

Although the district courts have been active policy makers in several issue areas, perhaps the civil rights arena stands out above all others. Following the Supreme Court's school desegregation decision in 1954, federal district judges, especially in the South, were faced with the problem of applying to local communities the general ruling that racially defined dual school systems were in violation of the Constitution. It has been pointed out, too, that the district judges have a good deal of discretion in developing desegregation policies to fit specific local needs. [65] As the judges develop policy in this area, they often make decisions that are not only unpopular but go against the tide of prevailing local opinion, as these extreme examples indicate:

[Some] Southern judges suffered ... social indignities after decisions favorable to civil rights, among them Judge Skelly Wright of the Louisiana eastern district and Judge Frank Johnson of the middle district of Alabama. Graves of their relatives were desecrated, crosses burned on home lawns, dynamite blasts set off near relatives' homes, and professional ostracism was inflicted by local bar groups.[66]

While incurring various atrocities, a federal district judge may at the same time invite further litigation and thus increase his or her opportunities as a policy maker:

Judge Skelly Wright's record in favor of civil liberties cases, particularly race relations cases, undoubtedly encouraged litigation in his court. Litigants unable to secure favorable decisions elsewhere in Louisiana regarded the federal district court in New Orleans as a haven to which they might turn for favorable judgments on civil liberties problems.

As evidence that Judge Wright did indeed have ample opportunity to be involved in the policy-making process, the study noted that in the 1956-1961 period he handled nearly twice as many labor and civil liberties cases as any other judge in the Fifth Circuit.[67]

Examinations of civil rights policy making by lower federal judges have indicated that a surprisingly large number of liberal decisions have come from judges sitting in southern cities.[68] Although noting that their civil rights and liberties category is broader than the ones used in the 1960s, the authors of a more recent analysis say that:

southern cities are well represented among the most liberal metropolitan areas. Four of the six most liberal cities are clearly from the Deep South: New Orleans, Houston, Atlanta, and Miami. None of the cities in the least liberal civil rights and liberties category is a traditional southern community.[69]

## State Court Systems

Earlier in this chapter we noted that state courts were already in existence when the Judiciary Act of 1789 created the federal court system. With the passage of that Act a dual court system was established in the United States: one system of courts for the states and one for the federal government.

As colonists moved from England to settle in this country they naturally brought with them the various customs and traditions with which they were familiar. For this reason, American law borrowed heavily from English common law. Likewise, common law traditions became important factors in shaping the state court systems. Ohio and Pennsylvania, for example, still call their major trial courts the court of common pleas, a title whose origin may be traced to England. Some traditions die hard; nonetheless, state courts have undergone major changes over the years.

## The Colonial Period

During the colonial period political power was concentrated in the hands of the governor, who was appointed by the King of England. Since the governors performed executive, legislative, and judicial functions, there was no need for an elaborate court system. Thus, the courts of this period were rather simple institutions which borrowed their form from the English judiciary. However, the colonists greatly simplified the English procedures to suit their own needs.

The lowest level of the colonial judiciary consisted of local judges called justices of the peace or magistrates. They were appointed by the colony's governor. At the next level in the system were the county courts, the general trial courts for the colonies. These courts "were at the heart of colonial government." [70] In addition to deciding cases, they also performed some administrative functions. Appeals from all courts were taken to the highest level—the governor and his council. Grand and petit juries were also introduced during this period and remain prominent features of the state judicial systems.

By the early eighteenth century the legal profession had begun to change. Lawyers trained in the English Inns of Court became more numerous, and as a consequence, colonial court procedures were slowly replaced by more sophisticated English common law. In addition, common commercial needs and a common language helped to make colonial and English legal practices more similar. As one judicial scholar notes, "In a relatively short time—between 1760 and 1820—a rather backward colonial legal framework was transformed into a very English common law system." [71]

## Early State Courts

Following the Revolution, the powers of the government were not only taken over by legislative bodies, but also greatly reduced. The former colonists were not eager to see the development of a large, independent judiciary since many of them harbored a distrust of lawyers and the common law. The state legislatures carefully watched the courts and in some instances removed judges or abolished specific courts because of unpopular decisions. However, the basic structure of the state judiciaries was not greatly altered.

Increasingly, a distrust of the judiciary developed as courts declared legislative actions unconstitutional. Conflicts between legislatures and judges, often stemming from opposing interests, became more prominent. Legislators seemed more responsive to policies that favored debtors while courts generally reflected the views of creditors. These differences were important, however, because "out of this conflict over legislative and judicial power . . . the courts gradually emerged as an independent political institution." [72]

## Modern State Courts

Moving beyond the Civil War and into the early twentieth century we find the state courts beset by still other problems. Increasing industrialization and the rapid growth of urban areas created new types of legal disputes and resulted in longer and more complex court cases. The state court systems, largely fashioned to handle the problems of a rural, agrarian society, were now faced with a crisis of backlogs as they struggled to adjust.

One typical response was to create new courts to handle the increased volume of cases. Often, courts were simply piled on top of each other. Another strategy involved the addition of new courts coupled with a careful specification of their jurisdiction in terms of a specific geographic area. Still another response was to create specialized courts to handle one particular type of case. Small claims courts, juvenile courts, and domestic relations courts, for example, became increasingly prominent.

The result of all this activity was a confusing array of courts, especially in the major urban areas. Additional problems were created as well. One observer notes that:

> each court was a separate entity; each had a judge and a staff. Such an organizational structure meant there was no way to shift cases from an overloaded court to one with little to do. In addition, each court produced political patronage jobs for the city political machines.[73]

Chicago provides an appropriate example of such problems. By the early 1930s there were over 550 independent courts in the city, primarily justice of the peace courts which handled minor cases.[74]

The largely unplanned expansion of state and local courts to meet specific needs led to a situation many have referred to as fragmentation. A multiplicity of trial courts was only one aspect of fragmentation, however. Many of these courts had very narrow jurisdiction. Furthermore, the jurisdiction of the various courts often overlapped. This meant that a case could be tried in a number of courts depending on the advantages each one offered. Court costs, court procedures, court delays, and last but certainly not least, the reputation of the judge all entered into the decision. For example, a strict, law-and-order district attorney prosecuting a criminal case might choose a court that had a reputation for handing out stiff sentences. An attorney filing a civil suit in behalf of a client might seek a court known for its complex procedures in order to draw the other side into a confusing web of legal technicalities. Political considerations were also involved in the choice of a court. The justice of the peace courts were especially political since many of them operated on a fee basis.

Justices of the peace (J. P.'s) were often willing to trade favorable decisions for court business. In fact, the initials J. P. were often said to stand for "Justice for the Plaintiff." [75]

Beginning early in the twentieth century a number of people have spoken out against the fragmentation in the state court systems. The program of reforms they have offered is generally known as the court unification movement. The first well-known legal scholar to speak out in favor of court unification was Roscoe Pound, dean of the Harvard Law School.[76] Pound and others called for the consolidation of trial courts into a single set of courts or two sets of courts, one to hear major cases and one to hear minor cases.

There has, of course, been a good deal of opposition to court unification. Many trial lawers who are in court almost daily become accustomed to existing court organizations and therefore are opposed to change. Knowledge of the local courts is the key to their success, so they naturally are not eager to try cases in strange new courts.

Also, judges and other personnel associated with the courts are sometimes opposed to reform. Their opposition often grows out of fear—of being transferred to new courts, or of having to learn new procedures, or of having to decide cases outside their area of specialization. Nonlawyer judges, such as justices of the peace, often oppose court reform because they see it threatening their jobs.

The court unification movement, then, has not been as successful as many would like. On the other hand, proponents of court reform have secured victories in some states. With this battle over court unification in mind, we next examine the basic organization of the state courts in a contemporary setting.

## State Court Organization

We should note at the outset that no two states are alike when it comes to the organization of courts. Furthermore, the organization of state courts is not as clear cut as the three-tier system found at the federal level. Some states have moved in the direction of a unified court system while others still operate within a bewildering complex of courts with overlapping jurisdiction. However, the variety of state courts may be placed into four general categories or levels: trial courts of limited jurisdiction, trial courts of general jurisdiction, intermediate appellate courts, and courts of last resort.

### Trial Courts of Limited Jurisdiction

Trial courts of limited jurisdiction handle the bulk of litigation in this country each year and constitute about 90 percent of all courts in the

United States.[77] They go by a variety of names: justice of the peace courts, magistrate courts, municipal courts, city courts, county courts, juvenile courts, domestic relations courts, and metropolitan courts, to name the more common ones.

The jurisdiction of these courts is limited to minor cases. In criminal matters, for example, they handle the lesser offenses such as misdemeanors and traffic violations. They may impose only limited fines (usually no more than $1,000) and jail sentences (generally no more than one year). In civil cases these courts are usually limited to disputes under a certain amount, such as $500. In addition, these types of courts are often limited to certain kinds of matters: traffic violations, domestic relations matters, or cases involving juveniles, for example. Another difference from trial courts of general jurisdiction is that in many instances these limited courts are not courts of record. Since their proceedings are not recorded, appeals of their decisions usually go to a trial court of general jurisdiction for what is known as a *trial de novo* (new trial).

Yet another distinguishing characteristic of trial courts of limited jurisdiction is that the presiding judges of such courts are often not required to have any formal legal training. Many, in fact, are only part-time judges who are sometimes unfamiliar with basic legal concepts.[78]

Many of these courts suffer from a lack of resources. Often, they have no permanent courtroom, meeting instead in grocery stores, restaurants, or private homes. Clerks are frequently not available to keep adequate records. The results are informal proceedings and the processing of cases on a mass basis. Full-fledged trials are rare and cases are disposed of quickly.

Finally, we should note that trial courts of limited jurisdiction are used in some states to handle preliminary matters in felony criminal cases. They often hold arraignments, set bail, appoint attorneys for indigent defendants, and conduct preliminary examinations. The case is then transferred to a trial court of general jurisdiction for such matters as hearing pleas, holding trials, and sentencing.

## Trial Courts of General Jurisdiction

Most states have one set of major trial courts which handles the more serious criminal and civil cases. In addition, in many states special categories, such as juvenile criminal offenses, domestic relations cases, and probate cases are under the jurisdiction of the general trial courts.

In the majority of states these courts also have an appellate function. They hear appeals in certain types of cases that originate in trial courts of limited jurisdiction. As we noted above, these appeals are often de novo, or tried again in the court of general jurisdiction.

General trial courts are usually divided into judicial districts or circuits.

Although the practice varies by state, the general rule is to use existing political boundaries such as a county or a group of counties in establishing the district or circuit. In rural areas the judge may literally ride circuit and hold court in different parts of the territory according to a fixed schedule. In urban areas, on the other hand, judges hold court in a prescribed place throughout the year. In larger counties the judges may be divided into specializations. Some may hear only civil cases while others try criminal cases exclusively.

The courts at this level go by a variety of names. The most common are district, circuit, and superior. As we noted earlier, Ohio and Pennsylvania still cling to the title court of common pleas. New York is undoubtedly the most confusing of all: it calls its trial court of general jurisdiction the supreme court.

The judges at this level are required by law in all states to have law degrees. These courts also maintain clerical help because they are courts of record. In other words, there is a degree of professionalism at this level that is often lacking in the trial courts of limited jurisdiction.

## Intermediate Appellate Courts

The intermediate appellate courts are relative newcomers to the state judicial scene. Only thirteen such courts existed in 1911, whereas thirty-six states had created them by 1986.[79] Their basic purpose is to relieve the workload of the state's highest court.

In most instances these courts are called courts of appeals, although other names are occasionally used. Most states have one court of appeals with statewide jurisdiction. Other states, such as Ohio and Texas, have created regional appellate courts to hear appeals from trial courts in a specific area. Alabama and Tennessee have separate intermediate appellate courts for civil and criminal cases.

The size of these intermediate appellate courts varies widely. The court of appeals in Alaska, for example, has only three judges. At the other extreme we find eighty courts of appeals judges in Texas.[80] In some states the intermediate appeals courts sit en banc, while in other states they sit in permanent or rotating panels.

Generally speaking, the jurisdiction of intermediate appellate courts is mandatory since Americans hold to the view that parties in a case are entitled to at least one appeal. In numerous instances, then, these are the courts of last resort for litigants in the state court system.

## Courts of Last Resort

Every state has a court of last resort. In fact, the states of Oklahoma and Texas have two highest courts. Both states have a supreme court with jurisdiction limited to appeals in civil cases and a court of criminal appeals for criminal cases. Most states call their highest courts supreme courts; other designations are the court of appeals (Maryland and New York), the supreme judicial court (Maine and Massachusetts), and the supreme court of appeals (West Virginia).

The courts of last resort range in size from three to nine judges (or justices in some states). They typically sit en banc and usually, although not necessarily, in the state capital.

The highest courts have jurisdiction in matters pertaining to state law and are, of course, the final arbiters in such matters. In states that have intermediate appellate courts, the supreme court's cases come primarily from these mid-level courts. The supreme court typically is allowed to exercise discretion in deciding which cases to review. Where there is no intermediate court of appeals, cases generally go to the state's highest court on a mandatory basis.

In most instances, then, the state courts of last resort resemble the U.S. Supreme Court in that they have a good deal of discretion in determining which cases will occupy their attention. Most state supreme courts also follow procedures similar to the U.S. Supreme Court. That is, when a case is accepted for review the opposing parties file written briefs and later present oral arguments. Then, upon reaching a decision, the judges issue written opinions explaining the court's decision.

## Summary

This chapter offers a brief historical review of the development of the federal and state judiciaries. Since preconstitutional times there has been a perennial concern for independent court systems.

At the federal level, our focus was on the three basic levels created by the Judiciary Act of 1789. We noted, however, that Congress has periodically created both constitutional and legislative courts. Still, the bulk of federal litigation is handled by U.S. district courts, courts of appeals, and the Supreme Court. We also briefly examined the role of the federal courts in the American political system as a whole.

No two state court systems are alike. However, there are four basic levels within each state: trial courts of limited jurisdiction, trial courts of general jurisdiction, intermediate appellate courts, and courts of last resort. Our discussion examined the work of each of these four levels.

## Notes

1. Charles Evans Hughes, *The Supreme Court of the United States* (New York: Columbia University Press, 1966), 1.
2. Ibid., 2.

3. Charles Warren, *The Supreme Court in United States History*, vol. 1 (Boston: Little, Brown, 1924), 4.
4. Fred Rodell, *Nine Men* (New York: Random House, 1955), 47.
5. See Warren, *The Supreme Court in United States History*, vol. 1, 44.
6. John P. Frank, *Marble Palace* (New York: Knopf, 1968), 9.
7. Warren, *The Supreme Court in United States History*, vol. 1, 51.
8. *Chisholm v. Georgia*, 2 Dallas 419 (1793).
9. *Champion and Dickason v. Casey*, U.S. District Court for the District of Rhode Island, June 2, 1792.
10. *Hayburn's Case*, 2 Dallas 409 (1792).
11. Robert J. Steamer, *Chief Justice: Leadership and the Supreme Court* (Columbia: University of South Carolina Press, 1986), 232.
12. Frank, *Marble Palace*, 79.
13. See Sheldon Goldman, *Constitutional Law and Supreme Court Decision-Making* (New York: Harper & Row, 1982), 41.
14. *Marbury v. Madison*, 1 Cranch 137 (1803).
15. See Lawrence Baum, *The Supreme Court*, 2d ed. (Washington, D.C.: CQ Press, 1985), 19.
16. *Gibbons v. Ogden*, 9 Wheaton 1 (1824).
17. *McCulloch v. Maryland*, 4 Wheaton 316 (1819).
18. Goldman, *Constitutional Law and Supreme Court Decision-Making*, 249.
19. See *National Labor Relations Board v. Jones and Laughlin Steel Corp.*, 301 U.S. 1 (1937); *Steward Machine Co. v. Davis*, 301 U.S. 548 (1937); and *West Coast Hotel Co. v. Parrish*, 300 U.S. 379 (1937).
20. *Brown v. Board of Education*, 347 U.S. 483 (1954).
21. See *Gideon v. Wainwright*, 372 U.S. 335 (1963); *Mapp v. Ohio*, 367 U.S. 643 (1961); *Miranda v. Arizona*, 384 U.S. 436 (1966); *Baker v. Carr*, 369 U.S. 186 (1962); and *Engel v. Vitale*, 370 U.S. 421 (1962), respectively.
22. Robert H. Birkby, *The Court and Public Policy* (Washington, D.C.: CQ Press, 1983), 1.
23. *Plessy v. Ferguson*, 163 U.S. 537 (1896).
24. See Baum, *The Supreme Court*, 115.
25. *Stanley v. Georgia*, 394 U.S. 557 (1969).
26. Stephen T. Early, Jr., *Constitutional Courts of the United States* (Totowa, N.J.: Littlefield, Adams, 1977), 100.
27. See Warren, *The Supreme Court in United States History*, vol. 1, 85, 86.
28. Richard J. Richardson and Kenneth N. Vines, *The Politics of Federal Courts* (Boston: Little, Brown, 1970), 27.
29. J. Woodford Howard, Jr., *Courts of Appeals in the Federal Judicial System: A Study of the Second, Fifth, and District of Columbia Circuits* (Princeton, N.J.: Princeton University Press, 1981), 75-76.
30. See *Douglas v. California*, 372 U.S. 353 (1963).
31. See Richard J. Richardson and Kenneth N. Vines, "Review, Dissent and the Appellate Process: A Political Interpretation," *Journal of Politics* 29 (August 1967): 597-616.
32. See Howard, *Courts of Appeals in the Federal Judicial System*, 42.
33. *Office of Communications of the United Church of Christ v. F.C.C.*, 359 F. 2d 994 (D.C. Cir. 1966).
34. *United States v. City of Parma, Ohio*, 661 F. 2d 562 (6th Cir. 1981). Also see the excellent discussion of this case in Phillip J. Cooper, *Hard Judicial Choices* (New York: Oxford University Press, 1988), 47-84.

35. Howard, *Courts of Appeals in the Federal Judicial System,* 79.
36. See Anthony Partridge and Allan Lind, *A Reevaluation of the Civil Appeals Management Plan* (Washington, D.C.: Federal Judicial Center, 1983).
37. See *The Third Branch* 15 (December 1983): 5.
38. See Early, *Constitutional Courts of the United States,* 112-113, for the specifics of Judge Cameron's charges.
39. See *The Third Branch* 15 (July 1983): 5.
40. *Tinker v. Des Moines Independent Community School District,* 393 U.S. 503 (1969).
41. See *Annual Report of the Administrative Office of the United States Courts* (Washington, D.C.: Government Printing Office, 1987), 106.
42. Stephen Wermeil, "Full-Court Review of Panel Rulings Becomes Tool Often Used by Reagan Judges Aiming to Mold Law," *Wall Street Journal,* March 22, 1988, 60.
43. Richardson and Vines, *The Politics of Federal Courts,* 21.
44. See Dwight F. Henderson, *Courts for a New Nation* (Washington, D.C.: Public Affairs Press, 1971), 27.
45. Ibid., 28.
46. Ibid., 29-30.
47. Ibid., 30-31.
48. See Herbert Jacob, *Justice in America,* 4th ed. (Boston: Little, Brown 1984), chap. 2.
49. Ibid., 37.
50. Robert A. Carp and C. K. Rowland, *Policymaking and Politics in the Federal District Courts* (Knoxville: University of Tennessee Press, 1983), 3.
51. See *Wyatt v. Stickney,* 325 F. Supp. 781 (1971) and 344 F. Supp. 373 (1972).
52. *Texas Government Newsletter,* April 27, 1981, 2.
53. Ibid. The amendment was later removed by the Texas Senate.
54. The decision of the three-judge district court may be found in *Roe v. Wade,* 314 F. Supp. 1217 (1970) and the Supreme Court decision in *Roe v. Wade,* 410 U.S. 113 (1973).
55. See *Northern Pipeline Construction Co. v. Marathon Pipe Line Company,* 6 B.R. 928 (1981) and 12 B.R. 946 (1981).
56. *Northern Pipeline Construction Co. v. Marathon Pipe Line Company,* 458 U.S. 50 (1982).
57. See *The Third Branch* 15 (January 1983): 1 and 8, for a chronology of events in this matter.
58. Robert A. Dahl, "Decision-Making in a Democracy: The Supreme Court as a National Policy-Maker," *Journal of Public Law* 6 (Fall 1957): 285, 294.
59. See, for example, David Adamany, "Legitimacy, Realigning Elections, and the Supreme Court," *Wisconsin Law Review* (September 1973): 790-846; Richard Funston, "The Supreme Court and Critical Elections," *American Political Science Review* 69 (September 1975): 795-811; Bradley C. Canon and S. Sidney Ulmer, "The Supreme Court and Critical Elections: A Dissent," *American Political Science Review* 70 (December 1976): 1215-1218; Jonathan D. Casper, "The Supreme Court and National Policy Making," *American Political Science Review* 70 (March 1976): 50-63; and Roger Handberg and Harold F. Hill, Jr., "Court Curbing, Court Reversals, and Judicial Review: The Supreme Court versus Congress," *Law and Society Review* 14 (Winter 1980): 309-322.
60. See Adamany, "Legitimacy, Realigning Elections, and the Supreme Court."

61. Funston, "The Supreme Court and Critical Elections," 808-809. It should be noted that the Funston study was criticized, primarily on methodological grounds, in Canon and Ulmer, "The Supreme Court and Critical Elections."

62. See Casper, "The Supreme Court and National Policy Making," 59.

63. Handberg and Hill, "Court Curbing, Court Reversals, and Judicial Review," 321.

64. Kenneth M. Dolbeare, "The Federal District Courts and Urban Public Policy: An Exploratory Study (1960-1967)," in *Frontiers of Judicial Research*, ed. Joel B. Grossman and Joseph Tanenhaus (New York: Wiley, 1969), 395.

65. See, for example, Jack W. Peltason, *Fifty-Eight Lonely Men* (New York: Harcourt, Brace & World, 1961), and Michael W. Giles and Thomas G. Walker, "Judicial Policy-Making and Southern School Segregation," *Journal of Politics* 37 (May 1975): 917-936.

66. Richardson and Vines, *The Politics of Federal Courts*, 98-99.

67. Ibid., 101.

68. See Richardson and Vines, *The Politics of Federal Courts*. Also see Dolbeare, "The Federal District Courts and Urban Public Policy"; Kenneth N. Vines,. "Federal District Judges and Race Relations Cases in the South," *Journal of Politics* 26 (May 1964): 337-357; and Kenneth N. Vines, "The Role of Circuit Courts of Appeals in the Federal Judicial Process: A Case Study," *Midwest Journal of Political Science* 7 (November 1963): 305-319.

69. Carp and Rowland, *Policymaking and Politics in the Federal District Courts*, 141.

70. Lawrence M. Friedman, *A History of American Law*, 2d ed. (New York: Simon & Schuster, 1985), 43.

71. Harry P. Stumpf, *American Judicial Politics* (San Diego: Harcourt Brace Jovanovich, 1988), 73.

72. David W. Neubauer, *America's Courts and the Criminal Justice System*, 2d ed. (Monterey, Calif.: Brooks/Cole, 1984), 37.

73. Ibid., 38.

74. See Albert Lepawsky, *The Judicial System of Metropolitan Chicago* (Chicago: University of Chicago Press, 1932), 19-23.

75. Henry J. Abraham, *The Judicial Process*, 3d ed. (New York: Oxford University Press, 1975), 139.

76. See Roscoe Pound, "The Causes of Popular Dissatisfaction with the Administration of Justice," *Journal of the American Judicature Society* 20 (1937): 178-187.

77. Stumpf, *American Judicial Politics*, 75.

78. See Allan Ashman and Pat Chapin, "Is the Bell Tolling for Nonlawyer Judges?" *Judicature* 59 (1976): 417-421.

79. See Council of State Governments, *The Book of the States*, 1986-1987 (Lexington, Ky.: Council of State Governments), 157-158.

80. Ibid.

# 3    Administrative and Staff Support in the Judiciary

The previous chapter discussed the function and organization of the courts. A closely related topic is judicial administration, or the concern for day-to-day operation of the courts, which includes a wide range of activities—some would say anything having to do with the judicial process. At the least, judicial administration involves "two broad areas: the management of court organization and personnel and the processing of litigation." [1] Because those charged with managing the courts and overseeing the flow of litigation are obviously interested in improving the methods by which their tasks may be accomplished, reform has historically been closely associated with court management.

In this chapter we focus on the daily operation of federal and state courts, a task that requires a myriad of personnel. Although judges are the most visible actors in the judicial system, a large supporting cast is also at work. Their efforts help free judges to perform their most important job—to decide cases. Some members of the support team, such as law clerks, may work specifically for one judge. Others—for example, U.S. magistrates—are assigned to a particular court. Still others may be employees of an agency, such as the Administrative Office of the United States Courts, that serves the entire judicial system. The chapter will look at the judicial reform movement first and then examine the administrative and policy-making agencies of the court system. It will conclude with a discussion of major judicial support staffs.

## The Judicial Administration Movement

To understand the problems associated with the development of an effective administrative system for the courts we must consider the nature of the judicial system. Historically, the judiciary has been characterized by three important characteristics: independence, decentralization, and individualism. [2]

Independence of judges is apparent both in the state courts and at the federal level, where the judiciary is established as one of the three separate branches of government. It is perhaps more readily apparent at the federal level, where judges of the constitutional courts serve during a period of good behavior (in reality, life tenure) and cannot have their salaries reduced while they hold office. However, it is also encouraged in the state courts, regardless of whether judges are popularly elected or chosen by a merit plan (discussed more fully in Chapter 8). In states that use a merit plan the judges periodically run on their records, not against an opponent, while judges in states that use an elective system have historically encountered little or no opposition. Furthermore, many states provide for the appointment of judges to fill vacancies or newly created positions. These judges then run for reelection, often unopposed, at the next general election. In short, although state judicial elections give the appearance of being competitive, they traditionally have not been. These factors have helped promote the administrative autonomy of individual judges.

Decentralization has also been the rule in both the federal and state court systems. The Judiciary Act of 1789 created a three-tier federal court system, and the two lower levels were set up in a manner that instilled a high degree of decentralization. The geographic jurisdiction of the three original circuit courts coincided with the boundaries of several states, while the district courts consisted of two members of the Supreme Court and one district judge residing within the circuit. The district judge assumed the major responsibility for developing the agenda of these courts. Further, the role of the Senate in the appointment process has meant that lower federal court judges are likely to be recruited from the area in which they will eventually serve. Once on the bench they may continue to be influenced to some extent by local customs and traditions.[3]

Both the elective and the merit systems for choosing state judges also contribute to decentralization. In both methods the judges of the lower courts are generally recruited from the region of the state in which they will eventually serve. Furthermore, senatorial courtesy (the tradition that permits senators to veto the appointments of residents of their districts) may also be a factor, since governors often are compelled to consult with state senators of the region before filling judicial vacancies.

Independence and decentralization both contribute to individualism among judges. As noted above, judges simply do not face the political and electoral pressures that often confront legislators and executives. As a result, judges often are freer than legislators and executives to express their individual views. The geographic separation of the courts also promotes autonomy.

Thus, the nature of the judiciary itself was the primary obstacle to the formation of an administrative system in the nineteenth century. However, events taking place outside the courtroom provided the chief impetus for reform in the twentieth century.

## The Move Toward Reform

Throughout the 1800s the judicial heritage of independence, decentralization, and individualism reigned supreme. By the end of the nineteenth century, however, America had changed. Industrialization helped transform the United States from a small, rural society to a large, urban, technologically complex one. The changes created new legal relationships: between landlords and tenants, merchants and consumers, and employers and workers. The uncertainties over these new legal relationships more and more frequently found their way into court in the form of lawsuits. Attorneys and judges were often forced to become specialists in specific subject areas. Thus, social and economic development in the early twentieth century "helped produce a greater sense of professionalism and heightened specialization within the legal community." [4]

The early 1900s also saw a major reform effort known as the Progressive movement, which addressed a variety of societal problems brought about by urbanization and industrialization. Judicial reform was one aspect of the Progressive movement and "attention to judicial administration throughout this century has been influenced heavily by this early Progressive legacy." [5]

The Progressive movement attracted many famous Americans. Among them were Roscoe Pound, a leading advocate of judicial reform and dean of the Harvard Law School; William Howard Taft, a former U.S. president who became chief justice of the U.S. Supreme Court in 1921; and Arthur T. Vanderbilt, a president of the American Bar Association and later chief justice of the New Jersey Supreme Court.

Pound, recognized as one of the founders of the judicial administration movement, was critical of court organization and procedures for handling civil cases. Cumbersome procedures and defective judicial administration were only part of the problem, however. A growing number of federal regulations created new litigation for the already congested federal courts. As a result, case backlogs developed and judicial reformers became increasingly alarmed at what they called "delayed justice." Reformers such as Pound and Taft stepped up their demands for efficiency, integration, unification, and coordination in the federal judicial system. These "slogans of the judicial-reform movement . . . were part of a broader campaign for the adoption of 'businesslike' methods in government." [6] More specifically, judicial reformers have focused on two major objectives: changes in the organization of courts and the development of auxiliary agencies within the judicial branch.

Taft worked tirelessly for these objectives. He was successful in obtaining congressional creation of an auxiliary agency: the Conference of Senior Circuit Judges (later to become the Judicial Conference of the United

States). Taft was also instrumental in the passage of the Judiciary Act of 1925, which established the basic scheme of appellate review under which our federal courts now operate.

While serving as president of the American Bar Association during the 1930s, Vanderbilt emphasized the need to reform the state judiciaries. To further this goal he appointed John J. Parker to chair a new American Bar Association section on judicial administration. The section, composed of seven committees, was to establish standards that would ultimately be adopted by state and local bar associations. Later, as chief justice of the New Jersey Supreme Court, Vanderbilt continued his efforts at judicial reform. In fact, he was able to implement many of his ideas; as a result, New Jersey became the first state to completely revamp its judiciary to bring its courts into line with the reform mood of the time.

Perhaps following the precedent established by Taft, more recent chief justices have also accepted a responsibility to help meet the administrative needs of the federal courts. Earl Warren, for example, was involved in the creation of the Federal Judicial Center in 1967. Prior to his retirement, Warren said that the "most important job of the courts today is not to decide what the substantive law is, but to work out ways to move the cases along and relieve court congestion." [7] Former chief justice Warren Burger, had a keen interest in judicial administration, frequently addressing both the legal profession and the general public on a wide variety of topics such as court congestion, the creation of new courts, legal training, and prison reform. Given these developments, it is understandable that one judicial scholar would say, "The most important change in the judicial branch of the federal government during the past half century has been the creation of a number of administrative structures linked to, but not part of, the federal courts." [8]

As noted above, 1967 was an important year for the federal court system because it marked the creation of the Federal Judicial Center. With the release of the president's task force report on the courts it also became an important year for the state courts. The report offered numerous recommendations for improving the state judicial systems.[9] The task force advocated adoption of single, unified state court systems. Also recommended were centralized administrative responsibility and the use of experts to handle business management. Finally, the report suggested efficient clerical and administrative management techniques to ensure the proper functioning of criminal courts. One student of judicial reform says, "It was this report, perhaps more than any other, that served as the impetus for states to revise and reform what can only be termed as extremely outdated and archaic judicial systems." [10]

## Major Administrative Support Structures

### Judicial Conference of the United States

The central administrative policy-making organization of the federal judicial system is the Judicial Conference of the United States. The conference—composed of the chief justice of the Supreme Court as the presiding member, the chief judges of each of the judicial circuits, one district judge from each of the twelve regional circuits, and the chief judge of the court of international trade—meets semiannually for two-day sessions. A variety of topics are dealt with, such as establishing policy on the temporary assignment of judges within circuits, recommending new judgeships, increasing judicial salaries, and developing budgets for court operations. Recommendations generally take the form of proposed legislation that is approved by the Supreme Court and then transmitted to Congress for ultimate approval. The conference's "most important function is the promulgation and revision of the various rules of federal civil and criminal procedure." [11] A number of judges, law professors, and lawyers are given the opportunity to offer input in the development of these rules. For example, the Advisory Committee on Criminal Rules of Practice and Procedure of the Judicial Conference of the United States announced in the January 1988 issue of *The Third Branch* that it planned to revise rule 32 of the Federal Rules of Criminal Procedure due to new sentencing guidelines (discussed in Chapter 5); the committee solicited written comments in advance of its May meeting. [12] In some instances public hearings are held to allow interested persons to state their views about federal rules of procedure. Concerning these public hearings, one law professor has stated, "Sometimes they provide very valuable insights, insights as to whether a given rule is effectively drafted, or has caused confusion, or needs some brushing up." [13]

Quite obviously, a group of judges meeting twice a year for two days cannot hope to accomplish a great deal. Therefore, a network of about twenty-five committees has been established to perform the substantive work of the conference. In addition to the Committee on Rules of Practice and Procedure mentioned above, groups such as the Judicial Conference Committee on the Budget and the Judicial Conference Committee on Court Administration meet for several days throughout the year. Working on its particular specialty, each committee submits a report on its findings or recommendations to the full conference.

The chief justice appoints the members of each committee from among judges and lawyers throughout the twelve circuits. In spite of the long hours and unpaid labor involved, positions on the committees are coveted.

A committee appointment is seen as a status symbol through which judges gain esteem among their peers.[14]

Thus judges themselves play the major role in developing policy for the federal judiciary. Because the Judicial Conference of the United States involves district and circuit judges in the process of national judicial administration, the system has not moved significantly toward the type of centralized administration favored by many judicial reformers.

## Administrative Office of the U.S. Courts

The administration of the federal judicial system as a whole is managed by the Administrative Office of the U.S. Courts, an agency established by Congress in 1939 as a consequence of President Franklin D. Roosevelt's attacks upon the Supreme Court two years earlier. The federal courts generally lost prestige and political support during the great depression of the 1930s. The problem was aggravated by the fact that the conservative Supreme Court declared unconstitutional much of Roosevelt's New Deal legislation. Following his reelection in 1936, Roosevelt put forth his famous plan to "pack" the Court with additional justices who, presumably, would rule in favor of congressional legislation. He also accused the High Court of administrative inefficiency, a criticism that carried over to the entire federal judiciary.

As a solution to the problem of administrative inefficiency, FDR proposed new legislation to transfer judicial administration from the Department of Justice (an agency of the executive branch) to the courts themselves. The Roosevelt proposal called for the creation of a national court administrator who would be appointed by the chief justice and would have absolute authority to manage the judicial system.

Given the judiciary's heritage of independence, decentralization, and individualism, it is understandable that most judges objected to the plan for national control of judicial administration. Still, the judges were dissatisfied with the old system of court management and what they perceived as the Justice Department's failure to represent their interests in Congress.[15] A movement developed among federal judges and national court reformers to clean their own house, and a compromise plan for judicial administration was offered. The Administrative Office Act of 1939 was "the judiciary's substitute for the Court bill introduced by President Roosevelt in 1937." The legislation created the Administrative Office as an agency of the Judicial Conference, although its director is appointed by the Supreme Court (more realistically, by the chief justice) and holds office at its pleasure. The Administrative Office's director, who answers to the Judicial Conference, is not at all like the powerful court adminisrator envisioned in the Roosevelt proposal. Neither the director nor the Administrative Office itself serves the function of policy making; that duty still belongs to the Judicial Conference. Instead, the Administrative Office has been described as "the judiciary's housekeeping agency." [16]

The initial organization of the Administrative Office lends some insight into the functions that Congress expected the new agency to fulfill. First, it was expected to carry out the administrative duties then being performed by the Department of Justice. Second, it was expected to collect and report judicial statistics. Consequently, two divisions were created: the Division of Business Administration and the Division of Procedural Studies and Statistics. The former became the business or managerial agency of the federal judiciary, serving a number of staff functions for both the courts and the Judicial Conference. Several sections were established within this division to perform such specialized duties as (1) allotting authorized funds and supervising their expenditure, (2) providing estimates for judicial appropriations, (3) auditing the accounts of court personnel, (4) distributing supplies, (5) negotiating with other government agencies for court accommodations in federal buildings, and (6) maintaining judicial personnel records.

The Division of Procedural Studies and Statistics took on the job of collecting data on cases in federal courts. Initially, the division amassed data only on civil and bankruptcy cases, while the U.S. attorneys gathered data on criminal cases. Beginning in 1941, however, the Administrative Office assumed responsibility for collecting data on criminal cases as well.[17] This division was able to provide "case flow" statistics showing the relationship between the number and types of cases commenced and terminated. It also began to keep records on such matters as length of trials, causes of delay, selection and use of jurors, methods and effect of pretrial proceedings, and comparative times spent by judges in disposing of cases. These statistics, along with personal inspections, were used to prepare a picture of judicial business conditions in each district.

In the more than forty years of its existence the Administrative Office has revised the initial organization to reflect its expanded duties for the federal judiciary. There has been a considerable increase in the number of divisions. It should also be noted that some restructuring of the two original divisions has taken place.

The Administrative Office also serves a staff function for the Judicial Conference. In addition to providing statistical information to the conference's many committees, it acts as a reception center and clearinghouse for information and proposals directed to the Judicial Conference.

Closely related to the staff function is the Administrative Office's role as liaison for both the federal judicial system and the Judicial Conference. The Administrative Office serves as advocate for the judiciary in its dealings with Congress, the executive branch, individual judges, professional groups, and the general public. Especially important in this regard is the fact that the Administrative Office acts as the Judicial Conference's official representative in Congress and, along with judges, presents the judiciary's budget proposals, requests for additional judgeships, suggestions for changes in court rules, and other key measures. Although the literature indicates that some early supporters of the Administrative Office envisioned it as the nucleus of a lobbying effort, it generally "has not been particularly powerful in obtaining money for the courts or congressional support for court proposals." [18]

One final service once performed by the Administrative Office deserves brief mention. It has, from time to time, arranged seminars and institutes to help orient new judges. This function, however, is now primarily carried out by the Federal Judicial Center.

## The Federal Judicial Center

In 1967 Congress created the Federal Judicial Center as the research and development arm of the federal judiciary. The legislation made it clear that the new agency was not a part of the Administrative Office. Instead, it was established as a distinct institution within the judicial branch of the government. It was vested with an independent status so that it might more effectively, and objectively, carry out its responsibilities. Those duties fall generally into three categories: (1) conducting research on the federal courts, (2) making recommendations to improve the administration and management of the federal courts, and (3) developing educational and training programs for personnel of the judicial branch.

The board of the Federal Judicial Center constitutes an advisory body for the center. It consists of the chief justice of the United States, who serves as permanent chair; the director of the Administrative Office, who also serves as a permanent member; two judges of the U.S. courts of appeals; three judges of the U.S. district courts; and a bankruptcy judge. The judges who serve on the board are elected for four-year terms by the Judicial Conference. The Federal Judicial Center is managed by a director appointed by the board.

The activities of the Federal Judicial Center are wide ranging, as we noted above. Let us consider its research role for a moment. The Research Division is given some responsibility for study of the federal courts. [19] The staff includes sociologists, social psychologists, political scientists, and lawyers. The Research Division resembles a small think tank, with its group of scholars bringing different areas of expertise to the division's work. Recent topics for study have included investigations of court-annexed arbitration, reviews of the psychological literature dealing with a jury's competency to evaluate complex fact situations, evaluations of the various management styles found in metropolitan district courts, and an analysis of the roles of magistrates in the district courts.

In addition to using its own staff, the Federal Judicial Center may negotiate with private firms, law schools, and other government agencies for research on various judicial operations and problems. For example, the Mitre Corporation engaged in a study of court congestion for the center. Specific judges were given cases that differed in complexity; the technique was analyzed with an eye toward determining what effects this practice had on the court's calendar.[20]

The studies conducted by, and for, the Federal Judicial Center are made available to judges and other judicial personnel. Announcements of new publications are made in *The Third Branch*, the bulletin of the federal courts published monthly by the Administrative Office and the Federal Judicial Center. In addition, *The Third Branch* recommends to judicial personnel books and articles from a wide variety of legal and professional journals. The center also publishes an annual catalog of its publications. The objective is to make available to judges and court employees the most current research findings and suggestions for improving the administration and management of the federal courts. In the final analysis, however, the Federal Judicial Center can only suggest and recommend—it has no direct supervisory power.

As we noted, the center plays a role in developing educational and training programs for judicial branch personnel. First, there is a conscious effort to help newly appointed judges by presenting regional orientation seminars for small groups of new district judges. These seminars

> are devoted to the basic sentencing, procedural, and case management tasks the new judges will soon face. A second, week-long orientation seminar attended in the first year of service presents the basic contours of substantive law in major areas of federal litigation, such as antitrust, civil rights, employment discrimination, and securities. Annual regional workshops, very much in the tradition of continuing legal education and shaped by the participants' expressed interests, deal mainly with updates on judicial and statutory changes in the law.[21]

How helpful are these seminars for new judges? A study of twenty-eight federal district judges who attended one of the seminars says that twenty-three reported that they had benefited from the experience.[22] The same study concludes that there appear to be two key elements that make the seminars helpful: the specific contents of the lectures and papers presented, and the opportunity to meet, talk, and exchange notes with other judges. The seminars may also have a specific impact on the novice judges' work. One researcher found, for example, that judges who attend seminars on civil litigation were more productive in handling civil cases than colleagues who had not attended the seminars.[23]

The center also assists new judicial personnel by publishing manuals for judges, clerks, and magistrates. *The Bench Book for United States District Court Judges*, for example, contains information on various federal court procedures and may serve as a checklist for a judge unfamiliar with a certain procedure. Training programs are not aimed solely at new judicial personnel, however. The Division of Continuing Education and Training organizes or sponsors a large number of seminars and workshops annually; during fiscal year 1982, for instance, the division was responsible for 192 seminars and workshops.[24]

A closer look at the Federal Judicial Center's activities in fiscal 1982 gives us valuable insight into the breadth of its educational and training effort. In keeping with its goals of providing every district judge an opportunity to attend at least one center-developed course each fiscal year, twenty-eight seminars, workshops, and institutes were offered, including two sentencing institutes (also attended by some chief probation officers), three conferences for metropolitan district chief judges, and eleven mini-seminars or video orientation programs for groups of newly appointed district judges.

District judges are not the only ones to benefit from the center's programs. In fiscal 1982 the Division of Continuing Education and Training presented five workshops and seminars for bankruptcy judges; five orientations and advanced seminars for U.S. magistrates; and twenty programs for U.S. probation officers, including a teleconference on white-collar crime that was held simultaneously in twenty different cities via satellite-beamed closed-circuit television. The division also serves the needs of clerks of court. In fiscal 1982 there were thirteen programs for these officials. Federal public defenders were the recipients of three programs, while two programs were designed for federal public defender investigators. Finally, a wide variety of in-court training programs are also provided. In fiscal 1982 the Division of Continuing Education and Training offered eighty-eight such sessions.

One of the Federal Judicial Center's major goals in offering its continuing education programs is to keep court personnel abreast of recent developments. Let us look at a timely example. In 1984 Congress passed the Comprehensive Crime Control Act and the Criminal Fine Enforcement Act, which provided for major changes in federal criminal law and procedure. In January 1985 the center broadcast a four-hour live video seminar by satellite to acquaint judicial personnel with the new developments. About 170 judges and some 2,000 supporting personnel in thirty major cities viewed the live telecast, while many others viewed videotapes of the broadcast. The videos featured circuit and district judges, a magistrate, and prosecution and defense attorneys who offered brief presentations and answered questions telephoned in by the viewing audience.[25]

The Judicial Conference of the United States, the Administrative Office of the U.S. Courts, and the Federal Judicial Center all serve the entire federal court system. We will now look at two agencies that operate on a regional, rather than national, scope.

## Circuit Judicial Conferences

Each circuit has its own judicial conference, as is required by statute, that meets at least once a year. Conferences are attended by all district and appellate judges in the circuit, the Supreme Court justice assigned to the circuit, and a number of special guests such as lawyers and law school professors. Although the specific program varies from circuit to circuit, a general pattern can be described. The agenda usually includes (1) papers and panels presented by judges, lawyers, law professors, and administrative personnel; (2) panels and conferences that allow for interchange between district and appellate judges; and (3) structured and unstructured social contact between the conference's participants. Although all the activities of the circuit judicial conferences are to a certain extent social gatherings, they provide a forum for the exchange of ideas. Furthermore, they establish communication links between judges within and between the circuit and lawyers who practice in the region.

## Circuit Judicial Councils

Each circuit also has a Judicial Council, consisting of some or all judges of that circuit's court of appeals and varying numbers of district judges. Federal legislation requires that each judicial council have at least two district judges as members; councils with more than six court of appeals judges as members must have at least three district judges on the council. Table 3-1 shows the current membership of the Circuit Judicial Council of each of the twelve circuits. The Administrative Office Act of 1939 authorizes the councils to order the judges within the circuit to comply with policies established by it, by the Judicial Conference of the United States, and by Congress.

Much of the council's work is an effort to see that the district courts operate as effectively as possible. In this regard the council monitors district court caseloads, judge assignments, the conduct of district judges, the utilization of jurors, the assignment of magistrates, and the use of court reporters. Traditionally, the major weapons at the disposal of the council have been persuasion, peer group pressure, and publicity directed at those judges who are reluctant to comply with circuit policy. Although formal council orders may be issued to district judges in an effort to gain compliance with council policy, such orders usually concern the more mundane aspects of judicial administration. For example, orders directing that a judge receive no new cases until his or her docket has been cleared are occasionally issued.[26]

Not everything the circuit judicial council does is routine, however. In fact, some council actions have a far-reaching effect. One good example concerns the Fifth Circuit Judicial Council in 1980. For many years the Fifth Circuit, which then contained the states of Alabama, Florida,

**Table 3-1**   Membership of the Circuit Judicial Councils

| Circuit | Circuit judges | District judges |
|---------|---------------|-----------------|
| D.C. | 11 | 6 |
| First | 4 | 3 |
| Second | 11 | 6 |
| Third | 10 | 5 |
| Fourth[a] | 5 | 4 |
| Fifth | 14 | 9 |
| Sixth | 11 | 5 |
| Seventh | 8 | 4 |
| Eighth | 9 | 5 |
| Ninth[a] | 5 | 4 |
| Tenth[a] | 6 | 4 |
| Eleventh | 12 | 3 |

Source: *The Third Branch* 16 (October 1984): 7.
[a] These circuits do not have all appellate judges in the circuit as members of the council.

Georgia, Louisiana, Mississippi, and Texas as well as the Canal Zone, had been plagued by heavy caseloads and a developing backlog. Innovative techniques in docket management and decision making, increases in authorized judgeships, and the aid of visiting judges served only to postpone what was seen as an inevitable disaster. However, the Omnibus Judges Act of 1978 authorized circuits with more than fifteen judges to divide themselves administratively and to set their own rules for the number of judges in *en banc* proceedings. Two years later the Fifth Circuit Judicial Council proposed that Congress create a Fifth Circuit composed of Louisiana, Mississippi, and Texas and a new Eleventh Circuit including Alabama, Florida, and Georgia. Meanwhile, the court would operate as two administrative units, but with the judges serving circuitwide.[27] As we noted in Chapter 2, Congress did divide the old Fifth Circuit according to the recommendation, effective on October 1, 1981.

Recently, the Committee on Juries of the Second Circuit Judicial Council invited trial judges in the circuit to adopt one or more experimental jury procedures. The district judges were asked to choose from seven procedures and use them for at least six trials in both civil and criminal cases. The experimental procedures included allowing attorneys, in addition to the judge, to question prospective jurors; allowing judges to ask detailed questions of potential jurors in their chambers after asking general questions of all jurors; allowing jurors to submit questions (screened by the judge) to witnesses, and allowing jurors to take notes. The committee issued a report that evaluated responses to the experimental jury procedures. Although the Second Circuit Judicial Council did not recommend that any of the procedures be made mandatory, it encouraged their discretionary use.[28]

It should be noted that the traits of independence, decentralization, and individualism that are characteristic of the federal judiciary in general are clearly reflected in the organization and actual operation of the circuit judicial councils. As a part of the middle tier of the judicial administrative system, the councils fit nicely into the scheme of local or decentralized control of the courts. Moreover, the appeals court judges on the circuit judicial councils generally see themselves as professional colleagues of the district judges rather than as supervisors directing their work. This relationship accounts in large part for the use of persuasion and compromise instead of direct orders to bring about administrative changes.

## Administering Individual Federal Courts

Our discussion of federal judicial administration would not be complete without noting that the chief justice of the Supreme Court and the chief judges of the courts of appeals and district courts have general administrative responsibility for their specific courts. The chief justice is, of course, specifically appointed to that position by the president with the approval of the Senate. Chief judges of the circuit and district courts, on the other hand, are determined on the basis of seniority. Traditionally, the chief judge has been the most senior judge of the court under the age of seventy. Upon reaching seventy the judge must step down as chief. Legislation adopted several years ago, however, states that someone cannot become chief judge after his or her sixty-fourth year unless no one else is eligible. Even then the judge may serve for only seven years.

Among other chores, the chief judge has budgetary responsibilities for a specific court. The chief judge also acts as the ultimate supervisor for all nonjudicial personnel associated with that court. In addition, the chief judge has overall responsibility for assigning judges and, in the case of the courts of appeals, panels of judges to cases.

The chief justice has some administrative responsibilities in relation to the entire federal judicial system. For example, he or she serves as chair of the Judicial Conference of the United States and as chair of the board of the Federal Judicial Center. In addition, the chief justice in effect selects the director of the Administrative Office of the United States Courts.

The chief judge of the court of appeals also has administrative responsibilities beyond the specific court. This judge assumes some administrative duties in relation to the district courts within the boundaries of a particular circuit.

As might be expected, chief judges over the years have delegated some of their administrative duties to other judges and to professional administrators. Traditionally, the court clerk and the clerk's staff have played important roles in this regard. More recently, circuit and district executives have assumed major administrative duties in their domains. In spite of these recent trends, chief judges of the courts of appeals still say that they must spend a good portion of their working time on administrative matters.[29]

## State Court Administration

In 1967, when the president's task force report on the courts was issued, only about half of the states had operating offices of court administration. By 1977 each of the states had such an office in operation.[30] As one would expect, the heads of these offices carry a variety of titles throughout the fifty states. Among the more common are administrative director of courts, chief of court administration, and director of the administrative office of the courts. These officeholders are appointed by state courts of last resort, the chief justice or chief judge of courts of last resort, or state judicial councils. Each of the directors has a staff to help carry out the work of the administrative office. According to a recent survey, the size of the staff ranged from 2 persons in Mississippi to 315 persons in New York.[31]

The work of these administrative offices varies from state to state and is affected by the size of the staff and the office's budget, among other things. Generally speaking, however, they compile statistics on case filings and terminations and prepare reports on various aspects of the state judicial system. In some states they have also been given the task of developing in-state training sessions and educational seminars for employees of the various levels of the state court system.[32]

As is true at the federal level, a great deal of administrative power in the state judiciary is still vested in the judges. One recent study said that "a majority of state supreme courts have rule-making authority and general administrative and supervisory control over all courts within their state"[33] At the lower levels of the state judiciary the daily operations are usually the responsibility of one designated as chief judge or presiding judge. In some states this person is elected by the other judges within the district (or other regional unit), whereas in other states the chief may be the judge with the most seniority.

The chief or presiding judge's primary responsibility is to keep the cases moving as efficiently as possible. Toward this end, the chief judge may pressure other judges to dispose of cases to prevent backlogs and temporarily assign judges to certain courts to help dispose of backlogs. In some areas the presiding judge may initiate disciplinary actions against judges in the district. Also, he or she will generally preside over special ceremonies and other functions that involve the district.

## Personnel Support

### United States Magistrates

In an effort to help federal district judges deal with increased workloads, Congress passed the Federal Magistrates Act in 1968. The legislation created the office of U.S. magistrate to replace the former U.S. commissioners, who had performed limited duties for the federal trial courts for a number of years. The result was the creation of "a new first echelon of judicial officers in the federal judicial system." [34] The scope and authority of the U.S. magistrates has been clarified and expanded twice since 1968, by the Federal Magistrates Acts of 1976 and 1979.

As the duties of magistrates have expanded, so too has the number of full-time magistrates assigned to the district courts. Between 1970, when a pilot program was begun in five districts, and 1987, the number of full-time magistrates increased from 61 to 292, while the number of part-time magistrates declined from 449 to 165. [35] New magistrates' positions are authorized by the Judicial Conference (subject to funding by Congress) after it considers recommendations from the Administrative Office of U.S. Courts, the district courts, the circuit councils, and the Magistrates Committee of the Judicial Conference.

The judges of the district court appoint full-time magistrates for eight-year terms of office. However, they can be removed before the expiration of their term for "good cause." A full-time magistrate is required to be a lawyer and a member of the state bar. If a qualified person cannot be found, the judges may appoint a person competent to perform the duties as a part-time magistrate for a term of four years.

The magistrates system constitutes a structure that responds to each district court's specific needs and circumstances. Within guidelines set by the Federal Magistrates Acts of 1968, 1976, and 1979, the judges in each district court establish the duties and responsibilities of their magistrates. The 1968 legislation generally described the magistrates' duties as including all the powers and duties formerly exercised by U.S. commissioners, the trial and disposition of minor criminal offenses, and "additional duties" to assist the district judges. [36] Although some districts established local rules authorizing magistrates to perform "additional duties," controversies developed among courts as to what kinds of duties might be delegated to the magistrates.

As a consequence of this uncertainty, both the 1976 and the 1979 acts clarified and expanded the scope of the magistrates' authority. The

1976 act says that a magistrate may be designated to hear and determine certain kinds of pretrial matters brought before the court, to conduct hearings, and to submit proposed findings and recommendations on motions. The court can then accept, reject, or modify the recommendations in whole or in part. The 1979 legislation permits a magistrate, with the consent of the involved parties, to conduct all proceedings in a jury or nonjury civil matter and to enter a judgment in the case, and to conduct a trial of persons accused of misdemeanors (less serious offenses than felonies) committed within the district, provided the defendants consent.

In other words, Congress has given federal district judges the authority to expand the scope of magistrates' participation in the judicial process. However, because each district has its own particular needs, a magistrate's specific duties may vary from one district and from one judge to another. The decision to delegate responsibilities to the magistrate is still made by the judges; therefore, a magistrate's participation in the processing of cases may be considerably narrower than that permitted by statute. The author of a recent in-depth study of U.S. magistrates sums it up this way:

> Some judges may, as a matter of common practice, request a magistrate's assistance in hearing all discovery motions, request a magistrate's assistance in scheduling . . . "initial" pretrial conferences, or request a magistrate's assistance in settlement conferences. In contrast, other judges may request a magistrate's assistance on a selective (i.e., case-by-case) basis for each of these types of matters.[37]

A recent study of nine federal districts discovered that magistrates were basically being used in one of three ways by the judges in the district.[38] In some districts the magistrates are used as additional judges. This means simply that they hear and decide their own civil caseloads. In other areas the judges may use magistrates as specialists who hear and then recommend action on some special aspect of the law. Social Security and prisoner cases are the most common areas of specialization. Finally, it was discovered that some judges elect to have a magistrate act as a team player. That is, the magistrate might hear all pretrial matters (on either a regular or selective basis) and then determine when the case is ready for the judge. In short, the magistrate becomes, in practice, a pretrial judicial officer.

Perhaps the most important power magistrates now possess is the authority to conduct trials in civil cases, with the consent of the parties involved. Since they have held this power only since 1979, an important question has been raised: How likely are the parties to agree to having the case heard by a magistrate? Table 3-2, based on a 1983 study conducted by the Federal Judicial Center, indicates that there is little reluctance to allow a magistrate to handle the case.

**Table 3-2**    Frequency of Parties' Consent to Magistrates in Civil Suits

| Frequency | Participating magistrates | |
| --- | --- | --- |
| | Number | Percentage |
| Almost always | 74 | 60 |
| Frequently | 22 | 18 |
| Occasionally | 23 | 19 |
| Rarely | 4 | 3 |

Source: Carroll Seron, *The Roles of Magistrates in Federal District Courts* (Washington, D.C.: Federal Judicial Center, 1983), 65.

There is no doubt that the approximately 500 full-time and part-time magistrates are now vital cogs in the federal judicial system. Statistics reveal that "United States Magistrates disposed of 466,078 cases and other matters in 1987, an increase of 2 percent over [the previous] year." [39]

## Law Clerks

In this section we examine the work of another individual who is vital to the operation of our courts: the law clerk. The first use of law clerks by an American judge is generally traced to Horace Gray of Massachusetts. In the summer of 1875, while serving as chief justice of the Massachusetts Supreme Court, he employed, at his own expense, a highly ranked new graduate of the Harvard Law School. [40] Each year, he would employ a new clerk from Harvard. When Gray was appointed to the U.S. Supreme Court in 1882, he brought a law clerk with him to the nation's highest court.

One of Gray's law clerks at the Supreme Court, Samuel Williston, left a record of his clerkship that provides some details about the tasks of the first law clerks. [41] Williston served Justice Gray as both a sounding board and an editor. He was expected to review all the new cases and to formulate a recommended disposition that he would discuss with Justice Gray before the Supreme Court's conference. Williston was frequently asked to draft opinions in cases assigned to Justice Gray and to read the opinions circulated by the other justices and discuss them with his justice. Justice Gray and Samuel Williston became close friends during the clerkship, as indicated by the fact that Gray, then sixty years old, became engaged and sought the clerk's advice on an engagement ring. Gray also altered Williston's schedule and doubled his pay so that the young clerk, who was also engaged, could save more money for the marriage.

In spite of Gray's happy experiences with the young Harvard Law School graduates, his method was not quickly adopted by his colleagues, even after Congress assumed the cost in 1886. By 1888, all nine justices were employing assistants, but the typical pattern was to obtain a law clerk through friends or relatives or from the bar and law schools of the District of Columbia and to retain that assistant as long as possible.

Justice Gray's successor on the High Court was Oliver Wendell Holmes, like Gray a former chief justice of the Massachusetts Supreme Court. Holmes also adopted the practice of hiring annual honor graduates of Harvard Law School as his clerks. At first, Holmes's clerks were selected by Professor John Chipman Gray. Upon Gray's death in 1915, Holmes asked a young Harvard Law School professor named Felix Frankfurter (later a Supreme Court justice himself) to serve as procurer of law clerks. When he joined the Court in 1916, Louis Brandeis made the same request of Frankfurter. Professor Frankfurter, whose protégés were known as the "happy hot dogs," thus supplied clerks for Holmes, Brandeis, and Holmes's successor Benjamin Cardozo.

When William Howard Taft became chief justice, he secured a new law clerk annually from the dean of the Yale Law School. Harlan Fiske Stone, former dean of the Columbia Law School, joined the Court in 1925 and made it his practice to hire a Columbia graduate each year. Over time, then, the justices gradually shifted their views so that the short-term law professor protégé became the typical Supreme Court law clerk.

During the 1919-1939 period the use of law clerks flourished at the lower-court level. Congress authorized a law clerk for each circuit judge in 1930 and one for selected district judges in 1936. Recent decades have seen a steady growth in the use of law clerks by all federal and some state courts. Supreme Court justices, for example, now have three or four clerks; each circuit judge has two, or in some cases three; and each district judge has one or two. The number of clerks varies because there is some discretion in salaries that may be paid and also because of judges' preferences. Some judges, for example, prefer an additional secretary to another law clerk.

What sorts of tasks do law clerks perform? Obviously, the duties vary according to the type of court and the judge for whom the clerk works. Nevertheless, several tasks common to law clerks at any level may be identified.

The clerks earliest involvement in the litigation process comes when they review petitions and motions. Law clerks working for the Supreme Court spend a great deal of their time on the appeals and certiorari petitions filed with the Court. They digest information contained in the many petitions and lower-court records, and summarize the material for the justices. Since 1972, several justices have participated in a "certpool," whereby a single clerk is designated to prepare a memorandum for the mutual use of the participating justices.

As we saw in Chapter 2, the U.S. courts of appeals do not have the same discretion to accept or reject a case that the Supreme Court has. Nevertheless, the courts of appeals now use certain screening devices to differentiate between cases that can be handled quickly and those that require more time and effort. Law clerks are an integral part of this screening process.

Traditionally, the law clerk is selected by a particular judge and works exclusively for that individual. About 1960, however, some courts of appeals began to utilize a new concept: the staff law clerk.[42] The staff clerk, who works for the entire court, began to be used primarily because of the rapid increase in the number of *pro se* matters (generally speaking, those involving indigents) coming before the courts of appeals. In some circuits the staff law clerks deal only with pro se matters, while in others they review nearly all cases on the court's docket. As a result of the review process, a case may be dealt with in a truncated procedure—that is, without oral argument or full briefing.

Law clerks working for trial judges spend a good deal of their time examining the various motions filed in civil and criminal cases. They review each motion, noting the issues and the positions of the parties involved, research important points raised in the motions, and prepare written memoranda for the judge. Although a large part of the law clerk's work is devoted to the earliest stages of the litigation process, the work does not end there.

The information provided by law clerks continues to be important to the judges who must actually decide the cases. In the courts of appeals, for example, intensive analysis of the record by judges prior to oral argument or decision is not always possible. They seldom have time to do more than scan pertinent portions of the record called to their attention by law clerks. As one judicial scholar aptly put it, "To prepare for oral argument, all but a handful of circuit judges rely upon bench memoranda prepared by their law clerks, plus their own notes from reading briefs." [43]

Many judges expect their law clerks to serve as sounding boards for their views about how a particular case should be decided. Such exchanges between judge and clerk contribute to the sharpening of thought processes and to the quality of judicial decisions. The judge "considers it the job of his law clerks to prevent him from making mistakes." [44]

The law clerk often differs ideologically from his or her judge—a situation that allows the judge to get a very different perspective on a case. The following account of former Supreme Court justice Lewis Powell and one of his law clerks, Joel Klein, provides a good example of what we are talking about:

Powell quickly grasped that Klein's brash, outspoken style would be a perfect counterpoint to his own genteel Southern background. He prided himself on hiring liberal clerks. He would tell his clerks that the conservative side of the issues came to him naturally. Their job was to present the other side, to challenge him. He would rather encounter a compelling argument for another position in the privacy of his own chamber, than to meet it unexpectedly at conference or in a dissent.[45]

Once a decision has been reached, the law clerk will frequently participate in writing the order or opinion that accompanies the decision. A district judge, for example, said, "I even allow my law clerks to write memorandum opinions. I first tell him what I want and then he writes it up. Sometimes I sign it without changing a word."[46]

A similar practice occurs at the Supreme Court, where the writing of the Court's opinion may be a long-drawn-out process. Chief Justice William Rehnquist describes his procedure as follows:

> I sit down with the law clerk who is now responsible for the case, and go over my conference notes with him. After this discussion, I ask the law clerk to prepare a first draft of a court opinion, and to have it for me in 10 days or two weeks. When I receive a rough draft of a court opinion from a law clerk, I read it over, and to the extent necessary go back and again read the opinion of the lower court and selected parts of the parties' brief. I go through the draft with a view to shortening it, simplifying it and clarifying it. When I have finished my revisions of the draft opinion, I return it to the law clerk, and the law clerk then refines and on occasion may suggest additional revisions. We then send the finished product to the printer, and in short order get back printed copies with the correct formal heading for the opinion.[47]

We should note that there has been some debate about the influence of law clerks. Without doubt they have an effect on decisions such as whether certiorari should be granted and whether cases should receive a full hearing or be disposed of through a truncated procedure. One federal judge says, for example,

> However hard a judge tries, he cannot completely review everything that his law clerks do or learn all that they know. Inevitably they assist him not only in routine tasks but in the work of judging. They read briefs, study precedents, prepare proposed jury charges and findings, and in some instances draft opinions for the judge's review. Of necessity the judge must rely to some degree on their work.[48]

However, law clerks have strong incentives to provide accurate summaries for their judges rather than trying to deceive them. Also, judges are sensitive to the problem of potential loss of control should they delegate too much responsibility to their clerks. Chief Justice Rehnquist, himself a former law clerk for Justice Robert Jackson, provides a good example. In a 1957 magazine article he expressed concern that the ideological biases of law clerks could affect their work on petitions for Supreme Court hearings.[49] Although he argued in the article that law clerks generally play minor roles in the decision process, he was careful when he first became a member of the Supreme Court to write all first drafts of opinions himself.[50] Rehnquist now defends the use of law clerks and, as noted earlier, finds them quite helpful in preparing drafts of court opinions. He recently stated that the "law clerk is not off on a frolic of his own, but is instead engaged in a highly structured task which has been largely mapped out for him by the conference discussions and my suggestions to him." [51]

The issue of trust between justice and clerk has yet another dimension— secrecy about the Court's thinking prior to announcement of a final decision. Traditionally, the High Court does not provide information about conference discussions and votes or about ideas expressed in the various drafts of opinions. Still, the law clerks are in a position to know the views of their own justice and perhaps others as well. The Court is simply dependent upon the clerks to refrain from leaking information prematurely. Occasionally, a book such as *The Brethren* will provide a behind-the-scenes look at the Court, but traditionally the law clerks have not betrayed their trust.

## Court Administrators

The clerk of the court has traditionally handled the day-to-day routines of the court. This includes such things as making courtroom arrangements, keeping records of case proceedings, preparing orders and judgments resulting from court actions, collecting court fees and fines, and disbursing judicial monies. At the federal level these officials are appointed by the judges, whereas in the great majority of states they are elected and may be referred to by other titles.

The traditional clerks of court have been replaced in many areas by well-trained court administrators. Since 1971 each circuit judicial council has been authorized to hire a circuit executive to provide managerial expertise and assistance for the court. A small number of federal district courts also employ district executives. The picture at the state level is somewhat more mixed; however, an increasing number of state courts, especially the busier ones, are employing professional court administrators. Finally, we should note that the chief justice of the U.S. Supreme Court now has an administrative assistant.

## Probation Officers

These members of the judicial supporting cast are important at the trial court level. Probation officers at the federal level serve within the jurisdiction and under the direction of the district judges. One of the probation officer's main functions is to prepare a presentence investigation report which is used by the judge to help determine an appropriate sentence for a criminal defendant. The Administrative Office of the U.S. Courts fixes the salaries of probation officers and provides for their necessary expenses through its Probation Division; the Federal Judicial Center runs training programs for the probation officers. Probation officers are also found at the state level, where the vast majority of criminal cases are processed. Their functions in providing help for the judge in determining an appropriate sentence are basically the same as in the federal judiciary.

## Other Support Personnel

Many other people, of course, perform vital tasks for the federal and state court systems, including bankruptcy judges, special masters, marshals, bailiffs, court reportors, secretaries, and deputy clerks. Scattered throughout the judicial system, they enable the courts to function as efficiently as they do.

The bankruptcy judges, who were discussed in Chapter 2, are especially important elements of the federal judiciary. As of June 30, 1987, there were 252 such judges in active service.[52] Their importance to the system becomes quite obvious when one considers that for the twelve-month period which ended on June 30, 1987, there were 561,278 cases filed in bankruptcy courts, 481,351 cases terminated, and 808,504 cases still pending.[53]

Special masters have also become quite prominent in some courts. They are invariably used in cases handled by the Supreme Court under its original jurisdiction. Special masters are also used quite frequently in cases that have an extended impact. For example, when Chief Judge Frank Battisti of the U.S. District Court for the Northern District of Ohio found that the city of Parma, Ohio, had engaged in a practice of discrimination in violation of the Fair Housing Act he included a special master in his original remedial order.[54] The master was to gather data for the court; distribute information for the city, the Department of Justice, and the two remedial committees established by the judge; and refine minor issues for the benefit of the court.[55]

Marshals are responsible for providing security in courtrooms, delivering legal orders to litigants and witnesses, guarding and transporting prisoners, making arrests, and protecting witnesses. The bailiff, a familiar figure in the courtroom, announces the judge's arrival, keeps order in the court, and administers oaths to witnesses. Deputy clerks and secretaries maintain records on the thousands of cases filed annually and generally help the courts keep up with the numerous items that must be typed, copied, and recorded daily.

# Summary

This chapter has focused on the agencies and individuals that help the courts process cases. Our emphasis has been not so much on judges as on those who assist them. We began with a brief history of the judicial administration movement—a movement closely associated with government reform in general and court reform in particular. Judicial changes have not come easily, however, because of the constitutional heritage of judicial independence, decentralization, and individualism. Still, ever-growing caseloads have forced judges to look for help in handling their dockets by relying increasingly on law clerks, magistrates, and professional court administrators. Agencies such as the Administrative Office of U.S. Courts now aid the judges in dealing with administrative duties and in devising more efficient court procedures. The Federal Judicial Center offers training programs for a wide range of judicial personnel.

In spite of all these changes, however, the judges themselves still retain control over major decisions affecting the courts. The Judicial Conference of the United States remains the policy maker for the federal judiciary, and circuit conferences and circuit councils help to decentralize decision making. In short, while the court systems may look like a hierarchy, there is still a good deal of local control and independence and some variation in how the lower courts handle their cases.

# Notes

1. Henry R. Glick, *Courts, Politics, and Justice*, 2d ed. (New York: McGraw-Hill, 1988), 43.
2. Peter G. Fish, *The Politics of Federal Judicial Administration* (Princeton, N.J.: Princeton University Press, 1973), 7.
3. This point is perhaps best documented in the case of southern federal judges called upon to enforce the Supreme Court's school desegregation decisions. See Jack W. Peltason, *Fifty-Eight Lonely Men* (New York: Harcourt, Brace & World, 1961).
4. Russell R. Wheeler and Howard R. Whitcomb, eds., *Judicial Administration: Text and Readings* (Englewood Cliffs, N.J.: Prentice-Hall, 1977), 27.
5. Ibid., 28.
6. Ibid.
7. Fred P. Graham, "Warren, Justice 15 Years, to Seek Speed in Courts," *New York Times*, September 30, 1968, 1.
8. Carl Baar, "Federal Judicial Administration: Political Strategies and Organizational Change," in *Judicial Administration*, ed. Wheeler and Whitcomb, 97.
9. See President's Commission on Law Enforcement and Administration of Justice, *Task Force Report: The Courts* (Washington, D.C.: Government Printing Office, 1967).
10. Larry C. Berkson, "A Brief History of Court Reform," in *Managing the State Courts*, ed. Larry C. Berkson, Steven W. Hays, and Susan B. Carbon (St. Paul,

Minn.: West), 12.
11. Sheldon Goldman and Thomas P. Jahnige, *The Federal Courts as a Political System*, 2d. ed. (New York: Harper & Row, 1976), 99.
12. See *The Third Branch* 20 (January 1988): 2.
13. The quote is from an interview with Arthur R. Miller in *The Third Branch* 18 (November 1986): 8.
14. See Fish, *The Politics of Federal Judicial Administration*, 273.
15. See ibid., 121-123.
16. Ibid., 124, 166.
17. The discussion of the initial organization of the Administrative Office is drawn from Fish, *The Politics of Federal Judicial Administration*, 172-176.
18. Glick, *Courts, Politics, and Justice*, 44.
19. Our discussion of the research role is drawn from "The Federal Judicial Center," *Law and Society Newsletter* (March 1984): 5.
20. Ernest C. Friesen, Jr., Edward C. Gallas, and Nesta M. Gallas, *Managing the Courts* (Indianapolis: Bobbs-Merrill, 1971), 200.
21. Gordon Bermant and Russell R. Wheeler, "From within the System: Educational and Research Programs at the Federal Judicial Center," in *Reforming the Law*, ed. Gary B. Melton (New York: Guilford, 1987), 108.
22. See Robert A. Carp and Russell R. Wheeler, "Sink or Swim: The Socialization of a Federal District Judge," *Journal of Public Law* 21 (1972): 382.
23. See Beverly Blair Cook, "The Socialization of New Federal Judges: Impact on District Court Business," *Washington University Law Quarterly* (1971): 269-270.
24. See *The Third Branch* 15 (January 1983): 6. All the information and figures on the activities in fiscal 1982 are drawn from this source.
25. Bermant and Wheeler, "From within the System," 111.
26. See Fish, *The Politics of Federal Judicial Administration*, 418-419.
27. See J. Woodford Howard, Jr., *Courts of Appeals in the Federal Judicial System: A Study of the Second, Fifth, and District of Columbia Circuits* (Princeton, N.J.: Princeton University Press, 1981), 273.
28. See *The Third Branch* 16 (October 1984): 3.
29. See Russell R. Wheeler and Charles Nihan, *Administering the Federal Judicial Circuits: A Study of Chief Judges' Approaches and Procedures* (Washington, D.C.: Federal Judicial Center, 1982), 5.
30. Council of State Governments, *The Book of the States, 1978-79* (Lexington, Ky.: Council of State Governments, 1978), 84.
31. Council of State Governments, *The Book of the States, 1982-83* (Lexington, Ky.: Council of State Governments, 1982), 269.
32. Ibid., 269.
33. Ibid., 246.
34. Steven Puro, "United States Magistrates: A New Federal Judicial Officer," *Justice System Journal* 2 (Winter 1976): 141.
35. See Carroll Seron, *The Roles of Magistrates in Federal District Courts* (Washington, D.C.: Federal Judicial Center, 1983), 8.
36. See 28 U.S.C. 636.
37. Seron, *The Roles of Magistrates in Federal District Courts*, 8.
38. Carroll Seron, *The Roles of Magistrates: Nine Case Studies* (Washington, D.C.: Federal Judicial Center, 1985).
39. *Annual Report of the Director of the Administrative Office of the United States Courts*, 1987 (Washington, D.C.: Government Printing Office), 34.

40. Our discussion of the historical evolution of law clerks is drawn from John Bilyeu Oakley and Robert S. Thompson, *Law Clerks and the Judicial Process* (Berkeley: University of California Press, 1980), 10-22.
41. See Samuel Williston, *Life and Law* (Boston: Little, Brown, 1940), and Samuel Williston, "Horace Gray," in *Great American Lawyers*, ed. W. Lewis (Philadelphia: J. C. Winston, 1907-1909; South Hackensack, N.J.: Rothman Reprints, 1971).
42. See Steven Flanders and Jerry Goldman, "Screening Practices and the Use of Para-Judicial Personnel in a U.S. Court of Appeals," in *Judicial Administration*, ed. Wheeler and Whitcomb, 244.
43. Howard, *Courts of Appeals in the Federal Judicial System*, 198.
44. Oakley and Thompson, *Law Clerks and the Judicial Process*, 103.
45. Bob Woodward and Scott Armstrong, *The Brethren* (New York: Simon & Schuster, 1979), 354-355.
46. Quoted in Carp and Wheeler, "Sink or Swim," 379.
47. William H. Rehnquist, "How the Court Arrives at Its Decisions," *Houston Chronicle*, November 4, 1987, 4:2.
48. Alvin B. Rubin, "Bureaucratization of the Federal Courts: The Tension between Justice and Efficiency," in *Views from the Bench*, ed. Mark W. Cannon and David M. O'Brien (Chatham, N.J.: Chatham House, 1985), 67.
49. William H. Rehnquist, "Who Writes Decisions of the Supreme Court?" *U.S. News & World Report*, December 13, 1957, 74-75.
50. See Woodward and Armstrong, *The Brethren*, 269.
51. Rehnquist, "How the Court Arrives at Its Decisions," 2.
52. *Annual Report of the Administrative Office*, 1987, 49.
53. Ibid., 347.
54. See *United States v. City of Parma, Ohio*, 504 F. Supp. 913 (1980). Also see the case study of this litigation in Phillip J. Cooper, *Hard Judicial Choices* (New York: Oxford University Press, 1988), 47-48.
55. The court of appeals later removed the special master. See *United States v. City of Parma, Ohio*, 661 F. 2d 562 (6th Cir. 1981). Also see Cooper, *Hard Judicial Choices*, 348.

# 4 Lawyers, Litigants, and Interest Groups in the Judicial Process

In this chapter we lay the foundation for a detailed examination of the courts in action by focusing on three crucial actors in the judicial process: lawyers, litigants, and interest groups. Judges in the United States make decisions only in the context of cases that are brought to the courts by individuals or groups who have some sort of disagreement, dispute, or controversy with each other. These adversaries, commonly called litigants, sometimes argue their own cases in such minor forums as small claims courts, but are almost always represented by lawyers in the more important judicial arenas.

Given the importance of lawyers in our system of justice, the first part of our discussion will be devoted to an examination of the legal profession. Following that we will turn our attention to the role of individual litigants and interest groups in the judicial process.

## Lawyers and the Legal Profession

Our examination of lawyers focuses on the training and work of attorneys in the United States. In keeping with a basic theme of earlier chapters, we will first examine lawyers and the legal profession in a historical context.[1]

### Development of the Legal Profession

*The Colonial Period.* Lawyers were not at all popular during the early colonial years; there were, in fact, very few lawyers to be found among the early settlers. Eventually, however, lawyers became a necessary evil as a growing society posed problems that required their skills. Some who rendered legal services had been trained in England while others were laymen who had only a smattering of legal knowledge. In spite of constant complaints about those who practiced law, "there was a competent, professional bar, dominated by brilliant and successful lawyers . . . in all major communities by 1750."[2]

There were no law schools during this period to train those interested in the legal profession. Some young men, especially those who lived in the South, where there were no colleges, went to England for their education and attended the Inns of Court. The Inns were not formal law schools, but were part of the English legal culture and allowed students to become familiar with English law.

Americans who aspired to the law during this period generally went through some form of clerkship or apprenticeship with an established lawyer. In other words, the student paid a fee to the lawyer, who promised to train him in the law. As might be expected, some found this to be a fruitful experience while others complained that it was of little or no value.

Each colony established its own standards for admission to the bar (the entire group of lawyers permitted to practice law in the courts of that colony). In some instances the colony's highest court was given control over licensing and admission to the bar. In Massachusetts each court admitted its own lawyers; in Rhode Island any court could admit lawyers, but admission by one court automatically meant admission to all the courts in the colony.

The impact of lawyers on the American political system was evident during this early period. Of the fifty-six signers of the Declaration of Independence, twenty-five were lawyers, and thirty-one of the fifty-five delegates to the Constitutional Convention were lawyers.[3] Among the leading founders of the Republic who were lawyers, one finds John Marshall, John Adams, Thomas Jefferson, James Wilson, John Jay, and George Wythe, to name a few.

*The Revolution to the Mid-Nineteenth Century.*   After the Revolution the number of lawyers increased rapidly since neither legal education nor admission to the bar was very strict. During the first half of the nineteenth century there were no large law firms. However, there were some lawyers who garnered wealth by representing rich clients and prosperous merchants. Other lawyers simply eked out a living by handling petty claims in minor courts.

It seems that the right social background was as important then as it is today. As one American legal historian says:

> There is evidence, indeed, that the bar, after the first Revolutionary generation, drew even more heavily than before upon children of professionals, as compared to children of farmers or laborers. Between 1810 and 1840, it seems, more than half the lawyers, who were college graduates and were admitted to the bar in Massachusetts, were sons of lawyers and judges; before 1810 the figure was about 38 percent.[4]

The apprenticeship method continued to be the most popular way to receive legal training, but law schools were coming into existence. The first law schools grew out of law offices that had begun to specialize in training clerks or apprentices. The earliest such school was the Litchfield School, founded by Judge Tapping Reeve in 1784. This school, which taught by the lecture method, placed primary emphasis on commercial law.

Eventually, a few colleges began to teach law as part of their general curriculum. William and Mary College was the first to establish a chair of law, with George Wythe being appointed to the professorship. Professorships were also established at the University of Virginia, the University of Pennsylvania, and the University of Maryland during the late eighteenth and early nineteenth centuries.

A chair of law was established at Harvard in 1816, and the first professor, Isaac Parker, worked to bring about a professional, independent law school. A major gift from Nathan Dane in 1826 helped to make this goal possible. He gave Harvard $10,000 to support a professorship and suggested that the first Dane professor be Joseph Story. Story was an associate justice of the United States Supreme Court when he accepted the position in 1829.[5] Harvard awarded an LL.B. (Bachelor of Laws) degree to students who completed the law school course. Harvard was to become the model for all newer schools.

*The Second Half of the Nineteenth Century.* During the second half of the nineteenth century the number of law schools increased dramatically. In 1850 only 15 law schools were operating, but by 1900 there were 102.[6]

There were two major differences between law schools of that time and those of today. First, law schools did not usually require any previous college work. Second, in 1850 the standard law school curriculum could be completed in one year. Later in the 1800s many law schools instituted two-year programs.

In 1870 major changes began at Harvard and were to have a lasting impact on legal training. In that year Christopher Columbus Langdell was appointed dean of the law school. As a start, Langdell instituted stiffer entrance requirements. If the student did not have a college degree, he was required to pass an entrance test. Langdell also made it more difficult to graduate. The law school course was increased to two years in 1871 and to three years in 1876. Another hurdle was the requirement that a student pass first-year final examinations before he could proceed to the second-year courses.

Without doubt, however, the most lasting change attributed to Langdell was the introduction of the case method of teaching. This method replaced lectures and textbooks with casebooks. The casebooks (collections of actual case reports) were designed to show the principles of law, what they meant, and how they developed. Teachers then used the Socratic method to guide the students to a discovery of legal concepts found in the cases. Students initially resisted this new method of teaching law, but other schools eventually adopted the Harvard approach. In fact, it remains the accepted method in many law schools today.

As the demand for lawyers increased during the late 1800s, there was a corresponding acceleration in the creation of new law schools. It was not really expensive to open a law school, and a number of night schools, using lawyers and judges as part-time faculty members, sprang into existence. Standards were often lax and the curriculum tended to emphasize local practice. These schools' major contribution lay in making legal training more readily available to poor, immigrant, and working-class students.

Naturally, then, the legal profession itself changed dramatically during this time. Lawyers no longer came solely from the upper rungs of society. Bar associations became interested in legal education as a way of controlling entry into the profession. Around the turn of the century the Association of American Law Schools was created and, along with the American Bar Association, became involved in the accreditation of law schools.

**The Twentieth Century.** This century has seen some major changes in the legal profession. For one thing, there has been a dramatic increase in the number of people wanting to study law. By the 1960s the number of applicants to law schools had grown so large that nearly all schools became more selective. The more prestigious schools were especially able to accept only the best students. In response to social pressure and litigation, many law schools began actively recruiting female and minority applicants.

During the first half of the twentieth century the case method of instruction continued to dominate the legal education process. By the 1920s, however, the legal realist movement (discussed more completely in Chapter 9) began to have an impact on the law school curriculum. Two new courses, administrative law and taxation, started to find their way into the schedule. Some schools also began to add clinical training to the curriculum.

By the 1960s the curriculum in some law schools had been expanded to include social concerns such as civil rights law and law-and-poverty issues. Foreign law courses were also added in some schools. In spite of these alterations and additions, however, the core law school curriculum has been highly resistant to radical changes.

The twentieth century has been an active period for the organized bar. The American Bar Association adopted in 1908 a canon of ethics to guide the conduct of lawyers. Most states followed suit by adopting the ABA canon or one of their own.

Another twentieth-century development is the integrated bar. This simply means that all lawyers in the state belong to a single bar association, pay dues to it, and are disciplined by it. The move toward an integrated bar began about the middle of the century and still continues.

Finally, we should note that the increasing use of advertising by lawyers has had a profound impact on the legal profession. In a 1977 decision the U.S. Supreme Court struck down Arizona's ban on advertising.[7] Today, on television stations across the country one can see lawyers appealing for clients. Furthermore, legal "clinics" have spread rapidly to handle the business generated by the increased use of advertising.

## The Practice of Law Today

The number of lawyers has risen sharply over the years. In 1980, the number of attorneys in the United States stood at just over 542,000, and by 1984 it had increased to 649,000. If annual admissions to the bar continue at this level, we can expect about 750,000 lawyers by 1990 and a full one million by the turn of the century.[8] This means that the number of attorneys has been increasing faster than the general population in this country.

Where do all these lawyers work? A recent study that analyzed the legal profession as it stood in 1980 reported that 68 percent of the country's lawyers were in private practice, 10 percent worked for private industry, 10 percent were employed by the government, 5 percent were retired or inactive, 4 percent were associated with the judiciary, and 3 percent fell into the "other" category.[9]

In short, America's lawyers choose to apply their professional training in a variety of settings. As one might expect, some environments are more prestigious and profitable than others. This situation has led to what is known as professional stratification.

**Stratification of the Legal Profession.** Lawyers and academicians identify three distinct levels within the legal profession. Stratum I is composed of the elite law firms. These are the Wall Street firms—the venerable firms originally situated on New York City's Wall Street—and other large national law firms. Corporate attorneys comprise stratum II. These lawyers represent the Fortune 500 firms and other large corporations. All other lawyers fall into stratum III. These are the solo practitioners, members of small law firms, attorneys for small corporations, and government attorneys.

The basic pattern followed by the large national firms was established early in the twentieth century by Paul D. Cravath, the head of a Wall Street law firm. The ideal candidate for Cravath's firm was a member of Phi Beta Kappa and editor of the law review at Harvard, Yale, or Columbia. Those recruited served a kind of internship during which they performed general work for a number of the firm's partners.[10] Later they moved into an area of specialization and by the tenth year were evaluated for a partnership with the firm. Some lawyers were rewarded with partnerships while others left for another job.

The Cravath approach was used by other New York firms; collectively the attorneys working for such firms came to be known as the Wall Street lawyers. These attorneys are totally dedicated to the interests of their clients and work long, hard hours on their behalf. The Wall Street lawyers have traditionally been known less for court appearances than for the counseling they provide their clients. The clients must be able to pay for this high-powered legal talent, and thus tend to be major corporations rather than individuals. It should be noted, however, that many of these large national firms often provide *pro bono* (free) legal services to further civil rights, civil liberties, consumer, and environmental causes.

The large national firms are comprised of partners and associates. The associates are paid salaries and in reality work for the partners. The partners, on the other hand, typically share the profits in proportion to their seniority and the amount of work they bring in. The Wall Street law firms compete for the best graduates from the most prestigious law schools, and starting salaries may range as high as $80,000 per year. In addition, bonuses may be paid if the associate has served as a law clerk for a judge. It was recently reported, for example, that the New York law firm of Cravath, Swaine, and Moore provided each associate who had clerked for a judge with a $10,000 bonus for each year of the clerkship.[11]

The most prestigious law firms have 200 or more lawyers working for them. They also employ hundreds of other people as paralegals, administrators, librarians, and secretaries. Besides New York City, prestigious firms may also be found in other major cities, such as Chicago, Houston, Los Angeles, San Francisco, and Washington, D.C. The current trend is for major law firms to have branches in several U.S. cities, and even abroad.

A notch below those who are partners or associates in the large national law firms are those who serve as attorneys for large corporations. As noted above, many corporations employ national law firms as *outside counsel.* Increasingly, however, such corporations are hiring their own salaried attorneys as *in-house counsel.* In fact, the legal staff of some corporations rivals those of the national law firms in size. Further, the corporations often compete with the major firms for the best law school graduates.

The legal division of a typical large corporation is headed by a senior-level official known as the general counsel. Rather than representing the corporation in court (this is usually handled by outside counsel when necessary), the legal division handles the multitude of legal problems associated with the modern corporation. For example, the legal division monitors the company's personnel practices to ensure compliance with federal and state regulations concerning hiring and removal procedures. The corporation's attorneys may also offer assistance in strategic planning by advising the board of directors about such things as contractual agreements, mergers, stock sales, and other business practices. The company lawyers may also help educate other employees about the laws that apply to their specific jobs and make sure that they are in compliance with such laws. Finally, the legal division of a large company serves as liaison to outside counsel.

Most of the nation's lawyers toil in stratum III, the lowest level of the legal profession in terms of prestige. One recent study aptly noted that

> the Manhattan megafirm with scores of highly paid associates may command headlines for the moment, but the truth is that most lawyers (70.2 percent) work in firms of fewer than 20 lawyers. Fully 21.3 percent, in fact, are in solo practice, and the median size of the American law firm is 6.3 lawyers.[12]

Generally speaking, the lawyers in this stratum do not command the high salaries associated with large national law firms and major corporations. In 1985, for example, the median starting salary for American lawyers was $25,000.[13]

While the attorneys in stratum I and stratum II are primarily involved in representing corporate clients, the lawyers who work in the lower stratum are engaged in a wide range of activities. They are much more likely to be found, day in and day out, in the courtrooms of the United States. These are the attorneys who represent clients in personal injury suits, who prosecute and defend persons accused of crimes, who represent husbands and wives in divorce proceedings, who help people conduct real estate transactions, and who help people prepare wills, to name just a few activities.

As might be expected, many attorneys, especially those in a solo practice, handle many types of cases. Others tend to specialize in one or two areas. Some charge a flat hourly rate for their activities, while those representing plaintiffs in a personal injury suit often work under a contingency fee arrangement. Under this arrangement the attorney receives no compensation in advance. Instead, if the suit is successful and the plaintiff is awarded monetary damages, the lawyer receives a certain percentage for his or her services.

As noted earlier, attorneys who work for the government are generally included in stratum III. While some, such as the U.S. attorney general and the solicitor general of the United States, occupy quite prestigious positions, many toil in rather obscure and poorly paid positions. A number of attorneys opt for careers as judges at the federal or state level. The judges will be dealt with more extensively at various points throughout the remainder of this book.

Since the remainder of this book focuses on the work of the federal and state courts, it seems appropriate to look more extensively at the lawyers who handle cases in these courts. In some instances the litigants are private individuals and are thus represented by attorneys who are engaged in private practice. In other cases one of the parties involved in the suit may be the state or federal government. When that occurs a government attorney as well as a private lawyer may be involved in the case.

## Government Attorneys in the Judicial Process

Government attorneys work at all stages of the judicial process, from trial courts to the highest state and federal appellate courts. Since the bulk of the cases never move beyond the trial courts, our discussion will begin with the government lawyers most commonly associated with this level of the judicial system.

**Federal Prosecutors.** Although the exact origins of the public prosecutor are uncertain, the prosecution of criminal cases in colonial America became the responsibility of a district attorney (or a person with an equivalent title) who was appointed by the governor and assigned to a specific region. The practice persisted, and by the end of the American Revolution every state had passed legislation creating a public prosecutor. In most instances he was an elected county official. The Judiciary Act of 1789 also provided for a United States attorney to be appointed by the president for each federal district court. Since these beginnings, "the prosecutor has become the most powerful figure in the criminal justice system." [14]

Today each federal judicial district has a *U.S. attorney* and one or more assistant U.S. attorneys. The number of assistants varies from district to district, with larger urban areas, such as the Southern District of New York (New York City), having over a hundred.

U.S. attorneys are appointed by the president and confirmed by the Senate. Nominees must reside in the district to which they are appointed and must be attorneys. They serve a formal term of four years but can be reappointed indefinitely or removed at the president's discretion.[15] The appointment of a U.S. attorney is often a political reward.[16] Overwhelmingly, only lawyers who belong to the president's party are considered; it has become customary for U.S. attorneys to resign their position when the opposition party wins the presidency. Since each nominee must be confirmed by the Senate, the senator or senators of the president's party in the state where the vacancy exists become important actors in the appointment process. The assistant U.S. attorneys are formally appointed by the U.S. attorney general, although in actual practice they are chosen by the U.S. attorney, who forwards the selection to the attorney general for ratification. Assistant U.S. attorneys may be fired by the attorney general.

The basic tasks handled by U.S. attorneys and their assistants are to prosecute defendants in the federal district courts and to defend the United States when it is sued in a federal trial court. Primarily, then, they function as prosecutors for the federal government, with considerable discretion in deciding which criminal cases to prosecute. In civil cases the U.S. attorneys have the authority to determine which cases to try to settle out of court and which ones to take to trial. The U.S. attorney is in a very good position to influence the federal district court's docket.

The other major federal participants in prosecution or litigation, federal district judges, are in a position to exert both direct and indirect influence over U.S. attorneys and their assistants.[17] Judges may decide which types of cases U.S. attorneys will prosecute and how they will actually argue their cases in court. One judicial scholar writes that U.S. attorneys and assistant attorneys "inevitably shape their behavior to conform to the predilections of the judge hearing the case." [18]

Since U.S. attorneys and judges within a district must work together on an ongoing basis, their relationship is extremely important. In some districts the relationship may be close and informal, while in other districts the atmosphere may be more businesslike. Although many factors play a role, one leading study notes that a close rapport between the judge and the U.S. attorney is most likely in a small district because of the close physical proximity of their offices. At the other extreme, "large districts must institutionalize procedures for scheduling cases and arranging the docket, cutting the occasions for informal contact." [19] Regardless of the working arrangement, U.S. attorneys engage in more litigation in the federal district courts than anyone else. Therefore, they and their staffs are vital participants in the policies fashioned in the federal trial courts.

**Prosecutors at the State Level.** Those who prosecute persons accused of violating state criminal statutes are commonly known as *district attorneys*. In most states they are elected county officials; however, in a few states they are appointed. The district attorney's office usually employs a number of assistants who do most of the actual trial work. Most of these assistant district attorneys are recent graduates of law school and are using the position to gain trial experience. Many will later enter private practice, often as criminal defense attorneys. Others will seek to become district attorneys or perhaps judges after a few years.

The district attorneys' office is characterized by a great deal of discretion in the handling of cases. Given budget and personnel constraints, not all cases can be afforded the same amount of time and attention. Therefore, some cases are dismissed, others are not prosecuted, and still others are prosecuted vigorously in court. Most cases, however, are subject to plea bargaining. This means that the district attorney's office agrees to accept the defendant's plea of guilty to a reduced charge or to drop other charges against the defendant. (Plea bargaining will be discussed at greater length in Chapter 6.)

District attorney's offices are organized in different ways. Some use what is known as the horizontal, or zone, model. This model, often found in heavily populated areas, assigns assistants to different steps in the judicial process. Some will screen cases as they enter the prosecutor's office. Others will be assigned to courts to deal with bond hearings, probable-cause hearings, misdemeanor cases, or felony cases. Still others will specialize in presenting cases to the grand jury. Those assigned to a particular courtroom become a part of the courtroom work group and interact more with other courtroom work group members than with the assistant prosecutors who have other assignments.[20]

A second organizational model, found frequently in smaller jurisdictions, is the vertical prosecution model. In this scheme each assistant is fully responsible for an assigned caseload. This means that one person receives the case when it is filed and follows it through to a final disposition.

Finally, some jurisdictions use a mixed model, which attempts to combine the best features of the other two models. Routine cases are likely to be handled in a horizontal model, and certain types of cases call for the vertical mode. For instance, the district attorney's office may establish bureaus to deal with organized crime, repeat offenders, drug trafficking, or other special problems. Such bureaus are staffed with persons having special training or experience in the particular areas.

*Public Defenders.*   Quite often the person charged with violating a state criminal statute is unable to pay for the services of a defense attorney. In some areas a government official known as a *public defender* bears the responsibility for indigent defendants. Thus, the public defender is a counterpart of the prosecutor. Unlike the district attorney, however, the public defender is usually appointed rather than elected.

In some parts of the country there are statewide public defender systems; in other regions the public defender is a local official, usually associated with a county government. In New York City an independent organization known as the Legal Aid Society represents all indigent criminal defendants except those charged with murder.[21] New York's Legal Aid Society also has a civil division.

Like the district attorney, the public defender employs assistants and investigative personnel. Furthermore, there is a great deal of similarity to the prosecutor's office in the organizational scheme used by public defenders. Some are organized horizontally, some vertically, and some in a mixed model.

*Other Government Lawyers.*   At both the state and federal levels there are government attorneys who are better known for their work in appellate courts than in trial courts. For example, each state has an attorney general who supervises a staff of attorneys that are charged with the responsibility of handling the legal affairs of the state. At the federal level the Department of Justice has similar responsibilities on behalf of the United States.

*The U.S. Department of Justice.*   Although the Justice Department is an agency of the executive branch of the government, it has a natural association with the judicial branch. Many of the cases heard in the federal courts involve the national government in one capacity or another. Sometimes the government is sued, while in other instances the government initiates the lawsuit. In either case, an attorney must represent the government. Most of the litigation involving the federal government is handled by the Justice Department, although a number of other government agencies have attorneys on their payrolls.

The Justice Department has several key divisions. The Office of Solicitor General is extremely important in cases argued before the Supreme Court. There are also seven legal divisions within the Justice Department: Antitrust, Civil, Civil Rights, Criminal, Internal Security, Land and Natural Resources, and Tax; each has a staff of specialized lawyers and is headed by an assistant attorney general. The seven legal divisions supervise the handling of litigation by the U.S. attorneys, take cases to the courts of appeals, and aid the solicitor general's office in cases argued before the Supreme Court.

*U.S. Solicitor General.* The solicitor general of the United States, the third-ranking official in the Justice Department, is assisted by five deputies and about twenty assistant solicitors general. The solicitor general's primary function is to decide, on behalf of the United States, which cases will and will not be presented to the Supreme Court for review. Whenever an executive branch department or agency loses a case in one of the courts of appeals and wishes a Supreme Court review, that department or agency will formally request that the Justice Department seek certiorari. The solicitor general will determine whether to appeal the lower-court decision.

Naturally, there are many factors to be taken into account when making such a decision. A former solicitor general, Wade H. McCree, Jr., explained what he thought was the most important consideration:

> I have to be aware of the fact that when I am asked to seek certiorari there is a limit to the number of cases that the Supreme Court can hear. I have to ask myself, "Is this one of the 250 most important cases that the Supreme Court will be asked to hear this year?"

McCree went on to say that in the previous year the Supreme Court had received 3,715 petitions for certiorari, only 68 of which were submitted by the Justice Department. Furthermore, he noted that 72 percent of the Justice Department's petitions for certiorari were granted, whereas only 6 percent of the total 3,715 petitions were granted.[22]

In addition to deciding whether to seek Supreme Court review of a particular lower-court decision, the solicitor general personally argues most of the government's cases heard by the High Court. However, there are some kinds of cases that the solicitor general may feel are more appropriately argued by a person who holds a particular office in government.

Another former solicitor general, Rex E. Lee, pointed out that the "tradition has been that the hardest cases—the most important cases— usually are argued by the Solicitor General." [23]

Although the solicitor general works for the attorney general and serves at the pleasure of the president, it has traditionally been argued that this official "must have the independence to exercise his craft as a lawyer on behalf of the institution of government without being a mouthpiece for the President." [24] During the Reagan administration, however, some suggested that the solicitor general's office became more politicized and, under Reagan's appointee Charles Fried, tried to press for the Reagan social and political agenda. [25]

State Attorneys General. Each state has an attorney general who serves as its chief legal official. In most states this official is elected on a partisan statewide ballot. The attorney general oversees a staff of attorneys who primarily handle the civil cases involving the state. Although the prosecution of criminal defendants is generally handled by the local district attorneys, the attorney general's office often plays an important role in investigating statewide criminal activities. Thus, the attorney general and his or her staff may work closely with the local district attorney in preparing a case against a particular defendant.

The attorney general does not usually control appeals in the state courts as the solicitor general does in the federal courts. Furthermore, the state attorney general normally argues cases before the state supreme court only when a state agency is involved in the case.

The state attorneys general also perform the important function of issuing advisory opinions to state and local agencies; many of these agencies simply cannot afford their own legal staff. Quite often, the attorney general's opinion will interpret an aspect of state law not yet ruled on by the courts. Although the advisory opinion might eventually be overruled in a case brought before the courts, the attorney general's opinion is important in determining the behavior of state and local agencies.

### Private Lawyers in the Judicial Process

In criminal cases in the United States the defendant has a constitutional right to be represented by an attorney. As we noted above, some jurisdictions have established public defender's offices to represent indigent defendants. In other areas, there will be some method of assigning a private attorney to represent a defendant who cannot afford to hire one. Those defendants who can afford to hire their own lawyer will of course do so.

In civil cases neither the plaintiff nor the defendant is constitutionally entitled to the services of an attorney. However, in the civil arena the legal issues are often so complex as to demand the services of an attorney. Various forms of legal assistance are usually available to those who need help.

*Assigned Defense Counsel.* In many jurisdictions throughout the country, especially rural areas, some method of appointing a private lawyer to represent an indigent defendant is the standard procedure. Usually the assignment is made by an individual judge on an ad hoc basis. Local bar associations or lawyers themselves often provide the courts with a list of attorneys who are willing to provide such services. Compensation for providing representation for an indigent defendant is generally based on a flat rate for hours spent in and out of court. The fee varies from area to area, and often according to the case's complexity. At any rate, it is usually a good deal less than an attorney would earn for providing services to a private client.

*Private Defense Counsel.* Some attorneys in private practice specialize in criminal defense work. Such lawyers are more often found in solo practices or in small firms than in the large law firms. Although the personal and private lives of criminal defense attorneys are depicted as rather glamorous on television, the average real-life criminal defense lawyer works long hours for low pay and low prestige.[26]

One of the major worries of the criminal defense attorney is getting paid. The clients are usually poor and often not very trustworthy; therefore, the criminal defense lawyer generally requires payment of a part of the fee in advance. Often, this is all the lawyer will collect. So the average criminal defense attorney must handle a large number of cases in order to survive. The large volume of cases in turn means that the attorney must spend a great deal of time in court and in the office juggling cases. All told, the lawyer who specializes in criminal defense work typically leads a rather hectic life.

## Legal Aid Services

Although criminal defendants are constitutionally entitled to be represented by a lawyer, those who are defendants in a civil case or who wish to initiate a civil case do not have the right to representation. That means, then, that those who do not have the funds to hire a lawyer may find it difficult to obtain justice.

In order to deal with this problem, legal aid services of one sort or another are now found in many areas. Legal aid societies were established in New York and Chicago as early as the late 1880s, and many other major cities followed suit in the twentieth century. Although some legal aid societies are sponsored by bar associations, most are supported by private contributions. There are also legal aid bureaus associated with charitable organizations in some areas. In addition, many law schools operate legal aid clinics to provide both legal assistance for the poor and valuable training for law students.

As part of President Lyndon B. Johnson's War on Poverty, Congress in 1965 authorized federal funding for legal aid for the poor through the Office of Economic Opportunity. Under this legislation neighborhood law offices were established to provide legal services for indigents. By 1973 there were some 5,000 lawyers working at over 900 legal services offices throughout the country.[27]

Among other things, these lawyers were successful in forcing local and federal agencies to pay welfare benefits to poor persons as mandated by law; in forcing public schools to admit children of illegal aliens; in forcing public hospitals to provide free abortions to indigent women; and in forcing officials to improve jail conditions. While some applauded the work of the legal services attorneys, others were less than thrilled with their activities.

In 1974 Congress created the Legal Services Corporation, which administers grants to a number of local agencies that provide legal help to the poor. Generally, these local agencies establish law offices to which clients can come for help. The work of the Legal Services lawyers seems to be concentrated in five main areas: family, consumer, housing, landlord-tenant relationships, and welfare.[28] Shortly after becoming president in 1981, Ronald Reagan began to move to have Congress cut off funding for the Legal Services Corporation. Although Congress refused, it did significantly cut the corporation's budget.

One other source of legal help for indigents deserves mention. Many lawyers provide legal services *pro bono publico* ("for the public good") because they see it as a professional obligation.

What about people who are not indigent but are still too poor to hire a competent private attorney? Two relatively low cost methods are available: legal clinics and prepaid legal plans.

A legal clinic is "simply a high-volume, high-efficiency law firm."[29] These clinics depend upon advertising and publicity to generate clients and keep costs down by relying on standard forms and delegating most of the routine work to paralegals (nonlawyers who are specifically trained to handle many of the routine aspects of legal work). The legal clinics concentrate on such fairly common legal problems as divorces, traffic offenses, personal bankruptcies, and wills.

Prepaid legal plans, also referred to as legal insurance plans, may be financed in two ways. One method is to enroll a group of people such as a labor union. A second method is simply to sign up individuals. Some plans make available a designated lawyer or group of lawyers from whom the client may choose. Other plans allow the client to choose any lawyer; however, there is usually a limit on how much of the attorney's fee will be covered.

Labor unions have been most active in organizing prepaid legal plans. A plan established by the United Auto Workers, which covers 150,000 Chrysler employees, retired employees, and their families, is probably the largest currently operating in the United States.[30]

Although legal insurance is often compared with medical insurance, the growth of the former will probably never rival that of the latter. Individuals in the United States simply do not consider their need for legal insurance to be as critical as their need for medical protection.

## Litigants

In this section we take a brief look at the parties who are involved in the cases taken before the courts. In some instances the litigants are individuals, whereas in other cases one or more of the litigants may be a government agency, a corporation, a union, an interest group, or a university. In short, almost any individual or group has the potential to become a litigant in the courts.

What motivates a person or group to take a grievance to court? In criminal cases the answer to this question is relatively simple. A state or federal criminal statute has allegedly been violated and the government prosecutes the party charged with violating the statute. In civil cases the answer is not quite so easy, however. While some persons readily take their grievances to court, many others avoid this route because of the time and expense involved. Still, enough cases are filed annually to cause concern about how the federal and state courts can manage their dockets.

In his recent study of the U.S. Supreme Court, Lawrence Baum concludes that the motives of litigants before that tribunal take two general forms: "ordinary" litigation and "political" litigation.[31] Baum's conclusions apply to other courts as well.

Political scientist Phillip Cooper points out that judges are called upon to resolve two kinds of disputes: private law cases and public law controversies. Private law disputes are those in which one private citizen or organization sues another. Public law controversies involve the government more directly. In these situations a citizen or organization contends that a government agency or official has violated a right established by a constitution or statute. Cooper goes on to state that "legal actions, whether public law or private law contests, may either be policy oriented or compensatory." [32]

A classic example of private, or ordinary, compensation-oriented litigation occurs when a person injured in an automobile accident sues the driver of the other car in an effort to win monetary damages to compensate him for the medical bills he had to pay. Quite obviously, this type of litigation is personal and is not aimed at changing governmental or business policies.

Some private law cases, however, are policy oriented or political in nature. Personal injury suits and product liability suits may appear on the surface to be simply compensatory in nature, but in reality may also be used to change the manufacturing or business practices of the private firms being sued. A good example may be found in *Greenman v. Yuba Power Products, Inc.*, a case decided by the California Supreme Court.[33] In that case, the plaintiff was injured while using a Shopsmith (a combination power tool that can be used as a saw, a drill, or a wood lathe) that his wife had given him as a Christmas present. He had used the lathe several times without difficulty, when a piece of wood suddenly flew out of the machine and struck him on the forehead, causing serious injuries. Substantial evidence was introduced at the trial to indicate that the plaintiff's injuries were caused by defective design and construction of the Shopsmith. The plaintiff was awarded damages in the amount of $65,000, and the verdict was upheld on appeal. In short, not only was the plaintiff compensated for his injuries, but the manufacturer was also forced to reconsider the design and construction of the product.

Most political or policy-oriented lawsuits, however, are public law controversies. That is, they are suits brought against the government primarily to stop allegedly illegal policies or practices. They may, of course, also seek damages or some other specific form of relief. A case decided by the Oregon Supreme Court, *Thornburg v. Port of Portland*, provides a good example.[34] The plaintiffs, who lived close to the Portland International Airport, complained that the noise from jet aircraft made their land unusable. They contended that since their land was no longer usable it had in effect been taken by the government agency and they should be compensated for their loss. The Oregon Supreme Court agreed with this contention.

Political or policy-oriented litigation is more prevalent in the appellate courts than in the trial courts and is most common in the Supreme Court. Ordinary compensatory litigation is often terminated early in the judicial process because the litigants find it more profitable to settle their dispute or accept the verdict of a trial court. On the other hand, litigants in political cases generally do little to advance their policy goals by gaining victories at the lower levels of the judiciary. Instead, they prefer the more widespread publicity that is attached to a decision by an appellate tribunal. Pursuing cases in the appellate courts is expensive; therefore, many lawsuits that reach this level are supported in one way or another by interest groups.

## Interest Groups in the Judicial Process

Although interest groups are probably better known for their attempts to influence legislative and executive decisions, they also pursue their policy goals in the courts. In fact, some groups have found the judicial branch to be far more receptive to their efforts than either of the other two branches of government. Interest groups that do not have the economic resources to mount an intensive lobbying effort in Congress or a state legislature may find it much easier to hire a lawyer and find some constitutional or statutory provision upon which to base a court case. Likewise, a small group with few registered voters among its members may lack the political clout to exert much influence on legislators and executives. Large memberships and political clout are not prerequisites for filing cases in the courts, however.

Interest groups may also turn to the courts because they find the judicial branch more sympathetic to their policy goals than the other two branches. The National Association for the Advancement of Colored People (NAACP) provides an excellent example. This group, which dates from the early twentieth century, soon realized that Congress and the executive branch were not very sympathetic to the struggle for civil rights of black citizens. Seeing the courts as potentially more sympathetic, the NAACP started to focus its efforts on litigation as a means of achieving its goals. As the Supreme Court became more favorable to civil rights after 1937, the NAACP began to realize the value of the judiciary as a forum for its activities and eventually established the Legal Defense Fund, a separate organization, to engage in litigation.

Following the pattern established by the NAACP, other minority group organizations began to use the courts. Cases dealing with the rights of Hispanics and women came to be pursued vigorously by groups such as the Mexican-American Legal Defense and Education Fund and the National Organization for Women.

Throughout the 1960s interest groups with liberal policy goals fared especially well in the federal courts. In addition, the public interest law firm concept, attributed to Ralph Nader, gained prominence during this period. The public interest law firms pursue cases that serve the public interest in general—including cases in the areas of consumer rights, employment discrimination, occupational safety, civil liberties, and environmental concerns.

With the coming of the 1970s and the increasing conservatism of the federal courts stemming from President Nixon's appointment strategy, some major changes began to take place in the interaction between interest groups and the judiciary. For one thing, conservative interest groups have become more frequent users of the federal courts than they were.[35] This is in part a reaction to the successes of liberal interest groups. It is also due, of course, to the increasingly favorable forum that the federal courts provide for conservative viewpoints. This latter trend has persisted throughout the 1980s because of President Reagan's success in placing judges on the federal bench who shared his conservative policy views.

The 1970s and 1980s have also seen predominantly liberal interest groups seeking forums other than the federal courts in which to pursue their policy goals. Some take their battles to the legislative branch while others now prefer to file their cases in state courts rather than in the federal courts. For instance, at a recent conference on the mentally retarded citizen and the law it was suggested that lawyers might explore the state courts in future suits on behalf of the mentally retarded.[36]

Interest group involvement in the judicial process may take several different forms depending upon the goals of the particular group. However, two principal tactics stand out: involvement in test cases and presentation of information before the courts through *amicus curiae* briefs.

## Test Cases

Since the judiciary engages in policy making only through decisions in specific cases, one favorite tactic of interest groups is to make sure that a case appropriate for obtaining its policy goals is brought before the court. In some instances this means that the interest group will initiate and totally sponsor the case by providing all the necessary resources. Undoubtedly, the best-known example of this type of sponsorship is to be found in the *Brown v. Board of Education* case.[37] In that case, although the suit against the Board of Education of Topeka, Kansas, was filed by the parents of Linda Brown, the NAACP supplied the legal help and money necessary to pursue the case all the way to the Supreme Court, where Thurgood Marshall (currently a U.S. Supreme Court justice) argued the case on behalf of the plaintiff and the NAACP. The result was certainly a personal victory for the Browns, who wanted their daughter to be able to attend a desegregated public school. However, the NAACP gained a much broader victory through the Supreme Court's decision that segregation in the public schools violates the equal protection clause of the Fourteenth Amendment.

Interest groups may also provide assistance in a case initiated by someone else, but which nonetheless raises issues of importance to the group. A good example of this situation may be found in a famous freedom of religion case, *Wisconsin v. Yoder*.[38] That case was initiated by the state of Wisconsin when it filed criminal complaints charging Jonas Yoder and others with failure to send their children to school until the age of sixteen as required by state law. Yoder and the others, members of the Amish faith, believed that education beyond the eighth grade led to the breakdown of the values they cherished and to "worldly" influences on their children.

An organization known as the National Committee for Amish Religious Freedom (NCARF), which had been formed in 1965 by non-Amish ministers, bankers, lawyers, and professors to defend the right of the Amish to pursue their way of life, came to the defense of Yoder and the others. The NCARF provided William R. Ball as defense attorney, as well as a number of expert witnesses who testified on behalf of the Amish.

Following a decision against the Amish in the trial court, the NCARF appealed to a Wisconsin circuit court, which upheld the trial court's decision. An appeal was made to the Wisconsin Supreme Court, which ruled in favor of the Amish, saying that the compulsory school attendance law violated the free exercise of religion clause of the First Amendment. Wisconsin then appealed to the U.S. Supreme Court, which on May 15, 1972, sustained the religious objection that the NCARF had raised to the compulsory school attendance laws.

Thus, even though the NCARF did not initiate the litigation, it found its test case and pursued it through four courts to obtain its objective. Without the actions of the NCARF the religious freedom interests of the Amish might not have been adequately presented, especially at the appellate level, since the Amish generally refused to defend themselves in litigation.

As the above examples illustrate, the bulk of the literature on interest group involvement in litigation has focused on cases involving major constitutional issues that have reached the Supreme Court. Since only a small percentage of cases ever reach the nation's highest court, however, most of the work of interest group lawyers deals with more routine work at the lower levels of the judiciary. Rather than fashioning major test cases for the appellate courts, attorneys may simply be required to deal with the legal problems of their groups' clientele.

A recent study of the routine activities of three litigation-oriented civil rights groups active in Mississippi in the mid-1960s provides some interesting insights.[39] For one thing, the authors found that although the lawyers associated with the Lawyers Committee for Civil Rights under Law, the Lawyers Constitutional Defense Committee, and the NAACP Legal Defense Fund evidently preferred to litigate in the federal courts, a majority of their work took place in the state and local tribunals. However, most of the cases involving issues at the heart of the civil rights movement, such as demonstrations, school desegregation, voting rights, and public accommodations, were litigated in the federal courts. The activities of these attorneys covered a wide variety of needs. In addition to litigating major civil rights questions, they also defended blacks and civil rights workers who ran into difficulties with the local authorities. These interest groups, then, performed many of the functions of a specialized legal aid society: they provided legal representation to those involved in an important movement for social change. Furthermore, they performed the all-important function of drawing attention to the plight of black citizens by keeping cases before the courts.

## Amicus Curiae Briefs

Submission of amicus curiae ("friend of the court") briefs is the easiest method by which interest groups can become involved in cases. Consequently, it is also the most common form of group involvement. This method allows a group to get its message before the court even though it does not control the case. Provided it has the permission of the parties to the case or the permission of the court, an interest group may submit an amicus brief to supplement the arguments of the parties.

Sometimes these briefs are aimed at strengthening the position of one of the parties in the case. When the Wisconsin v. Yoder case was argued before the U.S. Supreme Court, the cause of the Amish was supported by amicus curiae briefs filed by the General Conference of Seventh Day Adventists, the National Council of Churches of Christ in the United States, the Synagogue Council of America, the American Jewish Congress, the National Jewish Commission on Law and Public Affairs, and the Mennonite Central Committee.[40] All supported exemption of the Amish from the compulsory school attendance laws.

As might be expected, some cases attract amicus briefs supporting both parties in the case. For example, when the abortion cases were argued before the Supreme Court in 1973, there were forty-seven amicus curiae briefs filed, some of which could be classified as proabortion and others as antiabortion.[41] Another case that attracted an unusually large number of amicus briefs was Regents of the University of California v. Bakke, in which medical school admissions policies reserving a certain percentage of seats for minority applicants were declared unconstitutional.[42] Of the 120 amicus curiae briefs filed in that case, 32 were in opposition to the admissions policy and 83 were in favor of it; 5 dealt with other issues.[43]

Sometimes "friend of the court" briefs are used not to strengthen the arguments of one of the parties but to suggest to the court the group's own view of how the case should be resolved. A classic example of this occurred in Mapp v. Ohio.[44] When that case was presented to the Supreme Court the argument by the parties focused (1) on the issue of whether someone should be convicted for "mere possession" of obscene material and (2) on the "shocking" nature of the search that led to the discovery of the material. However, the defendant's lawyer did not urge a change in the ruling that improperly seized evidence could still be used in the trial. Instead, the exclusionary issue was raised in the amicus curiae brief filed by the American Civil Liberties Union and the Ohio Civil Liberties Union.[45] The Supreme

Court, without dealing with the obscenity issue, handed down a landmark constitutional decision excluding illegally seized evidence from trials in state courts (the exclusionary rule). Thus, it was the interest group's argument that provided the policy view adopted by the Supreme Court.

Scholars have recently begun to pay more attention to the fact that amicus curiae briefs are often filed in an attempt to persuade an appellate court to either grant or deny review of a lower-court decision. A recent study of the U.S. Supreme Court found, for instance, that the presence of amicus briefs significantly increased the chances that the Court would give full treatment to the case and concluded that "interested parties can have a significant and positive impact on the Court's agenda by participating as amici curiae prior to the Court's decision on certiorari or jurisdiction." [46]

We also need to pay special attention to the role of the government as a "friend of the court." Unlike private interest groups, all levels of the government can submit briefs without obtaining permission. The solicitor general of the United States is especially important in this regard. One study says that in recent years the solicitor general has filed an amicus brief in about one-third of all Supreme Court cases.[47] In some instances the Supreme Court may invite the solicitor general to present an amicus brief. It seems clear, then, that the Supreme Court values the input of the solicitor general's office.

As we noted earlier, the solicitor general is far more successful than private litigants in getting acceptance for certiorari petitions. It also appears that the solicitor general's amicus briefs in support of others' certiorari petitions are quite successful.[48]

We should note in closing our discussion of amicus curiae briefs that the filing of such briefs is a tactic used in appellate rather than trial courts. Furthermore, the literature on "friend of the court" participation deals almost exclusively with the federal courts although amicus briefs may be used in state appellate courts as well.

## Summary

This chapter has laid the groundwork for later chapters, which deal more extensively with the steps involved in the judicial process. Here, our focus has been on three important actors in the judicial process: lawyers, litigants, and interest groups.

The development of the legal profession was traced from its beginnings in colonial days to the contemporary practice of law. Our discussion focused on the stratification of the legal profession and the various types of lawyers who practice in the United States. Singled out for special emphasis were the government lawyers who are primarily involved in handling cases in the state and federal trial and appellate courts.

We next turned our attention to those who become litigants in our nation's courts. In some cases the adversaries are ordinary litigants who are primarily concerned with being compensated for their losses. At other times, the combatants are involved in political litigation and have as their major goal influencing public policy. Still other cases feature litigants who are interested in both personal compensation and exerting some influence over public policy.

The chapter concluded with an examination of the role of interest groups in the judicial process. Following a brief look at the reasons groups become involved in litigation we turned our attention to the major strategies and tactics used by interest groups in the judicial arena: involvement in test cases and the use of amicus curiae briefs.

## *Notes*

1. Our discussion draws heavily upon Lawrence M. Friedman, *A History of American Law*, 2d ed. (New York: Simon & Schuster, 1985).
2. Ibid., 97.
3. Ibid., 101.
4. Ibid., 306.
5. Ibid., 321.
6. Ibid., 607.
7. *Bates v. State Bar*, 433 U.S. 350 (1977).
8. Barbara A. Curran, "American Lawyers in the 1980s: A Profession in Transition," *Law and Society Review* 20 (1986): 49.
9. Ibid., 27.
10. See Erwin O. Smigel, *The Wall Street Lawyer: Professional Organization Man* (Glencoe, Ill.: Free Press, 1964).
11. *ABA Journal*, August 1, 1986, 28.
12. "Law Poll," *ABA Journal*, September 1, 1986, 44.
13. *ABA Journal*, August 1, 1986, 28.
14. Howard Abadinsky, *Law and Justice* (Chicago: Nelson Hall, 1988), 121.
15. For a good case study of the firing of a U.S. attorney, see Howard Ball, *Courts and Politics: The Federal Judicial System* (Englewood Cliffs, N.J.: Prentice-Hall, 1980), 202-206.
16. For an in-depth analysis of the appointment process for U.S. attorneys, see James Eisenstein, *Counsel for the United States: U.S. Attorneys in the Political and Legal Systems* (Baltimore: Johns Hopkins University Press, 1978), chap. 3.
17. A detailed study of the relationship between U.S. attorneys and federal district judges may be found in Eisenstein, *Counsel for the United States*, chap. 7.
18. Ibid., 133.
19. Ibid., 147.
20. See James Eisenstein and Herbert Jacob, *Felony Justice* (Boston: Little, Brown, 1977).
21. Abadinsky, *Law and Justice*, 129.
22. "Interview with Solicitor General Wade H. McCree, Jr.," *The Third Branch* 12 (August 1980): 3.

23. For a fuller discussion of this matter, see "Interview with Solicitor General Rex E. Lee," *The Third Branch* 14 (May 1982): 5.

24. Lincoln Caplan, "The Tenth Justice," pt. 1, *New Yorker*, August 10, 1987, 40.

25. See Caplan, "The Tenth Justice," pt. 1, 41-58, and pt. 2, *New Yorker*, August 17, 1987, 30-62. Also see Stephen L. Wasby, *The Supreme Court in the Federal Judicial System*, 3d ed. (Chicago: Nelson Hall, 1988), 146-147.

26. See Paul Wice, *Criminal Lawyers: An Endangered Species* (Beverly Hills, Calif.: Sage, 1978).

27. Abadinsky, *Law and Justice*, 133.

28. Steven Vago, *Law and Society*, 2d ed. (Englewood Cliffs, N.J.: Prentice-Hall, 1988), 277.

29. Ibid.

30. Ibid., 278.

31. Lawrence Baum, *The Supreme Court*, 2d ed. (Washington, D.C.: CQ Press, 1985), 73-75.

32. Phillip J. Cooper, *Hard Judicial Choices* (New York: Oxford University Press, 1988), 13.

33. 59 Cal. 2d 57 (1963).

34. 233 Or. 178 (1962).

35. See Karen O'Connor and Lee Epstein, "The Rise of Conservative Interest Group Litigation," *Journal of Politics* 45 (May 1983): 479-489, and Lee Epstein, *Conservatives in Court* (Knoxville: University of Tennessee Press, 1985).

36. See Ronald K. L. Collins, "Reliance on State Law: Protecting the Rights of People with Mental Handicaps," in *The Legal Rights of Citizens with Mental Retardation*, ed. Lawrence A. Kane, Jr., Phyllis Brown, and Julius S. Cohen (Lanham, Md.: University Press of America, 1988), 170-187. Also see Edward A. Kopelson, "State Law, Judicial Review and the Rights of People with Disabilities," in ibid., 188-204.

37. 347 U.S. 483 (1954).

38. 406 U.S. 205 (1972). Also see the excellent discussion of this case in Richard C. Cortner, *The Supreme Court and Civil Liberties Policy* (Palo Alto, Calif.: Mayfield, 1975), 153-182. Our discussion is based on this study.

39. See Joseph Stewart, Jr., and Edward V. Heck, "The Day-to-Day Activities of Interest Group Lawyers," *Social Science Quarterly* 64 (March 1983): 173-182.

40. See Cortner, *The Supreme Court and Civil Liberties Policy*, 169-170.

41. Ibid., 53-54.

42. 438 U.S. 265 (1978).

43. Henry R. Glick, *Courts, Politics, and Justice*, 2d ed. (New York: McGraw-Hill, 1988), 151.

44. 367 U.S. 643 (1961).

45. See Wasby, *The Supreme Court in the Federal Justice System*, 151-152.

46. Gregory A. Caldeira and John R. Wright, "Organized Interests and Agenda Setting in the U.S. Supreme Court," *American Political Science Review* 82 (December 1988): 1122.

47. Glick, *Courts, Politics, and Justice*, 156.

48. See Robert Scigliano, *The Supreme Court and the Presidency* (New York: Free Press, 1971), 176.

# 5 Jurisdiction, Workload, and Policy-Making Boundaries of Federal and State Courts

In setting out the jurisdictions of courts, Congress and the U.S. Constitution—and their state counterparts—mandate the types of cases each court can hear. Our examination of the courts' legal boundaries includes a discussion of a related topic: a court's workload, or the number of cases a court hears and the types of dispositions available to it. In Chapter 2 we began our survey with the supreme courts and proceeded to the appeals and trial courts. In this chapter we shall reverse the order, since the flow of litigation is in the opposite direction—from the bottom layer, the trial courts, upward through the appellate levels.

Because the role of legislative bodies in setting courts' jurisdictions is an ongoing one, we will consider how Congress in particular can influence judicial behavior by redefining the types of cases judges can hear. The chapter will close with a discussion of judicial self-restraint; we will examine ten principles, derived from legal tradition and constitutional and statutory law, that govern a judge's decision about whether to review a case.

## Federal Courts

### U.S. District Courts

In the United States Code Congress has set forth the jurisdiction of the federal district courts. These tribunals have *original jurisdiction* in federal criminal and civil cases—that is, by law, the cases must be first heard in these courts, no matter who the parties are or how significant the issues.

*Criminal Cases.* For the twelve-month period ending June 30, 1985, some 38,245 criminal cases were commenced in the federal district courts, up 21 percent over the past twenty years. These were cases for which the local U.S. attorneys had reason to believe that a violation of the U.S. Penal Code had occurred.

After first obtaining an indictment from a federal grand jury, the U.S. attorney files charges against the accused in the district court in which he or she serves. Criminal activity as defined by Congress covers a wide range of behavior, including interstate theft of an automobile, failure to register with Selective Service, illegal importation of narcotics, assassination of a president, conspiracy to deprive persons of their civil rights, and even the killing of a migratory bird out of season. For the past decade or so the most numerous types of criminal code violations have been embezzlement and fraud, larceny and theft, drunk driving and other traffic offenses, drug-related offenses, and forgery and counterfeiting. Some federal crimes, such as robbery, are comparatively uniform in occurrence in each of the ninety-four U.S. judicial districts, whereas others are endemic to certain geographic areas. For example, those districts next to the U.S. borders get an inordinate number of immigration cases, and districts in the southern states have had more than their share of criminal violations of the civil rights laws.

For fiscal 1987, the government reported that there was a 4 percent increase in criminal filings over the previous year. This increase resulted primarily from additional prosecutions for fraud, drunk driving, traffic offenses, and drug violations. Fraud prosecutions were up by 10 percent, due primarily to increases in postal fraud and fraud relating to lending institutions. Drunk driving and traffic offenses rose 8 percent, after declining 9 percent in 1986. Prosecutions under the Drug Abuse Prevention and Control Act jumped 12 percent, to 8,869 cases, and accounted for 21 percent of all criminal case filings. Such cases involved 17,120 defendants, or approximately 30 percent of all criminal defendants.[1]

After charges are filed against an accused, and if there is no plea bargain, a trial is conducted by a U.S. district judge. In court the defendant enjoys all the privileges and immunities granted in the Bill of Rights (such as "the right to a speedy and public trial") or by congressional legislation or Supreme Court rulings (for instance, a twelve-person jury must render a unanimous verdict). As noted in Chapter 2, defendants may waive the right to a trial by a jury of their peers. A defendant who is found not guilty of the crime is set free and may never be tried again for the same offense (the Fifth Amendment's protection against double jeopardy). If the accused is found guilty, the district judge determines the appropriate sentence within a range set by Congress. The length of a sentence is not appealable so long as it is within the range prescribed by Congress. A verdict of not guilty may not be appealed by the government, but convicted defendants may appeal if they believe that the judge or jury made an improper legal determination.

*Civil Cases.* The lion's share of the district court caseload is of a civil nature—that is, suits between private parties or between the U.S. government, acting in its nonprosecutorial capacity, and a private party. In 1985 a whopping 273,670 civil cases were commenced in the district courts, representing more than 87 percent of their total caseload. As Table 5-1 reveals, the size of the civil docket has increased dramatically—not only in comparison with criminal cases but in absolute terms. The increase in civil filings increased more than 73 percent in the years between 1965 and 1975, and

Table 5-1   Cases Commenced in the U.S. District Courts: 1965, 1975, and 1985

|  | 1965 | 1975 | 1985 | Percent change 1965-1975 | Percent change 1975-1985 |
|---|---|---|---|---|---|
| U.S. civil | 19,092 | 26,732 | 111,226 | 40.0 | 316.1 |
| Private civil | 40,698 | 71,281 | 128,976 | 75.2 | 80.9 |
| Prisoner petitions |  |  |  |  |  |
| Federal | 2,559 | 5,047 | 6,262 | 97.2 | 24.0 |
| State | 5,329 | 14,260 | 27,206 | 167.6 | 90.8 |
| Total Civil | 67,678 | 117,320 | 273,670 | 73.4 | 133.3 |
| Criminal | 31,569 | 43,282 | 38,245 | 37.1 | −11.6 |
| Total | 99,247 | 160,602 | 311,915 | 61.9 | 94.2 |
| Number of authorized judgeships | 288 | 396 | 571 | 37.5 | 44.2 |

Source: *Annual Report of the Director of the Administrative Office of the U.S. Courts,* 1965, 1975, and 1985 (Washington, D.C.: Government Printing Office).

then jumped 133.3 percent between 1975 and 1985. By comparison criminal filings actually declined by more than 11 percent in the most recent ten-year period.

Civil cases that originate in the U.S. district courts may be placed in one of several categories. The first covers litigation involving the interpretation or application of the Constitution, acts of Congress, or U.S. treaties in which at least $50,000 is at stake. Examples of cases in this category would include the following: a petitioner claims that one of his federally protected civil rights has been violated, a litigant alleges that she is being harmed by a congressional statute that is unconstitutional, or a plaintiff argues that he is suffering injury from a treaty that is improperly affecting him. The key point is that a *federal* question must be involved in order for the U.S. trial courts to have jurisdiction. It is not enough to say that the federal courts should hear a case "because there is an important issue involved" or "because an awful lot of money is at stake." Unless one is able to invoke the Constitution or a federal law or treaty, the case must be litigated elsewhere (probably in the state courts).

The jurisdictional amount of $50,000 is waived if the case falls into one of several categories which by law must be adjudicated by the federal courts regardless of the dollar amount in controversy. For example, an alleged violation of a civil rights law, such as the Voting Rights Act of

1965, must be heard by the federal rather than the state judiciary. Other types of cases in this category are patent and copyright claims, passport and naturalization proceedings, admiralty and maritime disputes, and violations of the U.S. postal laws.

Another broad category of cases over which the U.S. trial courts exercise general original jurisdiction are known as diversity of citizenship disputes—that is, the parties are from different states, or the dispute is between an American citizen and a foreign country or citizen. Thus if a citizen of New York were injured in an automobile accident in Chicago by a driver from Illinois, the New Yorker could sue in federal court, since the parties to the suit were of "diverse citizenship." The requirement that at least $50,000 be at stake in diversity cases does not appear to be much of a barrier to the gates of the federal judiciary: even if actual injuries come to less than $50,000, one can always ask for "psychological damages" to push the amount in controversy above the jurisdictional threshold.

Federal district courts also have jurisdiction over petitions from convicted prisoners who contend that their incarceration (or perhaps their denial of parole) is in violation of their federally protected rights. In the vast majority of these cases prisoners ask for what is termed a *writ of habeas corpus*—that is, an order issued by a judge to determine whether a person has been lawfully imprisoned or detained. The judge would demand that the prison authorities either justify the detention or release the petitioner.

Prisoners convicted in a state court must take care to argue that a *federally protected* right was violated—for example, the right to be represented by counsel at trial. Otherwise the federal courts would have no jurisdiction. Federal prisoners have a somewhat wider range for their appeals, since all their rights and options are within the penumbra of the U.S. Constitution. Petitions from state and federal prison inmates constituted about 12 percent of the total civil caseload in 1985—2 percent from federal prisoners and 10 percent from those hosted by state institutions.

Finally, the district courts have the authority to hear any other cases that Congress may validly prescribe by law. For example, while the Constitution grants to the U.S. Supreme Court original jurisdiction to hear "Cases affecting Ambassadors, other public Ministers and Consuls," Congress has also authorized the district courts to have concurrent original jurisdiction over cases involving such parties.

## U.S. Courts of Appeals

The U.S. appellate courts have no original jurisdiction whatsoever: every case or controversy that comes to one of these intermediate-level panels has been first argued in some other forum. As indicated in Chapter 2, these tribunals, like the district courts, are the creations of Congress, and their structure and functions have varied considerably over time. As Table 5-2 reveals, in 1965 only 6,766 cases found their way into one of the regional circuit courts, whereas by 1975 this figure had jumped to 16,658 cases—an increase of more than 146 percent. During the past decade the number of filings has continued to mount but at a somewhat slower rate. In 1985, 33,360 cases were commenced in one of the twelve U.S. appellate courts. As with the district courts, the increase in civil cases has outstripped those of a criminal nature. During the past decade the number of criminal cases was up 19.2 percent, whereas the number of civil cases climbed by more than 90 percent.

Basically there are two general categories of cases over which Congress has granted the circuit courts appellate jurisdiction. The first of these are ordinary civil and criminal appeals from the federal trial courts, including the U.S. territorial courts, the U.S. Tax Court, and some District of Columbia courts. In criminal cases the appellant is the defendant because the government is not free to appeal a verdict of "not guilty." (However, if the question in a criminal case is one of defining the legal right of the defendant, then the government may appeal an adverse trial court ruling.) For civil cases it is usually the party that lost in the trial court that is the appellant, although it is not unheard of for the winning party to appeal if it is not satisfied with the lower-court judgment. The U.S. government, acting in its private capacity, is a party to about 18 percent of the civil appeals, while 42 percent are between totally private parties. Prisoners' petitions also constitute a significant portion of the appeals from adverse rulings of trial jurists. In 1985, 23 percent of the civil appeals from the lower federal courts were centered on prisoners' petitions.

The second broad category of appellate jurisdiction centers on appeals from certain federal administrative agencies and departments and also from the important independent regulatory commissions, such as the Securities and Exchange Commission and the National Labor Relations Board. In 1985, 11 percent of the civil docket consisted of administrative appeals. Because so many of the administrative and regulatory bodies have their home base in Washington, the appeals court for that circuit gets an inordinate number of such cases.

## U.S. Supreme Court

The U.S. Supreme Court is the only federal court mentioned by name in the Constitution, which spells out the general contours of the High Court's jurisdiction. Although we usually think of the Supreme Court as an appellate tribunal, it does have some general *original* jurisdiction. Proba-bly the most important area of such jurisdiction is a suit between two or more states. For example, every so often the states of Texas and Louisiana spar in the Supreme Court over the proper boundary between them. By

Table 5-2   Cases Commenced in the U.S. District Courts: 1965, 1975, and 1985

|  | 1965 | 1975 | 1985 | Percent change 1965-1975 | Percent change 1975-1985 |
|---|---|---|---|---|---|
| U.S. civil | 803 | 1,426 | 5,234 | 77.6 | 267.0 |
| Private civil | 2,255 | 5,631 | 11,805 | 149.7 | 109.6 |
| Prisoner petitions | | | | | |
| Federal | 584 | 1,555 | 1,510 | 166.3 | −2.9 |
| State | 422 | 880 | 5,022 | 108.5 | 470.7 |
| Bankruptcy | 217 | 246 | 1,046 | 13.4 | 325.2 |
| Administrative appeals | 1,106 | 2,290 | 3,179 | 107.1 | 38.8 |
| D.C. Court of Appeals | 8 | — | — | — | — |
| Original proceedings | 148 | 443 | 575 | 199.3 | 29.8 |
| Total civil | 5,543 | 12,471 | 28,371 | 127.6 | 90.3 |
| Criminal | 1,223 | 4,187 | 4,989 | 242.4 | 19.2 |
| Total | 6,766 | 16,658 | 33,360 | 146.2 | 100.3 |
| Number of authorized judgeships | 78 | 97 | 156 | 24.4 | 60.8 |

Source: *Annual Report of the Director of the Administrative Office of the U.S. Courts,* 1965, 1975, and 1985 (Washington, D.C.: Government Printing Office).

law the Sabine River divides the two states, but with great regularity this effluent changes its snaking course, thus requiring the Supreme Court (with considerable help from the U.S. Army Corps of Engineers) to determine where Louisiana ends and the Lone Star State begins.

In addition the High Court shares original jurisdiction (with the U.S. district courts) in certain cases brought by or against foreign ambassadors or consuls, in cases between the United States and a state, and in cases commenced by a state against citizens of another state or against aliens. In situations such as these, where jurisdiction is shared, the courts are said to have *concurrent jurisdiction.*

Cases over which the Supreme Court has original jurisdiction are often important, but they do not represent a sizable portion of the overall caseload. In 1985 the High Court's docket consisted of 5,158 cases, but only 10 of these (a mere one-fifth of 1 percent) were heard on original jurisdiction.

The U.S. Constitution declares that the Supreme Court "shall have appellate Jurisdiction . . . under such Regulations as the Congress shall make." Over the years Congress has passed much legislation setting forth the "Regulations" under which cases may appear before the nation's most august judicial body. In essence, there are two main avenues through which appeals may reach the Supreme Court. First, there may be appeals from all lower federal constitutional and territorial courts and also from most, but not all, federal legislative courts. Second, the Supreme Court may hear appeals from the highest court in a state—as long as there is a "substantial federal question" involved.

When Congress passed the Judiciary Act of 1925, it gave the Supreme Court a great deal of discretion over which cases to hear on appeal. Nevertheless, Congress still required the Court to decide a number of specific cases that it believed were of primary national importance—for instance, when a court of appeals found that a state law was invalid because it conflicted with the U.S. Constitution or a federal law or treaty. Since 1925 many Supreme Court justices have lobbied the Congress to give the Court complete and total discretion over its appellate docket. In 1988 the justices were successful, when Congress passed Public Law 100-352, which completely abolished the Supreme Court's mandatory appellate jurisdiction. (In May of 1988 Chief Justice Rehnquist wrote that the elimination of the Supreme Court's mandatory jurisdiction was "the primary legislative goal of the Court.") [2]

Today most of the High Court's docket consists of cases in which it has agreed to issue a writ of certiorari—a discretionary action. Such a writ (which must be supported by at least four justices) is an order from the Supreme Court to a lower court demanding that it send up a complete record of a case so that the Supreme Court can review it. Historically the Supreme Court has agreed to grant the petition for a writ of certiorari in only a tiny portion of cases—usually less than 10 percent of the time.

There is another method by which the Supreme Court exercises its appellate jurisdiction: *certification*. This procedure occurs when one of the appeals courts asks the Supreme Court for instructions regarding a question of law. The justices may choose to give the appellate judges binding instructions, or they may ask that the entire record be forwarded to the Supreme Court for review and final judgment.

All in all, roughly half the litigation that arrives on the Supreme Court's doorstep are "paid cases"—that is, cases for which the appellant was able to pay the cost of the filing fee and of the multiple copies of required documents. The other half are in the form of paupers' petitions filed by indigent persons for whom the filing fee and the multiple-copy requirements are waived. Over three-quarters of the paupers' petitions are filed by inmates in federal and state prisons.

The overall caseload of the Supreme Court is high by historical standards, although since about 1975 the rate of increase seems to be declining (see Table 5-3). In 1965, 2,774 cases filled the Court's docket; this

Table 5-3    Cases Commenced in the U.S. Supreme Court: 1965,
1975, and 1985

|  | 1965 | 1975 | 1985 | Percent change 1965-1975 | Percent change 1975-1985 |
|---|---|---|---|---|---|
| Appellate docket | 1,188 | 2,398 | 2,571 | 101.9 | 7.2 |
| Miscellaneous docket | 1,578 | 2,324 | 2,577 | 47.3 | 10.9 |
| Original docket | 8 | 8 | 10 | 0.0 | 25.0 |
| Total | 2,774 | 4,730 | 5,158 | 70.5 | 9.1 |
| Number of authorized judgeships | 9 | 9 | 9 | 0.0 | 0.0 |

Source: Annual Report of the Director of the Administrative Office of the U.S. Courts, 1965, 1975, and 1985 (Washington, D.C.: Government Printing Office).

number jumped by over 70 percent, to 4,730 cases, by 1975. However, the number of cases commenced in the High Court was 5,158 ten years later—an increase of just over 9 percent.

One student of the trend in Supreme Court caseloads has speculated about the causes of the leveling off in workload after 1973. He concluded that

there is no way to determine if this marks a fundamental (long-term) change in caseload pattern or not. However, it does stand out as a variation and there may be some significance to it in the long term. What may have caused this fluctuation is certainly not apparent. Perhaps economic and social conditions changed in such a way that filings were dampened. People may have found alternative arenas in which to settle some kinds of disputes, which the Court did not appear amenable to hearing. . . . It may also be that potential litigants perceived that the Court would not be persuadable to their particular policy demands. Thus, the Court was not a viable policymaking body for these groups and interests. Certainly the Burger Court has been relatively conservative on some matters that would have received a liberal treatment by the Warren Court. Thus, these interests may have been "forced" to seek alternative remedies. It is possible that many of the social and civil liberties demands that were raised in the 1950s and 1960s have been resolved favorably and fewer such demands are being made on the Court now that the essential foundation of rights and liberties has been established. This explanation does not seem intuitively correct as many interests would normally seek to build on the foundation begun in the Warren Court, expand on these initial victories to reach new rights for new segments of the population, and thus have to litigate a large variety of claims—perhaps more specific than during the Warren years.[3]

Perhaps the key point to remember about the workload of the Supreme Court is that for all practical purposes the tribunal has time to consider on the merits only a few hundred cases per year and to write full opinions in only about 150. These figures have remained fairly constant for well over fifty years. What this means is that most appeals to the Supreme Court will never be considered by the high tribunal; in fact, the number of signed opinions constitutes less than 3 percent of all cases presented to the Court. Many angry litigants may exclaim, "I'll take my case all the way to the Supreme Court." Maybe so, but the odds are against it.

## Jurisdiction and Workload of State Courts

The lion's share of the nation's judicial business exists at the state, not the national, level. The fact that federal judges adjudicate over 300,000 cases a year is impressive; the fact that state courts handle well over 60 *million* is overwhelming, even if the most important cases are handled at the federal level. It is true that justice of the peace and magistrate courts at the state level handle relatively minor matters. However, the largest court judgment in recorded history—over $10 billion in the Texaco-Pennzoil case—was decided by an ordinary state trial court.

Table 5-4 presents the best guess of the eminent National Center for State Courts about the workload of our state judiciaries in a recent year; concrete, reliable figures for the state courts are somewhat hard to come by. Recordkeeping by some states is much better than others, and there is great variation among the justice of the peace courts, which are ordinarily not courts of record. Likewise, comparability between states is a problem. For example, in State X the request by an attorney for lawyer's fees may be considered as merely another motion in the case that is being litigated. However, in State Y such a motion may be recorded as a separate issue and hence as a separate case. Still, it is clear that our state judiciaries handle an enormous number of cases: they process over 99 percent of all litigation in the United States in any given year. As with the federal courts, the vast majority of the cases are civil, although it is often the criminal cases that receive more publicity. Two-thirds of all cases at the state level deal with traffic offenses.

One also needs to emphasize that much public policy making in the United States is done by state judges; put another way, the decisions of state jurists frequently have a great impact on public policy. For example, during the 1970s a number of suits were brought into federal court challenging the constitutionality of a state's spending vastly unequal sums on the education of its school children. (This occurred because poorer

Table 5-4   Number of Cases Filed in the State Courts, 1984

| Court | Cases |
|---|---|
| Trial Courts | |
| Civil | 13,580,067 |
| Criminal | 7,367,219 |
| Traffic | 39,847,432[a] |
| Juvenile | 1,172,750[b] |
| Total | 61,967,468 |
| Appellate Courts | |
| Courts of last resort | 55,977 |
| Intermediate appellate courts | 119,021 |
| Total, all state courts | $62,142,466 |

Source: National Center for State Courts, State Court Caseload Statistics: Annual Report, 1984 (Williamsburg, Va.: National Center for State Courts, 1986), tables 1, 8, 12, and 13.
[a] Data from sixteen states and Puerto Rico not included.
[b] Figure omits data from eight states.

school districts could obviously not raise the same amount of money as could wealthy school districts.) The litigants claimed that children in the poorer districts were victims of unlawful discrimination in violation of their equal protection rights under the U.S. Constitution. The Supreme Court said not, however, in a conservative-dominated five-to-four decision.[4] But the matter did not end there. Litigation was then instituted in many states arguing that unequal educational opportunities were in violation of various clauses in the state constitutions. As this is written, the courts in the states of Arizona, California, Kansas, Michigan, Minnesota, New Jersey, and Texas have agreed and have rendered decisions that have pushed their respective state legislatures in the direction of reforming their methods of financing state education. Indeed there is considerable evidence that in recent years many minority groups and supporters of liberal causes, unable to obtain relief in the face of conservative Burger and Rehnquist Court majorities, have turned their litigation efforts toward the state judiciaries. For the constitutional guarantees in most states are just as supportive of the rights of minorities as is the U.S. Constitution, and the judiciaries in many states are dominated by liberal and progressive judges who are every bit as much predisposed toward the claims of minorities and civil libertarians as any liberal justice who ever sat on the Warren Court of the 1950s and 1960s.

## Jurisdiction and Legislative Politics

In any discussion of the jurisdiction of the federal and state courts, there is one political reality that cannot be overemphasized: to all intents and purposes it is the Congress and the fifty state legislatures that determine what sorts of issues and cases the courts in their separate realms will hear. And equally important, what the omnipotent legislative branches give, they may also take away. It is true that some judges and judicial scholars argue that the U.S. Constitution (in Article III) and the respective state documents confer a certain inherent jurisdiction upon the judiciaries in some key areas, independent of the legislative will. Nevertheless, it is abundantly clear that the jurisdictional boundaries of American courts are a product of legislative judgments—determinations often flavored with the bittersweet spice of politics. We shall look at a few examples of this at the national level.

As we shall see in subsequent chapters, Congress may advance a particular cause by giving courts the authority to hear cases in a public-policy realm that theretofore had been forbidden territory for the judiciary. For example, when Congress passed the Civil Rights Act of 1968, it gave judges the authority to penalize individuals who interfere with "any person because of his race, color, religion or national origin and because he is or has been . . . traveling in . . . interstate commerce" (18 U.S.C.A., Sec. 245). Prior to 1968 the courts had no jurisdiction over incidents that stemmed from interference by one person with another's right to travel. Likewise Congress may consider withdrawing certain subject matters from judicial purview. For instance, in the more conservative mood in which the United States has bathed itself since the 1970s, Congress has passed legislation that has sought to remove the authority of judges to order busing as a means of achieving school integration.

Perhaps the most vivid illustration of congressional power over federal court jurisdiction occurred just after the Civil War, and the awesome nature of this legislative prerogative haunts the judiciary to this day. On February 5, 1867, Congress empowered the federal courts to grant habeas corpus to individuals imprisoned in violation of their constitutional rights. The Supreme Court was authorized to hear appeals of such cases. William McCardle was incarcerated by the military government of Mississippi for being in alleged violation of the Reconstruction laws. McCardle was alleged to have published "incendiary and libelous" articles that attacked his "unlawful restraint by military force." He sought relief in the circuit court but it was denied. He then appealed to the Supreme Court, which agreed to take the case.

After the arguments had been made before the High Court (but prior to a decision), Congress got into the act. Its antisouthern majority feared that the court would use the *McCardle* case as a vehicle to strike down all or part of the Reconstruction Acts—something Congress had no intention of permitting. And so, over President Andrew Johnson's veto, the following statute was enacted: "That so much of the act approved February 5, 1867 [as] authorized an appeal from the judgment of the Circuit Court to the Supreme Court of the United States, or the exercise of any such jurisdiction by said Supreme Court, on appeals which have been, or may hereafter be taken, [is] hereby repealed." Thus, while the court was in the very process of deciding the case, Congress removed the subject matter from the federal docket. And was all this strictly legal and constitutional? Yes, indeed. Stunned by Congress's action but obedient to the clear strictures of the Constitution, the Court limply ruled that McCardle's appeal must now "be dismissed for want of jurisdiction." [5]

In other words, while discussing what courts do or may do, we must not lose sight of the commanding reality that the jurisdiction of U.S. courts is established by "the United States of America in Congress assembled." Likewise at the state level, the jurisdictions of the courts in the states are very much governed by—and the political product of—the will of the state legislatures.

## Judicial Self-Restraint

We will now look at the other side of the coin—at the activities that judges are forbidden to do, or at least discouraged from doing. These forbidden activities deal not so much with technical matters of jurisdiction but with the broader term that courts call *justiciability*—that is, the question of whether judges in the system *ought* to hear or refrain from hearing certain types of disputes. It is only by exploring both sides of the demarcation line between prescribed and proscribed activity that we can acquire insight into the role and function of our federal and state courts. In the following sections we shall look at ten separate aspects of judicial self-restraint, ten principles that serve to check and contain the power of American judges. [6] These maxims originate in a variety of sources—the U.S. and state Constitutions, acts of Congress and of state legislatures, the common law tradition—and whenever possible we shall indicate their roots and the nature of their evolution. Some apply more to appellate courts than to trial courts, as we shall note. Although the primary examples provided will be illustrative of the federal judiciary, most apply to state judicial systems as well.

### A Definite Controversy Must Exist

The U.S. Constitution states that "the judicial Power shall extend to all Cases, in Law and Equity, arising under this Constitution, the Laws of the

United States, and Treaties made . . . under their Authority" (Article III, Section 2). The key word here is *cases*. Since 1789 the federal courts have chosen to interpret the term in its most literal sense—that is, that there must be an actual controversy between legitimate adversaries who have met all the technical legal standards to institute a suit. The dispute must involve the protection of a meaningful, nontrivial right or the prevention or redress of a wrong that directly affects the parties to the suit. There are two corollaries to this general principle that breathe a little life into its rather abstract-sounding admonitions.

The first is that the federal courts do not render advisory opinions—that is, rulings about situations that are hypothetical or that have not evoked an actual clash between adversaries. A dispute must be real and current before a court will agree to accept it for adjudication. Let us look at an example in which the Court refused to involve itself in a dispute because the facts and would-be parties were not considered "real." In 1902 Congress passed a law allocating certain pieces of land to the Cherokee Indians. Because such disbursements often stimulate a good deal of questions about property rights, Congress sought to head off any possible disputes over land by authorizing certain land recipients to bring suits against the U.S. government in the court of claims, with appeal to the Supreme Court. They were permitted to do so "on their own behalf and on behalf of all other Cherokee citizens" who received land "to determine the validity of any acts of Congress passed since the said act." Stripped of the legalese, the law thus said: "If you have any hypothetical questions about how the law might affect anyone, just sue the United States, and the courts will answer these questions for you." The Supreme Court politely but pointedly said, "We don't do that sort of thing; we settle only real, actual cases or controversies." The act of Congress was found to be nothing more

> than an attempt to provide for judicial determination, final in this court, of the constitutional validity of an act of Congress. [It] is true the United States is made a defendant to this action, but *it has no interest adverse to the claimants*. The object is not to assert a property right as against the government, or to demand compensation for alleged wrongs because of action on its part. . . . In a legal sense the judgement [amounts] to no more than an expression of opinion upon the validity of the [1902 act]. If such actions as are here attempted [are] sustained, the result will be that this court, instead of keeping within the limits of judicial power, and deciding cases or controversies arising between opposing parties, [will] be required to give opinions in the nature of advice concerning legislative action—a function never conferred upon it by the Constitution. [Emphasis added.][7]

A second corollary of the general principle is that the parties to the suit must have proper *standing*. This notion deals with the matter of *who* may bring litigation to court. While there are many aspects to the term *standing*, the most prominent component is that the person bringing suit must have suffered (or be immediately about to suffer) a direct and significant injury. As a general rule, a litigant cannot bring a claim on behalf of others (except for parents of minor children, or in special types of suits called *class actions*). In addition, the alleged injury must be personalized and immediate—not part of some generalized complaint.

In 1974 a case reached the Supreme Court in which a group of anti-Vietnam War protesters sued the secretaries of defense, the army, the navy, and the air force. They asked that members of Congress be enjoined from serving in the Armed Forces Reserve. Their claim was based on the constitutional stricture that "no Person holding any Office under the United States shall be a Member of either House during his continuance in Office" (Article I, Section 6). The members of Congress who were officers in the reserve were clearly in violation of the Constitution; no one ever seemed to question this fact. But where was the injury that would enable these particular litigants to make a court case out of the violation? The antiwar group contended that members of Congress who held a reservist position under control of the executive branch might be subject to undue influence by the president. Also, reserve membership was said to place upon members of Congress possible inconsistent obligations that might cause them to violate their duty faithfully to perform either or both of their two functions. As citizens, the protesters were concerned, and they asked the Court to grant them standing to sue. The court refused in a six-to-three ruling. Despite the fact that an apparent violation of both the letter and spirit of the Constitution was in progress, no one was directly or personally injured enough to create sufficient standing to sue. As the decision noted,

> the Court [has] held that whatever else the "case or controversy" requirement embodied, its essence is a requirement of "injury in fact." This personal stake is what the Court has consistently held enables a complainant authoritatively to present to a court a complete perspective upon the adverse consequences flowing from the specific set of facts undergirding his grievance. . . . [All] citizens, of course, share equally an interest in the independence of each branch of government. In some fashion, every provision of the Constitution was meant to serve the interests of all. [But the] proposition that all constitutional provisions are enforceable by any citizen simply because citizens are ultimate beneficiaries of those provisions has no boundaries.[8]

Thus we have one great principle of judicial self-restraint, of what most judges may not do. They may not decide an issue unless there is an actual case or controversy. From this it follows that they do not consider abstract, hypothetical questions, nor do they take a case unless the would-be litigants can demonstrate direct and substantial personal injury. This principle is an important one because it means that judges are not free to wander about the countryside like medieval knights slaying all the evil dragons they encounter. They may rule only on concrete issues brought by truly injured parties directly affected by the facts of a case.

Although federal judges do not rule on abstract, hypothetical issues, many state courts are permitted to do so in some form or other (such as those in Massachusetts, South Dakota, and Colorado).[9] Federal legislative courts (see Chapter 2) may give advisory opinions as well. Also, American judges are empowered to render what are termed *declaratory judgments*. Such judgments are made in actual controversies in which a court is called on to define the rights of various parties under a statute, a will, or a contract. The judgments do not entail any type of coercive relief. As Justice Rehnquist once put it, "A declaratory judgment is simply a statement of rights, not a binding order." [10] The federal courts were given the authority to act in this capacity in the Federal Declaratory Judgment Act of 1934, and about three-fourths of the states grant their courts this power. Although there is a real difference between an abstract dispute that the federal courts (at least) must avoid and a situation where a declaratory judgment is in order, in the real world the line between the two is often a difficult one for the jurists to draw.

## A Plea Must Be Specific

Another constraint upon the judiciary is that judges will hear no case on the merits unless the petitioner is first able to cite a specific part of the Constitution as the basis of the plea. For example, the First Amendment forbids government from making any laws "prohibiting the free exercise" of religion. Recently Robert Dale Callahan from Santa Rosa, California, won a lawsuit against state and federal authorities who insisted that a Social Security number be issued to Callahan's daughter. Social Security identification is required for those wishing to receive welfare benefits, which Callahan had requested for his child. The father, a man of fundamentalist religious beliefs, argued that any universal number used to designate human beings are "the mark of the beast" as described in the Bible's Book of Revelations. In other words, Callahan argued, the government regulation imposed an unreasonable burden on the free exercise of his religion. The government of course responded that an exemption for Callahan's daughter would "impede the goal of government efficiency." [11] Despite what we may think about the substantive wisdom of the court's ruling in favor of Callahan, there is little doubt that the specific criteria for securing judicial review had been met: the Constitution specifically forbids the government from prohibiting the free exercise of one's religion; the litigant in question held a "serious religious belief" that the government regulation struck at the very heart of the values and practices of his faith.

On the other hand, if one went into court and contended that a particular law or official action "violated the spirit of the Bill of Rights" or "offended the values of the Founders," a judge would dismiss the proceeding on the spot. For if judges were free to give concrete, substantive meaning to vague generalities such as these, there would be little check on what they could do. Who is to say what is the "spirit of the Bill of Rights" or the collective motivation of those who hammered out the Constitution? Judges who were free to roam too far from the specific clauses and strictures of the constitutional document itself would soon become judicial despots.

Despite what we have just said, we must also concede that in the real world this principle is not as simple and clear cut as it sounds, because the Constitution contains many clauses that are open to a wide variety of interpretations. For example, the Constitution forbids Congress from creating any law "respecting an establishment of religion," but few can agree exactly what the term *establishment* means. The Eighth Amendment prohibits "excessive bail" for criminal defendants, but what is *excessive?* The states are forbidden, in the Fourteenth Amendment, Section 1, from abridging "the privileges and immunities of citizens of the United States," but who is to say what these privileges and immunities are? The Constitution gives hardly a clue. Our point is that although petitioners must cite a particular constitutional clause as the basis for their plea— as opposed to some totally ambiguous concept—there are nevertheless enough vague clauses in the Constitution itself to give federal judges plenty of room to maneuver and make policy.

### Beneficiaries May Not Sue

A third aspect of judicial self-restraint is that a case will be rejected out of hand if it is apparent that the petitioner has been the beneficiary of a law or an official action that he or she has subsequently chosen to challenge. Let us suppose that Farmer Brown had long been a member of the Soil Bank Program (designed to cut back on grain surpluses); under the program he agreed to take part of his land out of production and periodically was paid a subsidy by the federal government. After years as a participant he learns that his lazy, ne'er-do-well neighbors, the Joneses, are also drawing regular payments for letting their farmland lie fallow. The idea that his neighbors are getting something for nothing starts to offend Farmer Brown, and he begins to harbor grave doubts about the constitutionality of the whole program. Armed with a host of reasons why Congress had acted illegally, Brown challenges the legality of the Soil Bank Act in the local federal district court. As soon as it is brought to the judge's attention that Farmer Brown had himself been a member of the program and had gained financially from it, the suit is dismissed: one may not benefit from a particular governmental endeavor or official action and subsequently attack it in court.

## Appellate Courts Rule on Legal— Not Factual—Questions

In the real world it is often very difficult to tell whether a particular legal dispute concerns who did what to whom (the facts of the case) or how one is to weigh and assess a series of events (the legal interpretation of the facts). Nevertheless a working proposition of state and federal appellate court practice is that these courts will not hear cases if the grounds for appeal are that the trial judge or jury wrongly amassed and identified the basic factual elements of the case. It is not that trial judges and juries always do a perfect job of making factual determinations. Rather, there is the belief that they are closer, sensorially and temporally, to the actual parties and physical evidence of the case. The odds are, so the theory goes, that they will do a much better job of making factual assessments than would an appellate body reading only a stale transcript of the case some months or years after the trial. On the other hand, legal matters—that is, which law(s) one is to apply to the facts of the case, or how one is to assess the facts in light of the prevailing law—are appropriate for appellate review. On such issues collegial, or multijudge, appellate bodies presumably have a legitimate and better capacity "to say what the law is," as Chief Justice John Marshall put it. Let us look at an illustration.

If X were convicted of a crime and the sole grounds for her appeal were that the judge and jury had mistakenly found her guilty (that is, incorrectly sifted and identified the facts), the appeals court would dismiss the case out of hand. However, let us assume that X provided evidence that she had asked for and been refused counsel during her FBI interrogation and that her confession was therefore illegal. At trial the district judge ruled that the Sixth Amendment (providing for "the Assistance of Counsel") did not apply to X's interrogation by the FBI. The defendant argued to the contrary. Such a contention would be appealable because the issue is one of legal—not factual—interpretation.

The fact that U.S. appellate courts are restricted to interpreting the law and not to identifying and assembling facts is one additional check on the scope of their decision making.

## The Supreme Court Is Not Bound by Precedents

If the High Court is free to overturn or circumvent past and supposedly controlling precedents when it decides a case, this might appear to be an argument for judicial activism—not restraint. In fact, however, this practice must be placed in the restraint column. If the Supreme Court were totally bound by the dictates of its prior rulings, it would have very little flexibility. It would not be free to back off when discretion advised a cautious approach to a problem; it would not have liberty to withdraw from a confrontation in which it might not be in the nation's or the Court's interest to engage. By occasionally allowing itself the freedom to overrule a past decision or to ignore a precedent that would seem to be controlling, the Supreme Court establishes a corner of safety to which it can retreat if need be. When wisdom dictates that the Court change direction or at least keep an open mind, this principle of self-restraint is readily plucked from the judicial kit bag.

## Other Remedies Must Be Exhausted

There is another principle of self-restraint that often frustrates the anxious litigant but is essential to the orderly administration of justice: courts in the United States will not accept a case until all other remedies, legal and administrative, have been exhausted. While this caveat is often associated with the U.S. Supreme Court, it is in fact a working principle for virtually all American judicial tribunals—namely, that one must work up the ladder with one's legal petitions. In its simplest form this doctrine means that federal cases must first be heard by the U.S. trial courts, then reviewed by one of the appellate tribunals, and finally heard by the U.S. Supreme Court. This orderly procedure of events must and will occur despite the "importance" of the case or of the petitioners who filed it. For instance, in 1952 President Truman seized the American steel mills in order to prevent a pending strike which he believed would imperil the war effort in the Korean conflict; both labor and management were suddenly told they were now working for Uncle Sam. The mill owners were furious and immediately brought suit, charging that the president had abused the powers of his office. A national legal-political crisis erupted. One might think that the Supreme Court would immediately grasp a case of this magnitude. Not so. In the traditional and orderly fashion of American federal justice, the controversy first went to the local district court in Washington, D.C., just as if it were the most ordinary dispute. After the district court had ruled, the case was appealed to the circuit court, and only after that did the nation's highest tribunal receive the chance to sink its teeth into this hearty piece of judicial meat.

Exhaustion of remedies refers to possible administrative relief as well as to adherence to the three-tiered judicial hierarchy. Such relef might be in the form of an appeal to an administrative officer, a hearing before a board or committee, or formal consideration of a matter by a legislative body. Let us consider a hypothetical illustration. Professor Ben Wheatley is denied tenure at a staunchly conservative institution. He is told that tenure was not granted because of his poor teaching record and lack of scholarly publications. He, however, contends it is in retaliation for his having founded the nearby Sunshine Socialist Society, a nudist colony for gay atheists. While he has the option of a hearing before the university's Grievance Committee, he declines it saying, "It would do no good; it would just be a waste of time." Rather, he takes his case immediately to the local federal district court, claiming that his Fourteenth Amendment rights have been violated. When the case is brought before the trial court, the judge will say in effect to Professor Wheatley: "Before I will even look at this matter, you must first take your case before the official, duly established Grievance Committee at your university. It doesn't matter whether you believe that you will win or lose your petition before the committee. You must establish your record there and avail yourself of all the administrative appeals and remedies that your institution has provided. If you are then still dissatisfied with the outcome, you may at that time invoke the power of the federal district courts."

Thus, judicial restraint means that judges do not jump immediately into every controversy that appears to be important or that strikes their fancy. The restrained and orderly administration of justice requires that before any court may hear a case all administrative and inferior legal remedies must first be exhausted.

## Courts Do Not Decide "Political Questions"

U.S. judges are often called upon to determine the winner of a contested election, to rule on the legality of a newly drawn electoral district, or to involve themselves in voting rights cases. How then can one say that political questions are out of bounds for the American judiciary? The answer lies in the narrow, singular use of the word *political*. To U.S. judges the executive and the legislative branches of government are political in that they are elected by the people for the purpose of making public policy. The judiciary, in contrast, was not designed by the Founders to be an instrument manifesting the popular will and is therefore not political. According to this line of reasoning, then, a political question is one that ought properly to be resolved by one of the other two branches of government (even though it may appear before the courts wrapped in judicial clothing). When judges determine that something is a political question and therefore not appropriate for judicial review, what they are saying in effect is this: "You litigants may have couched your plea in judicial terminology, but under our form of government, issues such as this ought properly to be decided at the ballot box, in the legislative halls, or in the chambers of the executive."

For example, when the state of Oregon gave its citizens the right to vote on popular statewide referendums and initiatives around the turn of the century, the Pacific States Telephone and Telegraph Company objected.[12] (The company feared that voters would bypass the more business-oriented legislature and pass laws restricting its rates and profits.) The company claimed that by permitting citizens directly to enact legislation, the state has "been reduced to a democracy," whereas Article IV, Section 4, of the Constitution guarantees to each state "a Republican Form of Government"—a term that supposedly means that laws are to be made only by the elected representatives of the people—not by the citizens directly. Pacific Telephone demanded that the Court take action. Opting for discretion rather than valor, the High Court refused to rule on the merits of the case, declaring the issue to be a political question. The Court reasoned that since Article IV primarily prescribes the duties of Congress, then it follows that the Founders wanted Congress—not the courts—to oversee the forms of government in the several states. In other words, the Court was being asked to invade the decision-making domain of one of the other (political) branches of government. And this it refused to do.

In recent decades an important political/nonpolitical dispute has been over the matter of reapportionment of legislative districts. Prior to 1962 a majority on the Supreme Court refused to rule on the constitutionality of legislative districts with unequal populations, saying that such matters were "nonjusticiable" and that the Court dared not enter what Justice Frankfurter called "the political thicket." According to traditional Supreme Court thinking, the Founders wanted legislatures to redistrict themselves—perhaps with some gentle prodding from the electorate. However, with the Supreme Court's decision in *Baker v. Carr*, the majority began to do an about-face.[13] During the past twenty-five years the Court has held in scores of cases that the equal-protection clause of the Fourteenth Amendment requires legislative districts to be of equal population size and furthermore that the courts would see to it that this mandate is carried out.

The refusal of the Supreme Court in recent decades to involve itself in foreign relations has likewise characterized its desire to ignore the siren call of the political realm. For example, during the years of the Vietnam War, the Court repeatedly declined many ardent pleas to rule on the constitutionality of U.S. involvement there.[14] Also, when President Carter acted on his own initiative to end the Mutual Defense Treaty between the United States and Taiwan, this action was challenged in the courts by a number of senators and representatives. The High Court, consistent with its traditions, refused to involve itself in this political question.[15]

Although the line between a taboo political question and a proper justiciable issue is not always a clear one, this doctrine provides the courts with still another opportunity and impetus to exercise restraint.

## The Burden of Proof Is on the Petitioner

Another weighty principle of self-restraint is the general agreement among the nation's jurists that an individual who would challenge the constitutionality of a statute bears the burden of proof. This is just a different way of saying that laws and official deeds are all presumed to be legal unless and until proven otherwise by a preponderance of evidence. The question of who has the burden of proof is of keen interest to lawyers because in effect it means: Which side has the biggest job to perform in the courtroom? and which party must assume the lion's share of the burden of convincing the court—or lose the case entirely? Thus, if one were attacking a particular statute, one would have to do more than demonstrate that it was "questionable" or "of doubtful constitutionality"; one must persuade the court that the evidence against the law was clear-cut and overwhelming—not often an easy task. In giving the benefit of the doubt to a statute or an executive act, judges have yet another area in which to exercise restraint.

## Laws Are Overturned on the Narrowest Grounds Only

Sometimes it becomes clear to a judge during a trial that the strictures of the Constitution have indeed been offended by a legislative or executive act. Even here, however, there is ample opportunity to proceed with caution. There are two common ways in which judges may act in a restrained manner even when they must reach for the blue pencil.

First, a judge may have the option of invalidating an official action on what is called statutory rather than constitutional grounds. Statutory invalidation means that a judge overturns an officials' action because the official acted beyond the authority delegated to him or her by the law. Such a ruling has the function of saving the law itself while still nullifying the official's misdeed.

Let us look at a hypothetical example. Suppose that Congress continues to authorize postal officials to seize all obscene nude photographs that are shipped through the mails. A photographer attempts to mail pictures taken at his "art studio," but the pictures are seized by postal officials. The photographer protests that the statute violates his First Amendment rights and the case is eventually taken to the federal courts. Assuming that the judges are generally sympathetic to the position of the photographer, they have two basic options. They may declare the statute to be in violation of the Constitution and thus null and void, or they may select another stance that permits them to have it both ways. They may decide that the law itself passed constitutional muster, but that the postal official in question mistakenly decided that the nude photos were obscene. Thus the statute is preserved and a direct confrontation between the courts and Congress is averted, but the court is able to give the petitioner virtually all of what he wants. This is an example of deciding a case on statutory rather than constitutional grounds.

There is a second method whereby restraint may be exercised under this general principle: judges may, if possible, invalidate only that portion of a law they find constitutionally defective rather than overturn the entire statute. For instance, in 1963 Congress passed the Higher Education Facilities Act, which provided construction grants for college buildings. Part of the law declared that for a twenty-year period no part of the newly built structures could be used for "sectarian instruction, religious worship, or the programs of a divinity school." Since church-related universities as well as public institutions benefited from the act, the entire law was challenged in court as being in violation of the establishment of religion clause of the First Amendment. The Supreme Court determined that the basic thrust of the law did not violate the Constitution, but it did find the "twenty-year clause" to be objectionable. After all, the Court reasoned, most buildings last a good deal longer than two decades, and a building constructed at public expense could thus house religious activities during the vast majority of its lifetime. Rather than strike down the entire act, however, the court majority merely inserted the word *never* for the phrase *twenty years*.[16] Thus the baby was not thrown out with the bath water and judicial restraint was maintained.

## No Rulings Are Made on the "Wisdom" of Legislation

This final aspect of judicial self-restraint is probably the least understood by the public, the most often violated by the courts, and yet potentially the greatest harness on judicial activism in existence. What this admonition means, if followed strictly, is that the only basis for declaring a law or an official action unconstitutional is that it literally violates the Constitution on its face. Statutes do not offend the Constitution merely because they are unfair, are fiscally wasteful, or constitute bad public policy. Official actions can be struck down only if they step across the boundaries clearly set forth by the Founders. If taken truly to heart, this means that judges and justices are not free to invoke their own personal notions of right and wrong or of good and bad public policy when they examine the constitutionality of legislation.

A keen expression of this phenomenon of judicial self-restraint is found in Justice Potter Stewart's dissenting opinion in the case of *Griswold v. Connecticut*. The Court majority had struck down the state's law which forbade the use of contraceptive devices or the dissemination of birth control information. Stewart said, in effect, that the law was bad, but that its weaknesses didn't make it unconstitutional.

Since 1897 Connecticut has had on its books a law which forbids the use of contraceptives by anyone. I think this is an uncommonly silly law. As a practical matter, the law is obviously unenforceable, except in the oblique context of the present case. . . . But we are not asked in this case to say whether we think this law is unwise, or even asinine. We are asked to hold that it violates the United States Constitution. And that I cannot do.[17]

Another spinoff of this principle is that a law may be passed that all agree is good and wise but that is nevertheless unconstitutional; conversely, a statute may legalize the commission of an official deed that all know to be bad and dangerous but that still does not offend the Constitution. Permitting the police to dispose of "known criminals" without benefit of trial would probably save taxpayers a good deal of money and also reduce the crime rate, but it would be a clear, prima facie violation of the Constitution. On the other hand, a congressional tax on every sex act might be constitutionally permissible but would be a very unwise piece of legislation—not to mention difficult to enforce. Thus when speaking of laws or official acts, the adjectives *goodness* and *constitutionality* are no more synonymous than are *badness* and *unconstitutionality*.

While few legal scholars would disagree with what we have just said, virtually all would point out that the principle of not ruling on the "wisdom" of a law is difficult to follow in the real world and is often honored in the breach. This is so because the Constitution, a rather brief document, is silent on many areas of public life and contains a number of phrases and admonitions that are open to a variety of interpretations—a theme that we shall touch upon continually throughout this text. For instance, the Constitution says that Congress may regulate interstate commerce. But what exactly is commerce, and how extensive does it have to be before it is of an "interstate" character? As human beings, judges have differed in the way they have responded to this question. The Constitution guarantees a person accused of a crime the right to a defense attorney. But does this right continue if one appeals a guilty verdict and, if so, for how many appeals? Strict constructionists and loose constructionists have responded differently to these queries.

Still in all, despite the inevitable intrusion of judges' personal values into their interpretation of many portions of the Constitution, virutally every jurist subscribes to the general principle that laws can be invalidated only if they offend the Constitution—not the personal fancies of the judges.

## Summary

The focus of this chapter has been on what federal and state courts are supposed to do and on what they must refrain from doing. They adjudicate cases that come within their lawful original or appellate jurisdiction. Federal district courts hear U.S. criminal cases and civil suits that deal with federal questions, diversity of citizenship matters, prisoners' petitions, and any other issues authorized by Congress. The appellate courts, having no original jurisdiction whatever, take appeals from the district courts and from numerous administrative and regulatory agencies. The U.S. Supreme Court has original jurisdiction over suits between two or more states and in cases where ambassadors or public ministers are parties to a suit. Its appellate jurisdiction, regulated entirely by Congress, permits it to hear appeals from the circuit courts and from state courts of last resort. Since 1988 Congress has delegated to the High Court the right to control its own appellate caseload. As for state courts, the previous chapter sketched the primary contours of their jurisdictions, but in this chapter we emphasized both the enormity of their caseloads and the great importance of the issues that are adjudicated at the state level.

Under our legal system federal courts are not to adjudicate questions unless there is a real case or controversy at stake, although many state courts may render advisory opinions. All pleas to the courts must be based on a *specific* portion of the Constitution. Judges are also to dismiss suits in which a petitioner is challenging a law from which he or she has benefited. Federal and state appellate courts may rule only on matters of law—not on factual questions. Not being bound entirely by its precedents, the Supreme Court is free to exercise flexibility and restraint if it wishes to do so. All courts insist that litigants exhaust every legal and administrative remedy before a case will be decided. Courts in the United States are to eschew political questions and insist that the burden of proof rests on those who contend that a law or official action is unconstitutional. If judges must nullify an act of the legislature or the executive, they are to do so on the narrowest grounds possible. Finally, courts ought not rule on the wisdom or desirability of a law but are to strike down legislation only if it clearly violates the letter of the Constitution.

## Notes

1. *Annual Report of the Director of the Administrative Office of the United States Courts,* 1987 (Washington, D.C.: Government Printing Office), 5.
2. "Congress Signs Supreme Court Docket Bill," *The Third Branch* 20 (July 1988): 5.
3. William P. McLauchlan, *Federal Court Caseloads* (New York: Praeger, 1984), 69.
4. *San Antonio Independent School District v. Rodriguez,* 411 U.S. 1 (1973).
5. *Ex Parte McCardle,* 74 U.S. (7 Wall.) 506 (1869).
6. For our discussion of the many aspects of judicial self-restraint we acknowledge our debt to Henry J. Abraham, on whose classic analysis of the subject we greatly relied. See *The Judicial Process,* 4th ed. (New York: Oxford University

Press, 1980), chap. 9.

7. *Muskrat v. United States*, 219 U.S. 346 (1911).

8. *Schlesinger v. Reservists Committee to Stop the War*, 418 U.S. 208 (1974).

9. Seven state constitutions expressly impose on their state supreme courts a duty to render advisory opinions (Colorado, Florida, Maine, Massachusetts, New Hampshire, Rhode Island, and South Dakota). In Alabama and Delaware state courts have upheld laws authorizing advisory opinions even in the absence of a constitutional mandate. In North Carolina the power to issue advisory opinions comes from a series of judicial decisions. For a general discussion of this topic, see "The State Advisory Opinion in Perspective," *Fordham Law Review* 44 (1975): 81-113.

10. *Steffel v. Thompson*, 415 U.S. 452 (1974) at 482.

11. William Overend, "Man Who Believes Social Security Numbers Devilish Wins Legal Appeal," *Houston Chronicle*, July 7, 1984, 1:5.

12. *Pacific States Telephone & Telegraph v. Oregon*, 223 U.S. 118 (1912).

13. *Baker v. Carr*, 369 U.S. 186 (1962).

14. *Massachusetts v. Laird*, 400 U.S. 886 (1970).

15. *Goldwater v. Carter*, 444 U.S. 996 (1979).

16. *Tilton v. Richardson*, 403 U.S. 672 (1971).

17. *Griswold v. Connecticut*, 381 U.S. 479 (1965).

# 6   The Criminal Court Process

We now begin the first of two chapters that examine our courts from a judicial process perspective. This chapter looks at the *criminal* process—from the stage when a law is first broken to subsequent stages such as arrest, indictment, trial, and appeal. The next chapter examines the *civil* process on the same step-by-step basis to provide the reader with a sense of how the system looks and feels to the ordinary litigant or observer.

## The Nature and Substance of Crime

"The way you treat me is a crime," a mother scolds her headstrong teenager, who has been rude to her for the umpteenth time that day. We hear comments such as this with some frequency in today's world; although we know what the mother is getting at, we also realize that in the literal sense there has been no crime committed. Being discourteous to one's parents may be wrong and immoral, but in the United States, at least, it is not a crime because it does not violate any specific law. And in realizing this we get a handle on the nature of criminality. An act is not automatically a crime because it is hurtful or sinful; after all, only about half of the Ten Commandments are enforced by criminal law. An action constitutes a true crime only if it specifically violates a criminal statute duly enacted by Congress, a state legislature, or some other public authority.

A good working definition of a *crime*, then, is that it is an offense against the state punishable by fine, imprisonment, or death. A crime is a violation of obligations due the community as a whole and can be punished only by the state. The sanctions of imprisonment and death cannot be imposed by a civil court or in a civil action (although a fine may be either a civil or criminal penalty).

In the United States crimes come in great variety. Most constitute sins of commission, such as aggravated assault and embezzlement; a few consist of sins of omission—failure to stop and render aid after a traffic accident or failure to file an income tax return. Some the state considers serious (such as murder and treason), and this seriousness is reflected in the corresponding punishments such as life imprisonment or the death penalty. Others the state considers only mildly reprehensible (such as double parking or disturbing the peace), and punishments of a light fine or a night in the local jail reflect the official slap on the wrist.

Some crimes constitute actions that virtually all the citizenry consider outside the sphere of acceptable human conduct (such as kidnapping or rape), while other crimes constitute actions on which opinion would be divided—a Nebraska statute that would forbid bingo games at church suppers or the North Carolina sodomy law that instructs couples (even married straights) about which parts of the human body may be touched and how. Other criminal statutes are plain silly. In Wisconsin it is illegal to sing in a bar, and in Louisiana it is forbidden to appear drunk at a meeting of a literary society.

The most serious crimes in the United States are called *felonies*. In a majority of the states a felony is any offense for which the penalty may be death or imprisonment in the penitentiary (a jail is not a penitentiary); all other offenses are misdemeanors or infractions. In other states (and under the U.S. Criminal Code) a felony is an offense for which the penalty may be death or imprisonment for a year or more. Thus, felonies are distinguished in some states according to the *place* where the punishment takes place; in some states and with the federal government the *length* of the sentence is the key factor. Examples of common felonies include murder, forcible rape, and armed robbery.

*Misdemeanors* are regarded as petty crimes by the state, and their punishment usually consists of confinement in a city or county jail for less than a year. Public drunkenness, small-time gambling, and vagrancy are common examples of misdemeanor offenses. Some states have a third category of offense known as infractions. Often they include minor traffic offenses (such as parking violations), and the penalty is usually a small fine. Fines may also be part of the penalty for misdemeanors and felonies.

## Categories of Crime

In thinking about various types of crime it is useful to sort them according to their public policy implications.[1] We shall look at five broad categories that take in the primary offenses against the state in the United States today: conventional, economic, syndicated, political, and consensual.

### Conventional Crimes

Property crimes make up the lion's share of the almost 13 million "conventional" crimes reported annually in the United States. In 1985 the Federal Bureau of Investigation (FBI) determined that 11,102,600 crimes of property were reported to the authorities.[2] Such crimes take in the offenses of burglary, larceny-theft, motor vehicle theft, and arson, the largest group of which was larceny-theft, with over 6 million reported occurrences. Property crimes are distinguished by the FBI from crimes of violence, although in reality the two often go hand in glove. The thief who breaks into a house and who inadvertently confronts a resistant owner is likely to be involved in more than just the property crime of burglary.

The less numerous, but more feared, group of conventional crimes are those against the person. These crimes of violence take in murder and nonnegligent manslaughter, forcible rape, robbery, and aggravated assault. The FBI indicates that in 1985 there were almost three quarters of a million personal assaults reported in the United States and that almost 19,000 persons died at the hands of their assailants.[3]

The overall trend of these conventional crime statistics has not been encouraging over the years. According to the FBI's tally of index crimes, the number of conventional crimes committed in the United States increased from 1,887.2 per 100,000 inhabitants in 1960 to 5,140.3 in 1978, and this jumped to 5,858.2 in 1981 but declined to 5,206.5 in 1985. Although the rate of serious conventional crimes per 100,000 population actually decreased by 1.5 percent between 1976 and 1985, the violent conventional crimes of rape and aggravated assault showed substantial increases.[4]

## Economic Crimes

Most of our thoughts about crime turn toward one of the categories in the above-mentioned lists of conventional criminal activity. We fear having someone break into our homes and hope that the kid who steals our hubcaps is "sent up for a long time." It is to combating these conventional, headline-making crimes that we want most of the nation's police resources devoted. Yet in dollars-and-cents terms, conventional crimes are not where the money is; it is the cost of *economic* crimes that robs the nation blind. In 1974 the Chamber of Commerce estimated that economic crimes cost Americans about $45 billion annually. Corrected for inflation in today's dollars, we are probably looking at an annual price tag of around $100 billion.

What are economic crimes? It would be too narrow to call them merely white collar crimes because such a definition does not take into consideration the fact that many such crimes are committed by persons *outside* their occupations—for example, a person filing a grossly inflated insurance claim. Harold J. Vetter and Leonard Territo list four broad categories of economic crimes that plague the nation.

1. *Personal crimes* consist of nonviolent criminal activity that one person inflicts on another with the hope of monetary gain. Examples include intentionally writing a bad check, cheating on one's income tax, and committing welfare frauds.

2. *Abuse of trust* occurs when business or government employees violate their fidelity to their employer or clients and engage in practices such as these: commercial bribery, theft and embezzlement from the workplace, and filling out false expense accounts.
3. *Business crimes* are crimes that are not actually part of the central purpose of the business enterprise but are rather incidental to (or in furtherance) of it. Misleading advertising, violations of the antitrust laws, and false depreciation figures computed for corporate income tax purposes are all business crimes.
4. *Con games* are white-collar criminal activity committed under the guise of a business. The "magic electric belt" that you can send away for to improve your sex life, or the Ph.D. diploma that you will receive for only $100 and an essay on your life experiences all fall into this category.[5]

Not only are economic crimes extremely costly to the American people, but they have two other characteristics that make them relevant to some of the broader themes of this chapter. First, economic crimes are harder to detect and prove in court than are the more conventional crimes. Convicting a thief who is caught red-handed running out of a jewelry store with a bag of watches and diamonds is a relatively easy and routine endeavor. Not so with most economic crimes. For example, in the fall of 1987 a Harris County (Houston), Texas, commissioner was accused of accepting an illegal gift from a contractor. The contractor, out of the goodness of his heart, had paved a mile-long driveway from the commissioner's home to a nearby highway. "It was just an anniversary gift to me and my wife," said the commissioner. It took two juries (one of them was hung) weeks of testimony and deliberation before the court could finally determine that a crime had in fact been committed.

Because most citizens do not regard economic crimes as serious as burglary or assault, fewer law enforcement resources are earmarked for these illegalities. Also, sentencing judges and juries look much more kindly on the stockbroker whose "misjudgment" caused her to engage in a little illegal insider trading (after all she didn't hurt anyone, did she?) than on the young pickpocket who was caught separating someone from his wallet.

## Syndicated, or Organized, Crimes

Syndicated crime differs from others addressed here in that it is engaged in by groups of people and is often run and directed on some type of hierarchical basis. It represents an ongoing activity that is inexorably entwined with fear and corruption. Organized crime may manifest itself in a variety of ways, but it tends to focus on several areas that are particularly lucrative, namely, trafficking in illegal drugs (such as cocaine or marijuana), gambling, prostitution, and loansharking. The latter is known for its exorbitant interest rates and high repayment rates. (Failure to pay may net the borrower a broken thumb or worse.) Figures are not readily available as to the costs of organized crime, but no one doubts that many billions of dollars are involved.

## Political Crimes

The usual meaning of "political crime" has been that it constitutes an offense against the government: treason, armed rebellion, assassination of public officials, and sedition. However, in recent decades legal scholars have come to use the word to include as well crimes committed *by the government* against individual citizens, dissident groups, and foreign governments or nationals. Examples of this murky category of political crime might include the following: illegal wiretaps and bugging by the FBI of politically dissident groups, much of the Watergate affair and the related "dirty tricks" against opposition candidates, and the illegal selling of weapons to Iran in 1987.

When we think of political crimes and of how judges and juries ought to, and actually do, respond to them, there are a couple of factors that complicate our analysis. One is that ordinary crimes can be committed to make a political point under the guise of what legal scholars call symbolic speech. When antiabortion activists are jailed for blocking the entrance to an abortion clinic, are they being punished for an ordinary act of criminal trespass or for their religious beliefs? When students occupy illegally a university president's office because the college holds investments in South Africa, are the protestors to be treated as mere vagrants or are they crusaders? It is questions such as these that often bedevil the judges and juries who must address the would-be political criminal.

In this same vein, the demarcation between the political crime and its conventional counterpart is often blurred when the government singles out unpopular persons or dissidents for meticulous application of a law that would not be enforced against ordinary folk. An unpopular group of protestors may suddenly find themselves under arrest for parading without a permit or for disorderly conduct, whereas a loud and drunken band of revelers had passed by an hour before without action by the authorities. A minority youth may be arrested for vagrancy or trespassing if he is found walking at night in an all-white neighborhood "where he clearly doesn't belong." The values and attitudes of American judges and juries are sorely tested when such cases appear before them in court.

## Consensual Crimes

A final category is the so-called victimless crime, such as prostitution, gambling, illegal drug use, and unlawful sexual practices between consenting adults. Such crimes are called consensual because both perpetrator and client desire the forbidden activity, but to call them all "victimless" sticks in the throats of many. The children whose parents spend their money and time on drugs rather than on properly caring for them may well regard themselves as victims. And tidy homeowners whose streets suddenly become part of a prostitution circuit and whose shrubbery begins to serve as both bedroom and bathroom may well gag when told that this activity is victimless. Nevertheless, because a great number of Americans question whether many of these consensual activities should in fact be proscribed by the criminal code, great problems are created for law enforcement officials, judges, and juries.

One of our primary themes is that a significant amount of discretion exists at all levels of the judicial process. We also demonstrate that the way in which decision makers exercise this discretion is a function of their values and attitudes. Because attitudes about consensual, or victimless, crimes vary significantly among police officers, the public at large (and the potential jurors they represent), and judges, it is not surprising that studies reveal great differences in the way our judicial system treats participants in consensual criminal activity.

## Elements of a Crime

In theory, at least, every crime contains several distinct elements. Furthermore, unless the state is able to demonstrate in court the existence of these essential elements there can be no conviction. While the judicial process in the courtroom may not focus separately and distinctly on each of these elements, they are at least implicit throughout the entire process of duly convicting someone of a criminal offense.

### A Law Defining
### the Crime and the Punishment

As we have previously indicated, if an act is to be prohibited or required by the law, a duly constituted authority (usually Congress or a state legislature) must properly spell out the matter so that the citizenry can know in advance what conduct is prohibited or required. The lawmakers must also set forth the penalties to be imposed upon the individual who engages in the harmful conduct. If there is no definition of the illegal act, and no penalty prescribed, there is no crime.

Several years ago one of the authors served on a state grand jury, and on several occasions a sheriff's deputy appeared before us to present evidence on a "pyramid club" scheme that he had been investigating. Persons, often elderly people living alone, were persuaded to buy membership shares in the club, and they were then asked to recruit other members. The original purchaser of the club membership would receive a percentage of the membership fees of all the new members, and so on. Obviously, some would make money from this scam, but ultimately most would be left holding the bag.

Before long a majority of us grand jurors were persuaded that an indictment was in order, and we so informed the district attorney. After a day or so of delay the D.A. appeared before us and said: "What this club is doing is wrong and shameful and people are being victimized, *but in this state there is no law against pyramid schemes*. You can do nothing." As the Latin maxim succinctly puts it, *nullum crimen sine lege—no crime without law.*

There are several corollaries to this general principle that also serve as grist for the criminal justice mill. One is that the U.S. Constitution forbids criminal laws that are *ex post facto*, that is, laws that declare certain conduct to be illegal *after* the conduct takes place. Past harmful or undesirable actions may not be declared criminal under our legal system. Likewise, the state may not pass what are termed bills of attainder. Those are laws that single out a particular person or group of persons and declare that something is criminal for them but legal for the rest of us. In the United States if an action (or inaction) is to be criminal, it must be so for all citizens.

A final corollary is that a law defining a crime must be precise so that the average person can determine in advance what conduct is prohibited or required. As the U.S. Supreme Court has put it, a statute defining a crime must be "sufficiently explicit to inform those who are subject to it what conduct on their part will render them liable to penalties." [6] Imagine the ease (and fun?) with which the Supreme Court struck down this Jacksonville, Florida, municipal vagrancy ordinance. Imagine, too, how many of us could go very many days without running afoul of at least some of its all-encompassing proscriptions. Criminal penalties were levied against

> rogues and vagabonds; dissolute persons who go about begging; common gamblers; persons who use juggling or unlawful games or plays; common drunkards; common night walkers, thieves, pilferers, or pickpockets; traders in stolen property; lewd, wanton, and lascivious persons; keepers of gambling places; common railers and brawlers; persons wandering or strolling around from place to place without any lawful purpose or object; habitual loafers; disorderly persons; persons neglecting all lawful business and habitually spending their time by frequenting houses of ill fame, gaming houses, or places where alcoholic beverages are sold or served; and persons able to work but habitually living on their wives or minor children. [7]

In addition to the law defining the crime, there must be a formal penalty attached to it. Traditional jurisprudence has always held that the punishment is an integral part of the crime. A number of years ago the State of Wyoming sought to convict a man for practicing medicine without a license. There was no question that the accused was actively prescribing medicines and even performing operations. During the course of his trial it was noticed that the law forbidding unlicensed medical practice said not a word about what would happen to someone who did it! The judge was forced to instruct the jury to bring in a verdict for the accused. (The "doctor" promptly decided to leave town, and the Wyoming legislature soon added a penalty clause to the statute.)

## The Actus Reus

Actus reus is the traditional Latin phrase meaning the criminal action committed by the accused that gives rise to the legal prosecution. The actus reus is the material element of the crime and will obviously vary from one offense to another. This element may be either the commission of an action that is forbidden (for instance, assault and battery), or it may be the failure to perform an action that is required (for instance, the refusal of an eighteen-year-old male to register with the Selective Service System).

## The Mens Rea

The mens rea is the essential mental element of the crime. An old legal axiom holds that "an act does not make the doer of it guilty, unless the mind be guilty; that is, unless the intention be criminal." Our legal system has always made a distinction between harm that was caused intentionally and harm that was caused by simple negligence or accident. "Even a dog," said Justice Oliver Wendell Holmes, "distinguishes between being stumbled over and being kicked." [8] Thus, if one person takes the life of another, the state does not always call it murder. If the killing was done with malice aforethought by a sane individual, it will likely be termed "murder in the first degree." But if the killing occurred in the passion of a barroom brawl, it would more likely be called "second degree murder"; that carries a lesser penalty. Reckless driving on the highway that results in the death of another would correspondingly be considered "negligent homicide"—a wrong, to be sure; but not as serious in the eyes of the state as the intentional killing of another.

Sometimes the judge or jury's determination of the mens rea actually defines the crime itself. Suppose that Police Officer Nelson comes upon Wino Willie lying inside a television warehouse on a cold winter's night. An arrest is made, but what is to be the charge and the crime for eventual conviction: burglary or simple criminal trespass? Burglary is defined as "entering a building without the consent of the owner with the intent to commit theft," while trespass means "to enter a building or habitation without the effective consent of the owner." Did Willie break into that warehouse to steal televisions or merely to keep warm while he drank? The determination of the *mens rea* here will influence whether Willie's time away from society is several years or only a few months.

## An Injury or Result

Except for regulatory crimes where a definition of the injury is rather abstract (for example, an illegal merger of two large airlines), a crime consists of a specific injury or a wrong perpetrated by one person against another. The crime may harm society at large, such as selling military secrets to the Soviet Union, or the injury may be inflicted upon an individual, and because of its nature considered to offend society as whole. In fact the nature of the injury, as with the *mens rea*, often determines the nature of the crime itself. For example, consider two hotheads who have been cutting each other off in traffic. Finally they both stop their cars and come out fighting. Suppose one of them actually hits the other so hard he dies; the crime may be "murder" (of some degree). If the man does not die but suffers serious bodily harm, the crime is "aggravated assault." If the injury is minor, the charge may be only "simple assault." Because the nature of the injury often determines the offense, it is frequently asserted that the nature of the injury is the key legal element of the crime.

It should be noted that some actions may be criminal even though no injury is actually inflicted. Most crimes of criminal conspiracy fall into this category. For instance, if several persons were to plan to assassinate a judge or to bribe jurors in an attempt to keep a criminal from being convicted, the crime would be "conspiracy to obstruct justice"; this would be a crime even if the judge went unharmed and no money was ever passed to the jurors. All that is required is that the crime be planned and intended and that some specific, overt act be taken by one of the conspirators in furtherance of their plan (such as the purchase of a weapon or possession of a map of the route that the judge takes between his home and the courtroom).

## A Causal Relationship Between
## the Action and the Resultant Injury

Before there can be a conviction for a criminal offense the state must prove that the accused's conduct constituted the "proximate cause" of the injury or result. This means that the defendant, acting in a natural and continuous sequence, produced the harmful situation. In other words, it must be clear that without the defendant's conduct, there would have been no harm or injury. Usually proving a causal relationship is not difficult. If A stabs B with a knife and inflicts a minor wound, there is no doubt that A is guilty of "assault with a deadly weapon." But what if B does not obtain proper medical care for the wound, develops an infection, and subsequently dies? Is A now guilty of manslaughter or murder? Or what if after being stabbed, B stumbles across a third party and causes injury to her? Is A to blame for this, too?

Resolution of questions such as these are often difficult for judges and juries. The law requires that all circumstances be taken into account. The accused can be convicted only if the state can prove that his or her conduct is the direct, immediate, or determining cause of the resultant harm to the victim. If other circumstances have come into play, the question becomes: Was the injury inflicted by the defendant sufficient to cause the result had the intervening factor(s) not occurred? Only if the harmful consequences were beyond the control of the accused or not a natural or probable consequence of his or her actions is the defendant free from criminal liability.

## Procedures Before a Criminal Trial

Before there can be a criminal trial, federal and state laws require a whole series of procedures and events. Some of these stages are mandated by the U.S. and state constitutions, some by court decisions, and others by legislative enactments; custom and tradition often account for the rest. Although the exact nature of these several procedural events varies from federal to state practice—and from one state to another—there are still some basic similarities throughout the country. We shall concentrate on the common patterns and indicate whenever possible where differences exist. We shall also provide further evidence for our thesis that these several procedures are not as automatic or routine as they might appear; rather, the decision makers exercise at all stages ample discretion according to their values, attitudes, and views of the world.

### The Arrest

There are over half a million police officers in the United States today—about one for every person in our jails and prisons. Each year these officers make almost 11 million arrests (not counting traffic offenses). The arrest is significant for our purposes here because it represents the first substantial contact between the state and the accused. The U.S. legal system provides for two basic types of arrest—those with a warrant and those without. A *warrant* is issued after a complaint, filed by one person against another, has been presented and reviewed by a magistrate who has found "probable cause" for the arrest. Arrests without a warrant occur when a crime is committed in the presence of a police officer or when an officer has probable cause to believe that someone has committed (or is about to commit) a crime. Such a belief must later be established in a sworn statement or testimony.

In the United States as many as 95 percent of all arrests are made without a warrant.

An officer's decision whether or not to make an arrest is far from simple or automatic. To be sure, the officer who witnesses a murder will make an arrest on the spot if possible. But most lawbreaking incidents are not that simple or clear-cut, and police officials possess—and exercise— wide discretion about whether to take someone into custody. There are simply not sufficient resources available to the police for them to proceed against all activities that Congress and the legislatures have forbidden. Consequently, discretion must be exercised in determining how to allocate the time and resources that do exist. To deny police discretion at the point of arrest, said Thurman Arnold, would be "like directing a general to attack the enemy on all fronts at once."

Criminal justice scholars have identified several areas in which police discretion is at a maximum: (1) minor or trivial offenses; (2) situations in which the victim will not seek prosecution; (3) cases in which the victim is also involved in misconduct; and (4) criminal conduct thought to reflect the mores of a community subgroup.

*Trivial Offenses.* Many police manuals advise their officers that when minor violations of the law are concerned, a warning is a more appropriate response than a formal arrest. Not only does this make common sense for borderline, trivial offenses, but it also has the effect of conserving law enforcement resources for more serious conduct. Traffic violations, misconduct by juveniles, drunkenness, gambling, vagrancy, and use of the services of a prostitute are all subjects that constitute less serious crime and that comprise a lot of close judgment calls by police. Let's look at a few illustrations.

The use of a warning rather than making an arrest or issuing a ticket is common in cases involving minor traffic violations. In fact, the officer's discretion in such situations is so well known to the motoring public that almost all of us have heard an errant driver plead, "Couldn't you just give me a warning this time, officer?" The following newspaper interview with former state director of the Texas Department of Public Safety Adrian Speir is instructive not only about discretion vis-à-vis traffic violations but about the allocation of police resources in general:

> "We just don't have enough manpower to have as much law enforce-
> ment as it takes to bring about voluntary compliance [with the speed
> limit laws] on a statewide level," Speir said. "On a typical day, 578
> highway patrol units are on duty, or an average of one for every 122
> miles. Troopers have other things to do besides clock speeders—chase
> drunk drivers, appear in court, enforce criminal laws, answer accident
> calls, and the like. So, choices must be made, limits drawn," says Speir.
> "Our people are instructed to enforce the law and to file a case in
> speeding when they are convinced there is a substantial violation of the

law," he said. What is a "substantial violation?" "We mean a degree that would get a person above the arguments of nominal speedometer error, tire slippage, human error in reading the radar. We do not encourage our people to be too technical. We are trying to get above the argumentative stage," he said. So when do you pass the argumentative stage?

"I am not going to tell you that they have got a three mile . . . tolerance or a five-mile tolerance. If I . . . [did], then people out in the state could drive that much above the limit," Speir said. He added that other factors might enter into a trooper's decision whether to write a speeding ticket, such as whether a driver was weaving in and out of traffic or using a car with defective equipment. Then, he said, "some counties are stricter about prosecution than others. If the county attorney feels five or six miles over the limit is not substantial, then that would indicate he would be batting his head against a brick wall if he filed cases under that limit." [9]

Another illustration of police discretion in the minor crime realm deals with gambling offenses. While an arrest might well be made for someone conducting a big-time, syndicated gambling operation, the "friendly little neighborhood poker game" is often ignored by police officials. Or, as a variation on this same theme, the former head of the Houston, Texas, vice squad once told a group of prospective grand jurors that "if respectable groups are engaged in gambling, such as church groups, only a warning is issued—and even then only after a complaint had been received. . . . If Sister Rosita is running a church bingo game, I'm sure not going to arrest her. I just wasn't raised that way."

Whether or not to arrest the "John" who procures the intimate favors of a prostitute also falls into the realm of police discretion and frequently places officers under pressure to turn a blind eye. Again, Houston's former vice squad head tells it like it is: "It is not the policy of the police department to enforce the law which makes it illegal for a man to be in the company of a prostitute. Why, the man might be someone with a family or a bank president! Also, we have a lot of big conventions here in town, and when the men come here . . . they like to have a little fun. If you start arresting these people, they wouldn't hold their conventions here any more, and then we'd have the mayor and all the restaurant and hotel owners on our backs." (Conventions in Houston bring in about $350 million annually.)

Finally, there is evidence that the deportment and demeanor of the accused may well influence the decision of the officer. The following quotation from an interview between one of the authors and an anonymous police officer is insightful, and its portrayal of reality is supported by much empirical evidence:

Q: In these minor sorts of cases how do you determine whether to make an arrest?

A: Well, lots of times it depends on whether the guy's got an attitude problem.

Q: A what?

A: An attitude problem. I mean if he's a smart ass and starts arguing with you and gets real lippy, we'll probably take him in. But if he's decent and admits he's wrong, we'll probably let him go. I mean, nobody enjoys filling out forms for hours on end that you got to do after you make an arrest.

*Victim Will Not Seek Prosecution.* Nonenforcement of the law is also the rule in situations where the victim of a crime will not expend his or her own time to help the state in a successful prosecution of a case. The reasons why a crime victim would not cooperate with the police in making an arrest are varied. In the instance of minor property crimes, the victim is often interested only in restitution; if that occurs, the victim may be satisfied. For example, when people are caught shoplifting, merchants frequently are unwilling to prosecute, asserting that they cannot afford the time away from the store to testify in court or that they do not want to risk a loss of goodwill. Unless the police have already expended considerable resources in investigating a particular property crime, they are generally obliged to abide by the victim's wishes.

When the victim of a crime is in a "continuing relationship" with the criminal, the police often decline to make an arrest. Such relationships include landlord and tenant, one neighbor and another (did X have a right to chop down Y's tree because its leaves continued to fall on X's yard?), and husband and wife. For example, the Detroit Police Manual provides: "When a police officer is called to a disturbance in a private home having family difficulties, he should recognize the sanctity of the home and endeavor diplomatically to quell the disturbance and create peace *without making an arrest*" (emphasis added).

Rape and child molestation constitute another major category of crimes for which there are often no arrests because the victims will not or cannot cooperate with the police. Oftentimes the victim is personally acquainted with, or related to, the criminal, and the fear of reprisals or of ugly publicity is sufficient to inhibit pressing a complaint. We know, for instance, that less than half of all rapes and considerably less than half of all cases of child molestation are even reported to the police. And for many cases that are reported, victims (or their parents) have second thoughts about prosecution and the charges are subsequently dropped.

*Victim Also Involved in Misconduct.* When police officers perceive that the victim of a crime is also involved in some type of improper or questionable conduct, the officers frequently opt not to make an arrest. Let us say that a Mr. Macho engages and pays for the services of a lady of the evening, but she fails to show up at the appointed place. Mr. Macho knows his rights and complains to the local officer on the beat. In such circumstances the officer may possibly detain the prostitute long enough to obtain a return of the victim's money, or he may merely tease the complainant and suggest that he has learned his lesson. In any case, it is not likely that an arrest will be made in any situation where the victim does not have clean hands, and officers well know that even if they do make an arrest, such cases are usually dropped by the prosecution.

*Criminal Conduct Thought to Reflect the Conduct of a Community Subgroup.* A final area of maximum police discretion regarding the matter of an arrest deals with lawbreaking that officers ignore because they regard it as normal and acceptable for members of racial minorities or members of the lower social classes. Studies have shown that police officers, usually white and from middle-class backgrounds, tend to regard the street violence, petty property crimes, and family altercations in minority and poor areas as just "normal for those kinds of people." On the other hand, such behavior in middle-and upper-middle-class neighborhoods is not seen as natural or acceptable, and the officer is more likely to make an arrest.

For example, if Officer Jones is summoned to a million dollar condominium on Chicago's exclusive Lake Shore Drive upon learning that a man has stabbed his socialite wife, there will likely be an arrest for assault with a deadly weapon; after all, people like that just oughtn't to behave in such a fashion, and if they do an arrest is definitely in order. However, if Officer Jones had been called to a ghetto neighborhood across town for an identical incident, his diary of events would more likely read as follows: "Called to scene of family disturbance in minority area. Woman hurt. Took her to the emergency ward to get her sewed up. Everything quiet. No arrest."

In sum, we see that the decision whether to make an arrest when a crime has been committed is not always simple and automatic for the police officer. Although no one would seriously doubt that officers must be given leeway to exercise their common sense and good judgment in close call situations, it is also clear that discretion may be arbitrary and subject to abuse. At the very least we know that to a substantial degree the decision making of police officers is the product of their own attitudes and values, community pressures, the "attitude" of the accused, and organizational constraints—a phenomenon that we shall subsequently see as well for prosecutors, judges, and other court personnel.

### Appearance Before a Magistrate

After a suspect is arrested for a crime, he or she is "booked" at the police station—that is, the facts surrounding the arrest are recorded and the accused may be fingerprinted and photographed. The next major step is for the accused to appear before a lower-level judicial official whose title may be judge, magistrate, or commissioner. Such an appearance is supposed to occur "without unnecessary delay;" while the meaning of this phrase varies from state to state, twenty-four hours is about the maximum delay permitted by law. In fact, in federal and most state jurisdictions if the appearance before a magistrate occurs more than six hours after an arrest, the court will likely question the voluntariness of any incriminating statements made by the accused.

This appearance is the scene of several important events in the criminal justice process. First, the accused must be informed of the precise charges and must be informed of all constitutional rights and guarantees. Among others, these rights include those of the now famous *Miranda* decision of the Warren Court handed down in 1966: that the accused "must be warned prior to any questioning that he has the right to remain silent, that anything he says can be used against him in a court of law, that he has the right to the presence of an attorney, and that if he cannot afford an attorney one will be appointed for him prior to any questioning." [10] (Such warnings must also be given by the arresting officer if the officer questions the suspect about the crime.) In some states the accused must be informed about other rights that are provided for in the state's Bill of Rights, such as the right to a speedy trial and the right to confront hostile witnesses.

Second, the magistrate will determine whether or not the accused is to be released on bail and, if so, what the amount of bail is to be. Constitutionally the only requirement for the amount is that it shall not be "excessive." If the magistrate believes that the accused will in fact appear for any future trial proceedings, no bail at all may be required and the accused may be released "on his own recognizance." Bail is considered to be a privilege—not a right—and it may be denied altogether in capital punishment cases for which the evidence of guilt is strong or if the magistrate believes that the accused will flee from prosecution no matter what the amount of bail.

The subject of bail has been riddled with controversy for a variety of reasons. One is that it is often used as a form of preventive detention when a judge intentionally sets bail at a level that is impossible for the defendant to make. A judge's decision to do this can be based on factors such as the defendant's prior criminal record, publicity the case may have generated, the recommendation of the prosecutor, and the defendant's previous conduct while out on bail. If a defendant cannot make bail (even $50 is prohibitive for those without means), he or she must remain in jail. This subjects legally innocent persons to punishment; it separates them from family, friends, and their jobs; it hinders their efforts to prepare for their defense in court; and it adds to the overcrowding that already bedevils most county jails.

An alternative to bail is to release the defendant "on recognizance" basically on a pledge by the defendant to return to court on the appointed date for trial. In some jurisdictions there are special programs designed to maximize the number of persons eligible for release on recognizance. Perhaps the best known, and often copied, of these is the Manhattan Bail Project. Here defendants are interviewed by pretrial investigators according to a special point system that takes into consideration such factors as the defendant's prior record, ties to the local community, and employment.

For minor cases the accused may be asked to plead innocence or guilt. If the plea is guilty, a sentence may be pronounced on the spot. If the defendant pleads not guilty, a trial date is scheduled. However, for the typical serious (felony) case the next primary duty of the magistrate is to determine whether or not the defendant requires a preliminary hearing. If such a hearing is appropriate, the matter is adjourned by the prosecution and a subsequent stage of the criminal justice process begins.

## The Grand Jury Process
## or the Preliminary Hearing

At the federal level all persons accused of a crime are guaranteed by the Fifth Amendment to have their cases considered by a grand jury. However, the Supreme Court has refused to make this right binding on the states, and indeed today only about half of the states even use grand juries; in some of these, they are used for only special types of cases. Those states that do not use grand juries employ what is called a preliminary hearing or an examining trial. (A few states use both procedures.) Regardless of which method is used, the primary purpose of this stage in the criminal justice process is to determine whether there is "probable cause" for the accused to be subjected to a formal trial.

**The Grand Jury.** Grand juries consist of sixteen to twenty-three citizens usually selected at random from the voter registration lists, and they render decisions by a majority vote.[11] Their terms may last anywhere between one month and one year, and some may hear over a thousand cases during their term. The prosecutor alone presents evidence to the grand jury; not only are the accused and his or her attorney absent from the proceedings, but usually they have no idea which grand jury is hearing the case or when. If a majority believes there is a "probable cause," then an indictment, or "true bill," is brought. Otherwise the result is a "no bill."

Fewer than 5 percent of all grand jury decisions result in no bills, and contrary to popular belief, no bills do not necessarily serve as a measure of grand jury independence vis-à-vis the prosecutor. Oftentimes the district attorney will ask the grand jury to render a no bill for personal reasons. Here is a statement made by a prosecutor to a state grand jury on which one of the authors served:

> Now here's a case where I'd like a little help from you all. There's a guy that's been after me every day for the past month because he says his brother-in-law borrowed his TV and some money and won't give 'em back. He wants me to file theft charges, but I keep telling him we're not a bill collection agency. I told him I would take the case to the grand jury, and I'm sure hoping you'll vote a no bill, and as soon as you do, I'm going to get on the phone and tell that guy that those "bleeding hearts" on the grand jury [laughs] wouldn't bring an indictment. That would sure get me off the hook.

Historically there have been two arguments in favor of grand juries. One is to serve as a check on a prosecutor who might be using the office to harass an innocent person for political or personal reasons. (Even though the innocent person might well eventually be found not guilty at trial, the cost and embarrassment of being tried for a crime is clearly a significant form of harassment.) Ideally an unbiased group of citizens would interpose themselves between an unethical prosecutor and the defendant.

A second justification for a grand jury is simply to make sure that the D.A. has done some homework and has in fact secured enough evidence to warrant the trouble and expense—for both the state and the accused—of a full-fledged trial. Sometimes in the haste and tedious routine of the criminal justice process persons are brought to trial when in fact there is insufficient evidence to justify this. Here is one true account of how a state grand jury served to prevent this from happening (albeit quite by accident):

> We had one case where the prosecutor tells us that several witnesses claim they saw this guy driving a stolen vehicle. So we vote a true bill—no questions asked. Then later on in the day when we were eating our sandwiches during lunch, one lady [also on the grand jury] was leafing through the files just for something to do. She says to us: "Hey, you know that guy we indicted this morning for auto theft. He claims he was on National Guard duty at the time a thousand miles away."
> Now we figured that that wasn't the sort of defense you'd lie about because it could be checked out so easily, so we called the D.A. back in. We asked him if he had called the guy's commanding officer on the WATS line to check out his story. The D.A. told us we weren't supposed to be trying this case and that there was probable cause because of the witnesses. But we made him call anyway, and sure enough there was a record that the guy was on guard duty the day the car was stolen. That day we did what a grand jury was supposed to be doing but, my God, it was only because that lady was bored with her baloney sandwich.

The evidence is pretty substantial that the prosecutor tends to dominate the grand jury process and that the jury's utility as a check on the motives and thoroughness of the district attorney is minimal.[12]

*The Preliminary Hearing.* In the majority of states that have abolished the grand jury system a preliminary hearing is used to determine whether there is probable cause for the accused to be bound over for trial. At this hearing the prosecution presents its case, and the accused has the right to cross-examine witnesses and to produce favorable evidence. Usually the defense elects not to fight at this stage of the criminal process; in fact, a preliminary hearing is waived by the defense in the vast majority of cases.

If the examining judge determines that there is probable cause for a trial or if the preliminary examination is waived, the prosecutor must file a "bill of information" with the court where the trial will be held. This serves to outline precisely the charges that will be adjudicated in the new legal setting. Usually about two weeks is allowed for the process.

## The Arraignment

*Arraignment* refers to the process in which the defendant is brought before the judge in the court where he or she is to be tried in order to respond to the grand jury indictment or the prosecutor's bill of information. The prosecutor or a clerk usually reads in open court the charges that have been brought against the accused. The defendant is informed that there is a constitutional right to be represented by an attorney and that a lawyer will be appointed without charge if necessary.

The defendant has several options about how to plead to the charges. The most common pleas, of course, are guilty and not guilty. But the accused may also plead not guilty by reason of insanity, former jeopardy (having been tried on the same charge at another time), or *nolo contendere* (no contest). *Nolo contendere* in effect means that the accused does not deny the facts of the case but claims that he or she has not committed any crime, or it may mean that the defendant does not understand the charges. The *nolo contendere* plea can be entered only with the consent of the judge (and sometimes the prosecutor as well). Such a plea has two advantages: it may help the accused save face vis-à-vis the public because he or she can later claim that technically there was no guilty verdict even though there may have been a sentence or a fine. Also, the plea may spare the defendant from certain civil penalties that might follow a guilty plea (for example, a civil suit that might follow from conviction for fraud or embezzlement).

If the accused pleads not guilty, the judge will schedule a date for a trial. If the plea is guilty, the defendant may be sentenced on the spot or at a later date set by the judge. Before the court will accept a guilty plea, the judge must certify that the plea was made voluntarily and that the defendant was aware of the implications of the plea. A guilty plea is to all intents and purposes the equivalent to a formal verdict of guilty.

## The Possibility of a Plea Bargain

Before we begin to talk about the procedures of a formal criminal trial we must dwell on the important fact that on both the state and federal levels *at least 90 percent of all criminal cases never go to trial.* That is because before the trial date a bargain has been struck between the prosecutor and the defendant's attorney concerning the official charges to be brought and the nature of the sentence that the state will recommend to the court. In effect, some form of leniency is promised in exchange for a guilty plea.

Under plea bargaining the role of the judges in the criminal justice system is much smaller than most of us assume. Most people believe that the courts operate under a pure adversary system in which the judge's role is to make a disinterested sentencing after hearing full arguments from both sides. But because plea bargaining virtually seals the fate of the defendant *before* trial, the role of the judge is simply to ensure that the proper legal and constitutional procedures have been followed.

Judicial scholars are not unanimous on why plea bargaining has become the norm rather than the exception, and indeed some have argued that in some form plea bargaining has always been with us. (That is, the state has always been more lenient to those who admit their guilt, are repentant, and cooperate with the government.) Nevertheless, there is evidence that the average felony trial is longer now than it was several decades ago and that defendants are filing more pretrial pleas and postconviction motions now than in the past. No doubt the changes are due at least in part to the Warren Court's many decisions favoring the rights of criminal defendants. But for whatever reasons the ever increasing caseloads of the past several decades have made the judicial system ever more dependant on the quick and simple plea bargain. There are three (not mutually exclusive) basic types of such bargains.

**Reduction of Charges.**    The most common form of agreement between a prosecutor and a defendant is a reduction of the charge to one less serious than that supported by the evidence. The defendant is thereby subject to a lower maximum sentence and is likely to receive a lighter sentence than would have been the case under a guilty verdict on the original charge. For example, a common plea bargain in many states for an individual accused of theft is to plead guilty to burglary with the intent to commit theft. This exposes the criminal to a substantially reduced range of sentence possibilities.

A second reason for a defendant to plead guilty to a reduced charge is to avoid a record of conviction for an offense that carries social stigma. The "good family man" and "pillar of the church" caught in the act of "indecency with a child" might be quite willing to plead guilty to the reduced charge of disorderly conduct.

Another possibility is that the defendant may wish to avoid a felony record altogether. A college student who hopes to be a lawyer or a public school teacher might be eager to plead guilty to almost any misdemeanor offered by the prosecutor rather than face a felony charge and risk being excluded from the legal and teaching professions.

*Deletion of Tangent Charges.* A second form of plea bargain involves the agreement of the district attorney to drop other charges pending against an individual. There are two variations on this theme. One is an agreement not to prosecute "vertically," that is, not to prosecute more serious charges filed against the individual. For example, it is common in many jurisdictions for individuals using credit cards illegally to be charged simultaneously with forgery and possession of a stolen credit card. A bargain may be made to drop the forgery indictment in exchange for a plea of guilty on the lesser charge. The second type of agreement is to dismiss additional indictments for the same crime ("horizontal" charges) pending against the accused. It is not unusual for several counts of burglary to be dropped following a confession to one other burglary indictment. (For an indictment to be dropped, most jurisdictions require the prosecutor to file a motion of *nolle prosequi*—"I refuse to prosecute"— with the court, but such motions are usually granted as a matter of course.)

Another variation of the type of plea bargaining that is concerned with dropping charges is the agreement in which a "repeater" clause is dropped from an indictment. In many states a person is considered a "habitual criminal" upon the third conviction for a violent felony anywhere in the United States. The mandatory sentence for the habitual criminal is life imprisonment. It is rather common for the habitual violent criminal charge to be dropped in exchange for a plea of guilty. For example, in Texas an individual convicted of theft as a habitual criminal must be sentenced to life imprisonment and will not be eligible for parole for at least twenty years. On the other hand, an individual who is offered the chance to plead guilty to "theft—second offense" must be given a sentence of ten years in prison but will be eligible for parole after serving only one-third of that sentence. The difference between twenty years of working on the rock pile and three years and four months is a keen incentive for a "three-time loser" to admit to being a "two-time loser."

A final wrinkle of this type of plea bargaining is the agreement in which indictments in different courts are consolidated into one court in order that the sentences may run concurrently. As indictments or preliminary hearing rulings are handed down in many jurisdictions, they are placed on a trial docket on a rotation system. (The first charge is placed on a docket of court 1, the second on court 2, and so on.) This means that a defendant charged with four counts of forgery and one charge of possession of a forged instrument might find herself on the docket of five different courts. Generally it is common practice in such multicourt districts to transfer all of a person's indictments to the first court listed. This gives the presiding judge the discretion of allowing all of the defendant's sentences to run concurrently. Although it is not often done, it is possible that an individual who refuses to plead guilty to any charges will simply not have the other indictments transferred, creating the likelihood of "stacked" (consecutive) sentences.

*Sentence Bargaining.*    A third form of plea bargaining concerns a plea of guilty from the defendant in exchange for a prosecutor's agreement to ask the judge for a lighter sentence.[13] At first blush it might seem that this type of plea negotiation is a weak substitute for either the reduction-of-charge or the dropping-of-charge form. After all, under sentence bargaining the state can make only a nonbinding recommendation to the court regarding the sentence, whereas under the other two types the state's concessions are concrete and not subject to doubt.

The strength of the sentence negotiation, however, is based upon the realities of the limited resources of the judicial system. At the state level, at least, prosecutors are able to promise the defendant a fairly specific sentence with confidence that the judge will accept the recommendation. If the judge were not to do so, the prosecutor's credibility would quickly begin to wane, and many of the defendants who had been pleading guilty would begin to plead not guilty and take their chances in court. The result would be a gigantic increase in court dockets that would literally overwhelm the judicial system and bring it to a complete standstill. Prosecutors and judges understand this reality, and so do the defense attorneys.

*Constitutional and Statutory Restrictions on Plea Bargaining.*    At both the state and federal levels the requirements of due process of law mean that plea bargains must be made voluntarily and with comprehension. This means that the defendant must be admonished by the court of the consequences of a guilty plea (for example, you waive all opportunities to change your mind at a later date), that the accused must be sane, and that, as one typical state puts it, "It must plainly appear that the defendant is uninfluenced by any consideration of fear, or by any persuasion, or delusive hope of pardon, prompting him to confess his guilt." It would appear from these requirements that the prosecutor's promise of a lighter sentence in exchange for a guilty plea would violate the letter, if not the spirit, of the due process clause. Not so, the courts have ruled. As long as judges tell the defendants that, at least in principle, they are subject to any sentence that is pronounced and the accused acknowledge this, the requirement of due process has been met. Thus when a state court certifies that a guilty plea was "knowingly and understandingly made," a form of legal fiction has often been in the works.

For the first two types of plea bargains there are some stricter standards that govern the federal courts. One is that the judge may not actually participate in the process of plea bargaining; at the state level judges may play an active role in this process. Likewise, if a plea bargain has been made between the U.S. attorney and the defendant, the government may not renege on the agreement. If the federal government does so, the federal district judge must withdraw the guilty plea. Finally, the Federal Rules of Criminal Procedure require that "the court shall not enter a judgment upon a plea of guilty unless it is satisfied that there is a factual basis for the plea." This means that before a guilty plea may be accepted, the prosecution must present a summary of the evidence against the accused, and the judge must agree that there is strong evidence of the defendant's guilt.

*Arguments for and Against Plea Bargaining.*    For the defendant the obvious advantage of the bargain is that he or she is treated less harshly than would be the case if the accused were convicted and sentenced under maximum conditions. Also, the absence of a trial often lessens publicity on the case, and because of personal interests or simple social pressures, the accused may wish to avoid the length and publicity of a formal trial. Finally, some penologists (professionals in the field of punishment and rehabilitation) argue that the first step toward rehabilitation is for a criminal to admit guilt and to recognize his or her problem. The idea is that a guilty plea is at least nominally the first step toward a successful return to society.

There are also some distinct advantages for the state and for society as a whole. The most obvious is the certainty of conviction, because no matter how strong the evidence may appear there is always the possibility of an acquittal as long as a trial is pending. (Evidence may be stolen or lost; important witnesses may die or drop out of sight; the prosecutor may make a key error in court that results in a mistrial.) Also, the district attorney's office and judges are saved an enormous amount of time and effort by their not having to prepare and preside over cases in which there is no real contention of innocence or which are not suited to the trial process. Finally, it is argued that when police officers are not required to be in court testifying in criminal trial, they have more time to devote to preventing and solving crimes.

Lest this all seem too good to be true, there is a negative side to plea bargains as well. The most frequent objection to plea bargaining is that the defendant's sentence may well be based upon nonpenological grounds. With the large volume of cases making plea bargaining the rule, the sentence often bears no relation at all to the specific facts of the case, to the correctional needs of the criminal, or to society's legitimate interest in vigorous prosecution of the case. A second defect is that if plea bargaining becomes the norm of a particular system, then undue pressure may be placed upon even innocent persons to plead guilty. Studies have shown that in some jurisdictions the less the chance for conviction, the harder the bargaining may be because the prosecutor wants to get at least some form of minimal confession out of the accused.

A third disadvantage of plea bargaining is the possibility of the abuse called *overcharging*—that is, the process whereby the prosecutor brings charges against the accused more severe than the evidence warrants, with the hope that this will strengthen his or her hand in subsequent negotiations with the defense attorney. One of us who served on a state grand jury had this exchange with a representative of the district attorney's office:

GRAND JUROR: In this case where one fellow killed another in that barroom fight, why do you want us to indict on a first-degree murder charge? There doesn't seem to be any premeditation here. You'll never get a conviction on that.

D.A.: Oh, I know. But it will strengthen our hand at the time when we talk with his attorney.

(The grand jury in question chose to indict on a lesser and more appropriate charge.)

Another flaw with the plea bargaining system is its very low level of visibility. This is really the flip side of flexibility. Bargains between prosecutor and defense attorney are not made in open court presided over by a neutral jurist and for all to observe; rather, they are more likely made over a cup of coffee in a basement courthouse cafeteria where the conscience of the two lawyers is the primary guide. In this same vein, when the defendant enters the guilty plea in open court and swears that no promise by the state has induced this plea, the prosecutor and defense counsel mutely corroborate the defendant's false statement. Meanwhile, the judge remains uninformed of the facts and is therefore unable to determine the fairness or validity of the agreement.

Finally, the system has the potential to circumvent key procedural and constitutional rules of evidence. Because the prosecutor need not present any evidence or witnesses in court, a bluff may result in a conviction even though the case might not be able to pass the muster of the due process clause. The defense may be at a disadvantage because the rules of discovery (the laws that allow the defense to know in detail the evidence the prosecution will present) in some states limit the defense counsel's case preparation to the period *after* the plea bargain has occurred. Thus the plea bargain may deprive the accused of basic constitutional rights.

## Procedures During a Criminal Trial

Assuming that there has been no plea bargain and the accused maintains his or her innocence, there will be a formal trial. This is a right guaranteed by the Sixth Amendment to all Americans charged with federal crimes and a right guaranteed by the various state constitutions—and by the Fourteenth Amendment—to all persons charged with state offenses. There are many constitutional and statutory rights that the accused is provided during the course of the trial. We shall not enumerate them all here, but the following are at least the primary rights that are binding on both the federal and state courts.

### Basic Rights Guaranteed During the Trial Process

The Sixth Amendment says, "In all criminal prosecutions, the accused shall enjoy the right to a speedy and public trial." The Founders emphasized the word *speedy* so that an accused would not languish in prison for a long time prior to the trial or have the determination of his or her fate put off for an unduly long period of time. But how soon is "speedy"? Although this word has been defined in various ways by the Supreme Court,[14] Congress gave new meaning to the term when it passed the Speedy Trial Act of 1974. The act mandated time limits, ultimately reaching 100 days, within which criminal charges must either be brought to trial or dismissed. Most states have similar measures on the statute books, although the precise time period varies from one jurisdiction to another. By "public trial" the Founders meant to discourage the notion of secret proceedings whereby an accused could be tried without public knowledge and whisked off to some unknown detention camp—a state of affairs still typical of totalitarian regimes today.

The Sixth Amendment also guarantees us the right to an impartial jury. At the very least this has meant that the prospective jurors must not be prejudiced one way or the other before the trial begins. For example, a potential juror may not be a friend or relative of the prosecutor or the crime victim; neither may someone serve who believes that anyone of the defendant's race or ethnic ancestry is "probably the criminal type." (We shall have more to say about the selection of the jury in a moment.) What the concept of an "impartial jury of one's peers" has come to mean in practice is that jurors are to be selected randomly from the voter registration lists—supplemented in some jurisdictions by lists based on automobile registrations, driver's licenses, telephone books, welfare rolls, and so on.[15] While this does not provide a perfect cross-section of the community, since not all persons are registered to vote, the Supreme Court has said that this method is good enough. The High Court has also ruled that no class of persons (such as blacks or women) may be systematically excluded from jury service. This does not mean that a black defendant, for example, has a right to have other persons of the same racial background on a jury; it means only that no racial category may be intentionally kept from jury service.

Besides being guaranteed the right to be tried in the same locale wherein the crime was committed and to be informed of the charges against us, we have the right to be confronted with the witnesses against us. We have the right to know who our accusers are and what they are charging so that a proper defense may be formulated. The accused is also guaranteed the opportunity "to have the Assistance of Counsel for his defence." Until recent decades this meant that one had this right (at the state level) only for serious crimes and only if one could pay for an attorney. However, because of a series of Supreme Court decisions it is now the law of the land that one is guaranteed an attorney if tried for any crime that may result in a prison term, and the government must pick up the tab for the legal defense for an indigent defendant. This is the rule at both the national and state levels.

With defense attorneys, as with many things in life, you usually get what you pay for. If money is no object, then you can afford to hire an experienced and highly competent defense lawyer who will be a superb advocate on your behalf. This does not automatically mean that you will be acquitted if you are guilty, but it may mean that you will obtain a more advantageous plea bargain or a lighter sentence if convicted. If you are not wealthy or have no means at all, you may be forced to rely on the services of a public defender appointed on your behalf by the state. Most public defenders are relatively young and inexperienced, and while some have a reputation for putting on a vigorous defense (such as those in Detroit), most are not or will never be within the top ranks of the legal profession.

Defense attorneys, whether paid by the defendant or the state, are often the subject of considerable criticism. It is said that they give too little time and effort to their clients' cases because of the limited resources of most public defenders' offices and because it is financially advantageous for private attorneys to turn cases over as rapidly as possible. Also, in many jurisdictions a public defender is given a fixed amount per case regardless of how much time the case takes. This may well encourage a public defender to pressure a client to plead guilty so that the case will take less time.

The Fifth Amendment to the U.S. Constitution declares that no person shall "be subject for the same offence to be twice put in jeopardy of life and limb." This is the famous "double jeopardy" clause and means in effect that no one may be tried twice for the same crime by any state government or by the federal government. It does not mean, however, that a person may not be tried twice for the same action if that action has violated both national and state laws. For example, someone who robs a federally chartered bank in New Jersey runs afoul of both federal and state law. It is possible and quite legal that that person could be tried and acquitted for that offense in a New Jersey court and then subsequently be tried for that same action in federal court: again, this clause means that the same level of government may not try you twice for the same crime.

Sometimes the question of which level of the judiciary has jurisdiction for a particular type of offense is a bit muddled. For instance, the Racketeer Influenced and Corrupt Organizations (RICO) section of the Organized Crime Control Act of 1970 authorizes prosecution in federal court for violations of certain state laws if the actions come under a certain special definition of "racketeering." Thus, beginning in 1985 a number of Cook County (Chicago), Illinois, state judges were prosecuted under RICO for accepting bribes.

Another important right guaranteed to the accused at both the state and federal level is not to "be compelled in any criminal case to be a witness against himself." This has also been interpreted to mean that the fact that someone elects not to testify on his or her own behalf in court may not be used against the person by judge and jury. This guarantee serves to reinforce the principle that under our judicial system the burden of proof is on the state; the accused is presumed to be innocent until the government proves otherwise beyond a reasonable doubt.

Finally, the Supreme Court has interpreted the guarantee of due process of law (in the Fifth Amendment, which binds the federal government, and in the Fourteenth, which binds the states) to mean that evidence procured in an illegal search and seizure may not be used against the accused at trial. The Court's purpose was to eliminate any incentive the police might have to illegally obtain evidence against the accused. Many have argued that this right does not in fact discourage improper police behavior and that it serves only as a technical loophole to free the guilty. Thus the more conservative Burger and Rehnquist Courts have taken steps to narrow the effect of the exclusionary rule. Civil libertarians have countered that this rule is a key element in the basic concepts of due process and fair play.

## Selection of Jurors

If the accused elects not to have a bench trial—that is, not to be tried and sentenced by a judge alone—his or her fate will be determined by a jury. At the federal level twelve persons must render a unanimous verdict. At the state level such criteria apply only to the most serious offenses. In many states a jury may consist of fewer than twelve persons and render verdicts by other than unanimous decisions. (Acceptable votes might be eleven to one, ten to two, or five to one.)

A group of veniremen (sometimes known as an array) is summoned from a panel of potential jurors to appear in a given courtroom. The veniremen are then questioned in open court about their general qualifications for jury service in a process known as *voir dire*. The prosecutor and the defense attorney ask general and specific questions of the potential jurors. Are they citizens of the state? Can they comprehend the English language? Have they or anyone in their family ever been tried for a criminal offense? Have they read about or formed any opinions about the case at hand?

In conducting the voir dire the state and the defense have two general types of goals. The first is to eliminate all members of the panel who have an obvious reason why they might not render an impartial decision in the case. Common examples might be someone who is excluded by law from serving on a jury, a juror who is a friend or relative of a participant in the trial, someone who openly admits a strong bias or prejudice in the case at hand. Objections to jurors in this category are known as challenges for cause, and the number of such challenges is unlimited. It is the judge who determines whether these challenges are valid.

There is a second goal that the opposing attorneys have in questioning the array of jurors: to eliminate those whom they believe would be unfavorable to their side even though there is no overt reason for the potential bias. This can be done because each side is given a number of what are termed peremptory challenges—requests to the court to exclude a prospective juror with no reason given. It is customary in most states to give the defense more peremptory challenges than the prosecution. At the federal level one to three challenges per juror are usually permitted each side, depending on the nature of the offense, although as many as twenty are allowed in capital cases. The use of peremptory challenges is more of an art than a science and is usually based on the hunch of the attorneys. For example, in a case where a poor person stole groceries from a supermarket, a prosecutor might use available challenges to exclude jurors of low economic status, thinking that they might be more sympathetic to the accused. Or in a case involving a sexual offender, a defense attorney might try to eliminate jurors who belong to fundamentalist religions, thinking that they would take a more judgmental stance in such matters than those of more "liberal" religious convictions.

The process of questioning and challenging prospective jurors continues until all those duly challenged for cause are eliminated, the peremptory challenges are either used up or waived, and a jury of twelve (six in some states) has been created. In some states alternate jurors are also chosen. They attend the trial but participate in deliberations only if one of the original jurors is unable to continue in the proceedings. Once the panel has been selected they are sworn in by the judge or the clerk of the court.

## Opening Statements

After the formal trial begins both the prosecution and the defense make an opening statement (although in no state is the defense compelled to do so). Long and detailed statements are more likely to be made in jury trials than in bench trials. Their purpose is to provide members of the jury—who lack familiarity with the law and with procedures of criminal investigation—with an outline of the major objectives of each side's case, the evidence that is to be presented, the witnesses that are to be called, and what each side seeks to prove from the evidence of the witnesses. If the opening statements are well presented, the jurors will find it easier to grasp the meaning and significance of the evidence and testimony, and ideally they will be less likely to get confused and bogged down in the complexities and technicalities of the case. The usual procedure is for the state to make its opening statement first and for the defense to follow with a statement about how it will refute that case.

## The Prosecution's Case

After the opening statements the prosecutor presents the evidence amassed by the state against the accused. Evidence is generally of two types—physical evidence and the testimony of witnesses. The physical evidence may include things such as bullets, ballistics tests, fingerprints, handwriting samples, blood and urine tests, and other documents or hard items that serve as physical aids. The defense may object to the admission of any of these tangible items and will if successful have the item excluded from consideration. If there is no successful defense objection, the physical evidence is labeled by one of the courtroom personnel and becomes part of the official record.

Most evidence at criminal trials takes the form of testimony of witnesses. The format is a question-and-answer procedure that may appear a bit stilted, but its purpose is to elicit very specific information in an orderly fashion. The goal is to present only evidence that is relevant to the immediate case at hand and not to give confusing or irrelevant information or illegal evidence that might result in a mistrial (for example, evidence that the accused had a prior conviction for an identical offense). The following hypothetical question and answer between a district attorney and a police officer is typical:

D.A.: Please state your name and occupation.

OFFICER: My name is Frank Benoit. I am employed as a police officer by the District of Columbia.

D.A.: Did you have reason to be at or near the corner of Massachusetts and Eighteenth about seven o'clock on the evening of March 5?

OFFICER: Yes, I was summoned to a liquor store at that address after a witness phoned the department and said she saw someone breaking into the building.

D.A.: What did you observe after you arrived on the scene?

OFFICER: I observed a white male with what appeared to be a crate of liquor under his arm.

D.A.: What was he doing at the time?

OFFICER: He was running away from the building.

D.A.: What did you do at that time?

OFFICER: I subdued the man and placed him under arrest.

D.A.: Is the person whom you saw running from the building and arrested sitting in this courtroom today?

OFFICER: Yes, sir.

D.A.: Would you point out that man?

OFFICER: He is sitting to the left of the defense attorney.

D.A.: Your Honor, may the record show that the officer pointed to the defendant in this case?

After each witness, the defense attorney has the right to cross-examine. The goal of the defense will be to impeach the testimony of the prosecution witness, that is, to discredit it. The attorney may attempt to confuse, fluster, or anger the witness, causing him or her to lose self-control and begin providing confusing or conflicting testimony. The prosecution's witness's testimony may also be impeached if defense witnesses who contradict the version of events suggested by the state are subsequently presented. Upon completion of the cross-examination, the prosecutor may conduct a "redirect examination" which serves to clarify or correct some telling point made during the cross-examination. After the state has presented all its evidence and witnesses, it rests its case.

## The Case for the Defense

The presentation of the case for the defense is similar in style and format to that of the prosecution. Tangible evidence is less common in the defense's case, and most of the evidence will be that of witnesses who are prepared to rebut or contradict the prosecution's arguments. The witnesses are questioned by the defense attorney in the same style as those in the prosecution case. Each defense witness may in turn be cross-examined by the district attorney, and then a redirect examination is in order.

The real difference between the case for the prosecution and the defense lies in their obligation before the law. The defense is not required by law to present any new or additional evidence or witnesses at all. The defense may consist merely of challenging the credibility or the legality of the state's evidence and witnesses. And as we have already noted, the defense is not obligated to prove the innocence of the accused; it need show only that the state's case is not beyond a reasonable doubt. The defendant need not even take the stand. (However, if he or she elects to do so, the accused faces the same risks of cross-examination as any other witness.)

After the defense has rested its case, the prosecution has the right to go back on the attack and present rebuttal evidence. In turn, the defense may offer a rejoinder known as a surrebuttal. After that point each side is ready for the closing arguments. Oftentimes this is one of the more dramatic episodes in the trial because each side seeks to sum up its case, condense its stongest arguments, and make one last appeal to the jury. New evidence may not be presented at this stage, and the arguments of both sides tend to ring with emotion and appeals to values that transcend the immediate case. The prosecutor may talk about the crime problem in general, about the need for law and order, and about the need not to let compassion for the accused get in the way of empathy for the crime victim. The defense attorney, on the other hand, may remind the jurors "how we have all made mistakes in this life," or that in a free, democratic society any doubt they have should be resolved in favor of the accused. The prosecution probably avoids emotionalism more than the defense attorney, however, because it is well known that many jury verdicts have been reversed on appeal after the district attorney injected prejudicial statements into the closing statements.

## Role of the Judge During the Trial

The judge's role in the trial, while very important, is a relatively passive one. He or she does not present any evidence or take an active part in the examination of the witnesses. The judge is expected to play the part of a neutral, disinterested party whose primary job is to see to it that both sides are allowed to present their cases as fully as possible within the confines of the law. The judge is called upon to rule on the many motions of the prosecutor and of the defense attorney regarding the types of evidence that may be presented and the kinds of questions that may be asked of the witnesses. In some jurisdictions the judge is permitted to ask substantive questions of the witnesses and also to comment to the jury about the credibility of the evidence that is presented; in other states the judge is constrained from such activity.

While judges do for the most part play a neutral and disinterested role, there is also evidence that the background and values of the jurists affect their decisions in the close calls, that is, when they are called upon to rule on a motion for which the arguments are about equally strong or on a point of law that is open to a variety of interpretations. Evidence for this discretion and the way it is influenced by the values of the judges comes from a variety of sources—a subject discussed in greater detail in Chapter 8. But to illustrate our point, let us look briefly at our data on the decisional patterns of federal trial judges, specifically, how they responded to motions made by a defendant's attorney before, during, and after trial and also on those cases where at a bench trial the judge alone could decide the fate of the accused.

First, our data (see Chapter 9) reveal that between 1933 and 1985 Republican judges responded favorably to the motions of the accused 39 percent of the time, whereas Democratic jurists did so in 47 percent of the reported cases. In other words, Democrats on the bench were 1.39 times more likely to support the motion of the criminal defendant than Republicans. Regional attitudes and values may also affect the judge's courtroom behavior. For instance, our data set reveals that between 1978 and 1985 judges in the eastern states supported motions of the accused in 28 percent of the reported cases while jurists in the West did so 35 percent of the time. Thus, judges in the East were only .72 times as likely to opt in favor of the defense attorney's motions than were his or her western colleagues. In sum, judges in a trial may be neutral, but as human beings they also have individual value sets, and in the close calls these value sets are discernible.

## Instructions to the Jury

An important function of the judge during the trial is to charge the jury after the prosecution and defense have rested their cases. Although the jury's job is to weigh and assess the facts of the case, it is the judge who must instruct the jurors about the meaning of the law and how the law is to be applied. The judge's instructions can be drafted in a way that favors one side or another. For example, if someone were accused of embezzlement and the judge favored acquittal, it might be possible to give the jury such a narrow legal definition of the word *embezzlement* that it would be difficult to bring in a guilty verdict. Likewise, if the judge were disposed toward conviction, a broader discussion of the laws on embezzlement might facilitate a conviction.

Both the prosecutor and the defense attorney know well that the nature of the instructions can nudge the jury in one direction or another. Consequently, it is often the practice for each side in the case to submit its own set of instructions to the judge asking that its version be the official one read to the jury. The judge may then select one of the two sets of instructions or, as often as not, develop one (perhaps based on selected parts of those offered or on a previously used set of instructions).

Because many cases are overturned on appeal due to faulty jury instructions, judges tend to take great care that the wording be technically and legally correct. The problem with this, however, is that although highly technical legal instructions may please an appellate court, they are often incomprehensible to individual jurors. Judges tend to decline the jury's subsequent pleas to clarify instructions or to put them into everyday language because to do so would risk saying something that will move one side or the other to appeal the instructions.

Whatever the thrust or bias of the instructions, they must all contain some basic elements. One is to define for the jurors the crime with which the accused is charged. This may involve giving the jurors a variety of options about what kind of a verdict to bring. For example, if one person has taken the life of another, the state may be trying the accused for first degree murder. Nevertheless, the judge may be obliged to acquaint the jury with the legal definition of second degree murder or manslaughter if they should determine that the defendant was the killer but did not act with malice aforethought. Or if the accused is pleading not guilty for reason of insanity, the judge must offer in the instructions the proper legal definition of insanity.

It is also incumbent upon the judge to remind the jury that the burden of proof is on the state and that the accused is presumed to be innocent. If after considering all the evidence, the jury still has a "reasonable doubt" as to the guilt of the accused, they must bring in a not guilty verdict. Jurors are often troubled by what this means. "How sure do we have to be," they often ask of themselves, "75 percent, 90 percent, 99 percent?" What is "reasonable" and how strong may the "doubt" be? One judge defined the matter as follows:

> It is such a doubt as would cause a juror, after careful and candid and impartial consideration of all the evidence, to be so undecided, that he cannot say that he has an abiding conviction of the defendant's guilt. It is such a doubt as would cause a reasonable person to hesitate or pause in the graver or more important transactions of life. However, it is not a fanciful doubt nor a whimsical doubt, nor a doubt based on conjecture.[16]

Despite this and other guidelines that the juror may be given to help determine reasonable doubt, in the final analysis each person has to decide alone at the moment when he or she votes to acquit or convict.

Finally, the judge usually acquaints the jury with a variety of procedural matters: how to contact the judge if they have questions, the order in which they must consider the charges if there are more than one, who must sign the official documents that express the verdict of the jury. After the instructions are read to the jury (and the attorneys for each side given an opportunity to offer objections), the jurors retreat into a deliberation room to decide the fate of the accused.

### The Jury's Decision

The jury deliberates in complete privacy: no outsiders observe or participate in its debate. During its deliberation it may request the clarification of legal questions from the judge, and it may look at items of evidence or selected segments of the case transcript, but it may consult nothing else—no law dictionaries, no legal writings, no opinions from experts. When it has reached a decision by a vote of its members, it returns to the courtroom to announce its verdict. If it has not reached a decision by nightfall, the jurors are sent home with firm instructions neither to discuss the case with others nor read about the case in the newspapers. In very important or notorious cases, the jury may be *sequestered* by the judge, which means that its members will spend the night in a local hotel away from the public eye.

If the jury becomes deadlocked and cannot reach a verdict, it may report that fact to the judge. In such an event the judge may insist that the jury continue its effort to reach a verdict, saying something like: "The state and the accused have spent a lot of time and money on this case, and if you can't agree, then another jury just like you folks is going to have to go through this whole thing again." (There's nothing like instilling a little guilt to motivate human behavior.) Or, if the judge is convinced that the jury is in fact hopelessly deadlocked, he or she may dismiss the jury and call for a new trial.

Research studies indicate that most juries dealing with criminal cases make their decisions fairly quickly. Almost all juries take a vote soon after they retire to their chambers ("just a nonbinding straw vote to see where we are"). In 30 percent of the cases it takes only one vote to reach a unanimous decision. In 90 percent of the remainder, the majority on the first ballot eventually wins out. Hung juries—those in which *no* verdict can be reached—tend to occur only when a large minority existed on the first ballot.

Scholars have also learned that juries often reach the same verdict that the judge would have had he or she been solely responsible for the decision. One large jury study asked judges to state how they would have decided jury cases over which they presided. It was found that judge and jury agreed in 81 percent of the criminal cases (about the same as in civil cases). In 19 percent of the criminal cases the judge and jury disagreed, with the judge showing a marked tendency to convict where the juries had acquitted. Most disagreement occurred over statutory rape cases and first-offense drunk-driving cases.[17] (The jury was likely to believe that the woman had encouraged the rape because of the way she was dressed or by where the rape occurred, for instance, in the back room of a sleazy bar. In drunk-driving cases many jurors apparently saw themselves in similar situations and had sympathy for the accused.)

Jurors, like police officers, prosecutors, grand jurors, and judges, reflect their personal values and backgrounds in their decision-making process. Studies have shown, for example, that men talk more than women in the jury deliberation process and have more influence in the final outcome. Likewise, and not surprisingly, well-educated people play a more significant role than those with weak educational backgrounds. There is also some evidence that ethnic or racial minorities carry some of their underdog values into the jury deliberation rooms, being more likely to favor the accused than are jurors with higher status. `

There is evidence that the demeanor and dress of the accused touch sensitive values in the jurors. For example, in a simulated study conducted at Michigan's Institute for Social Research, ninety-one individuals served as "jurors" in a mock automobile negligence trial during which they heard tape-recorded testimony. One group of jurors was shown pictures of a handsome male plaintiff and of an unattractive male defendant; another group was shown the reverse. A third, control, panel heard tape-recorded testimony only and was shown no pictures. Forty-nine percent of the jurors shown a picture of a good-looking plaintiff voted in his behalf, whereas only 17 percent of those shown a photo of an ugly plaintiff ruled for the plaintiff. (Of the control group, which saw no picture, 41 percent gave the plaintiff their vote.) The jurors were also asked to determine the degree of wrongdoing, and the unattractive individual was consistently rated as "more negligent." [18] As the famous trial lawyer Clarence Darrow said a half century ago, "Jurymen seldom convict a person they like or acquit one they dislike."

When the members of the jury do finally reach a decision, they return to the courtroom and their verdict is announced in open court, often by the jury foreman. It is commonplace at this time for either the prosecutor or the defense attorney to ask that the jury be polled, that is, each juror asked individually if the general verdict actually reflects his or her own opinion. The purpose of this is to determine whether each juror supports the overall verdict or whether he or she is just caving in to group pressure. If the polling procedure reveals that the jury is indeed not of one mind, it may be sent back to the jury room to continue deliberations; in some jurisdictions a mistrial may be declared. If a mistrial is declared, the case may be tried again before another jury. There is no double jeopardy because the original jury did not agree on a verdict. On the other hand, if the jury's verdict is not guilty the defendant is discharged on the spot and is free to leave the courtroom (unless, of course, there are other charges pending).

## Procedures After a Criminal Trial

At the close of the criminal trial there are generally two stages that remain for the defendant if he or she has been found guilty: sentencing and an appeal.

## Sentencing

Sentencing is the court's formal pronouncement of judgment upon the defendant, at which time the punishment or penalty is set forth. At the federal level and in most states sentences are imposed by the judge only. However, in several states the defendant may elect to be sentenced by either a judge or a jury, and in capital cases states generally require that no death sentence shall be imposed unless it is the determination of twelve unanimous jurors. Some states have a bifurcated procedure for determining innocence or guilt and then imposing a sentence for the guilty: that is, after a jury finds someone guilty, the jury deliberates a second time to determine the sentence. In fact, in several states a new jury is empaneled expressly for sentencing. At this time the rules of evidence are more relaxed, and the jury may be permitted to hear evidence that was excluded during the actual trial (for example, the previous criminal record of the accused).

When the judge pronounces the sentence, it is customary for several weeks to elapse between the time the defendant is found guilty and when the penalty is imposed. This interval permits the judge to hear and consider any posttrial motions that the defense attorney might make (such as a motion for a new trial) and to allow a probation officer to conduct a presentence investigation. As mentioned in Chapter 3, the probation officer is a professional with a background in criminology, psychology, or social work who makes a recommendation to the judge about the length of the sentence to be imposed. It is customary for the probation officer to examine factors such as the background of the criminal, the seriousness of the crime committed, and the likelihood that the criminal will continue to engage in illegal activity. Judges are not required to follow the probation officer's recommendation, but still it is a major factor in the judge's calculus as to what the sentence shall be. Judges are presented with a variety of alternatives and a range of sentences when it comes to punishment for the criminal. Many of these alternatives involve the concept of rehabilitation and call for the assistance of professionals in the fields of criminology and social science.

The lightest punishment that a judge can hand down is that of probation. This is often the penalty if the crime is regarded as minor or when the judge believes that the guilty person is not likely to engage in additional criminal activity. (For example, a woman with no prior criminal record who kills her husband after being beaten and maltreated for twenty years is unlikely to go on a rampage of bank robberies or additional killings.) If a probated sentence is handed down, the criminal may not spend any time in prison as long as the conditions of the probation are maintained. Such conditions might include staying away from bars or convicted criminals, not committing other crimes, and sometimes not engaging in certain other objectional activities. For example, in January 1988 a senior U.S. district court judge in Philadelphia ordered a convicted drug dealer not to have sex outside of marriage or to father any illegitimate children, saying that to do so would be considered probation violations. (The criminal, who was single, had fathered three children.) The judge's formal order listed "fornication" and "bastardy" as actions for which the criminal's probation could be revoked.[19] If a criminal serves out his or her probation without incident, the criminal record is usually wiped clean, and in the eyes of the law it is as if no crime had ever been committed.

If the judge is not disposed toward probation and feels that "hard time" is in order, he or she must impose a prison sentence that is within a range prescribed by law. For example, in a given state the penalty for aggravated assault may be a prison term of "no less than five but no more than fifteen years in the state penitentiary." The reason for a range of years rather than an automatic number is that the law recognizes that not all crimes and criminals are alike and that in principle the punishment should fit the crime. Thus a criminal with a prior record who held up a liquor store might be given a longer sentence than the person with no record who embezzled some money in order to pay for his child's life-or-death surgery.

Flexibility in the sentencing process thus has its advantages, but there is another side to this coin: sentencing disparities among judges are often great and frequently result in situations where sentences vary significantly for essentially the same crime and set of circumstances. That is, there is much empirical evidence that judges do not view similar sets of facts and come to the same determinations with regard to sentences. A former official of the Federal Bureau of Prisons anonymously provided us with an example of the injustice that can result:

> The first man has been convicted of cashing a check for $58.40. He was out of work at the time of his offense, and when his wife became ill and he needed money for rent, food, and doctor bills, he became a victim of temptation. He had no prior criminal record. The other man cashed a check for $35.20. He was also out of work, and his wife had just left him for another man. His prior record consisted of a drunk charge and a nonsupport charge. Our examination of these two cases indicates no significant difference for sentencing purposes. But they appeared before different judges, and the first man received fifteen years in prison and the second man received thirty days.

In an effort to eliminate gross disparities in sentencing for basically the same set of circumstances, the federal government and many states have attempted to develop sets of precise guidelines to create greater consistency among judges. At the national level this effort has been manifested by the enactment of the Sentencing Act of 1987, but congressional concern for this problem goes back many years. In October 1984 Congress passed the Comprehensive Crime Control Act, which among other things created a Sentencing Commission. This commission was authorized to study the problem of sentencing disparities among federal jurists and to develop a set of guidelines for sentences. It began its determination of guideline ranges "by estimating the average sentences now being served," and thus it expects that its suggested guidelines will "in many instances . . . approximate existing practice."

> The guidelines contain a Sentencing Table with 43 offense levels on the vertical axis and six categories of criminal history on the horizontal axis. Offenders in criminal history category 1 would likely have little or no criminal record, while those in category 6 would likely have extensive criminal histories.
>
> The judge would find the applicable guideline sentencing range, which the table expresses in months of imprisonment, by determining the offense level and then reading across the axis to the proper criminal history category. Offense level 4, for example, which could apply to an offender convicted of theft of $100 or less, prescribes a sentencing range of 0 to 4 months for an offender in criminal history category 1, and 6 to 12 months for an offender in criminal history category 6. Offense level 38, which could apply to an offender convicted of aircraft hijacking, prescribes a sentencing range of 235-293 months for offenders in criminal history category 1, and 360 months to life for offenders in both the 5th and 6th criminal history categories.[20]

Congress provided that judges may depart from the guidelines only if they find "an aggravating or mitigating circumstance" that the commission did not adequately consider. Although the congressional guidelines do not specify the kinds of factors that could constitute grounds for departure from the sentencing guidelines, Congress did state that such grounds could not involve race, sex, national origin, creed, religion, socioeconomic status, drug dependence, or alcohol abuse.[21]

While the effects of the Sentencing Reform Act remain to be seen, the immediate impact of the law was to stir up a storm of controversy among the trial judges themselves. They felt that their authority and discretion as judges were being undermined by the congressional legislation and, in fact, between 1987 and 1989 about 150 federal judges ruled the sentencing guidelines unconstitutional, most often saying that the membership and powers of the Sentencing Commission violated the Constitution's separation of powers doctrine.[22] As Reagan trial judge appointee Sam Hall grumbled after passage of the act: "While I was in Congress, I was always opposed to anything that would take away the discretion of judges. The judge sits there and listens to testimony. He's in a much better position to set the sentence. It takes away the judges' initiative." [23] Nevertheless, in an eight-to-one decision in January 1989, the U.S. Supreme Court declared that both the commission and the guidelines passed constitutional muster.[24]

The states, too, have a variety of programs for avoiding vast disparities in judges' sentences. In California, for example, the legislature in 1977 established very precise rules for felony sentences. A preferred length of imprisonment was set forth for each type of offense, and the judge's options for departing from the preferred sentences were narrowed. In Minnesota the legislature established sentence parameters with the provision that sentences handed down outside the guidelines were subject to appeal. How well have these attempts to mitigate sentencing disparities fared? Laurence Baum has noted that in California and Minnesota,

> variation in sentences for specific offenses had declined, but it has not been reduced as much as might have been expected. In Minnesota . . . there was a remarkable change in sentencing patterns in the first year under the guidelines, but in succeeding years the guidelines had less effect . . . as attorneys and judges have learned to adapt their practices to achieve sentencing outcomes they prefer. . . . And in California, judges have used their sentencing discretion to maintain a good deal of variation.[25]

All this would seem to indicate that legislatures can temper judicial sentencing discretion to some degree—at least initially—but that there are real limits on what can be accomplished in this realm.

Despite the enormous impact that judges have on the sentence, they do not necessarily have the final say on the matter. Whenever a prison term is set by the judge, it is still subject to the parole laws of the federal government and of the states. Thus parole boards (and sometimes the president and governors who may grant pardons or commute sentences) have the final say about how long an inmate actually stays in prison. Evidence collected by the Justice Department for the state level suggests that parole boards and governors have not been hesitant about exercising their prerogatives. In fact, the average prisoner serves less than half the court-ordered maximum sentence. In a survey of thirty-three states the Justice Department's Bureau of Justice Statistics found that the average prisoner released from confinement had been sentenced to three years but the median time served was seventeen months—only 45 percent of that sentence![26]

## An Appeal

At both the state and federal levels everyone has the right to at least one appeal upon conviction of a felony. About a third of all criminals avail themselves of this privilege. An appeal is based on the contention that an error of law was made during the trial process. Such an error must be "reversible" as opposed to "harmless." (An error is considered harmless if its occurrence had no effect on the outcome of the trial.) A reversible error, however, is a serious one that might have affected the verdict of the judge or jury. For example, a successful appeal might be based on the argument that evidence was improperly admitted at trial, that the judge's instructions to the jury were flawed, or that a guilty plea was not voluntarily made. As we stressed in Chapter 5, however, appeals must be based on questions of procedure and legal interpretations, not on factual determinations or the defendant's guilt or innocence as such. Likewise, under most circumstances one cannot appeal the length of one's sentence in the United States (as long as it was in the range prescribed by law). This is unlike the practice of most other Western democracies, which routinely permit criminals to contest in the appeals courts the length of their prison terms.

If an appeal is successful, the defendant does not usually just go free. The usual practice is for the appellate court to remand the case (send it back down) to the lower court for a new trial. At that point the prosecution must determine whether the procedural errors in the original trial can be overcome in a second trial and whether it is worth the time and effort to do so. A second trial is not considered double jeopardy, since the defendant has chosen to appeal the original conviction.

The media and champions of "law and order" often make much of appellate courts that turn loose obviously guilty criminals and of convictions reversed on technicalities. Surely this does happen, and indeed one might argue that this is inevitable in a democratic country whose legal system is based on fair play and the presumption of the innocence of the accused. But we need to keep in mind a few basic facts and figures. First, about 90 percent of all defendants plead guilty, and this plea virtually excludes the possibility of an appeal. Of the remaining group, two-thirds are found guilty at trial, and only about a third of these actually appeal. Of those who do appeal, only about 20 percent have their convictions reversed. (For example, in the famous case of *Miranda v. Arizona*,[27] which spearheaded the criminal rights emphasis of the Warren Court, Miranda's conviction was overturned by the High Court because tainted evidence had been used to convict him. Nevertheless at a subsequent trial—minus the tainted evidence—he was again convicted for the same crime.) Of those whose convictions are reversed, many are found guilty at a subsequent trial. Thus when we talk of the number of persons convicted of crimes who are subsequently freed because of reversible court errors, we are talking about a small fraction of 1 percent. Most of us would consider that an acceptable risk in a free society.

## Summary

We began this chapter by talking about the nature and substance of crime—at least as it is understood in twentieth-century America. We then walked through the myriad of procedures that constitute the judicial process at the federal and state levels. We noted the various aspects that lead to an arrest, the subsequent appearance before a magistrate, and the activity of the grand jury or the preliminary hearing. We also observed how plea bargaining enormously tempers the nature of the criminal court process. During the criminal trial we outlined the basic rights of the accused and looked at the vagaries of the jury selection process. We then examined the key players at the trial—the prosecutor, the defense attorney, and the judge. After discussing the work of the jury we discussed the posttrial procedures of sentencing and appeal. Throughout the chapter we stressed a theme that we shall develop throughout the text, namely that the backgrounds and attitudes of the criminal justice participants have as much to do with the nature and quality of justice as do the formal rules of the game. Whether we are talking about police officers, prosecutors, judges, or juries, our criminal justice system is much influenced by the role perceptions, mores, and values of the men and women who dispense justice in America.

## Notes

1. We wish to express our debt to the following, from whom we borrowed this categorization: Harold J. Vetter and Leonard Territo, *Crime and Justice in America* (St. Paul: West, 1984), chap. 1.
2. Federal Bureau of Investigation, *Crime in the United States, 1985* (Uniform Crime Reports) (Washington, D.C.: Government Printing Office 1985), 41.
3. Ibid.
4. Bureau of Justice Statistics, *Sourcebook of Criminal Justice Statistics, 1980* (Washington, D.C.: Government Printing Office), Table 3.51, 290, and FBI, *Crime in the United States, 1985*, 41.
5. Vetter and Territo, *Crime and Justice in America*, 11.
6. *Whitney v. California*, 274 U.S. 357 (1927).
7. Ordinance unanimously declared invalid in *Patachristou v. City of Jacksonville*, 405 U.S. 156 (1972).
8. Quotation in David W. Neubauer, *America's Courts and the Criminal Justice System*, 2d ed. (Monterey, Calif.: Brooks/Cole, 1984), 64.
9. "Trying to Enforce Unpopular Law Is Plaguing the Highway Patrol," *Houston Chronicle*, September 25, 1977, 1:18.
10. *Miranda v. Arizona*, 384 U.S. 436 (1966).
11. There are variations of this, however. In Texas, for example, grand juries consist of twelve persons chosen because they are friends or neighbors of judge-appointed jury commissioners. A vote of nine members is required for a decision.
12. For example, see Robert A. Carp, "The Behavior of Grand Juries: Acquiescence or Justice," *Social Science Quarterly* 55 (1975): 853-870.
13. Bargains on the sentence are primarily conducted at the state rather than the federal level because federal sentences are largely within the bailiwick of the judge with advice from the probation officer—with both acting under the newly written congressional sentencing guidelines.

14. In the case of *Barker v. Wingo*, 407 U.S. 514 (1972), the Supreme Court permitted a delay of as much as five years because it felt the various trial date postponements were justified.
15. Also, in many jurisdictions laws exempt persons in specific occupations (for example, doctors, members of the clergy, police officers) and in specific situations (for example, full-time students, persons over sixty-five years of age, mothers with young children at home).
16. *Moore v. U.S.*, 345 F. 2d 97 D.C. Cir. (1965).
17. For an excellent classic study of jury behavior, see Harry Kalven, Jr., and Hans Zeisel, *The American Jury* (Boston: Little, Brown, 1966).
18. "The Eyes Have It," *Newsweek*, December 3, 1973, 85.
19. "Judge Orders Convict to Halt Premarital Sex," *Houston Chronicle*, January 14, 1988, 3:15.
20. "News from the Sentencing Commission," *The Third Branch* 19 (May 1987): 3-4.
21. Ibid., 5.
22. Tom Moran, "High Court Rulings on Guidelines May Bury Federal Civil Lawsuits," *Houston Chronicle*, January 19, 1989, A7.
23. "Sentencing Rules Strip Discretion, Judges Say," *Beaumont Enterprise*, November 28, 1987, B1.
24. *Mistretta v. U.S.*, January 18, 1989.
25. Lawrence Baum, *American Courts* (Boston: Houghton Mifflin, 1986), 198-199.
26. "Study: Prisoners Serving 45% of Terms," *Houston Chronicle*, December 31, 1987, 1:9.
27. *Miranda v. Arizona*, 384 U.S. 436 (1966).

# 7  The Civil Court Process

This chapter continues our examination of courts from a judicial process perspective, focusing on the civil courts. After discussing how civil law differs from criminal law and describing the most important categories of civil law, we will proceed step by step through the civil trial process and then consider alternatives to trials.

## The Nature and Substance of Civil Law

The American legal system observes several important distinctions between criminal and civil law. As we saw in the last chapter, criminal law is concerned with conduct that is offensive to society as a whole. Civil law, on the other hand, pertains primarily to the duties of private citizens to each other. In civil cases the disputes are usually between private individuals, although the government may sometimes be a party in a civil suit. Just the opposite is true with criminal cases, which always involve government prosecution of an individual for an alleged offense against society.

Civil actions are completely separate and distinct from criminal proceedings. In a civil case the court attempts to settle a particular dispute between the parties by determining their legal rights. The court then decides upon an appropriate remedy, such as awarding monetary damages to the injured party or issuing an order that directs one party to perform or refrain from a specific act. In a criminal case the court decides whether the defendant is innocent or guilty. A guilty defendant may be punished by a fine, imprisonment, or both.

In some instances the same act may give rise to both a criminal proceeding and a civil suit. Suppose that Joe and Pete, two political scientists attending a convention in Atlanta, are sharing a taxi from the airport to their downtown hotel. During the ride they become involved in a heated discussion over the quality of President Reagan's appointees to the federal courts. By the time the taxi stops at their hotel, the discussion has become so heated that Joe suggests they settle their differences right then and there. If Pete strikes Joe in the ribs with his briefcase as he gets out of the taxi, Pete may be charged with criminal assault. In addition, Joe might file a civil suit against Pete in an effort to obtain a monetary award sufficient to cover his medical expenses.

Civil cases far outnumber criminal cases in both the federal and state courts, although they generally do not attract the same media attention as criminal trials. Still, they often raise important policy questions and cover a broad range of disagreements in society. One leading judicial scholar summarizes the breadth of the civil law field as follows:

> Every broken agreement, every sale that leaves a dissatisfied customer, every uncollected debt, every dispute with a government agency, every libel and slander, every accidental injury, every marital breakup, and every death may give rise to a civil proceeding.[1]

Thus, virtually any dispute between two or more persons may provide the basis for a civil suit. The number of suits is huge, but most of them fall into one of five basic categories.[2]

## The Main Categories of Civil Law

### Contract Law

Contract law is primarily concerned with voluntary agreements between two or more people. Some common examples familiar to us all include agreements to perform a certain type of work, to buy or sell goods, and to construct or repair homes or businesses. Basic to these agreements are a promise by one party and a counterpromise by the other party, usually a promise by one party to pay money for the other party's services or goods. For example, assume that Mr. Burns and Ms. Colder enter into an agreement whereby Colder agrees to pay Burns $125 if he will cut and deliver a cord of oak firewood to her home on December 10. If Burns does not deliver the wood on that date he has "breached" the contract and Colder may sue him for damages.

Although many contracts are relatively simple and straightforward, some rather complex fields also build on contract law or contract ideas. One such field is commercial law, which focuses primarily on sales involving credit or the installment plan. Commercial law also deals with checks, promissory notes, and other negotiable instruments.

Another closely related field—one that has become especially prominent in recent years—involves bankruptcy and creditors' rights. Bankrupt individuals or businesses may go through a process that essentially wipes the slate clean and allows the person filing for bankruptcy to begin again. The bankruptcy process is also designed to ensure fairness to creditors. As we noted in Chapter 2, bankruptcy law is a federal concern and is administered by special bankruptcy judges attached to the U.S. district courts.

One final area is the insurance contract, which is important because of its applicability to so many people. The insurance industry is regulated by government agencies and subject to its own distinct rules.

## Tort Law

Tort law may generally be described as the law of civil wrongs. It involves conduct that causes injury and fails to measure up to some standard set by society.

Actions for personal injury or bodily injury claims are at the heart of tort law. One law professor estimates that about 95 percent of all tort claims are for personal injury, and that automobile accidents are responsible for most of these claims.[3] In recent years one of the most rapidly growing subfields of tort law has involved product liability. This category has become an increasingly popular way to hold corporations accountable for their misdeeds. In the short span between 1963 and 1972, for example, the number of product liability suits increased from 50,000 to over 500,000 per year.[4] These figures include suits for injuries caused by defective foods, toys, appliances, automobiles, drugs, and a host of other products.

Perhaps one reason for the tremendous growth in product liability cases is a change in the standard of proof. Traditionally, negligence (generally defined as carelessness or the failure to use ordinary care, under the particular circumstances revealed by the evidence in the lawsuit) must be proven before one person is able to collect damages for injuries caused by someone else. However, it has been argued that for many years reliance on the negligence concept has been declining, especially in product liability cases. In its place, the courts often use a strict liability standard, which means that a victim can recover even if there was no negligence and even if the manufacturer was careful.

Another important development in this area of the law is the fact that some courts have extended liability beyond the manufacturer. Several years ago, for example, an American Airlines plane crashed as the result of an allegedly defective altimeter. When the case went to court, it was decided that the cause of action was against Lockheed, the manufacturer of the plane, not of the altimeter.[5]

In short, American courts have increasingly seen a need to protect consumers against defective products. While it has long been argued that consumers should have freedom of choice in the marketplace, there is now less freedom to make an unsafe choice.[6]

Still another rapidly growing subfield of tort law is the medical malpractice category. Ironically, the number of medical malpractice claims has increased while great advances have been made in medicine.

Yet two important problems in contemporary medicine are the increased risk from new treatments and the impersonal character of specialists and hospitals.[7] In other words, patients have high expectations, and when a doctor fails them their anger may lead to a malpractice suit.[8]

Courts generally use the traditional negligence standard rather than the strict liability doctrine in resolving medical malpractice suits. This means that the law does not attempt to make doctors guarantee successful treatment, but instead tries to make the doctor liable if the patient can prove that the physician failed to perform in a manner consistent with accepted methods of medical practice. The injured patient must demonstrate that the doctor's conduct was unreasonably negligent and that this negligence was the cause of the specific injury that occurred. The notion of acceptable practice is a rather slippery one which varies from state to state and must be resolved by the courts on a case-by-case basis. It should be noted, however, that there is customarily a presumption that the conduct of professionals, including doctors, is reasonable in nature. This means that to prevail against the doctor in court the injured patient needs at least the testimony of one or more expert witnesses stating that the doctor's conduct was not reasonable.[9]

Our discussion would not be complete without noting an interesting side effect of the increasing number of malpractice suits. The threat of a malpractice suit may lead some doctors to practice a sort of "defensive medicine," which calls for more tests, consultations, and diagnostic procedures than were used in the past.[10]

## Property Law

There has traditionally been a distinction between real property and personal property. The former normally refers to real estate, that is, land, houses, and buildings; traditionally it has also included growing crops. Basically everything else is considered personal property. Included, then, would be such things as money, jewelry, automobiles, furniture, and bank deposits.

All of us have some involvement with both real estate and personal property during our lives. Most of us are renters or homeowners, or we live with someone who is. However, for most Americans personal property—our possessions—means more to us. Yet, "as far as the law is concerned the word *property* means primarily real property; personal property is of minor importance." [11] In fact, there is no single special field of law devoted to personal property. Instead, personal property is generally considered under the rubric of contract law, commercial law, and bankruptcy law.

Property rights have always been important in this country. It has been argued, for instance, that the protection of property rights was the major motivation of the framers of the U.S. Constitution.[12] Another pertinent example is that in the early days of this country only male *landowners* were eligible to vote.

Today, property rights have reached the point of being far more complex than mere ownership of something. The notion of property now includes, among several other things, the right to use that property.[13]

One important branch of property law today deals with land use controls. Zoning is the most familiar type of land use restriction. Zoning ordinances are generally considered to have had their beginning about the time of World War I, and are now found in cities, towns, and villages throughout the country. The zoning ordinances divide a municipality into districts designated for different uses. For instance, one neighborhood may be designated as residential, another as commercial, and yet another as industrial.

Early zoning laws were challenged on the ground that restrictions on land use amounted to a "taking" of the land by the city in violation of the Fifth and Fourteenth amendments. A provision of the Fifth Amendment, made applicable to the states by the Fourteenth Amendment, says: "Nor shall private property be taken for public use without just compensation." In a sense, zoning laws do "take" from the owners of land the right to use their property in any way they see fit. Nonetheless, courts have generally ruled that zoning laws are not regarded as a "taking" in violation of the Constitution.[14]

Although the courts have given zoning authorities rather broad powers, they do not have unlimited powers. According to the Supreme Court, the regulations must "bear a substantial relation to the public health, safety, morals, or general welfare." [15]

Today, zoning is a fact of life in cities and towns of all sizes throughout the United States. City planners and other city officials recognize zoning ordinances as necessary to the planned and orderly growth of urban areas. In fact, it is a constant source of amazement to many that the nation's fourth largest city, Houston, does not have a comprehensive zoning ordinance.

## The Law of Succession

The law of succession considers how property is passed along from one generation to another. The American legal system recognizes a person's right to dispose of his or her property as he or she wishes. One common way to do this is to execute a will. If a person leaves behind a valid will, the courts will enforce it. However, if someone leaves no will (or has improperly drawn it up), then the person has died "intestate," and the state must dispose of the property.

The state's disposition of the property is carried out according to the fixed scheme set forth in the state statutes. By law, intestate property passes to the deceased person's heirs, that is, to his or her nearest relatives.

First in line are the spouse and children. If neither spouse nor children are left, then parents are next in line; then come brothers and sisters. Occasionally a person who dies intestate has no living relatives. In that situation the property *escheats*, or passes, to the state in which the deceased resided. State statutes often prohibit the more remote relatives, such as second cousins and great uncles and aunts, from inheriting.[16]

Increasingly, Americans are preparing wills to ensure that their property is disposed of according to their wishes, not according to a scheme determined by the state. A will is a formal document. It must be very carefully drafted, and in most states it must be witnessed by at least two persons. In some jurisdictions it is possible to execute a will without witnesses. Such a document is known as a holographic will, and it must be written by hand by the *testator*, the person whose will it is.

Generally speaking, if you have a valid will you may disinherit any relatives you choose, with the general exception of a husband or wife. Laws in most states allow the spouse to contest the will in court and receive up to one-half of the deceased's property.[17]

## Family Law

Family law concerns such things as marriage, divorce, child custody, and children's rights. It is, clearly, a field that touches the lives of a great number of Americans each year.

The conditions necessary for entering into a marriage are spelled out by state law. These laws traditionally cover the minimum age of the parties, required blood tests or physical examinations, mental conditions of the parties, license and fee requirements, and waiting periods.

The termination of a marriage was once very rare. In the early nineteenth century some states granted divorces only through special acts of the legislature; one state, South Carolina, simply did not allow divorce. Even in the other states, divorces were granted only when one party proved some grounds for divorce. In other words, divorces were available only to "innocent" parties whose spouses were guilty of such things as adultery, desertion, or cruelty.

The twentieth century has seen an enormous change in divorce laws. The movement has clearly been away from restrictive laws and toward a concept known as no-fault divorce. This trend is the result of two factors. First, for many years there has been an increasing demand for divorces. Second, the stigma once attached to divorced persons has all but disappeared.

The no-fault divorce system means that the traditional grounds for divorce have been eliminated. Basically, the parties simply explain that "irreconcilable differences" exist between them and that the marriage is no longer viable. In some states the defendant is not even required to appear in court. In short, the no-fault divorce system has put an end to the adversarial nature of divorce proceedings.

Not so easily solved are some of the other problems that may result from an ended marriage. Child custody battles, disputes over child support payments, and disagreements over visitation rights still find their way into court on a regular basis. In fact, custody disputes are probably more common and more contentious today than before the no-fault divorce. The child's needs come first, and courts no longer automatically assume that this means granting custody to the mother. Fathers are increasingly being granted custody, and it is also now common for courts to grant joint custody to the divorced parents.

## The Courts and Other Institutions Concerned with Civil Law

Disagreements are common in the daily lives of Americans. Usually these disagreements can be settled outside the legal system. Sometimes they are so serious, however, that one of the parties sees no alternative but to file a lawsuit. The decision whether to file a suit and the institutions involved in resolving such disputes are examined in this section.

### Deciding Whether to Go to Court

Every year thousands of potential civil cases are resolved without a trial because the would-be litigants settle their problems in another way or because the prospective plaintiff decides not to file suit. When faced with a decision to call upon the courts, to try to settle differences, or to simply forget the problem, many people resort to a simple cost-benefit analysis. That is, they weigh the costs associated with a trial against the benefits they are likely to gain if they win. Should a quick calculation indicate that the tangible and intangible costs in terms of such things as time, money, publicity, stress, and anxiety outweigh the benefits, then most people will opt for an alternative to a trial. On the other hand, if the prospective plaintiff perceives the costs to be low enough, then he or she might well file suit against the defendant.

One recent study of civil litigation patterns relied upon a telephone survey of approximately 1,000 households selected at random in each of the following five federal judicial districts: South Carolina, Eastern Pennsylvania, Eastern Wisconsin, New Mexico, and Central California.[18] The authors of the study tell us that about 40 percent of the households reported a grievance involving $1,000 or more during the previous three years, and approximately 20 percent reported two or more such grievances.

While many grievances are never pursued any further, some result in the plaintiff's initiating a claim. A claim may be accepted, partially accepted, or rejected. Claims that are met with a partial or total rejection move on to become disputes. The odds that a claim will become a dispute are quite high. In the survey under discussion, approximately 63 percent of the claims became disputes (met with partial or total rejection).

The authors of the study next focused on the extent to which disputants hired attorneys and took their cases to court. Overall, they found that attorneys were hired in fewer than one-fourth of the disputes and that only about 11 percent of the disputants reported taking their dispute to court. This finding should not be seen as minimizing the importance of lawyers and judges, however. Each party's understanding of everyone's legal position is based on the lawyer's advice, which is in turn based on an understanding of previous court decisions.

Disputes that become court cases may go into a variety of courts, depending upon the nature of the dispute and the type of damages being sought. Furthermore, most disputes do not go all the way through the trial process. Instead, they are dropped by the litigants or settled prior to trial.

## Specialized Courts

The state court systems are frequently characterized by a number of specialized courts that are set up to handle specific types of civil cases. Domestic relations courts are often established to deal with such matters as divorce, child custody, and child support. In many jurisdictions one also finds probate courts to handle the settlement of estates and the contesting of wills.

Perhaps the best known of the specialized courts are the small claims courts. These courts have jurisdiction to handle cases when the money being sued for is not above a certain amount. The amount varies by jurisdiction, but the maximum is usually $500 or $1,000. The first small claims court, established in Cleveland, Ohio, was characterized by a simplified process, a nominal filing fee, and no requirement that the parties be represented by a lawyer. By 1920 other major cities, including Chicago, Minneapolis, New York, and Philadelphia, as well as the state of Massachusetts, had set up small claims courts based on the Cleveland model.[19]

Today, small claims courts allow less complex cases to be resolved more informally than in most other trial courts. Filing fees are still low and the summons to the other party to appear in court can often be served by certified mail. Pleadings are often not required and the use of attorneys is often discouraged.

These courts are not without their problems, however. One complaint prevalent in a number of large cities is that collection agencies use these courts as a relatively cheap and efficient way to collect small debts. New York has enacted legislation to prohibit this use of small claims courts.[20] And because lawyers are often not used in small claims court, those who are not familiar with their legal rights and do not know much about preparing their cases may be at a disadvantage, especially when the other party is experienced in such courts.

### Administrative Bodies

A number of government agencies have also established administrative bodies with quasi-judicial authority to handle certain types of cases. At the federal level, for example, agencies such as the Interstate Commerce Commission, the Federal Trade Commission, and the Federal Communications Commission carry out an adjudication of sorts within their respective spheres of authority. As noted in Chapter 2, an appeal of the ruling of one of these agencies may be taken to a federal court of appeals.

At the state level a common example of an administrative body that aids in the resolution of civil claims is a workers' compensation board. This board determines whether an employee's injury is job related and thus whether the person is entitled to workers' compensation. Many state motor vehicle departments have hearing boards to make determinations about revoking driver's licenses. Another type of administrative board commonly found in the states rules on civil rights matters and cases of alleged discrimination.

## The Civil Trial Process

In this section we will describe the steps involved in a typical civil case. As with criminal cases, most civil cases are resolved by the parties without their actually going to trial; some are resolved after the trial has begun but before it is concluded. We will have more to say about the resolution of civil cases without trial in a later section.

Generally speaking, the adversarial process used in criminal trials is also used in civil trials, with just a few important differences. First, a litigant must have *standing*. This concept, which was discussed in detail in Chapter 5, means simply that the person initiating the suit must have a personal stake in the outcome of the controversy. Otherwise, there is no real controversy between the parties and thus no actual case for the court to decide.

A second major difference is that the standard of proof used in civil cases is a *preponderance of the evidence*, rather than the more stringent beyond-a-reasonable-doubt standard used in criminal cases. "A preponderance of the evidence" is generally taken to mean that there is sufficient evidence to overcome doubt or speculation. It clearly means that less proof is required in civil cases than in criminal cases.

A third major difference is the fact that many of the extensive due-process guarantees that a defendant has in a criminal trial do not apply in a civil proceeding. For example, neither party is constitutionally entitled to counsel. The Seventh Amendment does guarantee the right to a jury trial in lawsuits "where the value in controversy shall exceed twenty dollars." Although this amendment has not been made applicable to the states, most states have similar constitutional guarantees.[21]

## Filing a Civil Suit

The person initiating the civil suit is known as the *plaintiff*, and the person being sued is the *defendant* or the *respondent*. A civil action is known by the names of the plaintiff and the defendant, such as *Jones v. Miller*. The plaintiff's name appears first. In a typical situation, the plaintiff's attorney pays a fee and files a *complaint* or *petition* with the clerk of the proper court. The complaint states the facts on which the action is based, the damages alleged, and the judgment or relief being sought.

It is useful to understand how a decision is made about which court should actually hear the case. Such a decision involves the concepts of jurisdiction and venue: *jurisdiction* deals with a court's authority to exercise judicial power, and *venue* means the *place* where that power should be exercised.

Jurisdictional requirements are satisfied when the court has legal authority over both the subject matter and the person of the defendant. This means that it is possible for several courts to have jurisdiction over the same case. Suppose, for example, that you are a resident of Dayton, Ohio, and are seriously injured in an automobile accident in Tennessee when the car you are driving is struck from the rear by a car driven by a resident of Kingsport, Tennessee. Total damages to you and your car run about $60,000. A state trial court in Ohio has subject matter jurisdiction, and Ohio can in all likelihood obtain jurisdiction over the defendant. In addition, the state courts of Tennessee probably have jurisdiction, too. Federal district courts in both Ohio and Tennessee also have jurisdiction because diversity of citizenship exists and the amount in controversy is over $50,000. Assuming that jurisdiction is your only concern, you, as plaintiff, can sue in any of these courts.

Other questions are raised by this hypothetical example: Which of these courts is the proper one to handle the case? Which is the best place for this case to be tried? These questions bring up the problem of venue.

Venue is often a matter of convenience since improper venue can be waived. In other words, if a court has proper jurisdiction, and the party does not object to venue, then the court can render a valid judgment.

The determination of proper venue may be prescribed by statute, based on avoiding possible prejudice, or it may simply be a matter of convenience. The federal law states that proper venue is the district in which either the plaintiff or defendant resides, or the district where the injury occurred. State venue statutes vary somewhat, but usually provide that where land is involved, proper venue is the county where the land is located. In most other instances venue is in the county where the defendant resides.

Venue questions may also be related to the perceived or feared prejudice of either the judge or the prospective jury. Attorneys sometimes object to trials being held in a particular area for this reason and may move for a change of venue. Although this type of objection is perhaps more commonly associated with highly publicized criminal trials, it is also found in civil trials.

Still another ground for change of venue is the doctrine of *forum non conveniens*, which simply means that the place selected for trial is not convenient. In deciding whether to grant the change, the judge considers the relative cost and inconvenience to the parties and to the witnesses.

Once the appropriate court has been determined and the complaint has been filed, the court clerk will attach a copy of the complaint to a summons, which is then issued to the defendant. The summons may be served by personnel from the sheriff's office, a U.S. marshal, or a private process-service agency.

The summons directs the defendant to file a response, known as a pleading, within a certain period of time (usually thirty days). If the defendant does not do so, then he or she may be subject to a default judgment.

These simple actions by the plaintiff, clerk of the court, and a process server set in motion the civil case. What happens next is a flurry of activities that precedes an actual trial and may last for several months. Approximately 75 percent of cases are resolved *without a trial* during this time.[22]

## Pretrial Activities

*Motions.*  Once the summons has been served on the defendant, there are a number of motions that can be made by the defense attorney. A *motion to quash* requests that the court void the summons on the ground that it was not properly served. For example, a defendant might contend that the summons was never delivered to her personally as required by the law in her state.

Next we find two types of motions that are meant to clarify or to object to the plaintiff's petition. A *motion to strike* requests that the court excise, or strike, certain parts of the petition because they are prejudicial, improper, or irrelevant. Sometimes the defense attorney will file a *motion to make more definite*. This simply asks the court to require the plaintiff to be more specific about the complaints. For instance, the defendant's attorney may ask that the alleged injuries be described in greater detail.

A fourth type of motion often filed in a civil case is a *motion to dismiss*. This type of motion may argue, for example, that the court lacks jurisdiction. Or it may insist that the plaintiff has not presented a legally sound basis for action against the defendant even if the allegations are true. This action is called a *demurrer* in many state courts.

*The Answer.*  If the complaint survives the judge's rulings on the motions listed above, then the defendant submits an answer to the complaint. The response may contain admissions, denials, defenses, and counterclaims. When an *admission* is contained in an answer, there is no need to prove that fact during the trial. A *denial*, on the other hand, brings up a factual issue to be proven during the trial. A *defense* says that certain facts set forth in the answer may bar the plaintiff from recovery.

The defendant may also create a separate action by seeking relief against the plaintiff. This is known as a *counterclaim*. In other words, if the defendant thinks that a cause of action against the plaintiff arises from the same set of events, then he or she must present the claim to the court in response to the plaintiff's claim. Of course, the plaintiff may want to file a reply to the defendant's answer. In that reply, the plaintiff may admit, deny, or defend against the allegations of fact contained in the answer.

*Discovery.*  Although surprise was once a legitimate trial tactic, our present legal system provides "discovery" procedures that "take the sporting aspect out of litigation and make certain that legal results are based on the true facts of the case—not on the skill of the attorneys." [23] In other words, to prevent surprise at the trial and to encourage settlement, each party is entitled to information in the possession of the other. The term *discovery* "encompasses the methods by which a party or potential party to a lawsuit obtains and preserves information regarding the action." [24]

There are several tools of discovery. A *deposition* is testimony of a witness taken under oath outside the court. The same question-and-answer format as in the courtroom is used. All parties to the case must be notified that the deposition is to be taken so that their attorneys may be present to cross-examine the witness.

A second tool of discovery is known as *interrogatories*, written questions that must be answered under oath. Interrogatories can be submitted only to the parties in the case, not to witnesses. They are very useful in obtaining descriptions of evidence held by the opposing parties in the suit.

The *production of documents* is a third tool used in the discovery process. Often, one of the parties may request an inspection of documents, writings, drawings, graphs, charts, maps, photographs, or other items held by the other party.

Finally, when the physical or mental condition of one of the parties is at issue, the court may order that person to submit to an examination by a physician.

What happens if a party refuses to comply with discovery requests? The judge may compel compliance, deem the facts of the case established, dismiss the cause of action, or enter judgment by default.

*The Pretrial Conference.*   As a result of the discovery phase, surprise is no longer a major factor in civil cases; therefore, a large number of cases are settled without going to trial.[25] In the event the parties do not reach a settlement of their own accord, the judge may try to facilitate such an agreement during a pretrial conference.

Judges call such conferences to discuss the issues in the case informally with the opposing attorneys. The general practice is to allow only the judge and the lawyers to attend the conference, which is normally held in the judge's chambers. As federal district judge J. Skelly Wright put it, "If you bring the lawyer's litigants in there, the clients, well the lawyers will begin to act like thespians, in front of their clients."[26]

The judge and the attorneys use the conference to try to come to some agreement on uncontested factual issues, which are known as *stipulations*. The purpose of stipulations is to make the actual trial more efficient. The attorneys also share with each other a list of witnesses and documents that are a part of each case. In the words of Judge Wright, "We make each side disgorge completely and absolutely everything about its case. There can't possibly be surprise, if the lawyers know what they are doing."[27]

Lawyers and judges may also use the pretrial conference to try to settle the case. In fact, some judges actively work to bring about a settlement so the case does not have to go to trial. That Wright was such a judge is indicated by his own account of the pretrial conference:

> After we set the case for trial, we talk about settlement. I say, "Well have you exhausted the possibility of settlement?" Then I say to the plaintiff's lawyer: "You brought this suit, how much is it worth?" And then they begin to talk; and then I actually find out that they have discussed settlement, and they have reached a stand-off with reference to the offer of settlement: One having made an offer in X amount, and the other having countered in Y amount. So, if it's a personal injury case, I look at the doctor's reports—just the last paragraph, where they show the extent of injury—I tell them. "This case is worth $20,000 for the settlement," and I tell them why; and I tell them further to go tell their clients that I said so. And the funny thing is, the lawyers in our district want the judge to do that. They want to be able to go back to their clients and have some of the load taken off their shoulders. They say, "This is what I think, but the judge says this." And, by and large, these cases are settled.[28]

## The Civil Trial

*Selection of Jury.*   As we noted above, the right to a jury trial in a civil suit in a federal court is guaranteed by the Seventh Amendment. State constitutions likewise provide for such a right. A jury trial may of course be waived, in which case the judge decides the matter. Although the jury traditionally consists of twelve persons, today the number varies. Most of the federal district courts now use juries of fewer than twelve persons in civil cases. A majority of states also authorize smaller juries in some or all civil trials.

As we saw in Chapter 6, jurors must be selected in a random manner from a fair cross-section of the community. A large panel of jurors is called to the courthouse, and when a case is assigned to a court for trial, a smaller group of prospective jurors is sent to a particular courtroom.

Following the voir dire examination, which may include challenges to certain jurors by the attorneys, a jury to hear the particular case will be seated. Recall that lawyers may challenge a prospective juror for cause, in which case the judge must determine whether the person challenged is impartial or not. Each side may also exercise a certain number of peremptory challenges, that is, excusing a juror without stating any reason. Peremptory challenges are fixed by statute or court rule and normally range from two to six.

*Opening Statements.*   After the jury has been chosen, the attorneys present their opening statements. The plaintiff's attorney begins. He or she explains to the jury what the case is about and what the plaintiff's side expects to prove. The defendant's lawyer can usually choose either to make an opening statement immediately after the plaintiff's attorney finishes or to wait until the plaintiff's case has been completely presented. If the defendant's attorney waits, he or she will present the entire case for the defendant continuously, from opening statement onward. Opening statements are valuable because they outline the case and make it easier for the jury to follow the evidence as it is presented.

*Presentation of the Plaintiff's Case.*   In the normal civil case the plaintiff's side is first to present and attempt to prove its case to the jury and last to make closing arguments. In presenting the case, the plaintiff's lawyer will normally call witnesses to testify and produce documents or other exhibits.

When a witness is called, he or she will undergo direct examination by the plaintiff's attorney. Then the defendant's attorney will have the opportunity to ask questions or cross-examine the witness. Following the cross-examination, the plaintiff's lawyer may conduct a redirect examination, which may then be followed by a second cross-examination by the defendant's lawyer.

Generally speaking, witnesses may testify only about matters they have actually observed; they may not express their opinions. However, there is a very important exception to this general rule: expert witnesses are specifically called upon to give their opinions in matters within their areas of expertise.

In order to qualify as an expert witness, a person must possess substantial knowledge about a particular field. Furthermore, this knowledge must normally be established in open court. Both sides often present experts whose opinions are contradictory. When this happens, the jury must ultimately decide which opinion is the correct one.

Rule 706 of the Federal Rules of Evidence permits federal district judges to appoint experts to assist in deciding cases. A recent study by the Federal Judicial Center found that approximately one in five judges has appointed an expert under this rule's authority. Of this number, about half have appointed an expert more than once. When asked which types of cases most often required the assistance of an expert, the judges most frequently mentioned patent cases, followed by product liability and antitrust cases.[29]

When the plaintiff's side has presented all its evidence, the attorney rests the case. It is now the defendant's turn.

**Motion for Directed Verdict.** After the plaintiff's case has been rested, the defendant will often make a motion for a directed verdict. With the filing of this motion, the defendant is saying that the plaintiff has not proved his case and thus should lose. The judge must then decide whether the plaintiff could win at this point if court proceedings were to cease. Should the judge determine that the plaintiff has not presented convincing enough evidence, he or she will sustain the motion and direct the verdict for the defendant. Thus the plaintiff will lose the case.

The motion for a directed verdict is similar to the pretrial motion to dismiss, or demurrer. Essentially, each says "So what?" to the plaintiff— the former in court and the latter before trial.

**Presentation of the Defendant's Case.** Assuming that the motion for a directed verdict is overruled, the defendant then presents evidence. The defendant's case is presented in the same way as the plaintiff's case. That is, there is direct examination of witnesses and presentation of documents and other exhibits. The plaintiff has the right to cross-examine witnesses. Re-direct and re-cross questions may follow.

**Plaintiff's Rebuttal.** After the presentation of the defendant's case, the plaintiff may bring forth rebuttal evidence, which is aimed at refuting the defendant's evidence.

**Answer to Plaintiff's Rebuttal.** During this stage of the process the defendant's lawyer presents evidence to counter the rebuttal evidence. This rebuttal/answer pattern may continue until the evidence has been exhausted.

*Closing Arguments.*   After all the evidence has been presented, the lawyers make closing arguments, or summations, to the jury. The plaintiff's attorney speaks both first and last. That is, he or she both opens the argument and closes it, and the defendant's lawyer argues in between. In this stage of the process each attorney attacks the opponent's evidence for its unreliability and may also attempt to discredit the opponent's witnesses. In doing so, the lawyers often wax eloquent or deliver an emotional appeal to the jury. However, the arguments must be based upon facts supported by the evidence and introduced at the trial. In other words, they must stay within the record.

*Instructions to the Jury.*   Assuming that a jury trial has not been waived, the instructions to the jury follow the conclusion of the closing arguments. The judge informs the jury that it must base its verdict on the evidence presented at the trial. The judge's instructions also inform the jurors about the rules, principles, and standards of the particular legal concept involved. Recall that in civil cases a finding for the plaintiff is based on a preponderance of the evidence. This means that the jurors must weigh the evidence presented during the trial and determine in their minds that the greater weight of the evidence, in merit and in worth, favors the plaintiff.

*The Verdict.*   The jury retires to the seclusion of the jury room to conduct its deliberations. The members must reach a verdict without outside contact. In some instances the deliberations are so long and detailed that the jurors must be provided meals and sleeping accommodations until they can reach a verdict. The verdict, then, represents the jurors' agreement after detailed discussions and analyses of the evidence. It sometimes happens that the jury deliberates in all good faith but cannot reach a verdict. When this occurs, the judge may declare a mistrial. This means that a new trial may have to be conducted.

After the verdict is reached, the jury is conducted back into open court, where it delivers its verdict to the judge. The parties are informed of the verdict. It is then customary for the jury to be polled—the jurors are individually asked whether they agree with the verdict.

*Posttrial Motions.*   Once the verdict has been reached, a party not satisfied may pursue a variety of tactics. The losing party may file a motion for judgment notwithstanding the verdict. This type of motion is granted when the judge decides that reasonable persons could not have rendered the verdict the jury reached. Put another way, this decision says that the verdict is unreasonable in light of the facts presented at the trial and the legal standards to be applied to the case.

The losing party may also file a motion for a new trial. The usual basis for this motion is that the verdict goes against the weight of the evidence.

The judge will grant the motion on this ground if he or she agrees that the evidence presented simply does not support the verdict reached by the jury. A new trial may also be granted for a number of other reasons: excessive damages, grossly inadequate damages, the discovery of new evidence, and errors in the production of evidence, to name a few.

In some cases the losing party also files a motion for relief from judgment. This type of motion may be granted if the judge finds a clerical error in the judgment, discovers some new evidence, or determines that the judgment was induced by fraud.

*Judgment and Execution.*    A verdict in favor of the defendant ends the trial. However, a verdict for the plaintiff requires yet another stage in the process. There is no sentence in a civil case, but there must be a determination of the remedy or damages to be assessed. This determination is called the *judgment.*

In situations where the judgment is for money damages and the defendant does not voluntarily pay the set amount, the plaintiff can ask to have the court clerk issue an order to execute the judgment. The execution is issued to the sheriff and orders the sheriff to seize the defendant's property and sell it at auction to satisfy the judgment. An alternative is to order a lien, which is the legal right to hold property that may be used for the payment of the judgment.

*Appeal.*    If one party feels that an error of law was made during the trial, and if the judge refuses to grant a posttrial motion for a new trial, then the dissatisfied party may appeal to a higher court. Probably the most common grounds for appeal are that the judge allegedly admitted evidence that should have been excluded, refused to admit evidence that should have been introduced, or failed to give proper jury instructions.

An attorney lays the groundwork for an appeal by objecting to the alleged error during the trial. This objection goes into the trial record and becomes a part of the trial transcript, which may be reviewed by an appellate court. The appellate court decision may call for the lower court to enforce its earlier verdict or to hold a new trial.

## Alternative Dispute Resolution

As we have noted above, in practice very few persons make use of the entire judicial process. Instead, most cases are settled without resort to a full-fledged trial. In civil cases, a trial may be both slow and expensive. As the statistics on judicial workload presented in Chapter 5 indicate, most of our courts are hard pressed to keep up with their dockets. In many areas the backlogs are so horrendous that it takes three to five years for a case to come to trial.

Many civil suits today are also exceedingly complex. Although the following example is certainly not typical, we think it provides a vivid illustration of a complex case that will tax the resources of thousands of people before it is concluded:

> The [Judicial] Conference approved a recommendation that the trial of *In re Washington Public Power Supply Sys. Securities* Litig., No. MDL 551, be videotaped. The case, trial of which is expected to start in Tucson this year, involves more than 125,000 plaintiffs, multi-billion dollar claims, more than 200 defendants, and the expected presence in the courtroom of more than 100 attorneys. Since the trial will necessarily be protracted and some jurors or counsel may therefore miss a portion of it due to health reasons or emergencies, they will be given access to the videotapes for the times they were absent, but the videotapes will not be made public.[30]

Often, the expense of a trial is enough to discourage potential plaintiffs. There is always the possibility of losing; even if a plaintiff wins, there is always the possibility of a long wait before the judgment is satisfied—if indeed it is ever completely satisfied. In other words, a trial may simply create a new set of problems for the parties concerned. For all these reasons, we have recently begun to hear more and more about alternative methods of resolving disputes. These methods have been described as "a second major wave of judicial reform."[31] The first judicial reform wave, discussed in Chapter 3, emphasized structural and administrative changes in the federal and state judicial systems.

The alternative dispute resolution (ADR) movement is now well established in the United States. From major corporations to attorneys to individuals, support for alternative ways to resolve disputes has been growing. Corporate America is interested in avoiding prolonged and costly court battles as the way to settle complex business disputes. In addition, attorneys are more frequently considering alternatives such as mediation, arbitration, and rent-a-judge programs where there is a need for faster resolution of cases or confidential treatment of certain matters.[32] And individual citizens are increasingly turning to local mediation services for help in resolving family disputes, neighborhood quarrels, and consumer complaints.

Although various methods of resolving disputes have existed both formally and informally for a number of years, "what is perhaps most significant at present . . . is that the ADR movement appears to have captured the imagination of the courts."[33] Courts at all levels are now actively using alternative methods of resolving civil disputes such as arbitration and mediation.

One observer has described the use of alternative methods as a two-stage movement. During the first stage hundreds of local ADR programs were created throughout the country. The second stage has seen the "institutionalization" of many of these programs through official recognition, sponsorship (funding), or assimilation into the existing court system.[34]

In early 1987, for instance, the U.S. Claims Court and the U.S. Court of Appeals for the District of Columbia Circuit implemented programs using various ADR techniques.[35] The U.S. Claims Court decided to use two ADR techniques: settlement judges and minitrials. The D.C. Circuit Court of Appeals announced that it was implementing, on an experimental basis, a civil mediation program using distinguished senior members of the bar as mediators. All three of these ADR techniques, as well as some others, will be described in more detail in the sections that follow.

We begin with a look at two very popular techniques: mediation and arbitration. Although the two are different, there is often a good deal of confusion about them. In fact, one former U.S. magistrate who now serves as a mediator, an arbitrator, and a consultant in alternative dispute resolution says that "an amazing number of lawyers and business professionals are unaware of the differences between arbitration and mediation."[36] He explains that the confusion is understandable, however, because in the early development of the English language the two words were used interchangeably. Modern statutes in the labor relations area (which has long used these two techniques) perpetuate the confusion. Libraries can add to the confusion when a reader looking up "mediation" is referred to "arbitration."

*Mediation.* The mediation process calls upon an impartial intervenor to assist the disputants in reaching a voluntary settlement of their differences. The process is generally nonadversarial, and there is no attempt to determine right or wrong. Instead, the goals are reconciliation and a more harmonious relationship between the parties involved.

The mediation process generally includes the following eight steps: initiation, preparation, introduction, problem statement, problem clarification, generation and evaluation of alternatives, selection of alternative(s), and agreement.[37] The process may be initiated in two basic ways. In some instances parties voluntarily submit the argument to a dispute resolution organization or to a private mediator. At other times the matter may be referred to mediation by court order. Although the process is typically nonadversarial, the parties should seek counsel and have a lawyer present for advice if necessary.

The *introductory stage* may well be the most important stage in the mediation process, because it is in this stage that the mediator establishes credibility. Unlike a judge, or even an arbitrator, a mediator does not have the immediate trust and respect of the parties to the dispute. During this introductory stage the mediator will also explain the procedures to be followed throughout the process.

Once the actual mediation process begins, the complaining party will generally open by presenting his or her story. The mediator listens carefully, takes notes if necessary, and asks appropriate questions to clarify the issues. When the complaining party has finished, the mediator summarizes the presentation and then makes sure that the other party understands the complaining party's story. The responding party is then asked to present his or her story. Again, the mediator takes notes, clarifies, and summarizes.

The *problem clarification* stage comes next. During this phase of the process the mediator extracts the true underlying issues in the dispute. It may be necessary to confer separately with the parties in order to pull out information that may not have surfaced during the earlier presentation. It should be noted, however, that the mediator does not disclose information that has been given in confidence by either party. It is also during this stage that the parties are given assistance in grouping and prioritizing their issues and demands.

During the *generation and evaluation of alternatives* the mediator often accomplishes his or her task by "creating doubt in the minds of the parties as to the validity of their positions on issues; and suggesting alternative approaches which may facilitate agreement." [38]

The next stage involves the *selection of alternatives*. The parties are encouraged to eliminate unworkable solutions. The mediator also helps them determine which of the remaining workable solutions will produce the best results that each party can live with.

The final stage of the mediation process involves securing the *assent* of each party to the terms of the agreement. The mediator does not usually become involved in drafting the settlement agreement. Instead, this is left to the parties or to their attorneys. In short, the agreement is the parties' rather than the mediator's.

**Arbitration.** The arbitration process calls for one or more persons to hear the arguments in a dispute, review the evidence, and reach a decision. Arbitration has long been used in resolving labor disputes and is now becoming more widely used for settling disputes involving commercial transactions. Another fairly recent development is court-annexed arbitration, whereby judges refer civil suits to arbitrators who render prompt, nonbinding decisions. If the arbitrator's decision is not accepted by the losing party, then a trial de novo may be held in the court system. The arbitration process generally consists of the following six steps: initiation, preparation, prehearing conferences, hearing, decision making, and award. [39]

*Initiation* involves starting the process and choosing the arbitrator. There are several ways to initiate an arbitration proceeding. One way is for both parties to agree to submit the dispute to arbitration. This method is used where there is no previous agreement to arbitrate. The submission must be signed by both parties. In other instances, the parties may have agreed in advance to arbitrate certain types of disputes. When that is the case, then one party may unilaterally initiate arbitration by serving notice on the other party. In a court-annexed situation the dispute is referred to arbitration by a court order.

Generally speaking, the parties may choose between temporary and permanent arbitrators. They may also choose whether they wish to have single or multiple arbitrators. A number of directories list names of potential arbitrators from which the parties may choose.

The *preparation* stage is very important because arbitration, although less formal than a trial, nevertheless follows the standard adversary process. For example, prehearing discovery may be used in some cases, although usually in a more limited form than in a formal trial.

*Prehearing conferences* are the next order of business. The arbitrator may call for briefs to argue points made in motions attacking the validity of claims or of the proceeding. During this stage, *ex parte* (with one side only) conferences between the arbitrator and an individual party are not permitted.

Although the parties may waive an oral hearing and have the dispute resolved on the basis of written documents only, most cases go through an evidentiary-type hearing. As a general rule, arbitration hearings are closed to the public.

The *hearing* resembles a trial in that it consists of opening statements, presentation of evidence, and closing statements. In some instances the arbitrator may be authorized by law to subpoena witnesses and documents.

The *decision-making* stage comes next. In cases where the issues are not very complex, the arbitrator may hand down an immediate decision. The more complex cases may require several weeks of decision making. If an arbitration panel rather than a single arbitrator is used, it will usually be necessary for the panel to confer, thus making an immediate decision almost impossible.

The arbitrator determines the *award*, which is usually written and signed by the arbitrator(s). Such awards are normally short, definite, and final. An exception, of course, is in the court-annexed arbitration process, which guarantees that the dissatisfied losing party may obtain a trial de novo in court. Awards are occasionally accompanied by a short written opinion.

**Settlement Judges.**    As we noted above, the use of settlement judges is an ADR technique recently instituted by the U.S. Claims Court. When the parties agree to use this method they simply inform the presiding judge, who will consider the request. If it is deemed appropriate, the court clerk's office will assign the case to a judge who will preside over the procedure.

The settlement judge acts as a neutral adviser who provides a judicial assessment of the parties' settlement positions. In other words, the settlement judge is there to help facilitate a settlement of the case. Should settlement not be reached, the parties may then go to trial.

*Minitrials.*   The ADR technique of minitrials, also recently instituted by the U.S. Claims Court, is to be employed only in cases that involve factual disputes and are governed by well-established legal principles. The minitrial should normally be employed before significant discovery begins. In a minitrial each side presents an abbreviated version of its case to a neutral adviser (someone other than the presiding judge), who then assists the parties in negotiating a settlement. The minitrial procedures require that each party be represented by an attorney with the authority to settle the case. The parties meet with the minitrial judge for a prehearing conference, at which they exchange brief written summaries of their positions. They also use the pretrial conference to narrow the issues. Hearings are informal and are generally concluded in one day. The guidelines of the U.S. Claims Court direct that the entire minitrial process should conclude within one to three months. That is certainly quicker than most complete trials.

*"Private" Judicial Systems.*   One final form of alternative dispute resolution deserves attention because it is being used more and more extensively in minor cases. This method is referred to as a "private" judicial system because it is: the parties actually hire an arbitrator to resolve their dispute.

California is quite well known for its use of this dispute-solving method. Although the California legislature first provided for this approach in 1872, the law has been used extensively only since the 1970s.[40] In Los Angeles a large number of retired superior court judges are used as arbitrators. The great advantage to the litigants is the speed with which their dispute can be resolved. Another advantage, at least in California, is that the arbitrators have judicial authority and their decisions may be enforced by the state. A possible disadvantage is the fact that the parties pay for the services of the arbitrators, which "can range from $150 to $300 an hour or $750 a day."[41]

Without doubt, the most famous of these "private justice" judges is Joseph A. Wapner. Wapner, a retired presiding judge of the superior court in Los Angeles, is a past president of the California Judges' Association. For the past seven years he has been best known to American television viewers as the man who presides over "The People's Court." During that time, more than 2,000 cases have been resolved for the television audience in real disputes between real litigants who, according to Judge Wapner, are told nothing other than "where to stand."[42]

## Summary

This chapter has focused on the handling of civil cases. We began by looking at some of the important categories of civil law: contracts, torts, property, the law of succession, and family law.

Next we examined the process followed in resolving civil cases. Once a complaint has been filed in a civil case, a number of pretrial motions may narrow the scope of the dispute or lead to a settlement of the case. As in criminal cases, most civil cases never actually go to trial. The discovery process also is useful in narrowing the scope of the case and preventing surprises should the case proceed to trial.

The cases that are not settled prior to trial follow a fairly standard process, which was discussed step by step. Where appropriate, we pointed out the differences between a civil trial and a criminal trial.

Finally, we discussed in some detail the alternative dispute resolution movement, which has been around for quite some time but has only recently captured significant attention from the courts. We described several ADR techniques, focusing most on arbitration and mediation, which are now being used by federal and state courts to solve the problems of increasing caseloads and troublesome backlogs.

## Notes

1. Herbert Jacob, *Justice in America*, 4th ed. (Boston: Little, Brown, 1984), 210.
2. We are indebted to Lawrence M. Friedman, from whom we borrowed the classifications and on whose work our discussion is based. See his *American Law* (New York: Norton, 1984), 141-153.
3. Ibid., 144.
4. William T. Schantz, *The American Legal Environment* (St. Paul, Minn.: West, 1976), 557.
5. See *Goldberg v. Kollsman Instrument Corp.*, 12 N.Y. 2d 432, 240 N.Y.S. 2d 592, 191 N.E. 2d 81 (1963).
6. Schantz, *The American Legal Environment*, 565.
7. See L. Lander, *Defective Medicine* (New York: Farrar, Straus, & Giroux, 1978), chap. 1.
8. Mitchell S. G. Klein, *Law, Courts, and Policy* (Englewood Cliffs, N.J.: Prentice-Hall, 1984), 196.
9. See S. Law and S. Polan, *Pain and Profit: The Politics of Malpractice* (New York: Harper & Row, 1978), 7, 8.
10. Klein, *Law, Courts, and Policy*, 196.
11. Friedman, *American Law*, 146.
12. See Charles A. Beard, *An Economic Interpretation of the Constitution of the United States* (New York: Macmillan, 1913).
13. Klein, *Law, Courts, and Policy*, 183.
14. See *Village of Euclid v. Ambler Realty Co.*, 272 U.S. 365 (1926).
15. See *Nectow v. City of Cambridge*, 277 U.S. 188 (1928).
16. See Schantz, *The American Legal Environment*, 291.
17. Ibid., 292.
18. Richard E. Miller and Austin Sarat, "Grievances, Claims, and Disputes: Assessing the Adversary Culture," *Law and Society Review* 15 (1980-81): 525-566.
19. See Howard Abadinsky, *Law and Justice* (Chicago: Nelson-Hall, 1988), 183, and Christine B. Harrington, *Shadow Justice: The Ideology and Institutional-*

*ization of Alternatives to Court* (Westport, Conn.: Greenwood, 1985).
20. See Abadinsky, *Law and Justice*, 184.
21. See Jack H. Friedenthal, Mary Kay Kane, and Arthur R. Miller, *Civil Procedure* (St. Paul, Minn.: West, 1985).
22. See Abadinsky, *Law and Justice*, 180.
23. Schantz, *The American Legal Environment*, 169.
24. Friedenthal, Kane, and Miller, *Civil Procedure*, 380.
25. See Kenneth M. Holland, "The Federal Rules of Civil Procedure," *Law and Policy Quarterly* 3 (1981): 212.
26. J. Skelly Wright, "The Pretrial Conference," in *American Court Systems: Readings in Judicial Process and Behavior*, ed. Sheldon Goldman and Austin Sarat (San Francisco: Freeman, 1978), 120.
27. Ibid.
28. Ibid.
29. See *The Third Branch* 20 (April 1988): 2.
30. Ibid.
31. James J. Alfini, "Alternative Dispute Resolution and the Courts: An Introduction," *Judicature* 69 (February-March 1986): 252.
32. Ibid.
33. Ibid.
34. See Peter Edelman, "Institutionalizing Dispute Resolution Alternatives," *Justice System Journal* 9 (1984): 134.
35. See *The Third Branch* 19 (June 1987): 1, 9.
36. John W. Cooley, "Arbitration vs. Mediation—Explaining the Differences," *Judicature* 69 (February-March 1986): 263.
37. Ibid., 266. Our discussion of the steps in the mediation process draws heavily from this source.
38. Ibid., 267.
39. See ibid., 264-266. Our discussion of the arbitration process is drawn from this source.
40. Abadinsky, *Law and Justice*, 221.
41. Ibid.
42. Ann Hodges, "Wapner Calls 'Em as He Sees 'Em," *Beaumont Enterprise TV Week*, April 17, 1988, 13.

# 8 The Federal and State Judges

Previous chapters have explored the history, organization, and workload of the federal and state judiciaries and have identified those staff and support agencies that make the wheels of American justice spin with at least a modicum of efficiency. It is now time to focus upon the main actors in the federal and state court systems—the men and women who serve as judges and justices.

As we take an analytical look at the black-robed decision makers to whom most Americans still look with such reverence, we will keep several questions in mind: What characteristics do these people have that distinguish them from the rest of the citizenry? What are the qualifications—both formal and informal—for appointment to the bench? How are the judges selected and who are the participants in the process? Is there a policy link between the citizenry, the appointment process and, the subsequent decisions of the jurists? How are they socialized into their judicial roles—that is, how do judges learn to be judges?

Finally, we shall say a few words about how and when judges stop being judges—the retirement, discipline, and removal of jurists. Because data for state judges is sparse we will focus more on federal judges.

## Background Characteristics of Federal Judges

In the United States we still cling eagerly to the log cabin-to-White House myth of attaining high public office—that is, to the notion that someone born in the humblest of circumstances (like Abraham Lincoln) may one day grow up to be the president of the United States, or at least a U.S. judge. As with most myths, there is a kernel of truth to it. In principle virtually anyone can become a prominent public official, and there are in fact a few well-known examples of people who came from poor backgrounds yet climbed to the top of the heap of power and respectability. One example is Justice Thurgood Marshall, the great-grandson of a slave and the son of a Pullman car steward. Another is former chief justice Warren Burger, whose father earned his daily bread as a traveling salesman and as a railroad car inspector.

Despite these occasional exceptions, the normal pattern is usually quite different. For a long time uncontested data have clearly shown that America's federal judges, like other public officials and the captains of commerce and industry, come from a very narrow stratum of American society. As we shall momentarily see, while potential judges are not necessarily the sons and daughters of millionaires, it is at least helpful if they come from a special segment of the nation's middle- and upper-middle classes.

### District Judges

Before we can offer some generalizations about who U.S. trial judges are and where they come from, we need some facts and figures. Background data for all federal district judges for the past 200 years have never been collected, but about judges who have served in recent decades we know a good deal. Table 8-1 profiles some key factors for trial jurists appointed by Presidents Johnson, Nixon, Ford, Carter, and Reagan.

In terms of their primary occupation before assuming the federal bench, a plurality had been judges at the state or local level. About 28 percent of Nixon's judges had had extensive judicial experience, and as many as 45 percent of Carter's judicial team had previously worn the black robe. The next largest bloc had served in moderate-size law firms—that is, a firm with five to twenty-four partners or associates. Few had been professors of law.

Their educational background reveals something of their elite nature. All obviously graduated from college; about half attended either the costly Ivy League or other private universities to receive their college and law degrees. Most adult Americans have never gone to college, and of those who have, only a tiny portion could meet the admission requirements—not to mention the expense—of most private or Ivy League schools.

At least a third of the district judges had had some experience on the bench, and in the case of Carter's appointees, more than 54 percent had some taste of judicial duties. No fewer than a third had been former prosecutors; as many as half of Ford's judicial team had served in that capacity.

Judges differ in yet another way from the population as a whole. Among trial judges—and all U.S. judges for that matter—there is a strong tendency toward "occupational heredity"—that is, for judges to come from families with a tradition of judicial and public service.[1] A story about one of President Reagan's trial court appointees, Howell Cobb of Beaumont, Texas, is typical of this phenomenon. The nominee's hometown paper said of him:

**Table 8-1**  Background Characteristics of Presidents' District Court
Appointees (Percentage Having Characteristic)

| Characteristic | Reagan | Carter | Ford | Nixon | Johnson |
|---|---|---|---|---|---|
| *Occupation* | | | | | |
| Politics/government | 12.5 | 4.4 | 21.2 | 10.6 | 21.3 |
| Judiciary | 37.5 | 44.6 | 34.6 | 28.5 | 31.1 |
| Large law firm | | | | | |
| 100+ partners/associates | 3.1 | 2.0 | 1.9 | 0.6 | 0.8 |
| 50-99 partners/associates | 4.5 | 6.0 | 3.9 | 0.6 | 1.6 |
| 25-49 partners/associates | 6.7 | 6.0 | 3.9 | 10.1 | — |
| Moderate-size firm | | | | | |
| 10-24 partners/associates | 10.7 | 9.4 | 7.7 | 8.9 | 12.3 |
| 5-9 partners/associates | 9.4 | 10.4 | 17.3 | 19.0 | 6.6 |
| Small firm | | | | | |
| 2-4 partners/associates | 9.4 | 11.4 | 7.7 | 14.5 | 11.5 |
| solo practitioners | 2.7 | 2.5 | 1.9 | 4.5 | 11.5 |
| Professor of law | 2.7 | 3.0 | — | 2.8 | 3.3 |
| Other | 0.9 | 0.5 | — | — | — |
| *Experience* | | | | | |
| Judicial | 40.6 | 54.5 | 42.3 | 35.2 | 34.4 |
| Prosecutorial | 37.2 | 38.6 | 50.0 | 41.9 | 45.9 |
| Neither | 22.2 | 28.2 | 30.8 | 36.3 | 33.6 |
| *Undergraduate education* | | | | | |
| Public-supported | 34.4 | 57.4 | 48.1 | 41.3 | 38.5 |
| Private (not Ivy) | 51.3 | 32.7 | 34.6 | 38.5 | 31.1 |
| Ivy League | 14.3 | 9.9 | 17.3 | 19.6 | 16.4 |
| None indicated | — | — | — | 0.6 | 13.9 |
| *Law school education* | | | | | |
| Public-supported | 42.4 | 50.5 | 44.2 | 41.9 | 40.2 |
| Private (not Ivy) | 46.9 | 32.2 | 38.5 | 36.8 | 36.9 |
| Ivy League | 10.7 | 17.3 | 17.3 | 21.2 | 21.3 |
| *Gender* | | | | | |
| Male | 91.1 | 85.6 | 98.1 | 99.4 | 98.4 |
| Female | 8.9 | 14.4 | 1.9 | 0.6 | 1.6 |
| *Ethnicity or race* | | | | | |
| White | 92.9 | 78.7 | 88.5 | 95.5 | 93.4 |
| Black | 1.8 | 13.9 | 5.8 | 3.4 | 4.1 |
| Hispanic | 4.9 | 6.9 | 1.9 | 1.1 | 2.5 |
| Asian | 0.4 | 0.5 | 3.9 | — | — |

*(Table continues)*

**Table 8-1**   (Continued)

| Characteristic | Reagan | Carter | Ford | Nixon | Johnson |
|---|---|---|---|---|---|
| *ABA rating* | | | | | |
| Exceptionally | | | | | |
| well qualified | 5.4 | 4.0 | — | 5.0 | 7.4 |
| Well qualified | 46.4 | 47.0 | 46.1 | 40.2 | 40.9 |
| Qualified | 48.2 | 47.5 | 53.8 | 54.8 | 49.2 |
| Not qualified | — | 1.5 | — | — | 2.5 |
| *Party* | | | | | |
| Democratic | 4.9 | 92.6 | 21.2 | 7.3 | 94.3 |
| Republican | 93.8 | 4.4 | 78.8 | 92.7 | 5.7 |
| Independent | 1.3 | 2.9 | — | — | — |
| *Past party activism* | 60.3 | 60.9 | 50.0 | 48.6 | 49.2 |
| *Religious origin* | | | | | |
| *or affiliation* | | | | | |
| Protestant | 61.2 | 60.4 | 73.1 | 73.2 | 58.2 |
| Catholic | 30.4 | 27.7 | 17.3 | 18.4 | 31.1 |
| Jewish | 8.5 | 11.9 | 9.6 | 8.4 | 10.7 |
| Total number | | | | | |
| of appointees | 224 | 202 | 52 | 179 | 122 |
| Average age | | | | | |
| at nomination | 49.0 | 49.7 | 49.2 | 49.1 | 51.4 |

*Source:* Data from Sheldon Goldman, "Reagan's Second Term Judicial Appointments: The Battle at Midway," *Judicature* 70 (April-May 1987): 328.

The appointee is the fourth generation of a family of lawyers and judges. His great-grandfather, a Confederate officer, served as secretary of the Treasury under President James Buchanan and was governor of Georgia and speaker of the U.S. House of Representatives. Cobb's grandfather was a justice on the Georgia Supreme Court, and his father was a circuit judge in Georgia. Cobb's son, a lawyer in El Paso, also follows tradition. "Most trial lawyers aspire to a seat on the bench," Cobb said.[2]

Although the United States is about 51 percent female, it is clear that judging is still a man's business. Until Carter's presidency fewer than 2 percent of the lower judiciary were female, and even Carter was able to include only 14.4 percent women among his nominees to the trial bench. Being female is clearly not an asset if one covets a judicial robe.

The percentage of minorities on the trial bench has always been small, not only in absolute numbers but also in comparison with figures for the overall population. Only Jimmy Carter, who made affirmative action a cornerstone of his presidency, stands out as having appointed a significant number of non-Anglos to the federal bench—over 21 percent.[3]

The American Bar Association (ABA) ratings reveal that few make it to the federal bench who are not rated as "qualified" by this self-appointed evaluator of judicial fitness. More surprising, perhaps, is that precious few are dubbed "exceptionally well qualified" by the ABA. The difference in quality between the Republican and Democratic appointees is trivial.

About nine out of ten district judges have been of the same political party as the appointing president, and about half have had a record of active partisanship. The Carter and Reagan judges appear to have been more active party loyalists than those of their predecessors. More than half the jurists have been affiliated with Protestant religious denominations.

As for age, the typical judge has been forty-nine at the time of appointment. Much has been made of former President Reagan's supposed efforts to pack the bench with unusually young jurists so that his conservative legacy might last well beyond his administration. The data, however, do not bear out this speculation. The Reagan judge's average of 49.0 years is 1.7 years younger than the mean for Johnson's judicial team, but the differences between the Reagan cohorts and those of Nixon, Ford, and Carter are insignificant. (The Reagan appeals court judges—as we will show—are about two years younger than average, a notable but hardly impressive difference.)

### Appeals Court Judges

Because the statistics and percentages of the appellate court appointees of the five presidents from Johnson through Reagan are quite similar to those for the trial judges, we shall offer some commentary only on those figures that suggest a difference between the two sets of judges (see Table 8-2).

Appeals judges are much more likely to have had previous judicial experience than their counterparts on the trial court bench. Also, Presidents Carter and Reagan were more apt to look to the ranks of law school professors for their appeals court appointments than they were for their nominations to the district courts.

If the trend toward seeking out private school and Ivy League graduates was strong for trial judge appointments, it is even more pronounced for those selected for seats on the appeals courts. Compared with the population at large or even U.S. district judges, appellate court jurists appear to be true members of America's social and economic elite.

In terms of opposite-party selections, there is little difference between trial and appellate court appointments. However, there is a slight tendency

**Table 8-2**   Background Characteristics of Presidents' Appeals Court Appointees (Percentage Having Characteristic)

| Characteristic | Reagan | Carter | Ford | Nixon | Johnson |
|---|---|---|---|---|---|
| *Occupation* | | | | | |
| Politics/government | 4.8 | 5.4 | 8.3 | 4.4 | 10.0 |
| Judiciary | 50.8 | 46.4 | 75.0 | 53.3 | 57.5 |
| Large law firm | | | | | |
| 100+ partners/associates | 3.2 | 1.8 | — | — | — |
| 50-99 partners/associates | 3.2 | 5.4 | 8.3 | 2.2 | 2.5 |
| 25-49 partners/associates | 7.9 | 3.6 | — | 2.2 | 2.5 |
| Moderate-size firm | | | | | |
| 10-24 partners/associates | 4.8 | 14.3 | — | 11.1 | 7.5 |
| 5-9 partners/associates | 6.3 | 1.8 | 8.3 | 11.1 | 10.0 |
| Small firm | | | | | |
| 2-4 partners/associates | 1.6 | 3.6 | — | 6.7 | 2.5 |
| solo practitioners | — | 1.8 | — | — | 5.0 |
| Professor of law | 15.4 | 14.3 | — | 2.2 | 2.5 |
| Other | 1.6 | 1.8 | — | 6.7 | — |
| *Experience* | | | | | |
| Judicial | 48.0 | 53.6 | 75.0 | 57.8 | 65.0 |
| Prosecutorial | 18.7 | 32.1 | 25.0 | 46.7 | 47.5 |
| Neither | 33.3 | 37.5 | 25.0 | 17.8 | 20.0 |
| *Undergraduate education* | | | | | |
| Public-supported | 22.2 | 30.4 | 50.0 | 40.0 | 32.5 |
| Private (not Ivy) | 50.8 | 50.0 | 41.7 | 35.6 | 40.0 |
| Ivy League | 27.0 | 19.6 | 8.3 | 20.0 | 17.5 |
| None indicated | — | — | — | 4.4 | 10.0 |
| *Law school education* | | | | | |
| Public-supported | 34.9 | 39.3 | 50.0 | 37.8 | 40.0 |
| Private (not Ivy) | 42.9 | 19.6 | 25.0 | 26.7 | 32.5 |
| Ivy League | 22.2 | 41.1 | 25.0 | 35.6 | 27.5 |
| *Gender* | | | | | |
| Male | 93.7 | 80.4 | 100.0 | 100.0 | 97.5 |
| Female | 6.3 | 19.6 | — | — | 2.5 |
| *Ethnicity or race* | | | | | |
| White | 96.8 | 78.6 | 100.0 | 97.8 | 95.0 |
| Black | 1.6 | 16.1 | — | — | 5.0 |
| Hispanic | 1.6 | 3.6 | — | — | — |
| Asian | — | 1.8 | — | 2.2 | — |

Table 8-2  (Continued)

| Characteristic | Reagan | Carter | Ford | Nixon | Johnson |
|---|---|---|---|---|---|
| *ABA rating* | | | | | |
| Exceptionally | | | | | |
| well qualified | 15.9 | 16.1 | 16.7 | 15.6 | 27.5 |
| Well qualified | 39.7 | 58.9 | 41.7 | 57.8 | 47.5 |
| Qualified | 44.4 | 25.0 | 33.3 | 26.7 | 20.0 |
| Not qualified | — | — | 8.3 | — | 2.5 |
| *Party* | | | | | |
| Democratic | — | 82.1 | 8.3 | 6.7 | 95.0 |
| Republican | 98.4 | 7.1 | 91.7 | 93.3 | 5.0 |
| Independent | — | 10.7 | — | — | — |
| Other | 1.6 | — | — | — | — |
| *Past party activism* | 68.3 | 73.2 | 58.3 | 60.0 | 57.5 |
| *Religious origin* | | | | | |
| *or affiliation* | | | | | |
| Protestant | 55.6 | 60.7 | 58.3 | 75.6 | 60.0 |
| Catholic | 31.7 | 23.2 | 33.3 | 15.6 | 25.0 |
| Jewish | 12.7 | 16.1 | 8.3 | 8.9 | 15.0 |
| Total number | | | | | |
| of appointees | 63 | 56 | 12 | 45 | 40 |
| Average age | | | | | |
| at nomination | 49.9 | 51.9 | 52.1 | 53.8 | 52.2 |

*Source:* Data from Sheldon Goldman, "Reagan's Second Term Judicial Appointments: The Battle at Midway," *Judicature* 70 (April-May 1987): 331.

for appeals judges to be more active in their respective parties than their colleagues on the trial bench.

As with district judges, most appellate court appointees have been disproportionately white and male. Only the Carter team stands out: more than 21 percent of his appeals court judges were nonwhite, and more than 19 percent were women. Those bearing the "exceptionally well qualified" stamp of the American Bar Association are in much greater number in the appeals court camp than in the ranks of the trial court judges.

## Supreme Court Justices

Since 1789, 103 men and 1 woman have sat on the bench of America's highest judicial tribunal. If we have suggested that judges of the trial and appeals courts have been culled primarily from America's cultural elite, then members of the U.S. Supreme Court are truly the crème de la crème. Let's take a look at the Court's collective portrait.

Although perhaps 10 percent of the justices were of essentially humble origin, the remainder "were not only from families in comfortable economic circumstances, but were chosen overwhelmingly from the socially prestigious and politically influential gentry class in the late 18th and early 19th century, or the professionalized upper class thereafter." [4] A majority of the justices came from politically active families, and about a third were related to jurists and closely connected with families with a tradition of judicial service. Thus the justices were reared in far from commonplace American families.

Until the 1960s the High Court had been all white and all male, but in 1967 President Johnson appointed Thurgood Marshall as the first black member of the Court, and in 1981 the gender barrier was broken when President Reagan named Sandra Day O'Connor to the Court. In terms of religious background, the membership of the Court has been overwhelmingly Protestant, although during this century there has been a "Catholic seat" and (until Abe Fortas's resignation in 1969) a "Jewish seat" on the Court. Most Protestants have been affiliated with the more prestigious denominations (such as the Episcopal, Presbyterian, and Unitarian churches). Thus in terms of ethnicity, gender, and religious preference, the Court is by no means a cross-section of American society.

As for the nonpolitical occupations of the justices, all 104 had legal training and all had practiced law at some stage in their careers. An inordinate number had served as corporation attorneys before their appointments. Only 22 percent had state or federal judicial experience *immediately* prior to their appointments, although more than half had served on the bench at some time before their nomination to the Supreme Court. As with their colleagues in the lower federal judiciary, the justices were much more likely to have been politically active than the average American, and virtually all shared many of the ideological and political orientations of their appointing president.

### An Appraisal of the Statistics

Several conclusions are readily apparent from the summary data we have just presented. First, it is clear that federal judges in the United States are an elite within an elite. They come from upper- or upper-middle-class families that are politically active and that have a tradition of public and, often, judicial service. Is the narrow judicial selection process the result of pure chance? Has there been a sinister conspiracy for the past two centuries to keep women, blacks, Roman Catholics, the poor, and so on out of the U.S. judiciary, or are the causes more subtle and complex? We think the evidence points to the latter explanation. Let us look at a few variables indicative of the selection route to the federal bench—race, family background, and gender.

Legislation has never been passed that forbade non-Anglos to wear the black robe. But there have been laws, traditions, and unwritten codes that have kept them from entering the better law schools, from working in the more prestigious law firms and corporations, and from making the kind of social and political connections that may lead to nomination to judicial office. Likewise, no statutes have excluded the children of the poor from potential seats on the bench. But few youngsters from impoverished homes can afford expensive, good-quality colleges and law schools that would give them the training and the contacts they would need. Traditionally, too, many more young men than young women were encouraged to apply to law school. The process of exclusion, then, has not been part of a conscious, organized conspiracy; rather, it has been the inevitable consequence of more subtle social and economic forces in our society.

Another observation about the background profile of our federal judges is worthy of mention. Because they tend to come from the same kinds of families, to go to the same universities and law schools, and to belong to churches, clubs, and societies that uphold similar values, federal judges generally are much more alike than they are different. There may be Democrats and Republicans, former defense attorneys and former prosecutors on the bench, but to a significant degree virtually all play the game by the same rules. What one scholar has said about the recruitment process to the appeals courts is true for federal judgeships in general:

> Broadly speaking [the recruitment process] tends to reward supporters of the presidential party; weed out incompetents, mavericks, and ideological extremists; and ensure substantial professional and political experience among those who wield federal appellate power. Forged thereby are continuous links between judges and their political and professional surroundings. Restricted thereby are the types of persons inducted into Courts of Appeals. The multiple filters through which recruits must pass put a premium on moderate, middle-class, and political lawyers, successful people advantaged in life.[5]

The fact that the recruitment process produces a corps of jurists who agree on how the judicial game is to be played is the primary reason why the loosely organized judicial hierarchy, outlined in Chapter 2, does not come flying apart. It is a key explanation for the predictability of most judicial decisions, a subject that we shall explore in the next two chapters. The judicial machinery runs as smoothly and consistently as it does not because of outside watchdogs or elaborate enforcement mechanisms but because the principal participants largely share the same values and orientations and are working to further similar goals.

# Formal and Informal Qualifications of Federal Judges

## Formal Qualifications

Students often torture one another with horror stories of the hurdles to be overcome in order to achieve success in a particular profession. Would-be medical students are awed by the high grade-point averages and aptitude scores required for admission to medical schools; potential university professors shrink at the many years of work necessary to obtain a Ph.D., only to face the publish-or-perish requirements for a tenured position. It would be logical, then, to assume that the formal requirements for becoming a federal judge—and surely a Supreme Court justice—must be formidable indeed. Not so. There are in fact no constitutional or statutory qualifications for serving on the Supreme Court or the lower federal courts. The Constitution merely indicates that "the judicial Power of the United States, shall be vested in one supreme Court" as well as in any lower federal courts that Congress may establish (Article III, Section 1) and that the president "by and with the Advice and Consent of the Senate, shall appoint . . . Judges of the supreme Court" (Article II, Section 2). Congress has applied the same selection procedure to the appeals and the trial courts. There are no exams to pass, no minimum age requirement, no stipulation that judges be native-born citizens or legal residents, nor is there even a requirement that judges have a law degree. Despite the absence of formal qualifications for a federal judgeship, there are nevertheless some rather well-defined informal requirements.

## Informal Requirements

It is possible to identify at least four vital although informal factors that determine who sits on the federal bench in America: professional competence, political qualifications, self-selection, and the element of pure luck.

*Professional Competence.* Although candidates for U.S. judicial posts do not have to be attorneys—let alone prominent ones—it has been the custom to appoint lawyers who have distinguished themselves professionally—or at least not to appoint those obviously without merit. *Merit* may mean no more than an association with a prestigious law firm, publication of a few law review articles, or respect among fellow attorneys; a potential judge need not necessarily be an outstanding legal scholar. Nevertheless, one of the unwritten codes is that a judicial appointment is different from run-of-the-mill patronage. Thus while the political rules may allow a president to reward an old ally with a seat on the bench, even here tradition has created an expectation that the would-be judge have some reputation for professional competence, the more so as the judgeship in question goes from the trial to the appeals to the Supreme Court level.

A modern-day example of the unwritten rule that potential judges be more than just warm bodies with a law degree is found in President Nixon's nomination of G. Harrold Carswell to the Supreme Court in 1970. After investigations by the press and the Senate Judiciary Committee revealed that Carswell's record was unimpressive at best, his nomination began to stall on the floor of the Senate. To his aid came the well-meaning senator Roman Hruska of Nebraska, who stated in part: "Even if Carswell were mediocre, there are a lot of mediocre judges and people and lawyers. They are entitled to a little representation, aren't they, and a little chance? We can't have all Brandeises, and Frankfurters, and Cardozos and stuff like that there." [6] With such support Carswell must have wondered why he needed any detractors. In any case the acknowledgment by a friendly senator that the Supreme Court nominee was "mediocre" probably did more than anything else to prompt the Senate to reject Carswell. Although tradition may allow judgeships to be political payoffs and may not require eminence in the nominee, candidates for federal judicial posts are expected to meet a reasonable level of professional competence.

*Political Qualifications.* When at least 90 percent of all federal judicial nominees are of the same political party as the appointing president, it must strike even the most casual observer that there are certain political requirements for a seat on the bench. The fact that well over half of all federal judges were "politically active" before their appointments—in comparison with a 10 percent figure for the overall population—is further evidence of this phenomenon. What are the political criteria? In some cases a judgeship may be a reward for major service to the party in power or to the president or a senator. For example, when federal judge Peirson Hall (of the Central District of California) was asked how important politics was to his appointment, he gave this candid reply:

> I worked hard for Franklin Roosevelt in the days when California had no Democratic Party to speak of. In 1939 I began running for the Senate, and the party convinced me it would be best if there wasn't a contest for the Democratic nomination. So I withdrew and campaigned for Martin Downey. They gave me this judgeship as sort of a consolation prize—and one, I might add, that I have enjoyed.[7]

While examples like this are not uncommon, it would be a mistake to think of federal judgeships merely as political plums handed out to the party faithful. As often as not, a seat on the bench goes to a reasonably active or visible member of the party in power but not necessarily to someone who has made party service the central focus of a lifetime.

Political activity that might lead to a judgeship includes service as chair of a state or local party organization, an unsuccessful race for public office, or financial backing for partisan causes.

The reason why most nominees for judicial office must have some record of political activity is twofold. First, to some degree judgeships are still considered part of the political patronage system; those who have served the party are more likely to be rewarded with a federal post than those who have not paid their dues. Second, even if a judgeship is not given as a direct political payoff, some political activity on the part of a would-be judge is often necessary, because otherwise the candidate would simply not be visible to the president or senator(s) or local party leaders who send forth the names of candidates. If the judicial power brokers have never heard of a particular lawyer because that attorney has no political profile, his or her name will not come to mind when a vacancy occurs on the bench.

*Self-Selection.*   For those seeking the presidency or running for Congress, shyness doesn't pay. One needs to declare one's candidacy, meet a formal filing deadline, and spend considerable time and money to advertise one's qualifications. While Americans profess to admire modesty and humility in their leaders, *successful* candidates for elected office do well not to overindulge these virtues. With the judiciary, however, the informal rules of the game are a bit different. Many would consider it undignified and "lacking in judicial temperament" for someone to announce publicly a desire for a federal judgeship—much less to campaign openly for such an appointment.

We know, however, that some would-be jurists orchestrate discreet campaigns on their own behalf or at least pass the word that they are available for judicial service. While few will admit to seeking an appointment actively, credible anecdotes suggest that attorneys often position themselves in such a way that their names will come up when the powers-that-be have a vacant seat to fill. At judicial swearing-in ceremonies it is often said that "the judgeship sought the man (or woman) rather than vice versa," and surely this does happen. But sometimes the judgeship does its seeking with a little nudge from the would-be jurist.

*The Element of Luck.*   If all that were involved in the picking of a Supreme Court justice or a lower-court judge were professional and political criteria, the appointment process would be much easier to explain and predict. If, for instance, one wanted to know who was going to be appointed to a vacancy on the Sixth Circuit bench, one would need only to identify the person in the Sixth Circuit to whom the party was most indebted and who had a reputation for legal competence. The problem is that there would be hundreds of capable attorneys in the Sixth Circuit to whom the prevailing party owed much. Why should one of them be selected and several hundred not? Until judicial scholarship becomes more of a science and less of an art, we cannot make accurate predictions about who will wear the black robe; there are just too many variables and too many participants in the selection process. Let us look at the example of President Truman's appointment of Carroll O. Switzer to fill a vacant judgeship in 1949.

The story began in 1948 when Truman was seeking a full term as president. The campaign had not gone well from the start. Even the party faithful could barely muster a faint cheer when Truman proclaimed to sparse crowds, "We're gonna win this election and we're gonna make those Republicans like it. Just you wait 'n' see." Almost everyone predicted Truman would lose, and lose badly. Then one morning his campaign train stopped in the little town of Dexter, Iowa. An unexpectedly large number of farmers had put aside their milking chores and the fall corn harvest to see the feisty little man from Missouri "give those Republicans hell." Truman picked up a real sense of enthusiasm among the cheering crowd, and for the first time in the campaign he smelled victory.

On the campaign platform with Truman that morning was Carroll Switzer, a bright young Des Moines attorney who was the (unsuccessful) Democratic candidate for Iowa governor that year. No evidence exists that Truman met Switzer before or after that one propitious day. But when a vacancy occurred on the U.S. bench a year later, Truman's mind jumped like a spring to the name of his lucky horseshoe, Carroll Switzer. A longtime administrative assistant to an Iowa senator related the story as follows:

> I am sure that this day at Dexter was the first time President Truman and his staff were sure he could win—later proved right. I am sure that he recalled that day favorably when an appointment . . . came up in the Iowa judgeship. . . . Every time the Iowa judgeship came up, Truman would hear of no one but Switzer. Truman would say "That guy Switzer backed me when everyone else was running away, and, by God, I'm going to see that he gets a judgeship." [8]

That morning in Dexter was Switzer's lucky day. While he had the professional and political credentials for a judicial post, no one could have foreseen that he would happen to appear with Truman the day the national winds of political fortune began to blow in the president's favor. Had it been any other day, Switzer might never have been more than just a bright attorney from Des Moines.

This account illustrates the point that there is a good measure of happenstance involved in virtually all judicial appointments. Being a member of the right party at the right time or being visible to the power brokers at a lucky moment often has as much to do with becoming a judge as the length and sparkle of one's professional résumé.

## Qualifications and Backgrounds of State Judges

Although the selection process for state judges varies from that of the federal model, the men and women who are tapped for judicial service reflect a familiar profile. State jurists, like their counterparts on the federal bench, are overwhelmingly older, white, male, and Protestant. They tend to be home-grown fellows who are moderately conservative and staunchly committed to the status quo. They believe in the basic values and tradition of the legal and political communities from which they come. State judges, then, share with their federal colleagues the distinction of being local boys who made good.

Most state laws and constitutions provide few rigid conditions for being a state judge. The vast majority of the states do not require their justices of the peace or magistrates to have law degrees, but such degrees are virtually required (either formally or in practice) for trial and appellate judges. Some states require their judges to be U.S. citizens.

The informal qualifications for being a state jurist are reflected in the socioeconomic profile that seems to hold all throughout the United States. First, while women constitute a scant majority of the American population, this fact is of little use to them if they seek judicial service—still very much a man's game. Despite the upsurge in recent decades in the number of women in the legal profession, women are still rarely seen on the bench. In 1982 there were only 549 female state judges in the United States, and nearly all of these were serving on the lower trial courts rather than on the intermediate appellate or supreme courts. At the level of the state supreme courts only about 7 percent of the justices were women as of 1985. In this same vein, being non-Anglo is clearly not an asset if one yearns to wear a black robe: Fewer than 5 percent of all state judges are members of racial minorities.

State judges, like their federal counterparts, have never wandered far from the region in which they grew up and were educated. About three-fourths of all state jurists were born in the state in which they serve, and fewer than a third went out of state for their undergraduate degrees or even for their law degrees. This penchant for localism is also reflected in the patterns of work experience that state judges bring to the bench. For example, for those serving on the state supreme court bench only 13 percent have had any form of prior federal experience, whereas 93 percent have had some type of prior state experience.

Judges tend to be middle-aged when they assume the bench. State trial judges come to the bench at about age forty-six, which corresponds roughly to the figure of forty-nine for federal trial judges. State appellate court judges tend to be a tad older than their trial court colleagues when they become jurists—about fifty-three, which is approximately the same as their federal equivalents.

In terms of political party affiliation, state judges, whether they be elected or appointed, tend to mirror the party that dominates in the judge's particular state. Since more states are controlled by Democrats than by Republicans, this fact is reflected in the partisan affiliation of the judges. For example, 55 percent of state trial judges claim to be Democrats, 36 percent identify with the GOP, and 9 percent have no partisan affiliation. The South still seems to be solidly Democratic, at least at the state level, while the partisan distribution is more evenly divided in the rest of the nation. Perhaps the key point here is that the vast majority of state judges had been politically active before assuming the bench. Whether they were elected to the bench or whether a governor placed them there, state judges in America tend to know which way the political wind is blowing at any given moment.

Over half the state trial judges come to the bench from the private practice of law, and about a quarter were elevated from a lower-court judgeship, such as a magistrate's position. Of those who practiced law, most reported a general practice without specialization. About one in five were recruited from the ranks of district attorneys, and only 3 percent come from private criminal law practice. Of those serving on state supreme courts, almost two-thirds came from the ranks of the intermediate appellate courts or from the state trial courts.[9]

What one keen observer has said about state trial judges is true about state judiciaries as a whole:

> General trial judges, then, like their appellate brethren, represent a comparatively narrow group of legal professionals. White, middle-aged male lawyers in private practice (or sitting on lower courts or working in district attorney's offices) constitute the bulk of the pool. If you are young, female, a member of a racial minority, are of the wrong political party, or presumably have few contacts within the organized legal community in your state, the chances of making it to the trial bench are slight.[10]

## The Federal Selection Process and Its Participants

The skeletal framework of judicial selection is the same for all federal judges, although the roles of the participants vary depending on what level of the U.S. judiciary we are considering. All nominations are made by the president after due consultation with the White House staff, the attorney general's office, certain senators, and other politicos; it has been customary for the FBI to perform a routine security check. After the nomination is announced, various interest groups that believe they have a stake in the appointment may lobby for or against the candidate. Also, the candidate's qualifications will be evaluated by a committee of the American Bar Association. The candidate's name is then sent to the Senate Judiciary Committee, which conducts an investigation of the nominee's fitness for the post. If the committee's vote is favorable, the nomination is sent to the floor of the Senate, where it is either approved or rejected by a simple majority vote. In the next sections we will take a close look at the role of the various participants in the selection process.

## The President

Technically the chief executive nominates all judicial candidates, but history has shown that the president manifests greater personal involvement in appointments to the Supreme Court than to the lower courts. This is so for two major reasons. First, Supreme Court appointments are seen by the president—and by the public at large—as generally more important and politically significant than openings on the lesser tribunals. Presidents often use their few opportunities for High Court appointments to make a political statement or to set the tone of their administration. For example, during the period of national stress prior to U.S. entry into World War II, Democratic president Franklin D. Roosevelt elevated Republican Harlan Stone to chief justice as a gesture of national unity; in 1969 President Nixon used his appointment of the conservative Warren Burger to make good on his campaign pledge to restore "law and order"; and President Reagan hoped to dispel his reputation for being unsympathetic toward the women's movement by being the first to name a woman to the High Court. Because appointments to the lower judiciary are less newsworthy, they are less likely to command the personal involvement of the president, who will probably rely much more heavily on the judgment of the White House staff or the Justice Department in selecting and screening candidates for appeals and trial court benches.

A second reason why presidents are less likely to devote much attention to lower-court appointments is that tradition has allowed for individual senators and local party bosses to influence and often dominate such activity. In fact, the practice known as *senatorial courtesy* is a major restriction on the president's capacity to make district judge appointments. The conditions for this unwritten rule of the game are these: Senators of the president's political party who object to a candidate that the president wishes to appoint to a district judgeship in their home state have a virtual veto over the nomination. They exercise this veto through use of the "blue slip"—the printed form that a senator from the nominee's state is supposed to return to the Senate Judiciary Committee to express his or her views about the particular candidate.[11] So significant a restriction is this on the chief executive's appointing prerogatives that it caused one former assistant attorney general to quip: "The Constitution is backwards. Article II, Section 2 should read: 'The senators shall nominate, and by and with the consent of the President, shall appoint.' " [12] Many senators in fact regard their prerogatives in this realm to be ordained by the Founders. For example, when Texas senator Phil Gramm was recently asked to defend his key role in the appointment of district judges in his state, he said, "I'm given the power to make the appointment. . . . The people elected me to do that." [13] Senatorial courtesy does not apply to appellate court appointments, although it is customary for presidents to defer to senators of their party from states that make up the appellate court circuit. Thus in lower-court appointments presidents have less incentive to devote effort to a game in which they are not the star player.

The president also has authority "to fill up all Vacancies that may happen during the recess of the Senate, by granting Commissions which shall expire at the End of their next Session" (Article II, Section 2). One reason why a chief executive may wish to make a *recess appointment* is to fill a judicial vacancy in a court that has a large backlog of business. The other reason is more political. A president may find it easier to secure confirmation for a "sitting" judge than for a candidate named while the Senate is in session—that is, the Senate might be less likely to reject a *fait accompli*. For example, when President Kennedy selected Judge Irving Ben Cooper to fill an opening on the federal bench in New York State, the nomination stirred up great opposition in the Senate Judiciary Committee. Although Cooper enjoyed a good public image, he was not well liked by lawyers and other judges. [14] Most observers felt that the fact that Cooper was then serving an interim appointment was extremely useful, if not essential, to his subsequent confirmation. If the Senate had rejected Cooper, a new jurist would have had to be nominated, causing further delay in an urgent appointment.

During the presidency of Jimmy Carter a new wrinkle was added (but quickly ironed out by Reagan) to the appointment of appellate court judges. By executive order Carter created a U.S. Circuit Judge Nominating Commission. [15] The commission was split into thirteen panels, one for each circuit and two for each of the largest two circuits. The panels were instructed to review candidates for appellate vacancies and to make recommendations based on merit—not on political factors. Carter promised to appoint judges only from the panels' lists of best-qualified candidates. The Omnibus Judgeship Act of 1978 furthered this trend by giving the president the authority to recommend—but not to require—that similar panels be established to assist senators in their suggestions for trial bench appointments in their respective states. The effect of these commission panels is still the subject of controversy. They did indeed come up with candidates that reflected a broader spectrum of American society. (Tables 8-1 and 8-2 indicate the unprecedented number of women and blacks appointed by Carter.) It is doubtful, however, that the commissions took politics out of the selection process: 82.1 percent of Carter's appeals court judges and 92.6 percent of his trial judges somehow managed to be Democrats—most with a liberal bent. In any case on May 4, 1981, President Reagan signed an executive order quietly burying the nominating commission.

## The Department of Justice

Assisting the president and the White House staff in the judicial selection process are the two key presidential appointees in the Justice Department—the attorney general of the United States and the deputy attorney general. Their primary job is to seek out candidates for federal judicial posts who conform to general criteria set by the president. For example, if a vacancy were to occur on the Seventh Circuit appellate bench, the attorney general (or a staff member) might phone the U.S. attorneys in the states of Illinois, Wisconsin, and Indiana and ask, "Are there some attorneys in your district who would make good judges and who are members of our political party or who at least share the president's basic philosophy?" Once several names are obtained, the staff of the Justice Department will subject each candidate to further scrutiny. They may order an FBI investigation of the candidate's character and background; they will usually read copies of all articles or speeches the candidate has written or evaluate a sitting judge's written opinions; they might check with local party leaders to determine that the candidate is a party faithful and is in tune with the president's major public policy positions.

In the case of district judge appointments, where names are often submitted by home-state senators, the Justice Department's function is more that of screener than of initiator. But regardless of who comes up with a basic list of names, the Justice Department's primary duty is to evaluate the candidates' personal, professional, and political qualifications. In performing this role the department may work closely with the White House staff, with the senators involved in the nomination, and with party leaders who may wish to have some input on the potential nominee.

## State and Local Party Leaders

Regional party politicos have little to say in the appointment of Supreme Court justices, where presidential prerogative is dominant, and their role in the choice of appeals court judges is minimal. However, in the selection of U.S. trial judges their impact is formidable, especially when appointments occur in states in which neither senator is of the president's political party. In such cases the president need not fear that senatorial courtesy will be invoked against a district court nominee and thus will be more likely to consult with state party leaders rather than with the state's senators. For example, during the Kennedy and Johnson presidencies the Democratic mayor of Chicago, Richard J. Daley, personally approved every federal judge appointed in the Northern District of Illinois.

## Interest Groups

A number of pressure groups in the United States, representing the whole political spectrum from left to right, often lobby either for or against judicial nominations. Leaders of these groups—civil liberties, business, organized labor, civil rights—have little hesitation about urging the president to withdraw the nomination of someone whose political and social values are different from their own, or from lobbying the Senate to support the nomination of someone who is favorably perceived. When President Reagan nominated Sandra Day O'Connor for a Supreme Court position in 1981, a variety of interest groups clamored to make their views known. For example, the president of the National Organization for Women said her group was for the nomination, which she called "a major victory for women's rights." However, the conservative Moral Majority was not so pleased with Reagan's choice. Its leaders charged O'Connor with favoring abortion and objected to her support of the pending (later defeated) equal rights amendment. There is evidence that interest groups lobby for and against nominees at all levels of the federal judiciary. As one scholar has noted, pressure-group activity to influence the selection process "has long been characteristic of American politics." [16]

## Other Judges

It is not unknown for judges and justices to suggest names of individuals who they believe would make good judges or to lobby behind the scenes for or against a candidate who has been nominated by the president. Chief Justice William Howard Taft did not hesitate to suggest to the Harding and Coolidge administrations of the 1920s the names of men who were "of a sound judicial temperament"—that is, men of conservative ideology who would vote the right way if appointed to the bench. Soon after he became chief justice, Taft related to a confidant that he had "established a very pleasant relationship with the Attorney General and with the President. The Attorney General assures me that he expects to talk with me all the time about the selection of Judges, and I am very sure of what he says." Within weeks Taft was writing the attorney general on a "Dear Harry" basis, and as one scholar has noted: "Hardly a vacancy occurred anywhere on the federal bench without the Chief Justice actively intervening." [17] Most efforts by sitting judges to influence the selection process are more restrained than Taft's, and most jurists probably never enter the fray. But there is evidence at all levels that some judges do indeed lobby, albeit discreetly, to influence the composition of the federal judiciary.

## The American Bar Association

For more than four decades the Committee on the Federal Judiciary of the ABA has played a key role in evaluating the credentials of potential nominees for positions on the federal bench. The committee, composed of members from all the U.S. circuits, evaluates candidates on the basis of numerous criteria, including judicial temperament, age, trial experience, character, and intelligence. A candidate approved by the committee is rated "qualified," "well qualified," or "exceptionally well qualified." An unacceptable candidate is stamped with the "not qualified" label.

The traditional composition of the committee has made it the subject of some controversy. Because it has been made up largely of older, well-to-do, Republican, business-oriented corporation attorneys, some observers have argued that its evaluation of potential judicial candidates has been biased in favor of its peers. There is a strong suspicion that the committee has seen being wealthy and conservative as positive traits and being liberal and outspoken as uncharacteristic of "a sound judicial temperament." It should come as no surprise, then, that the ABA's committee has generally worked more closely with Republican presidents than with Democratic administrations.

Bucking the recommendations of the committee is a risky business, and presidents are likely to think long and hard before nominating a candidate tagged with the "not qualified" label.[18] President Kennedy in 1962 successfully pushed for the appointment of Sarah T. Hughes (of the Northern District of Texas) despite opposition from the ABA, which argued that she was too old. Nevertheless it required lobbying from none other than the vice president (Lyndon Johnson) and the Speaker of the House (Sam Rayburn) to ease the nomination through.[19]

Some presidents have gone back and forth in terms of their willingness to be bound by the pronouncements of the ABA committee. For example, when he first took office, President Nixon indicated that he would appoint no one who did not have the blessing of the ABA. However, after Senate defeat of two of Nixon's Supreme Court nominees, Clement Haynsworth and G. Harrold Carswell, the ABA began to cast a more critical eye on Nixon's choices. (The ABA had approved the Haynsworth and Carswell nominations and felt somewhat humiliated when investigations by the press and the Senate turned up a variety of negative factors overlooked by the committee.) Late in 1971, when he was trying to fill two vacancies on the Supreme Court, Nixon brought up the possibility of nominating

Senator Robert Byrd of West Virginia. Attorney General John Mitchell told Nixon that there would be a real problem securing ABA approval because Byrd had attended a "night law school" and had little experience as a practicing attorney. Nixon's reported reply to Mitchell indicates that the president's total confidence in the judgment of the ABA had waned. "Fuck the ABA," said Nixon. And indeed, from that time on, the president refused to submit names to the ABA committee until *after* he had already selected and publicized them.

Since President Nixon and Watergate, two changes seem to have occurred in the ABA. First, it appears to have severed some of its close ties to the conservative establishment and taken stands on public policy issues that offend traditional dogma. For instance, it has come out for federal support of legal aid for the poor. Second, its impact on the judicial selection process may be a bit less now than in past decades. President Carter's setting up of the U.S. Circuit Judge Nominating Commission was seen in part as a successful end run around the bar association, and when President Reagan appointed Sandra O'Connor to the Supreme Court, the ABA was not even consulted.

The most recent appointments to the High Court have, however, seen the ABA come back into the presidential graces. In 1987 when President Reagan nominated Robert H. Bork, a fifteen-member ABA panel supported Bork with some enthusiasm. Ten rated him well qualified, four said he was not qualified, and one member was "unopposed." (The Senate rejected Bork nevertheless by a vote of 58 to 42.) Reagan's next nominee was Douglas H. Ginsburg, but he withdrew from consideration before the ABA could decide on a rating. (After Ginsburg admitted that he had occasionally used marijuana during the 1960s and 1970s, Reagan's enthusiasm for his get-tough-on-crime nominee quickly evaporated, and Ginsburg was pressured to bow out.) The most recent appointee to the Supreme Court, Anthony M. Kennedy, was unanimously ranked "well qualified" by the ABA committee.

## The Senate Judiciary Committee

The rules of the Senate require its Judiciary Committee to pass on all nominations to the federal bench and to make recommendations to the Senate as a whole. Its role is thus to screen individuals who have already been nominated, not to suggest names of possible candidates. The committee by custom holds hearings on all nominations, at which time witnesses are heard and deliberations take place behind closed doors. In the case of district court appointments, the hearings are largely perfunctory because the norm of senatorial courtesy has for all intents and purposes already determined whether the candidate will pass senatorial muster. However, in the case of appeals court nominees—and surely in the instance of an appointment to the Supreme Court—the committee hearing is a serious proceeding.

Acting as a sort of watchdog of the Senate, the committee can affect the selection process in several ways. "First, it can delay Senate action on confirmation in the hope of embarrassing the president or to test his determination to make a particular appointment." As a general rule, the longer the delay, the poorer the nominee's chances are of securing approval. The Senate rejection of Nixon's two Supreme Court nominees, Haynsworth and Carswell, was the result, in part, of the elongated committee hearings, which permitted the opposition forces to gather negative data and flex their lobbying muscles. Second, the committee can simply recommend against Senate confirmation. Finally, committee opponents of the nomination might engage in an extensive Senate floor debate, which "affords still another opportunity for senators to seek to embarrass the administration by questioning the wisdom of a particular appointment." [20]

Historically the Judiciary Committee has had a distinctly southern and conservative flavor about it. As a result, it often did not look kindly upon appointees to the appeals courts and the Supreme Court who were thought to be too liberal—particularly on civil rights matters. Senator James Eastland of Mississippi, the powerful committee chair for many years, often exacted a terrible toll from presidents who sought to put integrationists on the upper federal courts. For example, when President Kennedy tried to secure the appointment of the black and liberal Thurgood Marshall for a seat on the appellate court bench, Senator Eastland refused to support the nomination unless he could get his old college chum, William Harold Cox, a seat on the federal district court in Mississippi. Cox, who on the bench referred to blacks as "niggers" and "chimpanzees," is regarded as the worst of several racist judges Kennedy was "forced" to appoint in the South. As one black civil rights leader put it: "The brothers had to pay a lot of dues" to get Thurgood Marshall appointed to the bench. [21]

In 1979 the formidable Senator Eastland retired and in his place—in accordance with the sacrosanct norm of seniority—stepped the liberal Senator Edward Kennedy of Massachusetts. The Senate Judiciary Committee immediately felt the impact of its new chair, and changes followed in the role and orientation of the committee. As one leading judicial scholar noted, "Senator Kennedy's ascendancy to the chairmanship of the Judiciary Committee at the start of the 96th Congress presaged increased scrutiny of judicial nominees as individual senators, the committee, and the Senate institution resolved to re-examine their advice and consent role." [22] In his opening remarks to the committee, Kennedy indicated the direction toward which he would marshal the power and prestige of his chairmanship:

The federal courts must become more representative of the people of this nation. Congress and the Administration must work together to insure that more women and more members of minority groups are appointed to the federal bench. . . . Excellence in the law is not restricted to candidates who by accident of birth are male or white. The sooner our judicial selection commissions and all other persons involved in the selection process accept this fact, remove their blinders, and expand their searches, the sooner we shall have a federal judiciary that truly meets all the tests of excellence in our society and that truly protects the rights of all citizens.[23]

Furthermore, Kennedy announced that as long as he was chairman, no judicial nomination would die because of the famous "blue slip" of senatorial courtesy. Rather, he insisted that all nominations must be considered by the full committee and that the committee as a whole would decide whether to make a recommendation to the full Senate.

But the Kennedy reforms on the Judiciary Committee were short-lived. In the 1980 election the Republicans gained control of the Senate, and this resulted in the elevation to the Judiciary chairmanship of Strom Thurmond, the conservative GOP senator from South Carolina. Even before he formally assumed that position, Thurmond made it clear that he favored returning to "traditional" methods of selecting federal judges.[24]

When Senate control returned to Democratic hands in 1986, Joseph Biden of Delaware became chair of the Judiciary Committee. An unabashed liberal, he has used his powerful role to tweak the noses of many conservative Reagan appointees to the federal bench. Indeed, when the most recent High Court appointee, Anthony Kennedy, appeared before the now more liberal Judiciary Committee, many observers believed that Kennedy muffled many of his conservative beliefs in order to pass the committee's muster. Republican senator Gordon Humphrey of New Hampshire described Kennedy's deference to the committee in a vivid use of "body language": "With the entrails of [recently defeated Reagan nominee] Robert Bork still strewn across the floor, still dangling from the chandeliers, I concluded Judge Kennedy didn't want his guts ripped out by senators on this committee."[25]

## The Senate

The final step in the judicial appointment process for federal judges is a majority vote by the Senate. As we have indicated, the Constitution states that the Senate must give its "advice and consent" to judicial nominations made by the president. Historically there have been two general views of the Senate's prescribed role. Presidents, from the time of George Washington, and a few scholars have taken the position that the Senate ought quietly to go along with the presidential choices unless there are overwhelmingly strong reasons to the contrary. Other scholars and, not unexpectedly, most senators have held to the views of Senator Birch Bayh of Indiana and Senator Robert Griffin of Michigan that the Senate "has the right and the obligation to decide in its own wisdom whether it wishes to confirm or not to confirm a Supreme Court nominee." [26] In practice the role of the Senate in the judicial confirmation process has varied, depending on the level of the federal judgeship that is being considered.

For district judges the norm of senatorial courtesy prevails. That is, if the president's nominee is acceptable to the senator(s) of the president's party in the state in which the judge is to sit, the Senate is usually happy to give its advice and consent with a quiet nod. For appointments to the appeals courts, as noted earlier, senatorial courtesy does not apply, since the vacancy to be filled covers more than just the state of one or possibly two senators. But it is customary for senators from each state in the circuit in which the vacancy has occurred to submit names of possible candidates to the president. An unwritten rule is that each state in the circuit should have at least one judge on that circuit's appellate bench, a practice often invoked when a vacancy involves a state's only representative on the circuit bench. As long as the norms are looked after and the president's nominee has reasonable qualifications, the Senate as a whole usually goes along with the recommendations of the chief executive.

It has been mainly with Supreme Court nominations that the Senate has been inclined traditionally to go toe-to-toe with the president if there is disagreement over the candidate's fitness for the High Court. Since 1789, presidents have sent the names of 140 persons to the Senate for its advice and consent. Of this number some 30 were either rejected or "indefinitely postponed" by the Senate, or the names were withdrawn by the president. Thus presidents have been successful about 79 percent of the time, and in fact their batting average seems to be improving, since as many as *one-third* of the nominations were rejected by the Senate in the last century. The record shows that presidents have met with the most success in getting their High Court nominations approved when (1) the nominee comes from a noncontroversial background and has middle-of-the-road political leanings, and (2) the president's party also controls the Senate, or at least there is a majority that shares the president's basic attitudes and values.

## The Selection Process for State Judges

As we have seen, at the federal level there is basically one method for choosing judges: They are nominated by the president with the advice and consent of the majority of the Senate. At the state level, however, there are a variety of methods used to select jurists, and each of these has many permutations. Basically there are five routes to a judgeship in any one of the fifty states: partisan election, nonpartisan election, merit selection, gubernatorial appointment, and appointment by the legislature. Tables 8-3 and 8-4 indicate how many states fall into each category, both for courts of general jurisdiction and for the appellate courts. Note that there is a rough regional pattern to the distribution. The South still has a penchant for selecting judges with a party label; the upper Midwest and the West seem to like nonpartisan selection schemes; states west of the Mississippi often opt for the merit selection plans; and the East is partial to appointments made by either the governor or the state legislature.

But as is often the case in the political world, things are not always what they seem. For instance, in states that officially choose their judges by partisan elections, the vast majority of judges may actually receive their initial position through gubernatorial appointment. This occurs because a sitting judge may die or resign or a new judicial vacancy may occur, and the position is filled by the governor in accordance with state law. The newly appointed judge may eventually have to run for another term in a general election, but most incumbent judges are easily reelected. Thus a state listed in the partisan election column may in reality be a "gubernatorial appointment state." Likewise in states which are officially in the nonpartisan election category—for example—Minnesota, it is often no secret which judicial candidate is the Democrat and which is the Republican, and the voters respond accordingly.

## Election of Judges

The election of judges, on either a partisan or a nonpartisan ballot, is the norm in the states. While it was almost unheard of in Colonial days, this method became popular during the time of President Andrew Jackson—an era when Americans sought to democratize the political process: "If only the average person in his simple innate wisdom could choose the judges, this would put an end to corruption and control of the government by the special (monied) interests." In practice things have not always worked this way, however. There is evidence that party bosses often regard judicial elections as indirect patronage to reward the party faithful. Also, judges who must run for election are often forced to solicit campaign contributions from the lawyers and law firms that will eventually appear before them in court—an obvious potential source of conflict of interest. Finally, the data overwhelmingly indicate that voter turnout in judicial elections is extremely low. Voters may know whom they prefer for president or member of Congress or state senator, but when presented with a long list of persons running for state judgeships, they often resort to the method used for so long by the grandmother of one of the authors: "I voted for the men who had honest-sounding names."

Table 8-3  Selection Processes for State Courts of General Jurisdiction

| Partisan election | Nonpartisan election | Merit selection | Gubernatorial appointment | Appointment by legislature |
|---|---|---|---|---|
| Alabama | Arizona | Alaska | California | South Carolina |
| Arkansas | Florida | Colorado | Maine[a] | Virginia |
| Illinois | Georgia | Connecticut | New Hampshire[b] | |
| Indiana | Idaho | Delaware[a] | New Jersey[a] | |
| Mississippi | Kentucky | Hawaii[c] | | |
| New Mexico | Louisiana | Iowa | | |
| New York | Michigan | Kansas | | |
| North Carolina | Minnesota | Maryland[a] | | |
| Pennsylvania | Montana | Massachusetts | | |
| Tennessee | Nevada | Missouri | | |
| Texas | North Dakota | Nebraska | | |
| West Virginia | Ohio | Rhode Island[a] | | |
| | Oklahoma | Utah | | |
| | Oregon | Vermont[a] | | |
| | South Dakota | Wyoming | | |
| | Washington | | | |
| | Wisconsin | | | |

Source: Council of State Governments, Book of the States, 1986-1987 (Lexington, Ky.: Council of State Governments, 1986), 161-163, as revised by data supplied by the American Judicature Society.

[a] Senate confirmation required.
[b] Gubernatorial nominees are approved by popularly elected council.
[c] Judges appointed by chief justice of the state with the assistance of Judicial Selection Commission.

During the Progressive movement at the turn of the century, reformers sought to take some of the raw partisanship out of judicial elections by having judges run on a nonpartisan basis. In principle they would run on their ideas and qualifications, not on the basis of which party they belonged to. But as with many a good idea, some little demon got hold of this one and ruined it in practice. One judicial scholar has noted that in about half of the "states that use nonpartisan judicial ballots, parties [still] play some role in the selection of judges." [27] That is, in these technically nonpartisan states the political parties still endorse individual judicial candidates and contribute toward their campaigns so that by the time of the election only a dullard would fail to distinguish the "nonpartisan" Republican from the "nonpartisan" Democrat.

**Table 8-4**   Selection Processes for State Appellate Courts

| Partisan election | Nonpartisan election | Merit selection | Gubernatorial appointment | Appointment by legislature |
|---|---|---|---|---|
| Alabama | Georgia | Alaska | California[a] | Rhode Island[b] |
| Arkansas | Idaho | Arizona | Maine[c] | South Carolina |
| Illinois | Kentucky | Colorado | New Jersey[c] | Virginia |
| Mississippi | Louisiana | Connecticut | New Hampshire[d] | |
| New Mexico | Michigan | Delaware[c] | | |
| North Carolina | Minnesota | Florida | | |
| Pennsylvania | Montana | Hawaii[c] | | |
| Texas | Nevada | Indiana | | |
| West Virginia | North Dakota | Iowa | | |
| | Ohio | Kansas | | |
| | Oregon | Maryland[c] | | |
| | Washington | Massachusetts | | |
| | Wisconsin | Missouri | | |
| | | Nebraska | | |
| | | New York | | |
| | | Oklahoma[e] | | |
| | | South Dakota | | |
| | | Tennessee[f] | | |
| | | Utah | | |
| | | Vermont | | |
| | | Wyoming | | |

*Source:* Council of State Governments, *Book of the States, 1986-1987* (Lexington, Ky.: Council of State Governments, 1986), 161-163, as revised by data supplied by the American Judicature Society.

[a] Gubernatorial nominees approved by Commission on Judicial Appointments.
[b] Intermediate appellate court judges appointed by the governor, confirmed by the Senate.
[c] Legislative confirmation required.
[d] Gubernatorial nominees approved by popularly elected council.
[e] Court of appeals judges selected in partisan election.
[f] Supreme Court judges elected on partisan ballot.

## Merit Selection

Undaunted, reformers have come up with a method other than nonpartisan elections to accomplish the goal of obtaining good quality state judges free from the taint of political bias. Merit selection, by whatever name, has been around since the early 1900s as a preferred method of selecting judges. The first state fully to adopt such a method was Missouri, in 1940, and ever since such schemes have come to be known as generic variants of "the Missouri Plan."

The states with Missouri-type plans use a combination of elections and appointments; in effect this type of plan provides for much greater influence from lawyers than any other selection method. In essence the governor appoints a judge from among several candidates recommended by a nominating panel of five or more people, usually including attorneys (often chosen by the local bar association), nonlawyers appointed by the governor, and sometimes a senior local judge. Either by law or by implicit agreement, the governor will appoint someone from the recommended list. After serving for a short period of time, often a year, the newly appointed judge must stand for a special election, at which time he or she in effect runs on his or her record. (The voters are asked, "Shall Judge X be retained in office?") If the judge's tenure is supported by the voters, as is virtually always the case, the judge will serve for a regular and fairly long term. Does a Missouri plan take politics out of the judicial selection process? Well, yes and no. After an exhaustive study of how the plan had operated in Missouri over a quarter century, two keen observers concluded:

> It is naive to suggest . . . that the Plan takes the "politics" out of judicial selection. Instead, the Plan is designed to bring to bear on the process of selecting judges a variety of interests that are thought to have a legitimate concern in the matter and at the same time to discourage other interests. It may be assumed that these interests will engage in the "politics" of judicial selection, that is, they will maneuver to influence who will be chosen as judges (1) because such judgeships constitute prestigious positions for aspiring lawyers, and (2) because, in the course of making decisions, judges inevitably affect the fortunes of persons and groups involved in the litigation process.[28]

Still, what Winston Churchill said about democracy (that it is the worst form of government—except for all the other forms) is probably true of plans for the merit selection of judges.

## Gubernatorial Appointment and Legislative Appointment

In the early days of American history judges were chosen either by the governor or by the state legislature, although at the present time such methods are used in only a handful of states. When judges are appointed by the governor, politics almost invariably comes into play. In the dozens of appointment opportunities that come their way governors tend to select individuals who have been active in state politics and whose activity has either benefited the governor personally or the governor's political party or allies. Also, in making judicial appointments the governor often bargains with local political bosses and/or with state legislators whose support he or she needs. A governor may also use a judgeship to reward a legislator or local politico who has given faithful political support in the past.

Only a few states still allow their legislators to appoint state judges. Although a variety of criteria may be used in choosing members of the state supreme courts, when it comes to filling the state trial benches, state legislators tend to turn to former members of the legislature—a whopping 80 percent of the time! [29] This does not mean that in these legislative-appointment states judges are merely political hacks in need of a job, but it is evidence that friends and colleagues do take care of their own when given the opportunity to do so.

## Policy Links Between the Citizenry, the President, and the Federal Judiciary

Because this book is about policy making, it is appropriate to examine the links between the policy values of the elected chief executive and the decisional propensities of federal judges. If in electing one presidential candidate over another, the citizenry expresses its policy choices, is there evidence that such choices spill over into the kind of judges presidents appoint and the way those judges decide policy-relevant cases? For instance, if the people decide in an election that they want a president who will reduce the size and powers of the federal bureaucracy, does that president subsequently appoint judges who share that philosophy? And, equally important, when those judges hear cases that give them the opportunity either to expand or reduce the extent of a bureaucrat's power, do they opt for the reduction of authority? While we are a long way from having complete answers to these questions, recent evidence suggests the existence of some policy links.

We shall look at this phenomenon by exploring two separate sets of questions. First, what critical factors must exist for presidents to be able to obtain a judiciary that reflects their own political philosophy? Second, what empirical evidence is there to suggest that judges' decisions to some degree carry the imprint of the presidents who selected them?

### The President and the Composition of the Judiciary

We suggest that there are four general factors that determine whether chief executives can obtain a fedeal judiciary that is sympathetic to their political values and attitudes.

*Presidential Support for Ideologically Based Appointments.* One key aspect of the success of chief executives in appointing a federal judiciary that mirrors their own political beliefs is the depth of their commitment to do so. Some presidents may be content merely to fill the federal bench with party loyalists and pay little heed to their nominees' specific ideologies. Some may consider ideological factors when appointing Supreme Court justices but may not regard them as important for trial and appellate judges. Other presidents may discount ideologically grounded appointments because they themselves tend to be nonideological; still others may place factors such as past political loyalty ahead of ideology in selecting judges.

Dwight D. Eisenhower was a chief executive in the first category—that is, he was an almost apolitical president for whom ideological purity counted little. While his judicial appointees were indeed primarily Republican, upper-middle-class types, there is no evidence to indicate that they were picked because their political philosophies matched Eisenhower's. As a result, the Eisenhower judges turned out to be a mixed bag; progressives and strong civil libertarians mingled with jurists of more conservative, law-and-order values.

As a president, Harry Truman had strong political views, but when selecting judges he placed loyalty to himself ahead of the candidate's overall political orientation. We noted earlier in this chapter how eager Truman was to appoint Carroll O. Switzer to fill the judicial vacancy in Iowa. Truman's premium on personal loyalty rather than ideology is generally reflected in the group of men he put on the bench. For example, there was scant linkage between Truman's personal liberal stance on civil rights and equal opportunity and his judicial selections: he appointed no blacks and no women at all, and at least three of his key Southern district court appointees have been identified as being very unfriendly toward the cause of civil rights.[30]

If Eisenhower and Truman exemplify presidents who eschewed ideological criteria, Ronald Reagan provides a good example of a chief executive who selected his judicial nominees with a clear eye toward their compatibility with his own conservative philosophy. During the first six years of his administration, Reagan appointed 287 judges to the district and appeals courts. Of these, 95 percent were Republicans, 94 percent were white, and 92 percent were males; the majority were well-off (45 percent had net worths of over $500,000 and more than one in five were millionaires); virtually all had established records as political conservatives and as apostles of judicial self-restraint. Indeed, as the Reagan administration's conservative programs began to bog down in the more liberal-minded Congress, the Reagan team looked more and more toward implementing their values through their judicial appointment strategy. As White House communications director Patrick J. Buchanan once put it, "[Our conservative appointment strategy] ... could do more to advance the social agenda—school prayer, anti-pornography, anti-busing, right-to-life and quotas in employment—than anything Congress can accomplish in 20 years." [31] In fairness to President Reagan it should be pointed out, however, that he was not the only modern president to pack the bench with those who shared his political and legal philosophies: Presidents Johnson and Carter both successfully appointed activist liberal judges.

*The Number of Vacancies to Be Filled.* A second element affecting the capacity of chief executives to establish a policy link between themselves and the judiciary is the number of appointments available to them. Obviously, the more judges a president can select, the greater the potential of the White House to put its stamp on the judicial branch. For example, George Washington's influence on the Supreme Court was significant because he was able to nominate ten individuals to the High Court bench. Jimmy Carter's was nil, on the other hand, because no vacancies occurred during his term as president.

The number of appointment opportunities depends, of course, on several factors: how many judges and justices die or resign during the president's term, how long the president serves, and whether or not Congress passes legislation that significantly increases the number of judgeships. Historically the last factor seems to have been the most important in influencing the number of judgeships available, and, as one might expect, politics in its most basic form permeates this whole process. A study of proposals for new-judges bills in thirteen Congresses tested these two hypotheses: (1) "proposals to add new federal judges are more likely to pass if the party controls the Presidency and Congress than if different parties are in power," and (2) "proposals to add new federal judges are more likely to pass during the first two years of the President's term than during the second two years." The author concluded that his "data support both hypotheses—proposals to add new judges are about 5 times more likely to pass if the same party controls the Presidency and Congress than if different parties control, and about 4 times more likely to pass during the first two years of the President's term than during the second two years." He then noted that these findings serve "to remind us that not only is judicial selection a political process, but so is the creation of judicial posts." [32] Thus the number of vacancies that a president can fill—a function of politics, fate, and the size of the judicial workloads—is another variable that helps determine the impact a chief executive has on the composition of the federal judiciary.

*The President's Political Clout.* Another factor is the scope and proficiency of presidential skill in overcoming any political obstacles. One such stumbling block is the U.S. Senate, as we have noted previously. If the Senate is controlled by the president's political party, the White House will find it much easier to secure confirmation than if opposition forces control the Senate. Sometimes when the opposition is in power in the Senate, presidents are forced into a sort of political horse trading to get their nominees approved. For example, when the Democrats controlled the Senate during the Nixon and Ford administrations, those two presidents had to make a political deal for the district judgeships in California: the state's two Democratic senators were permitted to appoint one of their own for every three Republicans that were put on the bench.

The Senate Judiciary Committee is another roadblock between the will and political savvy of the president and the men and women who sit on the federal bench. Some presidents have been more adept than others in easing their candidates through the jagged rocks of the Judiciary Committee rapids. Both Presidents Kennedy and Johnson, for example, had to deal with the formidable committee chairman James Eastland of Mississippi, but only Johnson seems to have had the political adroitness to get most of his liberal nominees approved. Kennedy lacked this skill, and we have mentioned the kinds of judges he was often obliged to appoint.

The president's personal popularity is another element in the political power formula. Chief executives who are well liked by the public and command the respect of opinion makers in the news media, the rank-and-file of their political party, and the leaders of the nation's major interest groups are much more likely to prevail over any forces that seek to thwart their judicial nominees. Personal popularity is not a stable factor and is sometimes hard to gauge, but there is little doubt that presidents' standing with the electorate helps determine the success of their efforts to influence the composition of the American judiciary. For example, in 1930, President Hoover's choice for a seat on the Supreme Court, John J. Parker, was defeated in the Senate by a two-vote margin. It is likely that had the nomination been made a year or so earlier, before the onset of the Depression took Hoover's popularity by the throat, Parker might have gotten on the Supreme Court. Likewise, in 1968 President Johnson's low esteem among voters and the powers-that-be may have been partially responsible for Senate rejection of Johnson's candidate for chief justice, Abe Fortas, and also for the Senate's refusal to replace Fortas with Johnson's old pal Homer Thornberry. As one observer commented, "Johnson failed largely because most members of the Senate 'had had it' with the lame-duck President's nominations." [33] Conversely, President Eisenhower's success in getting approval for an inordinately large number of nominees dubbed "not qualified" by the ABA (some 13.2 percent) may be attributed, in part at least, to Ike's great popularity and prestige.

   *The Judicial Climate the New Judges Enter.*   A final matter affects the capacity of chief executives to secure a federal judiciary that reflects their own political values: the current philosophical orientations of the sitting district and appellate court judges with whom the new appointees must interact. Since federal judges serve lifetime appointments during good behavior, presidents must accept the composition and value structure of the judiciary as it exists when they first come into office. If the existing judiciary already reflects the president's political and legal orientation, the impact of new judicial appointees will be immediate and substantial. On the other hand, if new chief executives face a trial and appellate judiciary whose values are radically different from their own, the impact of their subsequent judicial appointments will be weaker and slower to materialize. New judges must respect the controlling legal precedents and the existing constitutional interpretations that prevail in the judiciary at the time they enter it, or they risk being overturned by a higher court. Such a reality may limit the capacity of a new set of judges to get in there and do their own thing—at least in the short run.

When Franklin Roosevelt became president in 1933, he was confronted with a Supreme Court and a lower federal judiciary that had been solidly packed with conservative Republican jurists by his three GOP predecessors in the White House. A majority of the High Court and most lower-court judges viewed most of Roosevelt's New Deal legislation as unconstitutional, and indeed it was not until 1937 that the Supreme Court began to stop overturning virtually all of FDR's major legislative programs.

To make matters worse, his first opportunity to fill a Supreme Court vacancy did not come until the fall of 1937. Thus, despite the ideological screening that went into the selection of FDR's judges, it seems fair to assume that, at least between 1933 and 1938, Roosevelt's trial and appellate judges had to restrain their liberal propensities in the myriad of cases that came before them. This may explain in part why the voting records of the Roosevelt court appointees is not much more liberal than that of the conservative judges selected by his three Republican predecessors; the Roosevelt team just didn't have much room to move in a judiciary dominated by staunch conservatives.

The decisional patterns of the Eisenhower judges further serve to illustrate this phenomenon. Although the Eisenhower appointees were more conservative than those selected by Presidents Truman and Roosevelt, the differences in the rulings they made are pretty small. One major reason was that the Eisenhower jurists entered a realm that from top to bottom was dominated by Roosevelt and Truman appointees, who were for the most part liberals. Ike's generally conservative judges didn't have much more room to maneuver than did Roosevelt's liberal jurists in the face of a conservative-dominated judiciary.

President Reagan's impact on the judicial branch continues to be substantial. By the spring of his last year in office he had appointed an unprecedented 334 federal judges, 45 percent of those on the bench. When he entered the White House, the Supreme Court was already teetering to the right because of Nixon's and Ford's conservative appointments.

Although Carter's liberal appointees had places on the trial and appellate court benches, Reagan still found a good many conservative Nixon and Ford judges on the bench when he took office. Thus he has had a major role in shaping the entire federal judiciary for some time to come in his own conservative image even though his tenure as president has ended. The Bush judges should likewise have a much easier time making their impact felt since they are entering a judicial realm wherein well over half the judges already profess conservative, Republican values.

## Presidents' Values and Their Appointees' Decisions

We now know the conditions that must be met if presidents are to secure a judiciary in tune with their own policy values and goals. What evidence is there that presidents have in fact been able to do so? Or, to return to our original question, when the people elect a particular president, is there reason to believe that their choice will be expressed in the kinds of judges that are appointed and the kinds of decisions that those judges render?

To answer these questions we shall look at an investigation of the liberal-conservative voting patterns of the teams of district court judges appointed by thirteen presidents during this century. This comprehensive study is the only one that covers enough presidents, judges, and cases to allow us to make some meaningful generalizations. In essence we shall see whether liberal presidents appointed trial judges who decided cases in a more liberal manner and whether conservative chief executives were able to obtain district court jurists who followed their policy views.

To begin, we will offer some examples to define the sometimes slippery terms *liberal* and *conservative*. In the realm of civil rights and civil liberties, liberal judges would generally take a broadening position—that is, they would seek in their rulings to extend these freedoms; conservative jurists, by contrast, would prefer to limit such rights. For example, in a case in which a government agency wanted to prevent a controversial person from speaking in a public park or at a state university, a liberal judge would be more inclined than a conservative to uphold the right of the would-be speech giver. Or in a case involving school integration, a liberal judge would be more likely to take the side of the minority petitioners. In the area of government regulation of the economy, liberal judges would probably uphold legislation that benefited working people or the economic underdog. Thus, if the secretary of labor sought an injunction against an employer for paying less than the minimum wage, a liberal judge would be more disposed toward the labor secretary's arguments, whereas a conservative judge would tend to side with business, especially big business. Another broad category of cases often studied by judicial scholars is that of criminal justice. Liberal judges are, in general, more sympathetic to the motions made by criminal defendants. For instance, in a case in which the accused claimed to have been coerced by the government into an illegal confession, liberal judges would be more likely than their conservative counterparts to agree that the government had acted improperly.

Table 8-5 indicates the percent of liberal decisions rendered by the district court appointees of Presidents Wilson through Reagan. Fifty-one percent of the decisions of the Wilson judges are liberal, which puts these jurists almost on a par with those of Lyndon Johnson and Jimmy Carter for having the most liberal voting record. The liberal pattern of the Wilson judges is not surprising: Wilson was one of the staunchest liberal presidents of this century—particularly on economic issues. Moreover, he chose his judges on a highly partisan, ideological basis: 98.6 percent of his appointments to the lower courts were Democrats—still the record for any president in recent memory.

Succeeding Wilson in the White House were the three Republican chief executives of the 1920s, beginning with Harding's "return to normalcy" in 1921 and followed by the equally conservative Coolidge and Hoover. The right-of-center policy values of these three presidents (and the undisputed Republican domination of the Senate during their incumbencies) are mirrored in the decisional patterns of the trial judges they selected. The liberalism score drops by 10 points from Wilson to Harding, 51 to 41 percent, and stays around that same level for the Coolidge and Hoover judicial teams.

With Franklin D. Roosevelt's judges there is a shift back to left-of-center. At 47 percent liberal, the Roosevelt jurists are five points more liberal than those of his immediate predecessor, Herbert Hoover. We have good evidence that FDR used ideological criteria to pick his judges and that he put the full weight of his political skills behind that endeavor. He once instructed his dispenser of political patronage, James Farley, in effect to use the judicial appointment power as a weapon against senators and representatives who were balking at New Deal legislation: "First off, we must hold up judicial appointments in States where the [congressional] delegation is not going along [with our liberal economic proposals]. We must make appointments promptly where the delegation is with us. Second, this must apply to other appointments. I'll keep in close contact with the leaders." [34]

At first the comparatively conservative voting record of the Truman judges seems a bit strange in view of Truman's personal commitment to liberal economic and social policy goals. Only 40 percent of the Truman judges' decisions were liberal, a full seven points less than Roosevelt's-jurists—and even two points below the Hoover nominees. As we noted earlier, however, Truman counted personal loyalty much more heavily than ideological standards when selecting his judges, and as a result many

Table 8-5   Percentage of Liberal Decisions Rendered by District Court
Appointees of Presidents Wilson through Reagan, 1933-1986

| Appointing president | Percent | Number |
|---|---|---|
| Woodrow Wilson | 51 | 94 |
| Warren Harding | 41 | 538 |
| Calvin Coolidge | 43 | 630 |
| Herbert Hoover | 42 | 910 |
| Franklin D. Roosevelt | 47 | 2,828 |
| Harry S Truman | 40 | 3,273 |
| Dwight D. Eisenhower | 37 | 4,401 |
| John F. Kennedy | 41 | 5,065 |
| Lyndon B. Johnson | 52 | 7,577 |
| Richard Nixon | 38 | 6,872 |
| Gerald R. Ford | 45 | 1,311 |
| Jimmy Carter | 54 | 3,498 |
| Ronald Reagan | 36 | 702 |

Source:  Unpublished data collected by Robert A. Carp, Ronald Stidham, and C. K. Rowland.

conservatives found their way into the ranks of the Truman judges. Indeed, even Truman's Supreme Court nominees were of a rather nondescript, conservative ilk:

> Harry Truman's first [Supreme] court appointment was a Republican senator from Ohio, Harold Burton—the only Republican ever selected by a Democratic President. His three other nominees were high-ranking Democratic politicians—Chief Justice Fred Vinson had been his Secretary of the Treasury, Tom Clark had served as Attorney General, and Sherman Minton was an Indiana senator. Truman's men generally held to the modest "judicial restraint" defended so brilliantly by Frankfurter, the court's intellectual eminence. Three of Truman's appointees—Vinson, Burton, and Minton—were among eight justices rated as "failures" in the 1971 poll of professors.[35]

Because of Truman's lack of interest in making policy-based appointments, coupled with strong opposition in the Senate and lack of popular support throughout much of his administration, his personal liberalism was generally not reflected in the policy values of his judges. Eisenhower's judges were more conservative than Truman's, as expected, but the difference is not very great. But we have already noted that Eisenhower paid little attention to purely ideological appointment criteria; in addition, his judges had to work in the company of an overwhelming Democratic majority in the whole federal judiciary. These factors must have mollified many of the conservative inclinations of the Eisenhower jurists.

The 41 percent liberalism score of the Kennedy judges represents a swing to the left. This is to be expected, and at first blush it may appear strange that John Kennedy's team on the bench was not even more left of center. However, we must keep in mind Kennedy's problems in dealing with the conservative, southern-dominated Senate Judiciary Committee; his lack of political clout in the Senate, which often made him a pawn of senatorial courtesy; and his inability to overcome the stranglehold of local Democratic bosses, who often prized partisan loyalty over ideological purity—or even competence—when it came to appointing judges.

Lyndon Johnson's judges moved impressively toward the left, and, as we noted, his judges were as liberal as Wilson's and much more so than Kennedy's. We can account for this on the basis of the four criteria discussed earlier in this chapter that predict a correspondence between the values of chief executives and the orientation of their judges. Johnson knew well how to bargain with individual senators and was second to none in his ability to manipulate and cajole those who were initially indifferent or hostile to issues (or candidates) he supported; his impressive victories in Congress—for example, the antipoverty legislation and the civil rights acts—are monuments to his skill. Undoubtedly, too, he used his political prowess to secure a judicial team that reflected his liberal policy values. In addition, Johnson was able to fill a large number of vacancies on the bench, and his liberal appointees must have felt right at home ideologically in a judiciary capped by the liberal Warren Court.

If the leftward swing of the Johnson team is dramatic, it is no less so than the shift to the right made by the Nixon judges. Only 38 percent of the decisions of Nixon's jurists were liberal. Nixon, of course, placed enormous emphasis on getting conservatives nominated to judgeships at all levels; he possessed the political clout to secure Senate confirmation for most lower-court appointees—at least until Watergate, when the Nixon wine turned to vinegar; and the rightist policy values of the Nixon judges must have been prodded by a Supreme Court that was growing more and more conservative.

The 45 percent liberalism score of the Ford judges puts them right between the Johnson and Nixon jurists in terms of ideology. That Ford's jurists were less conservative than Nixon's is not hard to explain. First, Ford himself was much less of a political ideologue than his predecessor, as reflected in the way in which he screened his nominees and in the type of individuals he chose. (Ford's appointment of the moderate John Paul Stevens to the Supreme Court versus Nixon's selection of the highly conservative William H. Rehnquist illustrates the point.) Also, because Ford's circuitous route to the presidency did not enhance his political effectiveness with the Senate, he would not have had the clout to force highly conservative Republican nominees through a liberal, Democratic Senate, even if he had wished to.

With a score of 54 percent, Jimmy Carter holds the record as having appointed judges with the most liberal voting record of the thirteen presidents for whom we have data. Despite Carter's call for an "independent" federal judiciary based on "merit selection," it is clear that his judges were selected with a keen eye toward their potential liberal voting tendencies.[36] That there is a correspondence between the values of President Carter and the liberal decisional patterns of his judges should come as no surprise. Carter was clearly identified with liberal social and political values, and although his economic policies were perhaps more conservative than those of other recent Democratic presidents, there is little doubt about Carter's commitment to liberal values in the areas of civil rights and liberties and of criminal justice. Carter, too, had ample opportunity to pack the bench: The Omnibus Judgeship Act of 1978 passed by a friendly Democratic Congress created a record 152 new federal judicial openings for Carter to fill. Carter also possessed a fair degree of political clout with a Judiciary Committee and Senate controlled by Democrats. Finally, the Carter judicial team found many friendly liberals (appointed by Presidents Johnson and Kennedy) already sitting on the bench.

Reagan's judicial team has the distinction of having the most conservative voting record of all the judicial cohorts in our study. Only 36 percent of their decisions bear the liberal stamp. President Reagan's conservative values and his commitment to reshaping the federal judiciary in his own image were secrets to no one. Early in his first presidential campaign Reagan had inveighed against left-leaning activist judges, and he promised a dramatic change. As did his predecessor, Reagan had the opportunity, through attrition and newly created judgeships, to fill the judiciary with persons of his own inclinations. (At the end of his second term about half the federal judiciary bore the Reagan label.) This phenomenon was aided by Reagan's great personal popularity throughout most of his administration and a Senate that his party controlled during six of his eight years in office. Finally, the Reagan cohort entered the judicial realm with conservative greetings from the sitting right-of-center Nixon and Ford judges.

We have explored the degree to which presidents have been able to secure a judiciary that reflects their own policy values. The evidence indicates that if they are of a mind to, and have a little luck, chief executives can appoint judges who mirror many of the attitudes and values of the electorate. It is particularly significant that such data show up at the district court level, where presidential input is at its weakest because senatorial courtesy muddies the selection process. But even among district court jurists we see the imprint of policy links between the people's choice and the actions of their appointed judges! If this is the case, the potential policy ties at the appeals court and Supreme Court levels should be even stronger, because the president has a much freer hand in selecting those jurists than U.S. trial judges.

## President Bush and the Federal Judiciary

What kind of men and women will President Bush select for service on the federal bench, and what is the likelihood that their impact will be substantial? Using our previously discussed impact model and a little crystal ball gazing, this is what the future may hold.

We begin by noting that as of early 1989 the Court's conservatives hold a slim five-to-four edge over the liberals: Justices Rehnquist, Scalia, White, O'Connor, and Kennedy comprise the right wing of the Court while Justices Brennan, Marshall, Blackmun, and Stevens often lean left of center. However, the conservative coalition is a tenuous one. Kennedy, for example, has not been on the Court long enough to have a track record one way or the other, and Justices White and O'Connor (and occasionally even Rehnquist) sometimes confound the Court watchers with their "inconsistent" voting patterns. Also relevant to this discussion is the fact that three of the four liberals (Brennan, Marshall, and Blackmun) are over eighty years of age and not in the best of health. Thus the liberals are in a position of great vulnerability at the present time.

With this situation greeting his administration, President Bush has an enormous potential to move the Court in a significantly more conservative direction. If even one or two of the liberal justices resign or die and are replaced with conservatives, the Court will have a strong, working conservative coalition that could remain intact for decades. What is the evidence that President Bush will seize this opportunity?

In his actions and public statements President Bush appears to be a man of moderately conservative values. His appointees have been men and women with clear conservative credentials who are also pragmatists rather than diehard ideologues. And in a subtle attack on judicial liberalism (code named "activism"), Bush told the American Judicature Society, "I am firmly committed to appointing judges who are dedicated to interpreting the law as it exists, rather than legislating from the bench." [37] (The president obviously does not believe it possible to be a judicial activist for conservative causes—a position with which we respectfully disagree.)

What light does our model shed on Bush's capacity to mold the federal judiciary in his own image? First, President Bush does have an interest in making ideologically based appointments, and as we have seen, this desire is essential if the president is to alter the values of the judiciary. In terms of the number of vacancies to be filled, the potential seems great indeed for the Supreme Court, although it is more doubtful that a strong Democratic Congress is going to expand significantly the size of the lower judiciary so that Bush might fill its ranks with conservative Republicans. Regarding the president's political clout, the potential here is less in Bush's favor. Without a huge mandate in the popular election and in the face of a solidly Democratic-controlled Senate, there is little reason to believe that Bush could successfully appoint jurists that were too far right of the political mainstream. Finally, there is the matter of the judicial climate into which the new judges enter. Given that half of the judiciary bear the conservative Reagan stamp and that a fair number of Nixon and Ford judges still sit on the bench, Bush's conservative jurists should be able to swim with the tide rather than against it—all to the enhancement of his impact on the Court. In sum, President Bush has the desire to continue to move the federal judiciary in a moderately conservative direction, and our model suggests that his chances of success are very good indeed.

## The Judicial Socialization Process

The central focus of this chapter is on the judges and justices themselves. We continue our look at the judges by examining a critical period in their professional life—the judicial socialization process, the time during which new appointees learn to be judges.

When scholars use the term *socialization*, they are referring to the process whereby individuals acquire the values, attitudes, and behavior patterns of the ongoing social system. Factors that aid the process include family, friends, education, co-workers, religious training, political party affiliation, and the communications media. Social scientists also apply the term *socialization* to the process by which a person is formally trained to perform the specific tasks of a particular profession. It is the second meaning of the term, then, that will concern us.

Prior to looking at judges' on-the-job training, we must acknowledge that much significant socialization occurs *before* the judges first mount the bench. From their parents, teachers, exposure to the news media, and so on, future judges learn the rules of the American political game. That is, by the time they are teenagers they have absorbed key values and attitudes that will circumscribe subsequent judicial behavior: "the majority should rule on general matters of public policy, but minorities have their rights, too"; "judges ought to be fair and impartial"; or "the Constitution is an important document and all political leaders should be bound by it." In college and law school future judges acquire important analytic and communications skills, in addition to the basic substance of the law. After a couple of decades of legal practice, the preparation for a judgeship is in its final stage; the future judge has learned a good bit about how the courts and the law actually work and has specialized in several areas of the law. Despite all this preparation, sometimes called "anticipatory socialization," [38] most new judges in America still have a lot to learn even after donning the black robe.

In many other countries preparing to be a judge is like preparing to be a physician, an engineer, or a pharmacist—that is, one goes to a particular professional school in which one receives many years of in-depth training and perhaps an on-the-job internship. Since 1959 in France, for example, all new would-be judges are intensively trained for a minimum of twenty-eight months in the prestigious Ecole Nationale de la Magistrature; they enter judicial service only after passing rigorous, competitive examinations. Not only does the United States lack formalized training procedures for the judicial profession, but there is the naive assumption that being a lawyer for a decade or so is all the experience one needs to be a judge. After all, don't most lawyers, like judges, work in the courtroom? Isn't it enough for the lawyer-turned-judge just to mount the bench and put on a new hat? To the contrary, becoming a judge in America requires a good deal of *freshman socialization* (short-term learning and adjustment to the new role) and *occupational socialization* (on-the-job training over a period of years).

Let us examine what it is like to become a new judge and why socialization must continue well into the novice jurist's career. Typical new trial court appointees may be first-rate lawyers and experts in a few areas of the law in which they have specialized. As judges, however, they are suddenly expected to be experts on *all* legal subjects, are required to engage in judicial duties usually quite unrelated to any tasks they performed as lawyers (for example, sentencing), and are given a host of administrative assignments for which they have had no prior experience (for example, learning how to docket efficiently several hundred diverse cases.)[39] The following statements by U.S. trial judges reveal what it was like for them as the new kid on the judicial block. (Virtually all the judges who were interviewed for this book were promised anonymity, and thus no references will appear.)

> Before I became a federal judge I had been a trial lawyer dealing mainly with personal injury cases and later on with some divorce cases. Needless to say, I knew almost nothing about criminal law. With labor law I had had only one case in my life on this subject, and that was a case going back to the early days of World War II. In other words when I became a federal judge I really had an awful lot to learn about many important areas of the law.
>   My legal background and experience really didn't prepare me very well for the kind of major judicial problems I face. For instance, most lawyers don't deal with constitutional issues related to the Bill of Rights

and the Fourteenth Amendment; rather they deal with much more routine questions, such as wills and contracts. Civil liberties questions were really new to me as a judge, and I think this is true for most new judges.

At the appeals court level there is also a period of freshman socialization—despite the circuit judge's possible prior judicial experience—although former trial judges appear to make the transition with fewer scars. As a couple of appeals judges said of their first days on the circuit bench: "I was no blushing violet in fields I knew something about. How effective I was is another question." Even an experienced former trial judge recalled his surprise that "it takes a while to learn the job—and I'm not addressing myself to personal relationships. . . . That's a very different job." Another appeals judge, regarded by his peers as a leader from the beginning, said, "I don't know how I got through my first year." [40] During the transition time—the period of learning the appellate court ropes—circuit judges tend to speak less for the court than their more experienced colleagues; they often take longer to write opinions, defer more often to senior colleagues, or just wallow about in indecision.

The learning process for new Supreme Court justices is even harder—if the personal testimonies of justices as diverse as Benjamin Cardozo, Frank Murphy, Harlan F. Stone, Earl Warren, William Brennan, and Arthur Goldberg are to be believed. As one scholar has noted, "Once on the Court, the freshman Justice, even if he has been a state or lower federal court judge, moves into a strange and shadowy world." [41] Perhaps this is the metaphor that Chief Justice William Howard Taft had in mind when he confided that in joining the Court he felt that he had come "to live in a monastery." As with new appeals court judges, novice Supreme Court justices tend to defer to senior associates, to write fewer majority and dissenting opinions, and to manifest a good deal of uncertainty. New High Court appointees may have more judicial experience than their lower-court colleagues, but the fact that the Supreme Court is involved in broad judicial policy making—as opposed to the error correction of the appeals courts and the norm enforcement of the trial courts—may account for their initial indecisiveness.

Given the need on the part of all new federal jurists for both freshman and occupational socialization, where do they go for instruction? While there are many agents of socialization for novice judges, the evidence is pretty strong that the older, more experienced judges have the primary responsibility for this task: the system trains and nurtures its own. As one trial judge told us, "My prime sources of help were the two judges here in [this city]. They sent me various things even before I was appointed, and I was glad to get them." Another recalled, "I had the help I needed right down here in the corner of this building on this floor," pointing in the direction of another judge's chambers. One district judge gave a more graphic description of his "schooling":

> They [the other trial judges] let me sit next to them in actual courtroom situations, and they explained to me what they were doing at every minute. We both wore our robes and we sat next to each other on the bench. I would frequently ask them questions and they would explain things to me as the trial went along. Other times I would have a few free minutes and I would drop into another judge's courtroom and just sit and watch. I learned a lot that way.

For both the rotating appeals court judges and their trial court brethren, then, the lion's share of training comes from their more senior, experienced colleagues on the bench—particularly the chief judge of the circuit or district.[42] One scholar has noted that "the impact of chief judges was most noticeable on freshmen. . . . ('If all the judges are new, he'll pack a wallop out of proportion to one vote.')" [43] Likewise on the Supreme Court there is evidence that older associates, often the chief justice, play a primary part in passing on to novice justices the essential rules and values on which their very serious game is based.[44]

The training seminars provided by the Federal Judicial Center for newly appointed judges should also be mentioned again in this regard because over the years the center has played an ever increasing role in the training and socialization of new jurists. While some of these seminars are conducted by "outsider" specialists—subject matter experts in the law schools—the key instructors still tend to be seasoned judges whose real-life experience on the bench commands the respect of the new members of the federal judiciary.

The fact that judges in America still require socialization even after their appointments is interesting in and of itself, but we might well ask: What is the significance of all this for the operation of our judicial-legal system? First, the agents of socialization that are readily available to the novice jurists allow the system to operate more smoothly, with a minimum of down time. If new judges were isolated from their more experienced associates, geographically or otherwise, it would take them much longer to learn the fine points of their trade and presumably there would be a greater number of errors foisted upon hapless litigants.

There is a second consequence of the socialization process. As noted in Chapter 2, the judicial system is a rather loose hierarchy that is constantly subjected to centrifugal and centripetal forces from within and without. The fact that the system is able to provide its own socialization—that the older, experienced jurists train the novices—serves as a sort of glue that helps bond the fragmented system together. It allows the judicial values, practices, and orientations of one generation of judges to be passed on to another. It gives continuity and a sense of permanence to a system that operates in a world where chaos and random behavior appear to be the order of the day.

## The Retirement and Removal of Judges

We have reached the final stage in our look at the judges themselves—the time when they cease performing their judicial duties, by choice, by ill health or death, or by the disciplinary actions of others.

### Disciplinary Action Against Federal Judges

All federal judges appointed under the provisions of Article III of the Constitution hold office "during good Behavior," which means in effect for life or until they choose to step down. The only way they can be removed from the bench is by impeachment (indictment by the House of Representatives) and conviction by the Senate. In accordance with constitutional requirements (for Supreme Court justices) and legislative standards (for appeals and trial court judges), impeachment may occur for "Treason, Bribery, or other high Crimes and Misdemeanors." An impeached jurist would face trial in the Senate, which could convict by a vote of two-thirds of the members present.

The impeachment of a federal judge is a fairly rare event, although recently it has become a more familiar topic. Congress has moved to take such drastic action against several judges in the past several years, and at the present time U.S. District Judge Alcee L. Hastings is facing a Senate trial after the House of Representatives approved seventeen articles of impeachment by a vote of 413 to 3 in the fall of 1988. However, since 1789 the House has initiated such proceedings against only eleven jurists—although about an equal number of judges resigned just before formal action was taken against them. Of these eleven cases, only five resulted in a conviction, which removed them from office. Considering all the men and women who have sat on the federal bench during the past two centuries, that's not a bad record. (Four members of Congress have been convicted of felonies in a single session!)

Although outright acts of criminality on the bench are few, a gray area of misconduct may put offending judges somewhere in the twilight zone between acceptable and impeachable behavior. What to do with the federal jurist who hears a case despite an obvious conflict of interest, who consistently demonstrates biased behavior in the courtroom, who too often totters into court after a triple-martini lunch? A case in point is Judge Willis Ritter, who used to sit on the federal bench in Salt Lake City. One observer described Ritter as ecumenically mean, which is to say he seems to dislike most persons who come into his court, be they defendant, government lawyer, private trial attorney, or ordinary citizen. Ritter is also selective about his fellow judges. He was once so estranged from another Utah federal judge that they wouldn't ride on the elevator together, much less speak; for a while the court clerk divided cases so that they didn't have to appear in the courthouse on the same day. . . . . Ritter is one of the few federal judges in the nation who becomes so emotionally involved in his hearings that appeals courts often order him not to retry cases when they are reversed.[45]

One lawyer who had managed to fall from Judge Ritter's graces recalled an incident. As the lawyer was starting to present his case in open court, from out of the blue the judge began to hiss at him and continued to do so throughout the attorney's presentation. "Like a snake, he was going 'ssssss' all the time I was speaking," the astounded lawyer recounted later. "I never ever have been before a judge of this kind."[46]

But what to do with Judge Ritter and those of his ilk? Had Ritter committed impeachable offenses? Surely he had not been guilty of "Treason, Bribery, or other high Crimes and Misdemeanors," although one could well question whether he was indeed serving "during good Behavior." Historically, little was done in such cases other than issuance of a mild reprimand by colleagues (a useless gesture for a Judge Ritter) or impeachment (a recourse considered too drastic in most cases). In recent decades, however, actions have been taken to fill in the discipline gap. In 1966, for example, the Supreme Court upheld an action taken by the Tenth Circuit Judicial Council against U.S. District Judge Stephen S. Chandler of Oklahoma. The council had stripped him of his duties and authority (while permitting him to retain his salary and title) for a series of antics both on and off the bench that made Judge Ritter seem venerable by comparison.

In addition, on October 1, 1980, a new statute took effect on which Congress had labored for several years. Titled the Judicial Councils Reform and Judicial Conduct and Disability Act, the law contains two distinct parts.[47] The first authorizes the Judicial Council in each circuit, composed of both appeals and trial judges and presided over by the chief judge of the circuit, to "make all necessary and appropriate orders for the effective and expeditious administration of justice within its circuit." The second part of the act establishes a statutory complaint procedure against judges. Basically, it permits an aggrieved party to file a written complaint with the clerk of the appellate court. The chief judge then reviews the charge and may dismiss it if it appears frivolous, or for a variety of other reasons. If the complaint seems valid, the chief judge must appoint an investigating committee consisting of himself or herself and an equal number of trial and circuit judges. After an inquiry the committee reports to the council, which has several options: (1) the judge may be exonerated; (2) if the offender is a bankruptcy judge or magistrate, he or she may be removed; and (3) an Article III judge may be subject to private or public reprimand or censure, certification of disability, request for voluntary resignation, or prohibition against further case assignments. However, removal of an Article III judge is not permitted; impeachment is still the only recourse. If the council determines that the conduct "might constitute" grounds for impeachment, it will notify the Judicial Conference, which in turn may transmit the case to the U.S. House of Representatives for consideration.

In 1987 there were 232 judicial misconduct complaints filed, and some 244 were concluded during the fiscal year ending June 30. The circuit chief judges dismissed 198 complaints, an additional 35 were set aside by the judicial councils, 2 charges were withdrawn, 8 were terminated after some action was taken against the errant judge, and 1 was referred to the U.S. Judicial Conference. There is also some evidence that the direct or indirect threat of invoking the act may serve to curb some forms of unacceptable judicial deportment.[48] Because the Judicial Conduct Act has been on the books for only a short time, it is difficult to assess its true effectiveness. However, it appears to fill a wide gap in the disciplinary process between informal pressure on the one hand and outright impeachment on the other.

### Disability of Federal Judges

Perhaps the biggest problem has not been the removal of criminals and crackpots from the federal bench; rather, it has been the question of what to do with jurists who have become too old and infirm effectively to carry out their judicial responsibilities. As the former chief judge of the Fifth Circuit Court of Appeals John Brown tersely put it, "Get rid of the aged judges, and you get rid of most of the problems of the federal judiciary: drunkenness, incompetence, senility, cantankerous behavior on the bench." [49] For example, Justice William O. Douglas suffered a stroke while on the Supreme Court but refused afterward to resign, even when it was clear to all that he should do so. In 1974 Chief Justice Burger "believed Douglas was developing the paranoid qualities of many stroke victims. Douglas complained that there were plots to kill him and to remove him from the bench. Once he was wheeled in the Chief's chambers and maintained it was his. Rumors circulated among the staff that Douglas thought he was the Chief Justice." But he stayed on. A year later he was still interpreting the Constitution for over 200 million Americans although he "was in constant pain and barely had the energy to make his voice audible. He was wheeled in and out of conference, never staying the entire session, leaving his votes with Brennan to cast.

Powell counted the number of times Douglas fell asleep. Brennan woke him gently when it came time to vote." Eventually Douglas resigned, but surely he remained on the bench longer than he should have. On the Court at the same time as Douglas were Justices John Harlan and Hugo Black. The latter, at eighty-five, was in such poor health that Douglas was counseling *him* to resign. "But Black would not accept the advice." [50]

> In contrast to Black, Harlan continued to run his chambers from his hospital bed. Nearly blind, he could not even see the ash from his own cigarette, but he doggedly prepared for the coming term. One day a clerk brought in an emergency petition. Harlan remained in bed as he discussed the case with the clerk. They agreed that the petition should be denied. Harlan bent down, his eyes virtually to the paper, wrote his name, and handed the paper to his clerk. The clerk saw no signature. He looked over at Harlan.
> "Justice Harlan, you just denied your sheet," the clerk said, gently pointing to the scrawl on the linen. Harlan smiled and tried again, signing the paper this time. [51]

While the federal judiciary as a whole is not proportionally in the same state of ill health and advanced age as was the Supreme Court during the early 1970s, the problem of what to do with the aged or mentally disabled judge has not disappeared. Congress has tried with some success to tempt the more senior judges into retirement by making it financially more palatable to do so. Since 1984 federal judges have been permitted to retire with full pay and benefits under what is called "the rule of eighty"—that is, when the sum of a judge's age and number of years on the bench is eighty. Congress has also permitted judges to go on "senior" status instead of accepting full retirement: In exchange for a reduced caseload they are permitted to retain their office and staff and—equally important—the prestige and self-respect of being an active judge. Despite the congressional inducements to retire, "more vacancies occur as a result of death in harness, particularly at the higher levels, than in any other way." [52]

We conclude this discussion of federal judicial tenure on a more political note. There is some credible evidence that judges often time their resignations to occur when their party controls the presidency so that they will be replaced by a jurist of similar political and judicial orientation. As one researcher concluded, "Among the Appeals and District judges there is a substantial contingent who bring to the bench political loyalties that encourage them, more often than not, to maneuver their departure in such a way that will maximize the chance for the appointment of a replacement by a president of their party." [53] We catch the flavor of this phenomenon in this account of an Iowa district judge's decision about retirement:

By 1948 Iowa Southern District Federal Judge Charles A. Dewey had decided that the time had come for him to retire. The seventy-one year old jurist had served on the federal bench for two full decades, and he felt that he had earned the right to his government pension. As a good Republican, however, he felt that it would be best to withhold his resignation until after the November election when "President Thomas E. Dewey" would be in a position to fill the vacancy with another "right-minded" individual like himself. Much to Judge Dewey's chagrin, his namesake did not receive the popular mandate in the presidential election, and Judge Dewey did not believe that he could carry on for another four years until the American people finally "came to their senses" and put a Republican in the White House. Therefore, shortly after the November election, Judge Dewey tendered his resignation.[54]

A similar note is sounded by former chief justice William Howard Taft, who clung to his High Court position lest he be replaced with someone whose policy values were more progressive than his own: "As long as things continue as they are, and I am able to answer in their place, I must stay in the Court in order to prevent the bolsheviki [that is, American Communists] from gaining control."[55] And more recently the liberal black Supreme Court justice Thurgood Marshall vowed not to "retire from the Court as long as Reagan remains in the White House."[56] (One wonders whether he will be able to stick it out through the Bush presidency.)

These illustrations provide further evidence that many jurists view themselves as part of a policy link between the people, the judicial appointment process, and the subsequent decisions of the judges and justices.

## Tenure and Removal of State Judges

Being burdened with judges too old and unfit to serve seems to be less of a problem at the state level than at the federal level. This is so perhaps because a goodly number of states (thirty-five in all) have mandatory retirement plans. Minimum ages for retirement range from sixty-five to seventy-five, with seventy being the most common. Some states even go so far as to have declining retirement benefit plans for judges who serve beyond the desired tenure—that is, the longer you stay on the bench, the lower your retirement benefits. Observers say that such plans are often quite effective in getting old, workaholic jurists to start examining travel brochures.

Retirement plans, no matter how effective in getting the older judge to resign, are still of little use against the younger jurist who is incompetent or corrupt. Throughout American history the states have used procedures such as impeachment, recall elections, and concurrent resolutions of the legislature to rid themselves of the judge gone bad. The evidence suggests that these methods were only minimally effective, however, because such methods proved to be politically difficult to put into operation or because of their time-consuming, cumbersome nature. (Sometimes, however, recall elections can be keenly effective—particularly when there is an ideological motif behind them. For example, in California in 1986 three justices on the state supreme court, including its chief justice, Rose Bird, were turned out of office by a conserative wave of voters who objected to the justices' liberal voting record.)

More recently the states have begun to set up special commissions, often made up of judges themselves, to police their own members. Reformers have given such commissions only fair-to-poor marks, however. The reason is that the persons most familiar with the problem—the judges them-selves—are often loath to expose a colleague to public censure and discipline. One state judge anonymously told one of us about a fellow jurist who was alcoholic:

> We all know he's on the bottle and the [chief court] administrator no longer assigns him any real cases. He just signs grand jury indictments and stuff like that. The tragedy is that he was a great man and a very good judge before he turned to drink. He recently has had a lot of sorrow in his life, you see, and no one wants to be the one known as the mean bastard who went public with what we know. We [all the judges] just cover for him and hope he will either lay off the booze or resign.

Policing the state judiciaries remains a challenge that beckons champions of good government.

## Summary

This chapter began with a collective portrait of the men and women who have served in the federal and state judiciaries. We noted that despite the occasional maverick, the jurists have come from quite a narrow stratum within America's social and economic elite. The result is a core of judges who share similar values and who therefore strive, with minimal coercion, to keep the judicial system functioning in a relatively harmonious manner. Though formal qualifications for a seat on the bench are few, tradition has established several informal criteria, including a reasonable degree of professional competence, the right political affiliation and contacts, at least some desire for the job itself, and a bit of luck thrown in for good measure.

At the national level the judicial selection process includes a variety of participants, despite the constitutional mandate that the president shall do the appointing with the advice and consent of the Senate. If presidents are to dominate this process and name individuals of similar policy values to the bench, several conditions must be met: Chief executives must desire to make ideologically based appointments, they must have an ample number of vacancies to fill, they must be adroit leaders with political clout, and the existing judiciary must be attuned to their policy goals. If most of these conditions are met, presidents tend to get the kind of judges they want. In other words, there is an identifiable policy link between the popular election of the president, the appointment of judges, and the substantive contents of the judges' decisions.

At the state level, politics and the judiciary also go hand in glove. If the governor appoints the judges, then the script that applies at the national level is likely to prevail in the selection of state judges and in the interrelation of values between the governor and the judicial nominees. If judges are elected—even on "nonpartisan" ballots—the political and judicial processes are still inexorably intertwined. Judicial decisions by state judges, as with federal judges, reflect both the process by which the judges are chosen and the values of those who choose them.

Although much judicial socialization occurs before the judges don their black robes, a good deal of learning takes place after they assume the bench. Because both freshman socialization and occupational socialization are performed by senior colleagues, the values and practices of one generation of judges are smoothly passed on to the next. Thus continuity in the system is maintained.

The disciplining and removal of corrupt or mentally unfit judges is still a problem, although at the national level it may be eased somewhat if recent congressional legislation proves effective. The fact that so many judges time their resignations to allow a president (or a governor) of similar party identification and values to appoint a replacement is further evidence that the jurists themselves see a substantive link between the appointment process and the content of many of their decisions.

## Notes

1. For a more extensive study of this subject, particularly as it pertains to the U.S. appeals courts and the Supreme Court, see John R. Schmidhauser, *Judges and Justices: The Federal Appellate Judiciary* (Boston: Little, Brown, 1979), 55-58.
2. Debra Sharpe and Peggy Roberson, "Tower Backs Cobb for Federal Judge," *Beaumont Enterprise*, May 4, 1984, A1.
3. For a good discussion of President Carter's affirmative action policies for the federal judiciary, see Sheldon Goldman, "Should There Be Affirmative Action for the Judiciary?" *Judicature* 62 (1979): 488-496, and Sheldon Goldman, "Reagan's Judicial Appointments at Mid-Term: Shaping the Bench in His Own Image," *Judicature* 66 (March 1983): 335-347.
4. Schmidhauser, *Judges and Justices*, 49.
5. J. Woodford Howard, Jr., *Courts of Appeals in the Federal Judicial System* (Princeton, N.J.: Princeton University Press, 1981), 121.
6. Howard Ball, *Courts and Politics: The Federal Judicial System* (Englewood

Cliffs, N.J.: Prentice-Hall, 1980), 201-202.

7. As quoted in Joseph C. Goulden, *The Benchwarmers: The Private World of the Powerful Federal Judges* (New York: Weybright & Talley, 1974), 33.

8. As quoted in Robert A. Carp and C. K. Rowland, *Policymaking and Politics in the Federal District Courts* (Knoxville: University of Tennessee Press, 1983), 55.

9. The statistics for the background characteristics of the state judges are taken from these sources: Beverly Blair Cook, "Women Judges: The End of Tokenism," in *Women in the Courts*, ed. Winifred L. Hepperle and Laura Crites (Williamsburg, Va.: National Center for State Courts, 1978), 84-105; Bradley C. Canon, "Characteristics and Career Patterns of State Supreme Court Justices," *State Government* 45 (Winter 1972): 34-41; Susan Carbon, "Women in the Judiciary," *Judicature* 65 (1982): 285; Henry Glick and Craig Emmert, "Stability and Change: Characteristics of Contemporary State Supreme Court Judges," *Judicature* 70 (1986): 107-112; and John Paul Ryan et al., *American Trial Judges: Their Work Styles and Performance* (New York: Free Press, 1980).

10. Harry P. Stumpf, *American Judicial Politics* (San Diego: Harcourt Brace Jovanovich, 1988), 184.

11. As a standard procedure, the Senate Judiciary Committee sends to the senator(s) of the state in which a district court vacancy exists a request, printed on a blue form, to approve or disapprove the nomination being considered by the committee. If approval is not forthcoming, the senator simply retains the slip; but if there is no objection, the blue form is returned to the committee.

12. As quoted in Ball, *Courts and Politics*, 176.

13. Cragg Hines, "Dispensing Legal Plums," *Houston Chronicle*, April 21, 1985, 1:1.

14. Goulden, *The Benchwarmers*, 65. The reason Kennedy was under pressure to appoint Cooper in the first place was that Cooper was the choice of Rep. Emanuel Celler, titular leader of New York State's congressional delegation and chairman of the House Judiciary Committee.

15. For more information about the commission, see Larry C. Berkson and Susan B. Carbon, *The United States Circuit Judge Nominating Commission: Its Members, Procedure and Candidates* (Chicago: American Judicature Society, 1980).

16. John R. Schmidhauser, *The Supreme Court: Its Politics, Personalities, and Procedures* (New York: Holt, Rinehart and Winston, 1960), 21.

17. Walter F. Murphy, *Elements of Judicial Strategy* (Chicago: University of Chicago Press, 1964), 114.

18. The classic study of the role of the ABA is Joel B. Grossman, *Lawyers and Judges: The ABA and the Politics of Judicial Selection* (New York: Wiley, 1965).

19. For the humorous and interesting details of this controversy, see Goulden, *The Benchwarmers*, 61-62.

20. Harold W. Chase, *Federal Judges: The Appointing Process* (Minneapolis: University of Minnesota Press, 1972), 21, 23.

21. As quoted in Donald Dale Jackson, *Judges* (New York: Atheneum, 1974), 122.

22. Elliot E. Slotnick, "Federal Appellate Judge Selection during the Carter Administration: Recruitment Changes and Unanswered Questions," *Justice System Journal* 6 (1981): 283.

23. As quoted in Elliot E. Slotnick, "Reforms in Judicial Selection: Will They

Affect the Senate's Role?" pt. 2, *Judicature* 64 (1980): 116.
24. *Tallahassee Democrat*, November 7, 1980, 11A.
25. Judy Wiessler, "Panel Unanimously OKs Kennedy for Court Seat," *Houston Chronicle*, January 28, 1988, 1:4.
26. As quoted in Ball, *Courts and Politics*, 167.
27. Herbert Jacob, *Justice in America*, 4th ed. (Boston: Little, Brown, 1984), 124.
28. Richard A. Watson and Rondal G. Downing, *The Politics of the Bench and the Bar* (New York: Wiley, 1969), 331-332.
29. Herbert Jacob, "The Effect of Institutional Differences in the Recruitment Process: The Case of State Judges," *Journal of Public Law* 13 (1964): 104-119; Bradley C. Canon, "The Impact of Formal Selection Process on the Characteristics of Judges—Reconsidered," *Law and Society Review* 6 (1972): 575-593; and Henry R. Glick and Craig F. Emmert, "Selection Systems and Judicial Characteristics," *Judicature* 70 (1987): 228-235.
30. "Judicial Performance in the Fifth Circuit," *Yale Law Review* 73 (1963): 90-133.
31. Jack Nelson, "Courts Main Hope for Reagan Social Stand," *Houston Chronicle*, March 18, 1986, 1:6.
32. Jon R. Bond, "The Politics of Court Structure: The Addition of New Federal Judges," *Law and Policy Quarterly* 2 (1980): 182, 183, and 187.
33. Henry J. Abraham, *The Judicial Process*, 3d ed. (New York: Oxford University Press, 1975), 77.
34. James A. Farley, "Why I Broke with Roosevelt," *Collier's*, June 21, 1947, 13.
35. Jackson, *Judges*, 340.
36. See Jon Gottschall, "Carter's Judicial Appointments: The Influence of Affirmative Action and Merit Selection on Voting on the U.S. Courts of Appeals," *Judicature* 67 (1983): 165-173.
37. George Bush, "Candidates State Positions on Federal Judicial Selection," *Judicature* 72 (August-September 1988): 77.
38. Howard, *Courts of Appeals in the Federal Judicial System*, 107.
39. New federal district judges with prior state court experience have a somewhat easier time of it, particularly in terms of the psychological adjustment to the judgeship and in dealing with some of the administrative problems. However, prior state court experience seems to be of little help in the jurist's efforts to become expert in *federal* law. See Robert A. Carp and Russell R. Wheeler, "Sink or Swim: The Socialization of a Federal District Judge," *Journal of Public Law* 21 (1972): 367-374.
40. All quoted in Howard, *Courts of Appeals in the Federal Judicial System*, 224.
41. Murphy, *Elements of Judicial Strategy*, 50.
42. For the best discussion of this phenomenon, see Howard, *Courts of Appeals in the Federal Judicial System*, chap. 8.
43. Ibid., 229.
44. For examples of this, see Murphy, *Elements of Judicial Strategy*, 49-51.
45. Goulden, *The Benchwarmers*, 298.
46. Philip Hager, "Legal Leaders Seek Way to Unseat Unfit Federal Judges," *Houston Chronicle*, October 2, 1977, 1:6.
47. For a good recent discussion of this subject, see Collins T. Fitzpatrick, "Misconduct and Disability of Federal Judges: The Unreported Informal Responses," *Judicature* 71 (1988): 282-283.
48. Stephen B. Burbank, "Politics and Progress in Implementing the Federal Judicial Discipline Act," *Judicature* 71 (1987): 13-28.

49. As quoted in Goulden, *The Benchwarmers*, 292.
50. Bob Woodward and Scott Armstrong, *The Brethren* (New York: Simon & Schuster, 1979), 361, 392, 156.
51. Ibid., 157.
52. Henry J. Abraham, *The Judicial Process*, 4th ed. (New York: Oxford University Press, 1980), 43.
53. R. Lee Rainey, "The Decision to Remain a Judge: Deductive Models of Judicial Retirement" (Paper delivered at the annual meeting of the Southern Political Science Association, Atlanta, 1976), 16.
54. Robert A. Carp, "The Function, Impact, and Political Relevance of the Federal District Courts: A Case Study," Ph.D. dissertation, University of Iowa, 1969, 76.
55. As quoted in C. Herman Pritchett, *The Roosevelt Court: A Study of Judicial Votes and Values, 1937-1948* (New York: Macmillan, 1948), 18.
56. "Grading the Presidents," *Newsweek*, September 21, 1987, 33.

# 9   The Decision-Making Process

On what basis and for what reasons do judges in the United States rule the way they do on the motions, petitions, and judicial policy with which they must deal? We shall respond to this query by summarizing the theories and research findings of a large number of judicial scholars who have tried to find out what makes judges tick. (Chapter 10 will examine the special case of decision making on the *collegial* appellate courts at the state and federal levels.)

It is useful to begin with a brief discussion of the decision-making environment in which trial judges and their appellate colleagues operate. Because of the differing purposes and organizational framework of trial and appellate courts, judges of each type face particular kinds of pressures and expectations. As the chapter emphasizes, however, all jurists are subject to two major kinds of influences: the legal subculture and the democratic subculture. It is often difficult to determine, in any given case, the relative weight that any specific influence has on a judge. Studies have suggested, though, that when judges, especially trial judges, find no significant precedent to guide them—that is, when the legal subculture cupboard is bare—they tend to turn to the democratic subculture, an amalgam of determinants that include their own political inclinations.

At the base of the federal and state judicial hierarchies are the trial court judges who preside over the judicial process and who corporately make hundreds of millions of decisions each year. Some pertain to legal points and procedures raised by litigants even before a trial begins, such as a motion by a criminal defendant's lawyer to exclude from trial a piece of illegally obtained evidence. During the actual course of the trial a judge must rule on scores of motions made by the attorneys in the case—for example, an objection to a particular question asked of a witness or a request to strike from the record a contested bit of testimony. Even after a verdict has been rendered, a trial judge may be beset with demands for decisions—for instance, the request by a litigant to reduce a monetary award made by a civil jury.

Trial judges can and occasionally do take ample time to reflect on their more important decisions and may consult with their staff or other judges about how to handle a particular legal problem. Nevertheless, a significant portion of their decision making must be on the spur of the moment, without the luxury of lengthy reflection or discussion with staff or colleagues. As one trial judge told us: "We're where the action is. We often have to 'shoot from the hip' and hope you're doing the right thing. You can't ruminate forever every time you have to make a ruling. We'd be spending months on each case if we ever did that." (Again, virtually all of the judges interviewed for this study were promised anonymity.)

Decision making by members of the appeals courts and by supreme courts is different in several important respects. By the time a case reaches the appellate levels, the record and facts have already been established. The jurists' job is to review dispassionately the transcript of a trial that has already occurred, to search for legal errors that may have been committed by others. Few snap judgments are required. And while the appeals courts and a supreme court may occasionally hear oral arguments by attorneys, they do not examine witnesses and they are removed from the drama and confrontations of the trial courtroom. Another difference in the decision-making process between the trial and appellate levels is that the former is largely individualistic, while the latter is to some degree the product of group deliberation (discussed in Chapter 10).

Despite the acknowledged differences between trial and appellate judge decision making, there are many factors common to all American jurists, and we shall examine several studies that have sought to explain why judges in general think and act as they do. As we shall see, the thrust of these scholarly attempts at explanation has differed. Some view judges as judicial computers who take in a volume of facts, law, and legal doctrines and spew out "correct" rulings—determinations that are virtually independent of the judges' values and attributes as human beings. Other researchers tend to explain judicial decision making in terms of the personal orientations of the judges themselves. A decision is seen not so much as the product of some unbiased, exacting thought process that judges acquire in law school but rather as the effects of the judge's life experiences, prejudices, and overall social values. As with most explanatory theories of human behavior, each of these approaches contains its fair share of the truth, but none accounts for the whole story of the activity in question.

One simple but comprehensive model for explaining judicial decision making was developed by Professors Richardson and Vines more than a decade ago.[1] These two judicial scholars argued that judges are influenced in their decision making by two separate but overlapping sets of stimuli: the legal subculture and the democratic subculture. We shall use their basic analytic framework, with updated research findings, to offer an account of how and why judges make decisions the way they do.

# The Legal Subculture

In examining the legal subculture as a source of trial judge decision making, it is useful to focus on a number of specific questions. What are the basic rules, practices, and norms of this subculture? Where do judges learn these principles, and what groups or institutions keep judges from departing from them? How often and under what circumstances do judges respond to stimuli other than those from the traditional legal realm?

## The Nature of Legal Reasoning

In a popular television series of the 1970s, "The Paper Chase," the formidable Professor Kingsfield promises his budding law students that if they work hard and turn their mush-filled brains over to him, he will instill in them the ability "to think like a lawyer." How *do* lawyers and judges think when they deliberate in their professional capacities? In one classic answer to this question, we are told that "the basic pattern of legal reasoning is reasoning by example. It is a three-step process described by the doctrine of precedent as follows: (1) similarity is seen between cases; (2) the rule of law inherent in the first case is announced; and (3) the rule of law is made applicable to the second case." [2]

Let us look at an example. The cases of *Lane v. Wilson* and *Gomillion v. Lightfoot* contained similar arguments and factual situations. [3] In the former case a black citizen of Oklahoma brought suit in federal court alleging that he had been deprived of the right to vote. In 1916 the legislature of that state had passed a law, ostensibly designed to give formerly disenfranchised black citizens the right to vote, that required them to register—but the registration period was only *twelve days!* (White voters were for all practical purposes exempted from this scheme through the use of a "grandfather clause.") If blacks did not sign up within that short interval, never again would they have the right to vote. The Oklahoma legislature clearly realized that a twelve-day period was wholly inadequate for blacks to mount a voter registration drive and that the vast majority would not acquire the franchise. The plaintiff in this case did not get on the registration rolls in 1916. When he was thereafter forbidden from ever voting, he brought suit claiming the Oklahoma registration scheme to be unconstitutional. The Supreme Court agreed with the plaintiff; in striking down the statute, it set forth this principle, or rule of law: "The Fifteenth Amendment nullifies sophisticated as well as simple-minded modes of discrimination." [4]

Two decades later another black citizen, Charles Gomillion, brought suit in the federal courts alleging a denial of his right to vote as secured by the Fifteenth Amendment. Here an Alabama statute altered the Tuskegee city boundaries from a square to a twenty-eight-sided figure, allegedly removing "all save only four or five of its 400 Negro voters while not removing a single white voter or resident." While not denying the right of a legislature to alter city boundaries "under normal circumstances," the Court saw through this thinly disguised attempt by the Alabama legislature to deny the suffrage to the black citizens of Tuskegee. Reasoning that the situation in *Gomillion* was analogous to that in the Oklahoma case, the Court used the precedent of *Lane v. Wilson* to strike down the Alabama law: "It is difficult to appreciate what stands in the way of adjudging a statute having this inevitable effect invalid in light of the principles of which this Court must judge, and uniformly has judged, statutes that, howsoever speciously defined, obviously discriminate against colored citizens. 'The Fifteenth Amendment nullifies sophisticated as well as simple-minded modes of discrimination.' *Lane v. Wilson*." Here is one example of the judicial reasoning process—of thinking like Professor Kingsfield's lawyer. Two cases are compared because the facts or principles are similar; a rule of law gleaned from the first case is applied to the second. This step-by-step process is the essence of proper and traditional legal reasoning.

### Adherence to Precedent

A related value possessed by trial and appellate judges is a commitment to follow *precedents*—that is, decisions rendered on similar subjects by judges in the past. The sacred doctrine of *stare decisis* ("stand by what has been decided") is a cardinal principle of our common law tradition. In a series of interviews, William Kitchin asked federal district judges to rate the importance of "clear and directly relevant" precedents in their decision-making process. Precedent attained a score of 90.44 on a 100-point scale, whereas the judge's "personal, abstract view of justice in the case" was ranked at only 60.69.[5] As for appellate court judges, a recent study of appeals courts in the Second, Fifth, and District of Columbia Circuits concluded that "adherence to precedent remains the everyday, working rule of American law, enabling appellate judges to control the premises of decision of subordinates who apply general rules to particular cases."[6] The U.S. Supreme Court, while technically free to depart from its own precedents, does so very seldom, for when "the Court reverses itself or makes new law out of whole cloth—reveals its policy-making role for all to see—the holy rite of judges consulting a higher law loses some of its mysterious power."[7]

Ideally, adherence to past rulings gives predictability and continuity to the law and reduces the dangerous possibility that judges will decide cases on a momentary whim or on a totally individualistic sense of right and wrong. Not all legal systems have placed such emphasis on stare decisis, however. In early Greek times, for example, the judge-kings decided each case on what appeared fair and just to them at the moment. When a judge-king resolved a dispute, the judgment was assumed to be the result of direct divine inspiration.[8] The early Greek model is thus the antithesis of the common law tradition. As we shall momentarily see, however, strict adherence to past precedent may be something of a legal fiction. We have long known that judges can and do distinguish among various precedents in creating new law. This helps to keep the law flexible and to account for changing societal values and practices. Indeed, many scholars have argued that the readiness of common law judges occasionally to discard or ignore precedents that no longer serve the public has contributed to the very survival of the common law tradition.

## Constraints on Trial Judge Decision Making

Another significant element of the legal subculture—found under the heading of what one prominent scholar has called the "great maxims of judicial self-restraint" [9]—we have already examined, in Chapter 5. These maxims derive from a variety of sources—the common law, statutory law, legal tradition—but each one serves to limit and channel the decision making of state and federal judges. Because we have discussed these various principles in detail, we shall merely reiterate here a few of the major themes of judicial self-restraint.

First, before a judge will agree even to hear a case, there must exist a definite "case" or "controversy" at law or in equity between bona fide adversaries under the Constitution. The case must involve the protection or enforcement of valuable legal rights or the punishment, prevention, or redress of wrongs directly related to the litigants in the case. Allied with this maxim is the principle that U.S. judges may not render "advisory opinions"—that is, rulings on abstract, hypothetical questions. (As noted in Chapter 5, this rule is not followed as strictly in many state systems.) Also, all parties to a lawsuit must have "standing," or a substantial personal interest infringed by the statute or action in question.

The rules of the game also forbid jurists to hear a case unless all other legal remedies have been exhausted. In addition, the legal culture discourages the judiciary from deciding "political questions," or matters that ought to be resolved by one of the other branches of government, by another level of government, or by the voters. Judges are also obliged to give the benefit of the doubt to statutes and to official actions whose constitutionality is being questioned. A law or an executive action is presumed to be constitutional until proven otherwise (some judges adhere to this principle on economic issues but not on matters of civil rights and civil liberties, believing that on these matters the burden of proof is on the government). In this same realm judges feel bound by the norm that if they must invalidate a law, they will do so on as narrow a ground as possible or will void only that portion of the statute that is unconstitutional.

Finally, America's jurists may not throw out a law or an official action simply because they personally believe it to be unfair, stupid, or undemocratic. In order for a statute or an official deed to be invalidated, it must be clearly unconstitutional. Of course, judges do not always agree about what is a "clearly unconstitutional" act, but most acknowledge that broad matters of public policy should be determined by the people through their elected representatives—not by the judiciary.

## The Impact of the Legal Subculture: An Example

Because the principles that make up the legal subculture—reasoning, precedent, and restraint—tend to be abstract, it is useful to illustrate them with a real-life example. The 1964 case of *Evers v. Jackson Municipal Separate School District* is a case in point.[10] It was an uncomplicated school integration case in which a group of black children and their parents sought to enjoin the "district and its officials from operating a compulsory biracial school system." The facts and controlling precedents were clear enough: (1) Jackson, Mississippi, was overtly maintaining a segregated public school system; (2) the U.S. Supreme Court had ruled a decade previously in *Brown v. Board of Education* that such segregation was unconstitutional; and (3) the U.S. Court of Appeals for the Fifth Circuit, which has jurisdiction over Mississippi, had handed down a string of rulings ordering the integration process to go ahead.

The federal trial judge in this case, Sidney Mize, did not like the commands he heard from the legal subculture. Appointed to the federal bench back in 1937, Mize was an unabashed segregationist, as his written opinion in this case clearly shows. After discussing a score of alleged physical and mental differences between blacks and whites, Mize argued further that

> in the case of Caucasians and Negroes, such differences may be directly confirmed by comparative anatomical and encephalographic measurements of the correlative physical structure of the brain and of the neural and endocrine systems of the body. The evidence was conclusive to the effect that the cranial capacity and brain size of the average Negro is approximately ten per cent less than that of the average white person of similar age and size, and that brain size is correlated with intelligence.[11]

On an ostensibly more positive and benign note, Judge Mize also argued, "From the evidence I find that separate classes allow greater adaptation to the differing educational traits of Negro and white pupils, and actually result in greater scholastic accomplishments for both."[12]

It seems clear where this decision is headed. But wait: Enter the legal subculture. After fourteen single-spaced printed pages of argument against the integration of the Jackson schools, Mize yielded to the requirements of legal reasoning, respect for precedent, and judicial self-restraint. Almost sheepishly he concluded his decision with these unexpected words:

> Nevertheless, this Court feels that it is bound by what appears to be the obvious holding of the United States Court of Appeals for the Fifth Circuit that if disparities and differences such as that reflected in this record are to constitute a proper basis for the maintenance of separate schools for the white and Negro races it is the function of the United States Supreme Court to make such a decision and no inferior federal court can do so.[13]

Mize then quietly enjoined the school district and its officials from operating a compulsory biracial school system: The legal subculture tiptoed to victory.

## Wellsprings of the Legal Subculture

We have examined some of the major threads of the tapestry of America's legal subculture; we will now point briefly to the institutions that instill and maintain the legal values in this country—"the law schools, the bar associations, the judicial councils, and other groups that spring from the institutionalization of the 'bench and the bar.' "[14]

"The purpose of law school," we are told, "is to transform individuals into novice lawyers, providing them with competency in the law, and instilling in them a nascent self-concept as a professional, a commitment to the values of the calling, and that esoteric mental state called 'thinking like a lawyer.' "[15] The world just does not look the same to someone on whom law school has worked its indoctrinating magic. Facts and relationships in the human arena that had formerly gone unnoticed suddenly become "compelling" and "controlling" to the fledgling advocate. Likewise other facets of reality that previously had been important in one's world view are now dismissed as "irrelevant and immaterial."

Besides the indoctrination that occurs in law school, the values of the legal subculture are maintained by the state and national bar associations[16] and by a variety of professional-social groups whose members are from both bench and bar—for example, the honorary Order of the Coif. We have already documented in Chapter 8 how the values and practices of jurists are handed down from one generation to another. Thus the traditions and tenets of the American legal subculture are well tended by powerful support groups. They are rightly accorded ample deference if one is to understand judicial decision making in America.

## The Limits of the Legal Subculture

Despite the taut nature of judicial reasoning and the importance of stare decisis and of judicial self-restraint, the legal subculture does not totally explain the behavior of American jurists. If "objective facts" and "obvious controlling precedents" were the only stimuli to which jurists responded, then the judicial decision-making process would be largely mechanical and all judicial outcomes would be quite predictable. Yet even the legal subculture's most loyal apologists would concede that judges often distinguish among precedents and that some judges are more inclined toward self-restraint than others.

To understand the thinking of judicial decision makers and the evolution of the law, we must consider more than law school curricula and the canons of the bar associations. One of the first great minds to realize this was Justice Oliver Wendell Holmes, Jr., who over a century ago wrote that

> the life of the law has not been logic; it has been experience. The felt necessities of the time, the prevalent moral and political theories, intuitions of public policy, avowed or unconscious, even the prejudices which judges share with their fellow-men have had a good deal more to do than syllogism in determining the rules by which men should be governed. The law embodies the story of a nation's development through many centuries, and it cannot be dealt with as if it contained only the axioms and corollaries of a book of mathematics. In order to know what it is, we must know what it has been, and what it tends to become. . . . The very considerations which judges most rarely mention, and always with an apology, are the secret root from which the law draws all the juices of life. I mean, of course, considerations of what is expedient for the community concerned.[17]

By about the 1920s a whole school of thought had developed that argued that judicial decision making was as much the product of human, extralegal stimuli as it was of some sort of mechanical legal thought process. Adherents of this view, who were known as "judicial realists," insisted that judges, like other human beings, are influenced by the values and attitudes learned in childhood. As one of these "realists" put it, a judge's background "may have created plus or minus reactions to women, or blonde women, or men with beards, or Southerners, or Italians, or Englishmen, or plumbers, or ministers, or college graduates, or Democrats. A certain facial twitch or cough or gesture may start up memories, painful or pleasant."[18]

Since the late 1940s, the study of the personal, extralegal influences on decision making has become more rigorous. Often calling themselves "judicial behavioralists," modern-day advocates of the realist approach have improved on it in two ways. First, they have tried to test empirically many of the theories and propositions advanced by the realist school and, second, they have attempted to relate their findings to more scientifically grounded theories of human behavior. Thus, while a realist might have asserted that a Democratic judge would probably be more supportive of labor unions than a Republican jurist, a judicial behavioralist might go a step further by taking a generous random sample of labor union-versus-management decisions and statistically determining whether Democratic judges are significantly more likely to back the union position than their GOP counterparts. Thus it is one thing to intuitively ascribe a cause for human behavior; it is another to subject an assertion to careful empirical analysis.

In the next section we shall discuss the many extralegal stimuli that the realists and behavioralists have shown to impinge upon trial judge decision making. In the last section of the chapter, we shall explore questions such as these: Which is the more compelling explanation for judicial decision making—the one provided by the legal subculture model or the one offered by the realist-behavioralist school? Does the efficacy of the model depend on the type of case(s) we are attempting to analyze? Does the way that judges view their judicial role help to determine which mode of explanation is the more compelling?

## The Democratic Subculture

We know that the legal subculture has an impact on American jurists. There is evidence, too, that popular, democratic values—manifested in a variety of ways through many different mediums—have an influence as well. Indeed, some scholars have argued that the only reason courts have maintained their significant role in the American political system is that they have learned to bend when the democratic winds have blown—that is, that judges have tempered rigid legalisms with common-sense popular values and have maintained "extensive linkages with the democratic subculture":

> Very often, legal elites such as bar associations and judicial councils are more noticeable spokesmen for the federal judiciary than are the spokesmen of the democratic subculture. However, representatives of the democratic subculture, such as members of political parties, members of social and economic groups, and local state political elites, can also be observed commenting on controversial questions. In matters like staffing the courts, determining their structure and organization, and fixing federal jurisdiction, democratic representatives have access through Congress and through other institutions that are influential in establishing judicial policy. Although Congress provides a main channel to the federal courts, access for democratic values is also obtained through the President, the attorney general, and through nonlegal officials who deal with the judiciary. In addition, the location of federal courts throughout the states and regions renders them unusually susceptible to local and regional democratic forces.[19]

In our discussion of the democratic subculture, we shall focus on the influences most often observed by students of the American court system— political party identification, localism, public opinion, and the legislative and executive branches of government.

## The Influence of Political Party Affiliation

Do judges' political party affiliations affect the way they decide certain cases? The question is straightforward enough, but those who reply to it are by no means unanimous in their response. To most attorneys, judges, and court watchers among the general public, the question rings with outright impertinence, and their answer is usually something like this: After taking the sacred judicial oath and donning the black robe, a judge is no longer a Republican or a Democrat. Former affiliations are (or at least certainly should be) put aside as the judge enters a realm in which decisions are the product of evidence, sound judicial reasoning, and precedent rather than such a base factor as political identification. Or, as Donald Dale Jackson quipped in his perceptive book *Judges*, "Most judges would sooner admit to grand larceny than confess a political interest or motivation." [20]

Despite the cries of indignation from those who contend that the legal subculture explains virtually all judicial decision making, a mounting body of evidence strongly suggests that judges' political identification does indeed affect their behavior on the bench. Studies have shown that other personal factors—such as religion, sex, race, pre-judicial career, and the level of prestige of their law school education—may also play a role. However, only political party affiliation seems to have any significant and consistent capacity to explain and predict the outcome of judicial decisions. [21] One prominent student of American politics explains why there may be a cause-and-effect relationship between judges' party allegiance and their decisional patterns:

> If judges are party identifiers before reaching the bench, there would be a basis for believing that they—like legislators—are affected in their issue orientations by party. . . . Furthermore, judges are generally well educated and the vote studies show that the more educated tend to be stronger party identifiers, to cast policy preferences in ideological terms, to have clearer perceptions of issues and of party positions on those issues, to have issue attitudes consistent with the positions of the party with which they identify, and to be more interested and involved in politics. For judges, even more than for the general population, party may therefore be a significant reference group on issues. [22]

*Federal District Court Judges.*    In examining what we have learned about the relationship between party affiliation and court decision making, we can begin with an observation that should come as no suprise: As a whole, Democratic trial judges on the U.S. district courts are more liberal than their Republican colleagues. In a study of more than 37,000 published district court decisions between 1933 and 1985, it was determined that Democratic judges took the liberal position 47 percent of the time whereas Republican jurists did so in only 39 percent of the cases. Thus, for almost a half-century, the Democrats' ratio of liberal-to-conservative opinions has been 1.39 times greater (more liberal) than the Republican ratio has been.[23] Although the overall differences cannot be called overwhelming, neither can we dismiss them as inconsequential.

As the data in Table 9-1 suggest, differences between Republicans and Democrats depend considerably on what type of cases we are talking about.

Table 9-1 Liberal Decisions of Federal District Judges in Order of Magnitude of Partisan Differences for Twenty-Two Types of Cases, 1933-1985

| Type of case | Overall | Demo-crats | Repub-licans | Partisan difference | Odds ratio |
|---|---|---|---|---|---|
| Local economic regulation | 67% | 77% | 57% | 20% | 2.50 |
| Rights of the handicapped | 55 | 65 | 46 | 19 | 2.20 |
| Race discrimination | 50 | 57 | 39 | 18 | 2.19 |
| Secretary of labor or NLRB v. union | 56 | 63 | 45 | 18 | 2.09 |
| Criminal convictions | 38 | 44 | 30 | 14 | 1.91 |
| Women's rights | 52 | 59 | 44 | 15 | 1.81 |
| Freedom of religion | 53 | 58 | 44 | 14 | 1.80 |
| Fourteenth amendment | 41 | 46 | 34 | 12 | 1.67 |
| Freedom of expression | 56 | 61 | 50 | 11 | 1.56 |
| Employee v. employer | 40 | 44 | 34 | 10 | 1.55 |
| U.S. habeas corpus pleas | 27 | 30 | 22 | 8 | 1.54 |
| U.S. commercial regulation | 68 | 72 | 63 | 9 | 1.49 |
| Union v. company | 49 | 52 | 45 | 7 | 1.35 |
| Alien petitions | 40 | 42 | 36 | 6 | 1.30 |
| Environmental protection | 60 | 63 | 57 | 6 | 1.29 |
| Criminal court motions | 30 | 32 | 27 | 5 | 1.27 |
| State habeas corpus pleas | 25 | 26 | 22 | 4 | 1.23 |
| Indian rights and law | 50 | 52 | 47 | 5 | 1.22 |
| Rent control, excess profit | 59 | 61 | 58 | 3 | 1.14 |
| Voting rights cases | 49 | 49 | 48 | 1 | 1.06 |
| Union members v. union | 47 | 48 | 47 | 1 | 1.04 |
| Secretary of labor or NLRB v. employer | 68 | 66 | 73 | −7 | .72 |

Source: Unpublished data collected by Robert A. Carp, Ronald Stidham, and C. K. Rowland.
Note: The odds ratio, also called the cross-product ratio, is a measure of the relationship between two dichotomous variables. Specifically, it is a measure of the relative odds of respondents from each independent variable category being placed in a single dependent variables category.

In looking at partisan voting patterns in twenty-two separate case categories, we can see that differences between judges from the two parties were greatest for cases involving state and local government efforts to regulate the economic lives of their citizens, disputes involving the rights of handicapped persons, race relations cases, and legal disagreements between the secretary of labor (or the National Labor Relations Board, the NLRB) and a labor union.

On the other hand, partisan differences were almost totally absent in cases involving rent control and/or excess profits, voting rights cases, and suits between union members and their union. In disputes between the secretary of labor (or the NLRB) and an employer, the GOP jurists were actually more liberal than the Democrats by 7 percentage points. In all the other case types examined in this study, however, Republican judges tended to follow the traditional conservative views of their party. Partisan differences among federal trial judges also vary a good deal from one time period to another. Between 1933 and 1953, partisan differences among judges averaged 4 percentage points. This disparity dropped to a mere 1 percent between 1953 and 1969, then jumped to 11 percent between 1969 and 1977. (It reached a high of 17 percentage points in 1972.) In the most recent period studied, 1977 through part of 1985, the difference between Republican and Democratic judges has averaged 12 percentage points (going as high as 19 percent in 1984.) [24] Thus, it is fair to conclude that partisan differences have been much greater in the past twenty years than they were in the preceding thirty-five.

All these facts and figures would become more meaningful if we could enter into the minds of typical Republican and Democratic judges and view the world from their perspectives. The closest we can come is to report the partial contents of interviews with two lifelong members of their respective parties. The two jurists, sitting in the same city and on the same day, discussed a subject that in recent decades has divided Republican from Democratic judges—their philosophy of criminal justice and, more specifically, their views about sentencing convicted felons. The rank-and-file Democrat (appointed by Lyndon Johnson) said in part:

> You know, most of the people who appear before me for sentencing come from the poorer classes and have had few of the advantages of life. They've had an uphill fight all the way and life has constantly stepped on them. . . . I come from a pretty humble background myself, and I know what it's like. I think I take all this into consideration when I have to sentence someone, and it inclines me towards handing down lighter sentences, I think.

One hour later a lifelong Republican (appointed by Richard Nixon) addressed the same issue but with quite a different twist at the end:

When I was first appointed, I was one of those big law-and-order types. You know—just put all those crooks and hippies in jail and all will be right with the world. But I've changed a lot. I never realized what poor, pathetic people there are who come before us for sentencing. My God, the terrible childhoods and horrendous backgrounds that some of them come from! Mistreated when they were kids and kicked around by everybody in the world for most of their lives. Society has clearly failed them. As a judge there's only one thing you can do: *send them to prison for as long as the law allows because when they're in that bad a state there's nothing anyone can do with them. All you can do is protect society from these poor souls for as long as you can.* [Emphasis added.]

While we would not contend that all Republican and all Democratic trial judges think precisely in these terms, we believe that something of the spirit of partisan differences is captured in these two quotations.

*Federal Appeals Court Judges.*  As for partisan variations in the voting patterns of U.S. appeals court judges, here, too, there is evidence that the judges' (prior) party affiliation tempers their decision making to some degree.[25] In 1966 Sheldon Goldman's study exploring the decision-making process of circuit judges in all U.S. courts of appeals was published. Goldman found that party affiliation was "associated with voting behavior, notably when the issues involved economic liberalism," and that other background variables "such as religion, socio-economic origins, education, and age were found to be almost entirely unrelated to voting behavior." Goldman cautions us, however, not to believe that party identification explains more than a small portion of appellate court decision making. He stresses the point that we emphasized in the previous chapter—namely, that U.S. federal jurists are more alike than different, that they are not for the most part split into warring ideological camps. This first comprehensive survey concluded that "on balance, the findings underscore the absence of a sharp ideological party cleavage in the United States but also give support to the contention that the center of gravity of the Democratic party is more 'liberal' than that of the Republican party." [26]

About a decade later Goldman updated his earlier study, but the conclusions did not vary greatly. He found Republican appeals court judges to be more conservative than their Democratic colleagues and that "the party split was most pronounced on economic issues." (That is, GOP jurists were a bit more likely than their Democratic counterparts to oppose government efforts to regulate the economy and to support business in its judicial tussles with labor.) [27] Again, however, partisan differences were considered to be only a modest predictor of appellate court decision making.

*U.S. Supreme Court Justices.*  Does political party affiliation affect the way members of the U.S. Supreme Court decide some of their cases? Although scholars have found this to be a hard subject to investigate, the evidence suggests a mild but positive yes. The research hurdle stems, in part, from the fact that at any given time there are only nine justices on the Court, and it is virtually impossible to generalize about the behavior of groups this small. Moreover, numerous political parties have been represented on the Court in its nearly two-century history, and the definitions of *Federalist, Democrat, Whig, Republican, liberal,* and *conservative* have varied so over time that generalizations become very difficult. For example, prior to the 1920s most mainstream Democrats opposed civil rights for blacks; since that era most champions of the civil rights movement have been Democrats. In the jargon of the trade: The variables are so numerous and the *n*'s (number of justices) are so small that statistically significant observations are extremely difficult to make.

Despite the methodological problems involved, some judicial scholars have gone where even angels fear to tread and have sought to explore this subject. In a comprehensive study of the relationship between party affiliation and the liberal-conservative voting patterns of the justices in this century, one scholar found that between 1903 and 1939 party identification was "clearly a good cue for selecting judicial decision-makers with the proper values"—that is, on matters of support for the economic underdog, Democratic justices were more liberal than their Republican colleagues. Since 1940 the greater liberalism of Democratic Court members has extended as well to matters of civil rights and liberties, thereby reaffirming "the concept that judges are not random samples of their group." But even this scholar concedes, as did those who studied partisan voting by the appeals court and trial judges, that the relationships are weak:

> The inability to predict at high rates of probability is not surprising when one considers the assumptions that must be made and the variety of other influences on the Court such as political and environmental pressures, social change, precedent, reasoned argument [the "legal subculture" for these last two], intracourt social influences and idiosyncrasy.[28]

A more elaborate and revealing study of voting patterns over time of members of the Supreme Court was published in 1981.[29] It analyzed the voting behavior of twenty-five justices who had served on the Court between 1946 and 1978. The justices' decisional patterns on economic matters and on civil rights and liberties cases were related to some twenty possible explanatory variables. The study found strong correlations between liberal voting and the following attributes: (1) being a Democrat, (2) being appointed by a president other than Nixon or Truman, (3) having judicial rather than prosecutorial experience prior to becoming a justice, and (4) having had a long record of previous judicial service rather than a short tenure. The author was able to account for 87 percent of the variance in split decisions on civil liberties cases and 72 percent for economic regulation cases. (Both of these percentages are extraordinarily high for social science research.)

More recently, however, one leading scholar in the field has cautioned that studies that demonstrate a relationship between the justices' backgrounds and their subsequent voting patterns may in fact be time-bound. That is, during some time periods decisional differences among the justices might well be explained by background characteristics whereas during other time frames background is only a modest predictor of behavior.[30] When we are faced with such conflicting and tentative studies, it is clear that the final chapter of that book is yet to be written.

*Partisanship in State Courts.* The federal courts are not the only arena in which Republican and Democratic jurists sometimes square off against one another. There is evidence that state courts as well often see partisan voting patterns among the men and women who sit on the trial and appellate court benches. Still, the evidence at the state level is weaker, for two general reasons. First, the state courts have not been studied as extensively and systematically as have the federal courts. This may be either because political scientists have held the (mistaken) view that state judiciaries are less important than their federal counterparts or because many state court decisions are unpublished and therefore much more difficult to acquire and study. Second, we know for a fact that partisanship among state jurists is not strongly uniform across the country. In some states, for instance, judicial selection is truly bipartisan (or nonpartisan) and both political parties may support the same candidates. Also, many state judges do not have extensive relationships with a political party; though they may have partisan identifications, they might not see judicial questions as being reflective of their party's ideology. Finally, there are still quite a number of one-party states in America in which virtually all judges bear the same party label. Thus it would make little sense to study partisan differences among judges in states like Mississippi or South Carolina, where almost all the jurists are Democrats. Still, keen levels of partisanship have been documented in some jurisdictions—particularly in the states with big cities.

Michigan is a state in which partisan voting patterns among the judges, especially on the state supreme court, have been noteworthy. Studies have shown that on labor-management issues, for example, Democrats on the bench were significantly more likely to support the side of the worker in unemployment compensation cases and in issues dealing with workers' compensation (on-the-job injuries). Democratic judges are also more likely to support criminal defendants seeking a new trial, to favor government efforts to regulate business, and to side with persons who sue business enterprises—all consistent with the voting behavior of Democrats on the federal bench.[31]

In a recent study of partisan conflict on a California intermediate court of appeals, significant differences were found between Democrats and Republicans on both criminal and civil cases.[32] Studying issues such as votes in criminal justice cases, labor-management disputes, debtor/creditor disagreements, and consumerism issues, the author concluded that "as previous research . . . would have predicted, the results are in the expected direction, with Republican panels significantly more likely to reach conservative outcomes than Democratic panels."[33]

Illinois, Pennsylvania, Iowa, Maryland, and New York are examples of other states for which researchers have reported meaningful partisan differences between Republican and Democratic judges.[34]

*An Appraisal.*   Let us stop for a moment to look back on what we have said. Our basic point is that the political party affiliation of the judges and justices can well make a difference in the way they decide cases. Of all the background variables studied, it seems to be the most compelling and consistent. But a word of caution is in order, too. While evidence for partisan influence on judicial behavior is convincing, it by no means suggests that Democrats always take the liberal position on all issues while Republicans always opt for the conservative side. Rather, we are talking about tendencies—that is, where the decision is a close call, a Democrat on the bench tends to be more liberal than a GOP judge. When controlling precedents are absent or ambiguous or when the evidence in the case is about evenly divided, Democrats more than Republicans are inclined to be supportive of civil rights and liberties, to support government regulation that favors the worker or the economic underdog, and to turn a sympathetic ear toward the pleas of criminal defendants.

## The Impact of Localism

A wide range of influences are included in the term *localism*, and we shall regard it as a broad second category of factors that affect federal and state judicial decision making. First, let's examine localism at the federal level. An accumulating body of literature suggests that judges are influenced by the traditions and mores of the region in which their courts are located or, in the case of Supreme Court justices, by the geographic area in which they were reared. Indeed, for trial and appeals court judges geographical differences define both the legal and the democratic subcultures as well as the nature of the questions they must decide. Historically, such judges have had strong ties with the state and the circuit in which their courts are situated, and on many issues judicial decision making reflects the parochial values and attitudes of the region. As Richardson and Vines have noted:

A persistent factor in the molding of lower court organization has been the preservation of state and regional boundaries. The feeling that the judiciary should reflect the local features of the federal system has often been expressed by state officials most explicitly. Mississippi Congressman John Sharp Williams declared that he was "frankly opposed to a preambulatory judiciary, to carpetbagging Nebraska with a Louisianian, certainly to carpetbagging Mississippi or Louisiana, with somebody north of Mason and Dixon's line." [35]

Why should judges in one district or circuit decide cases differently from their colleagues in other localities? Why should a Supreme Court justice make decisions differently from colleagues who hail from other parts of the United States? [36] Richardson and Vines have put the matter succinctly:

> Since both district and appeals judges frequently receive legal training in the state or circuit they serve, the significance of legal education is important. If a federal judge is trained at a state university, he is exposed to and may assimilate state and sectional political viewpoints, especially since state law schools are training grounds for local political elites. . . . Other than education, different local environments provide different reactions to policy issues, such as civil rights or labor relations. Indeed, throughout the history of the lower court judiciary there is evidence that various persons involved in judicial organization and selection have perceived that local, state, or regional factors make a difference and have behaved accordingly.[37]

Moreover, as we noted in Chapter 8, trial and appellate judges tend to come from the district or state in which their courts are located, and the vast majority were educated in law schools of the state or circuit they work in. (For example, two-thirds of all district judges in one study were born in the same state as their court, and 86 percent of all circuit judges attended a law school in their respective circuits.) [38] Also, the strong local ties of many judges tend to develop and mature even after their appointment to the bench.[39]

In their identification with their regional base, judges in fact are similar to other political decision makers. We have long known that public attitudes and voting patterns on a wide range of issues vary from one section of America to another.[40] As for national political officials, there is evidence that regionalism affects the voting patterns of members of Congress on many important issues—for example, civil rights, conservation, price controls for farmers, and labor legislation.[41] Furthermore, sectional considerations have their impact within each political party—for instance, northern Democrats are more liberal than their southern counterparts on many significant issues.

*Regionalism at the Three Judicial Levels.* We noted in Chapter 2 that when President Washington appointed the first Supreme Court, half of its members were northerners and the other half were southerners.

Surely Washington's choice was more than just a symbolic gesture to give a superficial balance to the Court. Washington, who had successfully led a group of squabbling, dissident former colonies during the Revolutionary War, understood that the attitudes and mores of his fellow citizens differed widely from one locale to another and that justices would not be immune to these parochial influences. Indeed, studies of the early history of the High Court reveal that sectionalism did creep into its decision-making patterns—particularly along North-South lines. For example, from a study of Supreme Court voting patterns in the sectional crisis that preceded the Civil War, we note that the four justices who were most supportive of southern regional interests were all from the South, whereas those jurists from the northern states usually favored the litigants from that region.[42]

In this century, too, there is evidence for the belief that where the justices come from tempers their decision making to some degree.[43] A fairly dramatic manifestation of this principle is found in President Nixon's famous "southern strategy." After the appointment of Warren Burger as chief justice in 1969,

> pressure had been building on Nixon to name a southerner to the Court. Though he had never publicly promised a southern nominee, Nixon's intentions were never seriously doubted. Aware that a judge in the South enjoyed a prestige unrivaled in any other section of the country, Nixon advisors believed that he could do southerners no higher favor than to appoint one of their own to the highest court in the land. Even before Nixon assumed office, he had successfully identified with the southern cause. "The one battle most white southerners feel they are fighting is with the Court and Nixon has effectively identified himself with that cause," wrote election analyst Samuel Lubell. "Only Nixon can change the makeup of the Court to satisfy southern aspirations."[44]

Nixon then nominated Clement Haynsworth, Jr., of South Carolina, who was turned down by the Senate. Next he sent forth the name of G. Harrold Carswell of Florida, but this nomination met the same fate as Haynsworth's. An angry Nixon then stated, "As long as the Senate is constituted the way it is today, I will not nominate another southerner."[45]

Although political leaders and much of the general public believe that there is a relationship between the justices' regional backgrounds and their judicial decisions, scholars have had difficulty in documenting this phenomenon. First, links between the justices' regional heritage and their subsequent voting behavior are very difficult to pinpoint, and they exist at most for probably a few regionally sensitive issues. Also, there is reason to believe that after Supreme Court justices are appointed and move to Washington, over time they may take on a more national perspective, loosening to a significant degree the attitudes and narrow purview of the region in which they were reared and educated. For example, in his early days in Alabama, Hugo Black had been a member of the Ku Klux Klan, but after his judicial appointment in 1937, Justice Black became one of the most articulate advocates of civil rights ever to sit on the Supreme Court.

Some evidence exists that regionalism pervades the federal judicial system at the appeals court level as well. One recent study noted regional differences on such important questions as rights of the consumer, pleas by criminal defendants, petitions by workers and by blacks, public rights in patent cases, and immigration litigation. The author of this study concluded that "regionalism is an inescapable adjunct of adjudicating appeals in one of the oldest regional operations of federal power in existence." He observed that while the appeals courts may adhere to national standards, such norms are nevertheless "regionally enforced. In the crosswinds of office and constituencies, Courts of Appeals may mediate cultural values—national and local, professional and political—in federal appeals." [46]

Federal district judges appear to reflect their sectional heritage in decisional patterns even more distinctly than their colleagues on the appellate bench. In an analysis of trial judge decision making between 1933 and 1985, one research team compared the ratio of liberal to conservative opinions for northern and southern judges (see Table 9-2). They learned that the northerners were 1.23 times more liberal than their colleagues in the South. However, it was also learned that North-South differences have declined in recent years. Between 1969 and 1977 the ratio was 1.41, but in the interval between 1978 and 1985 it declined to a mere 1.08—the smallest ratio of all the time periods studied. East-West differences among the district judges have been almost negligible for all the time periods studied since 1933. On questions of criminal justice, judges in the North have historically been somewhat more liberal, although this trend has reversed itself since 1977. For cases that pertain to civil rights and liberties northern jurists have been on the liberal side more often since 1969, although this was not the case in earlier time spans. Finally, for issues involving government regulation of the economy and labor, judges in the North were more liberal prior to 1978, but since that time the North-South split has been negligible.

Regional differences within the parties have also been observed over the years—mainly between judges in the North and South. For the past half century northern Democrats have been the most liberal group of judges. This is followed by southern Democrats, northern Republicans, and then southern Republicans. The difference between southern Republicans and northern Democrats is 16 percentage points—that is, northern Democrats are 48 percent more liberal than southern Republicans.[47]

*Variances in Judicial Behavior Among the Circuits.* Not only does judicial decision making vary from one region of the land to another, but studies reveal that, for numerous reasons, each of the circuits has its own particular way in which its appellate and trial court judges administer the

Table 9-2  Liberal Decisions of Federal District Judges,
Controlled for Region, 1933-1985

|  | 1933-1953 | 1954-1968 | 1969-1977 | 1978-1985 | All years |
|---|---|---|---|---|---|
| *All cases* | | | | | |
| North (%) | 46 | 42 | 47 | 47 | 46 |
| South (%) | 43 | 37 | 38 | 45 | 41 |
| $\alpha$ | 1.14 | 1.22 | 1.41 | 1.08 | 1.23 |
| East (%) | 46 | 42 | 43 | 43 | 44 |
| West (%) | 44 | 39 | 44 | 48 | 44 |
| $\alpha$ | 1.08 | 1.08 | 0.90 | 0.82 | 0.95 |
| *Criminal justice* | | | | | |
| North (%) | 26 | 23 | 31 | 31 | 28 |
| South (%) | 27 | 21 | 24 | 35 | 27 |
| $\alpha$ | 0.93 | 1.12 | 1.40 | 0.85 | 1.14 |
| East (%) | 23 | 23 | 27 | 28 | 25 |
| West (%) | 29 | 23 | 30 | 35 | 29 |
| $\alpha$ | 0.66 | 0.94 | 0.89 | 0.72 | 0.81 |
| *Civil rights and liberties* | | | | | |
| North (%) | 39 | 39 | 53 | 50 | 45 |
| South (%) | 45 | 42 | 45 | 42 | 44 |
| $\alpha$ | 0.79 | 0.88 | 1.39 | 1.39 | 1.21 |
| East (%) | 39 | 39 | 51 | 46 | 44 |
| West (%) | 42 | 41 | 49 | 48 | 45 |
| $\alpha$ | 0.80 | 0.86 | 1.00 | 0.91 | 0.92 |
| *Labor and economic regulation* | | | | | |
| North (%) | 58 | 64 | 61 | 55 | 60 |
| South (%) | 49 | 55 | 55 | 56 | 54 |
| $\alpha$ | 1.48 | 1.40 | 1.30 | 0.95 | 1.24 |
| East (%) | 62 | 65 | 61 | 53 | 60 |
| West (%) | 51 | 58 | 58 | 57 | 56 |
| $\alpha$ | 1.59 | 1.32 | 1.08 | 0.87 | 1.16 |

*Source:* Unpublished data collected by Robert A. Carp, Ronald Stidham, and C. K. Rowland.

law and make decisions. One reason, of course, is that circuits tend to follow sectional lines that mark off historical, social, and political differences. Another reason is that the circuit courts of appeals tend to be idiosyncratic, and thus the standards and guidelines they provide the trial judges will reflect their own approach.[48] Let us look at an example. On October 1, 1981, the Eleventh Circuit Court of Appeals came into existence when Congress split the Fifth Circuit. One of the many decisions the new Eleventh Circuit faced was which law it would follow. In a recent interview Chief Judge John C. Godbold explained how this problem was solved:

> We selected a case where the law of the old Fifth was materially different from the law of some of the other circuits, and we voted it *en banc* to decide the question of choice of law. We heard the case *en banc* the morning of October 2, 1981, the second day we were in existence, because we had all been in New Orleans the day before closing down the old Fifth. We announced our decision later that day. In it we said, we choose the law of the old Fifth not only in this case but for all cases.[49]

Studies of liberal-conservative voting patterns over time have shown that trial judge decision making varies a good deal from one circuit to another. In the First Circuit, for example, which covers several New England states, 51 percent of the judges' decisions have been liberal. In the Fourth Circuit, on the other hand (Maryland, North and South Carolina, Virginia, and West Virginia), only 34 percent of the judges' decisions have been liberal. Also, "variances in judicial voting patterns from one circuit to another seem to have increased over time, and this trend appears to have accelerated." [50]

*Variances in Trial Judge Behavior Among the States.*   At first blush it may appear strange to argue that U.S. judicial decisions vary significantly state by state, since the state is not an official level of the federal judicial hierarchy, which advances from district to circuit to nationwide system. Still, direct and indirect evidence suggests that each state is unique in the way its federal judges administer justice. There are several reasons why this is so. First, a state, like a circuit or a region, is often synonymous with a particular set of policy-relevant values, attitudes, and orientations. One would automatically expect, for instance, that on some issues U.S. trial and appellate judges in Texas would act differently from Massachusetts jurists, not so much because they are from different states but because they are from different political, economic, legal, and cultural milieus. Second, many judges regard their states as meaningful boundaries and behave accordingly. For example, a U.S. trial judge in Louisiana told us: "One thing I frequently discuss with the other judges here is sentencing matters. Judge _____ has been a big help with this. I wouldn't want to hand down a sentence which is way out of line with what the other judges are doing here in this state for the same crime."[51] Comments from a jurist indicate that the same phenomenon occurs in the U.S. Eighth Circuit. For instance, in Iowa the federal trial judges

> were anxious that their sentencing practices be reasonably similar, particularly where the facts of a case were almost identical. They . . . believed that if a person committed a federal crime in Iowa, the criminal should expect nearly equal treatment regardless of whether he was tried in the Northern or Southern federal districts of the state. This mutual belief is nicely illustrated in these remarks made by Judge Graven to Judge Riley in 1954:
>
> "I have coming before me at Sioux City for sentencing on December 14 one . . . who apparently was splitting $20 [bills] and passing them. I am informed that there is a similar charge against him in the Southern District which is being transferred to this District under Rule 20 and that it is expected that that charge will also be disposed of at Sioux City on December 14th.
>
> "I note that you have two defendants who were associates of Mr. _____ coming up before you for sentencing. Since all the defendants committed the same crimes and presumably have much the same background, I would not want my sentence of Mr. _____ to be out of line with the sentence you impose. If you impose your sentences before December 14th at 10:00 a.m., I wish you would let me know what your sentences are."[52]

Third, we would note the impact upon federal judicial behavior of diversity of citizenship cases—suits that comprise a quarter of the district courts' civil business and about a sixth of civil appeals to circuit courts (see Chapter 5). Because the Supreme Court requires the lower courts to apply *state* rather than federal law in such cases, it behooves U.S. trial judges to keep abreast of and be sensitive to the latest developments in state law. The effect may be the same for circuit judges as well. For example, when three-judge appellate panels are appointed for diversity of citizenship cases, there is a tendency to name circuit judges from states whose law governs. As one scholar observed: "A 'slight local tinge' thus colored diversity opinions as part of a general tendency of members to defer to colleagues most knowledgeable about the subject."[53]

We would also note that quantitative studies of federal trial judges' voting behavior substantiate the proposition that there are meaningful differences on a state-by-state basis. In fact, such differences have been increasing since the late 1960s. Also, it has been observed that in both circuits that cross North-South boundaries, the Sixth and the Eighth, the district courts in the border and southern states are markedly more conservative than in the other states.[54] This suggests that local and regional values—as personified by the state—have a greater influence on trial judge decision making than the circuit as a whole.

*Urban-Rural Variances in Judicial Behavior.* We shall examine one final aspect of the impact of localism on federal court decision making: whether the judge grew up in, or now holds court in, a large city or a rural setting. There is good reason to believe that decision making by urban-oriented judges in America is somewhat more liberal than judicial behavior by small-town, rural-directed jurists. First, as documented by social scientists in attitude surveys of the overall population and in numerous studies of the voting behavior of legislators from urban and rural areas, the values and attitudes of urban areas tend to be more liberal.[55] Second, since, as we have noted, trial and appellate court judges often preside over courts in the same environments in which they were born and socialized, big-city jurists probably bring to the bench the liberalism they have grown up with, while their rural counterparts have been less exposed to the pluralism of metropolitan areas and thus have a more homogeneous, conservative view.

A third reason to associate liberal decision making in America's larger cities with the judges who sit there is the presence of articulate, well-financed liberal judicial lobbying groups. Whether they appear as litigants or as *amici* ("friends of the court"), liberal groups are more likely to be based in metropolitan areas, where they in turn sponsor a good deal of litigation. Labor unions, gay rights activists, the American Jewish Congress, the National Association for the Advancement of Colored People, and women's rights groups are examples of organizations that have strong bases in urban America. Just because these lobbying groups are more active in urban centers does not mean, of course, that the cities will automatically become centers of judicial liberalism. Still, there can be no victories for liberal causes until the appropriate cases are heard in court. Progressive-minded jurists in small towns would have little effect if they were not presented with cases through which they could express their liberal orientation. Likewise, conservative judges in the big cities would be under little intellectual pressure to render liberal decisions were they not often confronted with teams of well-organized attorneys representing liberal causes. Thus, while the mere presence of activist groups does not cause liberal decision making, their efforts at least create the opportunities for liberal decisions to be rendered.

Finally, the anonymity that the larger cities provide U.S. trial and appellate judges makes it psychologically easier for them to go out on a limb and render innovative, often unpopular, liberal decisions.[56] This was vividly illustrated by a district judge in Houston as he compared himself with a colleague in a small East Texas community not known for its progressive values:

> It's not so bad for us here when we have to hand down one of those bombshell rulings. The press covers it and some of the right wing groups squawk, and some people cuss you out on the local [radio] call-in shows

that night, but in a day or so it blows over and some other story comes along to take its place. . . . I mean, when I leave the courthouse at night, I step outside and nobody even knows who I am. But now with Judge _____ up in _____ city, it's different. Everyone in town calls him the "red judge." He's had death threats made on him, and at one time had to be under special guard. He can't even go into a supermarket without people pointing him out. It must be hell for him up there.

The propositions about urban versus rural decision making seem to be borne out by empirical studies. We have learned that since the turn of the century justices on the Supreme Court who were raised in larger cities have been more liberal on economic matters than their colleagues bred in more pastoral settings. This has also been true on the dimension of civil rights and liberties since the 1940s.[57] Although liberal-conservative differences on the urban-rural scale have not yet been systematically documented for appeals judges, there is evidence to show that judicial administration varies greatly depending on whether the circuit is rural or contains many urban centers.[58] For federal trial judges we have good cause to assert that urban jurists are more liberal than their colleagues in the smaller cities and towns. For instance, for the years 1933 to 1977, 41 percent of the decisions were liberal in rural districts with only one judge, whereas 46 percent were liberal in the larger cities where two judges presided. The phenomenon has been even more dramatic when one looks at the South. Here 38 percent of the decisions were liberal in districts where only one judge sat, while in cities with seven or more judges the liberal percentage was 49 percent.[59] Thus the urban-rural dichotomy is one final aspect of the effect of localism on the behavior of judges in the United States.

*Localism and the Behavior of State Judges.*   If regional factors leaven the bread of federal judicial decisions, there is every reason to believe that this phenomenon is even more pervasive for state jurists. As we noted in Chapter 8, state judges, even more than their federal counterparts, tend to be local folks—born, bred, educated, and socialized in the locale in which they preside. Whether they be elected directly by the people or appointed via their political connections with the governor or the local political machine, state judges are likely to mirror the values and attitudes of their environment. Let us look at an example from a study by Martin A. Levin, who compared and contrasted judges and justices in Minneapolis and Pittsburgh.[60]

In Minneapolis the state trial judges are elected on a nonpartisan ballot, and in practice the political parties have almost no role in the selection of judges. "The socialization and recruitment of [the] . . . judges reflect this pattern of selection. Most of these judges [as the majority of the local population] have Northern European-Protestant and middle-class backgrounds, and their pre-judicial careers have been predominantly in private legal practice. . . . Such career experiences seem to have stimulated these judges to be interested more in 'society' than in the defendant." Minneapolis's conservative, middle-class environment, from which its judges come, is reflected in the law-and-order, no nonsense grist of the judicial mill.

> This pre-judicial experience, reinforced by their lack of party or policy-oriented experiences and their middle-class backgrounds, seems to have contributed to the legalistic and universalistic character of their decision-making and their eschewal of policy and personal considerations. In their milieu, rules were generally emphasized, especially legal ones, and these rules had been used to maintain and protect societal institutions. Learning to "get around" involved skill in operating in a context of rules. The judges' success seems to have depended more on their objective achievements and skills than on personal relationships.[61]

The environment of the Pittsburgh jurists is in stark contrast. The highly partisan (Democratic) judges reflect the working-class, ethnic-group-based values of the political machine that put them on the bench. These jurists were likely to have held public office before becoming judges, and they were thus much more people oriented than their counterparts in Minneapolis. They often felt that their own "minority ethnic and lower-income backgrounds and these government and party experiences had developed their general attachment to the problems of the 'underdog' and the 'oppressed.'" Levin concludes this about the judicial behavior that is reflected by the local environment and recruitment process:

> Their political experiences and lack of much legalistic experience apparently contributed to the highly particularistic and nonlegalistic character of their decision-making, their emphasis on policy considerations, and their use of pragmatic criteria. . . . Personal relationships, expecially with constituents, were emphasized, and focused on particular and tangible entities. Success depended largely on the ability to operate within personal relationships. It depended on *whom* one knew, rather than on *what* one knew. Abstractions such as "the good of society as a whole" seem to have been of little concern.[62]

Although social science still needs to develop more systematic empirical evidence for the relationship between the local environment and the "output" of state courts, these two brief case studies are indicative of the kind of phenomena we are describing.

## The Impact of Public Opinion

If one were to approach a typical judge or justice and ask whether public opinion affected the decisions made from the bench, the jurist might well respond with a fair measure of indignation. We might hear an answer something like this: "Look, as a judge with a lifetime appointment, I'm expected to be free from the pressures of public opinion. That's part of what we mean when we say that we're a 'government of laws—not of men.' When I decide a case, I look at the law and the facts. I don't go out into the streets and take some sort of public opinion poll to tell me what to do."

Yet there is reason to believe that to some degree and on certain issues American judges do temper their decision making with public opinion. Before we look at the specific evidence for this, let us outline our intuitive reasons for asserting some role for public opinion. First, judges as human beings, as parents, as consumers, as residents of the community are themselves part of public opinion. Putting on a black robe may stimulate a greater concern for responsible, objective decision making, but it does not void a judge's membership in the human race. As one judicial scholar has noted, "Since judges often have been born and reared locally, and recruited from a local political system, it seems likely that public opinion would have an effect, especially in issues that are locally visible and controversial. Even with lifetime appointments . . . public opinion still might seep into judicial decisions via judges' personal experiences and attitudes." [63] A keen example of a judge's sensitivity to local public opinion was provided by a New Orleans jurist who related one aspect of a pending school integration case. He noted that he lives "in a white, middle class suburb and my neighbors feel pretty strongly against busing and I have to be careful not to express my thoughts on the matter in front of them." My wife gets this kind of 'static' from the neighbors all the time." [64] In another instance, when the media reported that the late U.S. district judge William Overton was involved in a decision that overturned Arkansas's creation-science law, the judge received over 500 letters, most of them highly critical. (The Arkansas law required that the teaching of evolution in schools be accompanied by the teaching of creation science, a theory that life is of recent, supernatural, sudden origin, as related in the book of Genesis; Overton's position was that the law violated the principle of separation of church and state.) The judge was so overwhelmed by the outpouring of negative public opinion that he took the unusual step of making the letters available to reporters and to the University of Arkansas at Little Rock. "How many monkeys are in your family tree?" asked one angry letter writer from Richmond, Virginia. "Repent!" And from Benton, Arkansas, came a clipping that included a picture of three persons who filed suit, and wrote: "I hope the souls of you and these 3 goons rot in Hell for eternity." [65]

A second reason for suggesting the influence of public opinion on judicial behavior is that in many instances it is actually supposed to be an official factor in the decision-making process. For example, when it came to implementing the famous *Brown v. Board of Education* school desegregation ruling, the Supreme Court refused to set strict national guidelines for how their ruling was to be carried out. Rather, it was left up to individual federal district judges to implement the High Court decision based on the judges' determination of local moods, conditions, and traditions.[66] Likewise, when the Supreme Court ruled that it was permissible for federal courts to hear cases involving malapportionment of state legislatures, it refused to indicate how its decision was to be carried out. Instead it was in effect left to the lower federal judiciary to implement the ruling in accordance with the way they viewed local needs, conditions, and the state political climate.[67] A further example may be found in the obscenity rulings of the Burger Court, in which the justices determined that the courts should use community values and attitudes in determining what materials are obscene.[68]

Thus, not only is it humanly impossible for judges to rid themselves of the influence of public opinion, but indeed for many important types of cases judges are obliged to consider the attitudes and values of the public. This does not mean they go out and take opinion polls whenever they face a tough decision, but it does mean that public opinion is often one ingredient in the decision-making calculus.

Third, both federal and state judges are surely aware that ultimately their decisions cannot be carried out unless there is a reasonable degree of public support for them. As Lawrence Baum has noted, "Presumably, the more favorably people view the Court and its work, the more likely they are to carry out the Court's policies rather than to impede them.[69] It has been an open secret for a long time that when the Court is about to hand down a bombshell decision likely to be unpopular among many groups of Americans, the author of the majority opinion takes great pains to word the decision in such a way as to generate popular support for it—or at least to salve the wounds of those potentially offended by it. Examples of High Court decisions in which the author is thought to have written as much for the public at large as for the usual narrow audience of lawyers and lower court judges include the following: *Marbury v. Madison*, in which the Court claimed for itself the right to declare acts of Congress unconstitutional; *Brown v. Board of Education*, which called for an end to racial segregation in the public schools; *Roe v. Wade*, in which the Court upheld a woman's right to an abortion; and *United States v. Nixon*—the Watergate case—in which the justices ordered the president of the United States to yield to the authority of the courts.[70]

The *empirical* evidence for the impact of public opinion is suggestive but hardly conclusive, in part because social scientists have only recently begun to examine this phenomenon and because the proposition is very difficult to prove. Nevertheless, several studies have provided some concrete evidence of a link between public opinion and judicial decision making. For example, during the war in Vietnam, some scholars tried to determine whether popular support for the war was related to the severity of federal sentences in draft evasion cases. Not all studies reached identical conclusions, but one found a close relation between public opinion that American involvement in Vietnam was a mistake and the tendency of judges to give probation rather than a prison term to draft evaders. Also, federal judges in states that generally are more liberal and innovative in policy making handed down lighter sentences in draft evasion cases.[71] Another study conducted during the Vietnam era found that as opposition to the war increased among the American people, federal judges were more and more likely to grant requests for conscientious objector status.[72]

Finally, a study of California state courts noted that sentencing in marijuana cases often changed in severity soon after a popular referendum was held on reducing criminal penalties for personal use of the drug. For example, judges who had given light sentences prior to the referendum sometimes gave harsher sentences if the local vote was in favor of maintaining criminal penalties. Conversely, harsh-sentencing jurists sometimes became more lenient when the vote indicated that the public favored reducing the penalties.[73]

Given the fact that in a majority of the states judges must periodically run for election (see Tables 8-3 and 8-4), there is good reason to believe that they are even more attuned to public opinion than federal judges with their lifetime tenure. Here is an example which we believe illustrates a state judge's greater grass-roots political awareness and also the greater degree to which elected jurists interact with the local environment.

On November 28, 1988, Jack Hampton, a state district court judge in Dallas, Texas, gave a thirty-year prison sentence to a defendant who had been convicted of murdering two gay men. The killer, Richard Bednarski, had testified in court that he and some friends went to a central Dallas park to "pester homosexuals" and ended up killing two of them in what authorities called an execution-style slaying. (Bednarski placed a gun in one victims' mouth and pulled the trigger; he then coldly shot the other man several times.) Because of the heinous and unprovoked nature of the crime and because Hampton is known as a "hanging judge" who usually gives life sentences for murder, the *Dallas Times Herald* decided to interview the judge about his lighter-than-usual sentence. During the course of the interview Judge Hampton said that the murder victims more or less got what they asked for since they were "queers" who "wouldn't have been killed if they hadn't been cruising the streets picking up teenage boys."[74]

Immediately after the interview was published, public protests began from human rights groups, local church leaders, and various gay rights organizations. Protest rallies were held, including one attended by 500 persons at the City Hall Plaza, where letters of support were read from Sen. Edward Kennedy of Massachusetts and Texas state treasurer Ann Richards.

Also, formal complaints were filed with the Texas Commission on Judicial Conduct, calling for Hampton to be disciplined. Realizing that he had perhaps bitten off more than he could chew, this elected judicial official issued a four-paragraph letter to a group of eight Methodist ministers. Judge Hampton said he wished "to apologize" for his "poor choice of words that appeared in a recent newspaper story. . . ." He promised that in his court "everyone is entitled to and will receive equal protection."

Was the judge's public apology in response, at least in part, to his perception of public opinion and the effect that it might have on his bid for reelection? This might well be surmised from a more recent statement made by the judge when he was asked about possible political fallout stemming from the incident: "If it makes anybody mad, they'll forget it by 1990" (when Judge Hampton is up for reelection).[75]

We are not suggesting that this particular incident is typical of the behavior of state judges, but we do believe that it demonstrates the degree to which locally elected judicial officials respond to the tides of public opinion. Very rarely indeed do *lifetime judicial appointees,* such as federal judges, feel the need to justify their sentencing behavior in the form of interviews with the local press or to issue public apologies when public opinion turns critical of their behavior. For better or worse, public opinion does affect judicial behavior, and this is particularly true when judges must be accountable directly to the electorate.

Thus, despite the traditional notion of the blindfolded justice weighing only the facts in a case and the relevant law, there is common-sense and statistical support for the assertion that jurists do keep their eyes (and ears) open to public opinion.

## The Influence of the Legislative and Executive Branches

We shall now look at one final set of stimuli that the democratic subculture may bring to bear on the behavior of American judges—the executive and the legislative branches. We shall first explore this phenomenon at the national level and then indicate how it is equally prevalent at the state and local levels.

*Congress and the President.*    Perhaps the most obvious link between the values of the democratic subculture and the output of the federal courts lies in the fact that the people elect the president and members of the Senate, and the president appoints judges and justices with the advice and consent of the Senate. We have already noted in Chapter 8 the substantial capacity of the chief executive and certain key senators to influence what kind of men and women will sit on the bench, but even after judges have been appointed, the president and the Congress may have an impact on the content and direction of judicial decision making.

First, as we discussed in Chapter 5, to a very large degree the jurisdiction of the federal trial and appellate courts is determined by the Congress of the United States. Congress has the authority to decide which types of issues may become appropriate matters for judges to resolve. For example, the Wagner Act, passed by Congress in 1935, prohibited employers from engaging in several unfair labor practices, all of which would have disrupted trade union organizing. In doing so Congress in effect expanded the jurisdiction of the federal courts to hear a large number of labor-management disputes that previously had been outside the purview of the federal judiciary. Conversely, Congress may restrict the jurisdiction of the federal courts. In response to popular dissatisfaction with many court rulings on busing, abortion, school prayer, and so on, Congress, with the indirect support of the president, has been considering passage of a number of bills that would restrict the right of the courts to render decisions on these subjects.[76] Even if Congress does not actually pass such legislation, one may speculate that the threat to do so may cause the federal courts to pull in their horns when it comes to deciding cases in ways that are not in accord with the will of the president or Congress.

Second, there is evidence that judicial decision making is likely to be bolder and more effective if it has the active support of at least one, and ideally both, other branches of the federal government.[77] School integration is a case in point. When the federal courts began to order desegregation of the public schools after 1954, we know that they met with considerable opposition—primarily from those parts of the country most affected by the Supreme Court ruling in the Brown case. It is doubtful whether the federal courts could have overcome this resistance without the support given them (sometimes reluctantly) by the president and Congress. For example, in 1957 Arkansas governor Orville Faubus sought to obstruct a district judge's order to integrate Little Rock's Central High School. President Eisenhower then mobilized the National Guard and in effect used federal bayonets to implement the judge's ruling. President Kennedy likewise used federal might to support a judge's decision to admit a black student to the University of Mississippi in the face of massive local resistance. Congress also lent its hand to federal desegregation rulings. For instance, it voted to withhold federal aid to school districts that refused to comply with district court desegregation decisions. Surely White House and congressional support emboldened the Supreme Court and the lower judiciary to carry on with their efforts to end segregation in the public schools.

Sometimes presidential and congressional actions may in fact lead rather than just implement judicial decision making. One study analyzed the impact on trial judge behavior of the 1937 Supreme Court decisions that permitted much greater government regulation of the economy.[78] As expected, federal district judge support for government regulation increased markedly after the Supreme Court gave its official blessing to the government's new powers. However, it was also learned that district court backing for labor and economic regulation had been building *before* the Supreme Court's decisions: proregulation decisions by U.S. trial judges went from 44 percent in 1936 to 67 percent in 1937—a change of 23 points. The authors attributed this at least in part to the fact that prior to 1937 the president and Congress were strongly pushing legislation in response to public opinion that favored an expanded federal role in labor and economic regulation.[79]

Another example is found in the willingness of the lower federal judiciary to support the petitions of those who sought classification as conscientious objectors. In 1965 the Supreme Court liberalized the definition of what constitutes a valid conscientious objector status. The Court ruled that for an individual to attain such status, it was no longer necessary to believe in a supreme being as such, but that one could possess any belief that occupied "a place in the life of its possessor parallel to that filled by the orthodox belief in God." [80] The district courts did not respond to this High Court ruling with any noticeable increase in proconscientious objector rulings: The percentage of decisions in favor of conscientious objectors, which was 40 percent in 1965, actually decreased to 18 percent in 1966 and remained at that same level throughout the following year. However, in 1967 Congress amended the Selective Service Act and deleted the statutory reference to a supreme being. Between 1967 and 1968—more than two years after the Supreme Court decision—the percentage of district court decisions in favor of conscientious objector petitions jumped from 18 to 59 percent.[81] There is reason to believe that this change in judicial decision making was spurred in part by the lead of Congress.

Thus the Supreme Court and the lower courts are not, and cannot be, immune to the will of Congress and of the chief executive as they go about their judicial business. Not only does the president, with the advice and consent of the Senate, select all members of the federal judiciary, but to a large degree the Congress prescribes the jurisdiction of the federal courts and often the qualifications of those who have standing to sue in these tribunals. Moreover, many court decisions cannot be meaningfully implemented without the support of the other two branches of government—a fact not lost on the judges and justices themselves. Sometimes, too, the courts appear to follow the lead of the president and Congress on various public policy matters. Whichever set of circumstances is the case, it is clear that the legislative and executive branches of government constitute an important source of nonjudicial influence on court behavior.

*The State Legislature and the Governor.*    Just as the legislative and executive branches affect judicial decision making at the national level, so, too, do their counterparts at the state and local levels. In almost half of the jurisdictions the popularly elected governor (or the state legislature) makes the selection of the state judges (see Tables 8-3 and 8-4), and there is every reason to suggest a policy link between the value sets of the voters, the appointing officials, and the judges who render subsequent decisions. More specifically, the authors of a recent study tell us that there are three major ways that the political branches affect the role of the state courts.[82]

First, legislation sponsored by the governor or passed by the legislature regulates the sorts of claims that can be adjudicated in state courts and also brought to the state appellate courts. For example, let us look at the ease with which class actions suits may be brought in state judicial tribunals. (Such suits facilitate access to the courts by allowing large numbers of potential litigants with individually small claims to band together, thereby reducing or eliminating entirely the financial costs of seeking redress.) Actions by the legislature determine who may bring such suits and under what circumstances. The evidence suggests that there is great variation from one state to another in this realm: some states make it very easy to initiate such suits while in others access to the courts in this fashion is very difficult.[83]

Second, actions by the legislature (which may or may not be part of the governor's political agenda) determine the authority of the state supreme court to regulate its workload and focus on important cases. For example, it is generally accepted that for most cases litigants should have the right to appeal trial court decisions. In states that have an ample number of intermediate appellate courts this right to appeal is readily available. However, in states without sufficient numbers of intermediate appeals courts or in states where the supreme court is forced by law to deal with a succession of relatively minor disputes, the chances of litigants having their cases heard by the supreme court are slim indeed. This fact is significant in itself in terms of the distribution of justice, but it is important for another reason. In states where the supreme court is forced by the legislature into overwork on judicial trivia, the court does not have time to devote much attention to cases that raise important policy questions. For instance, after the legislature in North Carolina created intermediate courts of appeals, a study concluded that such action enabled the state high court to assume "a position of true leadership in the legal development of the state." [84] Thus actions by the legislature (supported or opposed by the governor) may well determine whether the supreme court plays a major or minor role in policy questions important to the state.

Finally, because a prime function of courts is to enforce existing legal norms, the sorts of issues that state courts address depend to a large degree on the substantive law of the state. For instance, seventeen state constitutions contain "little ERA's" (equal rights amendments); ten states specifically protect the right to privacy; and in some states there is a provision guaranteeing a right to quality of the environment.[85] Thus, a judge in a state in which good air quality is guaranteed will have a much greater opportunity and right to issue an injuction against a polluter than one in a state where such a right is not legally provided for. The point here is that judges render decisions within the existing constitutional and legal environment of their respective states. Such an environment is largely the product of political decisions made by the governor and the legislature as representatives of the electorate.

In sum, the output of the state courts, as with federal tribunals, is to a significant degree the result of the political values and policy goals of the chief executive and the legislative branch of government.

## The Subcultures as Predictors

Earlier in the chapter we indicated that there is scholarly divergence over the question of whether judicial decision making is essentially the product of facts, laws, and precedent (the legal subculture), or whether the various extralegal factors we have examined carry more weight (the realist-behavioralist view). In other words, are court decisions better explained by understanding the facts and law that impinge upon a given case, or by knowing which newspaper the judge reads in the morning or how the judge voted in the last election?

The clue to answering the question lies in knowing what kind of case the judge is being asked to decide. In our discussion of the nature and scope of the federal judicial workload, in Chapter 5, we indicated that the vast majority of the trial judge's cases and much appellate judicial business involve routine norm enforcement decisions. In cases in which the law and the controlling precedents are clear, the victor will be the side that is able to marshal the best evidence to show that their factual case is stronger. In other words, in the lion's share of cases the legal subculture model best explains and predicts judicial decision making. When traditional legal cues are unclear, ambiguous, or absent, however, judges are obliged to look to the democratic subculture for guidance in their decision making. We will examine the types of situations in which the legal subculture model might give way to the democratic subculture as an explicator of judicial behavior.

## When the Legal Evidence Is Contradictory

It is probably fair to say that in a majority of cases the facts, evidence, and controlling precedents distinctly favor one side or another. In such instances the judge is clearly obliged to decide for the party with the stronger case. Not to do so would violate the judge's legal training and mores; it would subject a trial or appeals court judge to reversal by a higher court, an event most jurists find embarrassing; and it would render the

Supreme Court vulnerable to the charge that it was making up the law as it went along—an impression not flattering to the High Court justices. On the other hand, judges often find themselves in situations in which the facts and evidence are about equally compelling on either side, or in which there are about an equal number of precedents to sustain a finding for either party. As one U.S. trial judge in Houston told us:

> There are days when you want to say to the litigants, "I wish you guys would've settled this out of court because I don't know what to do with you." If I grant the petition's request, I can often modify the relief requested [in an attempt to even out the decision], but still one side has got to win and one side has got to lose. I could cite good precedents on either side, and it's no good worrying about the appeals court because there's no telling what they would do with it should the judge's decision be appealed.

In such situations the judge has little choice but to turn to his or her value set to determine how to resolve the case. We can assume that decision making is affected by local attitudes and traditions or by the judge's perception of the public mood or the will of the current Congress or state legislature or administration.

As we shall see in Chapter 10, since the advent of the Burger Court in 1969, and continuing throughout the Rehnquist Court since 1986, an inordinate number of the Supreme Court's decisions have been regarded as "ideologically imprecise and inconsistent," often sustained by weak, five-to-four majorities. This state of affairs has surely increased the likelihood that trial and appellate judges will respond to stimuli from the democratic rather than the legal subculture. That is, the confusion created by the Court in setting forth ambiguous or contradictory guidelines has meant that the lower federal and state courts—and perhaps even members of the Supreme Court—have been forced to rely on (or have felt free to give vent to) their own personal ideas about how the law should read. As one study concluded, "With the decline of the fact-law congruence after 1968 the . . . [lower courts] became more free to take their decision-making cues from personal-partisan values rather than from guidelines set forth by the Higher Court." [86]

## When a Case Involves New Areas of the Law

There is a second situation that causes researchers to set aside the legal subculture model and turn to the democratic subculture approach—when jurists are asked to resolve new types of policy questions for which statutory law and appellate court guidelines are virtually absent. Since about 1937 most new and uncharted areas of the law (at least at the federal level) have been in the realms of civil liberties and criminal justice rather than in the area of labor and economic regulation. As we noted in Chapter

2, since 1937 the federal courts have leaned toward self-restraint and deference to the elected branches when it comes to ordering the economic lives of the American people.[87] Moreover, in recent decades Congress has legislated, often with precision, in the areas of economic regulation and labor relations, and this has further restricted the discretion of judges in these fields. As a result, the noose of the legal subculture has been drawn tightly around trial judges' necks in this realm, and there is little room for creative decision making or for responding to the tug of the heart rather than to the clear command of the law. Thus, since New Deal days the legal rather than the democratic subculture has been the better predictor of trial and appellate judge decision making for labor and economic regulation cases.

Since the 1930s the opposite trend has been true for issues involving criminal justice and civil rights and liberties:

> The "great" and controversial decisions of the Stone, Vinson, Warren, and Burger Courts [and, one might add, the Rehnquist Court] focused primarily on issues of civil liberties and of the rights of criminal defendants, and it is precisely those sorts of issues which evoked the greatest partisan schisms among the justices. Research has shown that . . . [the lower courts] were by no means immune to the debates and divisions which racked the nation's High Court; they, too, seem to have split along "political" lines more often on criminal justice and on civil rights matters than they did with other sorts of cases.[88]

The ambiguity (or perhaps the constant state of flux) of the law on matters such as the rights of criminal defendants, First Amendment freedoms, equal protection of the law, and so on, has given the federal jurists greater opportunity to respond than in the labor and economic realms, where their freedom of action has been more circumscribed. Put another way, since the 1930s the democratic rather than the legal subculture model has become increasingly important as a predictor of judicial behavior on Bill of Rights matters.[89]

A series of interviews with a wide range of district and appellate court judges lends further credence to this notion. In Kitchin's study the trial judges were asked about their willingness to "innovate"—that is, their inclination to make new law in areas where appellate court or congressional guidelines were ambiguous or nonexistent. After asking why judges create new law through judicial innovation, Kitchen noted:

> One answer is that the courts innovate because other branches of government ignore certain significant problems which, to individual judges, cry out for attention. Accordingly, the individual district judge innovates in an attempt to fill a legal vacuum, as one judge commented, "The theory is that judges should not be legal innovators, but there are some areas in which they have to innovate because legislatures won't do the job. Race relations is one of these areas. . . ." Other areas mentioned as needing judicial innovation because of legislative inaction were

housing, equal accommodations, and criminal law (especially habeas corpus).[90]

Picking up on the thread of these interviews, a more recent study of decisional patterns and variations in U.S. district judge decision making showed that "the subjects that . . . [the Kitchin study] found to represent the greatest areas of freedom in judicial decision making are the very same subjects that we find to maximize partisan voting differences among the district judges. In situations where judges are more free to take their decision-making cues from sources other than appellate court decisions and statutes, they are more likely to rely on their personal-partisan orientations." [91]

A cross-section of federal appellate judges were recently asked: "When precedents are absent or ambiguous, what do you do?" Seventy-four percent replied that their own personal conception of the "dictates of justice" would be "very important" in their coming to grips with such a situation, and another 17 percent said that such personal dictates would be "moderately important." Not a single appeals judge indicated that such dictates would be "not important." The interviewer concluded that "when judges are free to choose, personalities, predilections, and group relations perforce fill the void." [92]

Let us look at a relatively new area of the law in which appellate court and congressional guidelines are few and thus lower-court judges must fend for themselves—the definition of obscenity. Prior to 1957 there were no Supreme Court decisions of note on the matter of obscenity. In that year the nation's High Court ruled that obscenity was not protected by the First Amendment and said that it could be defined as material that dealt with sex "in a manner appealing to prurient interest." [93] Seven years later the Supreme Court said that in determining what appealed to the prurient interest of the average person, hypothetical "national standards" were to be used,[94] but then nine years after that the Court changed its mind and ruled that "state community standards" could be employed." [95] But what is obscenity? No one seems to know with any greater certainty today than Justice Potter Stewart did in 1964 when he confessed that he could not intelligibly define obscenity but that "I do know it when I see it." [96] Given the reluctance or the inability of Congress and the Supreme Court to define obscenity, America's trial and appellate judges have little choice but to look to their own personal values and perceptions of the local public need in order to determine what kinds of books, films, and plays the First Amendment protects in their respective jurisdictions.

## The Judge's Role Conception

In our discussion of which better explains judicial decision making—the rules of the legal subculture or stimuli from the democratic subculture—

there is one additional factor to consider: how judges conceive of their judicial role. Judicial scholars often talk about three basic decision-making categories regarding whether judges should make law when they decide cases. "Lawmakers" are those who take a broad view of the judicial role. These jurists, often referred to as "activists" or "innovators," contend that they can and must make law in their decisions, because the statutory law and appellate or Supreme Court guidelines are often ambiguous or do not cover all situations and because legislative intent is frequently impossible to determine. In Kitchin's study of federal district judges, 14 percent were classified in this category, whereas in an investigation of appeals court judges 15 percent were associated with this role.[97]

At the other end of the continuum are the "law interpreters," who take a very narrow, traditional view of the judicial function. Sometimes called "strict constructionists," they don't believe that judges should substitute judicial wisdom for the rightful power of the elected branches of government to make policy. They tend to eschew making innovative decisions that may depart from the literal meaning of controlling precedents. In the Kitchin study, 52 percent of the U.S. trial judges were found to be "law interpreters," while only 26 percent of the appeals court judges were so designated.[98] This finding is consistent with our discussion in Chapters 2 and 5 that federal district judges are more concerned with routine norm enforcement, whereas the appellate judges' involvement—and their perception of it—is with broader questions of judicial policy.

Midway between the law interpreters and the lawmakers are judges known as "pragmatists" or "realists," who believe that on occasion they are indeed obliged to make law, but that for most cases a decision can be made by consulting the controlling law or appellate court precedents. Studies have indicated that a third of federal district judges assume this moderate role, while a full 59 percent of their appellate court colleagues do so.[99] Comparing federal jurists with state judges, one scholar has noted, "Federal judges appear to take the pragmatist or realist view more often, which may reflect their opportunities to make a larger number of innovative decisions."[100]

Thus, whether judicial decisions are better explained by the legal model or by the democratic model depends not only on the nature of the cases and the state of the controlling law and precedents; it also depends to some degree on how the individual judges evaluate these factors. In virtually every case that comes before them, judges have to determine how much discretion they have and how they wish to exercise it. This is obviously a subjective process, and, as one research team put it, "activist judges will find more discretion in a given fact situation than will their more restrained colleagues."[101]

## Summary

Federal and state judges make hundreds of millions of decisions each year, and scholars have sought to explain the thinking behind these decisions. Two schools of thought provide an explanation. One theory is based on rules and procedures of the legal subculture. Judges' decisions, according to this model, are the product of traditional legal reasoning and adherence to precedent and to judicial self-restraint. Another school of thought, the realist-behavioralist approach, argues that judges are influenced in their decision making by such factors as party affiliation, local values and attitudes, public opinion, and pressures from the legislative and executive branches. We asserted that in the vast majority of cases the legal subculture model is the more accurate predictor of judicial decision making. However, stimuli from the democratic subculture often become useful in accounting for judges' decisions (1) when the legal evidence is contradictory or equally compelling on either side; (2) if the situation involves new areas of the law and significant precedents are absent; and (3) when judges are inclined to view themselves more as activist lawmakers than as law interpreters.

## Notes

1. Richard J. Richardson and Kenneth N. Vines, *The Politics of Federal Courts* (Boston: Little, Brown, 1970). Although Richardson and Vines developed their model primarily for federal courts, we feel that their hypotheses and conclusions are equally true for state judges.
2. Edward H. Levi, *An Introduction to Legal Reasoning* (Chicago: University of Chicago Press, 1948), 1-2.
3. *Lane v. Wilson*, 307 U.S. 268 (1939), and *Gomillion v. Lightfoot*, 364 U.S. 339 (1960).
4. *Lane v. Wilson*, 307 U.S. 275 (1939).
5. William Kitchin, *Federal District Judges* (Baltimore: Collage Press, 1978), 71.
6. J. Woodford Howard, Jr., *Courts of Appeals in the Federal Judicial System: A Study of the Second, Fifth, and District of Columbia Circuits* (Princeton, N.J.: Princeton University Press, 1981), 187.
7. Walter F. Murphy, *Elements of Judicial Strategy* (Chicago: University of Chicago Press, 1964), 204.
8. Henry Sumner Maine, *Ancient Law* (Boston: Beacon Press, 1963), 3-19.
9. Henry J. Abraham, *The Judicial Process*, 4th ed. (New York: Oxford University Press, 1980), 373-400.
10. *Evers v. Jackson Municipal Separate School District*, 232 F. Supp. 241 (1964).
11. Ibid., 247.
12. Ibid., 249.
13. Ibid., 255.
14. Richardson and Vines, *The Politics of Federal Courts*, 8-9.
15. Steven Vago, *Law and Society*, 2d ed. (Englewood Cliffs, N.J.: Prentice-Hall,

1988), 307.

16. For a good, current bibliography on this subject, see Vago, *Law and Society*, 292-295.

17. Oliver Wendell Holmes, Jr., *The Common Law* (Boston: Little, Brown, 1881), 1-2.

18. Jerome Frank, *Courts on Trial: Myth and Reality in American Justice* (Princeton, N.J.: Princeton University Press, 1950), 151.

19. Richardson and Vines, *The Politics of Federal Courts*, 10.

20. Donald Dale Jackson, *Judges* (New York: Atheneum, 1974), 18.

21. Some studies suggest that age, socioeconomic status, and religion may influence some judges on some of their cases, but the associations are weak. For example, see Sheldon Goldman, "Voting Behavior on the United States Courts of Appeals Revisited," *American Political Science Review* 69 (1975): 491-506; John R. Schmidhauser, "The Justices of the Supreme Court: A Collective Portrait," *Midwest Journal of Political Science* 3 (1959): 1-57; and Donald Leavitt, "Political Party and Class Influences on the Attitudes of Justices of the Supreme Court in the Twentieth Century" (Paper delivered at the annual meeting of the Midwest Political Science Association, Chicago, 1972). Other studies suggest that these background factors have virtually no explanatory power—e.g., Howard, *Courts of Appeals in the Federal Judicial System*, chap. 6. For a more detailed discussion of this subject and a literature review, see Robert A. Carp and C. K. Rowland, *Policymaking and Politics in the Federal District Courts* (Knoxville: University of Tennessee Press, 1983), chap. 2.

22. David W. Adamany, "The Party Variable in Judges' Voting: Conceptual Notes and a Case Study," *American Political Science Review* 63 (1969): 59.

23. For a more extensive discussion of the "odds ratio" and methodology used in this study, see Carp and Rowland, *Policymaking and Politics in the Federal District Courts*, 33-34.

24. These figures are based on unpublished data collected by Robert A. Carp, Ronald Stidham, and C. K. Rowland.

25. For a good review of the literature on this subject, see Goldman, "Voting Behavior on the United States Courts of Appeals Revisited," 491, note 2. Also, see Howard, *Courts of Appeals in the Federal Judicial System*, chap. 6.

26. Sheldon Goldman, "Voting Behavior on the United States Courts of Appeals, 1961-1964," *American Political Science Review* 60 (1966): 384.

27. Goldman, "Voting Behavior on the United States Courts of Appeals Revisited," 505. Goldman's second article also found that the variable of the judge's age was of some significance: Older judges tended to be somewhat more conservative than their younger colleagues.

28. Leavitt, "Political Party and Class Influences on the Attitudes of Justices of the Supreme Court in the Twentieth Century," 18-19.

29. C. Neal Tate, "Personal Attribute Models of the Voting Behavior of U.S. Supreme Court Justices: Liberalism in Civil Liberties and Economic Decisions, 1946-78," *American Political Science Review* 75 (1981): 355-367.

30. S. Sidney Ulmer, "Are Background Models Time-Bound?" *American Political Science Review* 80 (1986): 957-967.

31. S. Sidney Ulmer, "The Political Party Variable in the Michigan Supreme Court," *Journal of Public Law* 11 (1962): 352-362; and Malcolm M. Feeley, "Another Look at the 'Party Variable' in Judicial Decision-Making: An Analysis of the Michigan Supreme Court," *Polity* 4 (1971): 91-104.

32. Philip L. Dubois, "The Illusion of Judicial Consensus Revisited: Partisan Conflict on an Intermediate State Court of Appeals," *American Journal of Political Science* 32 (1988): 946-967.
33. Ibid., 953-954.
34. For a good, current bibliography of the literature of partisan voting patterns among state judges, see Dubois, "The Illusion of Judicial Consensus Revisited," 965-967.
35. Richardson and Vines, *The Politics of Federal Courts*, 71.
36. For a more elaborate discussion of this phenomenon, see Carp and Rowland, *Policymaking and Politics in the Federal District Courts*, chap. 4.
37. Richardson and Vines, *The Politics of Federal Courts*, 73.
38. Ibid., 72.
39. For example, see Robert A. Carp and Russell Wheeler, "Sink or Swim: The Socialization of a Federal District Judge," *Journal of Public Law* 21 (1972): 359-393. Also, Robert A. Carp, "The Influence of Local Needs and Conditions on the Administration of Federal Justice" (Paper delivered at the annual meeting of the Southwestern Political Science Association, Dallas, 1971).
40. For example, see Angus Campbell et al., *The American Voter* (New York: Wiley, 1960); Everett Carll Ladd, Jr., and Charles D. Hadley, *Transformations of the American Party System*, 2d ed. (New York: Norton, 1978); V. O. Key, Jr., *Public Opinion and American Democracy* (New York: Knopf, 1967); and Samuel A. Stouffer, *Communism, Conformity, and Civil Liberties* (New York: Doubleday, 1955).
41. Barbara Hinckley, *Stability and Change in Congress* (New York: Harper & Row, 1978); Randall B. Ripley, *Congress: Process and Policy*, 2d ed. (New York: Norton, 1978); V. O. Key, Jr., *Politics, Parties, and Pressure Groups*, 5th ed. (New York: Crowell, 1964), especially chaps. 9 and 24; and J. H. Fenton, "Liberal-Conservative Divisions by Sections of the United States," *Annals* 344 (1962): 122-127.
42. John R. Schmidhauser, "Judicial Behavior and the Sectional Crisis of 1837-1860," *Journal of Politics* 23 (1961): 615-640. To be more precise, Schmidhauser found that justices' party affiliations and their geographic orientations were highly interrelated. Because the four justices who were most supportive of southern regional interests were all southern Democrats and since the two justices with the strongest pronorthern voting patterns were northern Whigs, Schmidhauser concluded that the effects of party and region were virtually inseparable.
43. Leavitt, "Political Party and Class Influences on the Attitudes of Justices of the Supreme Court in the Twentieth Century."
44. James F. Simon, *In His Own Image* (New York: David McKay, 1973), 103-104.
45. Ibid., 123.
46. Howard, *Courts of Appeals in the Federal Judicial System*, 55, 79, 156.
47. Carp and Rowland, *Policymaking and Politics in the Federal District Courts*, 98.
48. For example, see Sheldon Goldman, "Voting Behavior on the United States Courts of Appeals, 1961-1964," 370-385.
49. *The Third Branch* 15 (June 1983): 8. The formal opinion in the case, *Bonner v. City of Prichard, Alabama*, 661 F. 2d 1206, was released on November 3, 1981.
50. Carp and Rowland, *Policymaking and Politics in the Federal District*

*Courts*, 101, 102.
51. Carp and Wheeler, "Sink or Swim," 376.
52. Carp, "The Influence of Local Needs and Conditions on the Administration of Federal Justice," 17-18.
53. Howard, *Courts of Appeals in the Federal Judicial System*, 234.
54. For example, see Carp and Rowland, *Policymaking and Politics in the Federal District Courts*, 106-116.
55. For example, see Key, *Public Opinion and American Democracy*; Leon Epstein, "Size and Place and the Two-Party Vote," *Western Political Quarterly* 9 (1956): 138-150; and John Wahlke et al., *The Legislative System* (New York: Wiley, 1962).
56. We do not mean to suggest that it is impossible to render innovative *conservative* decisions. It is just that during the past several decades the vast majority of the highly unpopular judicial decisions have been of a liberal nature—e.g., the release of an obviously guilty criminal on a legal technicality, an order to a state university to grant recognition to a campus gay organization, a ruling that a local obscenity ordinance is too vague.
57. Leavitt, "Political Party and Class Influences on the Attitudes of Justices of the Supreme Court in the Twentieth Century," 19.
58. Howard, *Courts of Appeals in the Federal Judicial System*, chaps. 2 and 3.
59. Carp and Rowland, *Policymaking and Politics in the Federal District Courts*, 133, 137.
60. This discussion is based on material taken from Martin A. Levin, *Urban Politics and the Criminal Courts* (Chicago: University of Chicago Press, 1977).
61. Ibid., 136-142.
62. Ibid., 142-147.
63. Henry R. Glick, *Courts, Politics, and Justice*, 2d ed. (New York: McGraw-Hill, 1988), 264.
64. Carp and Wheeler, "Sink or Swim," 373.
65. "Arkansas Judge Who Struck Down Creation-Science Law Condemned in Hundreds of Letters," *Houston Chronicle*, August 6, 1982, 1:9.
66. *Brown v. Board of Education*, 349 U.S. 294 (1955).
67. *Baker v. Carr*, 369 U.S. 186 (1962).
68. *Miller v. California*, 413 U.S. 15 (1973).
69. Lawrence Baum, *The Supreme Court*, 2d ed. (Washington, D.C.: CQ Press, 1985), 128. For a good recent discussion of this subject, see David G. Barnum, "Supreme Court and Public Opinion: Judicial Decision Making in the Post-New Deal Period," *Journal of Politics* 47 (1985): 652-666.
70. The full citations are as follows: *Marbury v. Madison*, 1 Cranch 137 (1803); *Brown v. Board of Education*, 347 U.S. 483 (1954); *Roe v. Wade*, 410 U.S. 113 (1973); and *United States v. Nixon*, 418 U.S. 683 (1974).
71. For example, see Glen T. Broach et al., "State Political Culture and Sentence Severity in Federal District Courts," *Criminology* 16 (1978): 373-382.
72. Ronald Stidham and Robert A. Carp, "Trial Courts' Responses to Supreme Court Policy Changes: Three Case Studies," *Law & Policy Quarterly* 4 (1982): 215-235.
73. James H. Kuklinski and John E. Stanga, "Political Participation and Government Responsiveness: The Behavior of California Superior Courts," *American Political Science Review* 73 (1979): 1090-1099.
74. "Dallas Judge Apologizes for 'Poor Choice of Words,'" *Montrose Voice*,

December 23, 1988, 5.

75. "Overheard," *Newsweek*, January 2, 1989, 13.

76. However, many constitutional scholars argue that the right of the federal courts to hear such cases stems directly from Article III of the Constitution and that therefore Congress could not legally curtail court jurisdiction over these subjects except by initiating an amendment to the Constitution.

77. For example, see Stephen L. Wasby, *The Impact of the United States Supreme Court* (Homewood, Ill.: Dorsey Press, 1970), especially 255-256; Harrell R. Rodgers, Jr., and Charles S. Bullock III, *Coercion to Compliance* (Lexington, Mass.: Heath, 1976).

78. *National Labor Relations Board v. Jones and Laughlin Steel Corp.*, 301 U.S. 1 (1937) and *West Coast Hotel Co. v. Parrish*, 300 U.S. 379 (1937).

79. Stidham and Carp, "Trial Courts' Responses to Supreme Court Policy Changes," 218-222.

80. *United States v. Seeger*, 380 U.S. 166 (1965).

81. Stidham and Carp, "Trial Courts' Responses to Supreme Court Policy Changes," 222-227.

82. G. Alan Tarr and Mary Cornelia Aldis Porter, *State Supreme Courts in State and Nation* (New Haven, Conn.: Yale University Press, 1988), chap. 2.

83. Ibid., 45.

84. Roger D. Groot, "The Effects of an Intermediate Appellate Court on the Supreme Court Product: The North Carolina Experience," *Wake Forest Law Review* 7 (1971): 548-572.

85. Tarr and Porter, *State Supreme Courts in State and Nation*, 51.

86. Carp and Rowland, *Policymaking and Politics in the Federal District Courts*, 37.

87. However, on matters of *local* economic regulation, voting differences among judges are still sharp (see Table 9-1). Only at the national level have federal judges tended to refrain from substituting their own views for those of elected officials.

88. Carp and Rowland, *Policymaking and Politics in the Federal District Courts*, 39.

89. Of course, at the state level it varies from one jurisdiction to another whether High Court ambiguity is greater on civil rights and liberties issues or in the labor and economic realm. Note those several areas discussed in Chapter 5 under the heading of "Jurisdiction and Workload of State Courts" in which state courts have taken the lead in bringing about policy-making innovations.

90. Kitchin, *Federal District Judges*, 104.

91. Carp and Rowland, *Policymaking and Politics in the Federal District Courts*, 40.

92. Howard, *Courts of Appeals in the Federal Judicial System*, 165, 166-167.

93. *Roth v. United States* and *Alberts v. California*, 354 U.S. 476 (1957).

94. *Jacobellis v. Ohio*, 378 U.S. 184 (1964).

95. *Miller v. California*, 413 U.S. 15 (1973).

96. *Jacobellis v. Ohio*, 378 U.S. 197 (1964).

97. Kitchin, *Federal District Judges*, 107.

98. Ibid.

99. Ibid.

100. Glick, *Courts, Politics, and Justice*, 261.

101. Carp and Rowland, *Policymaking and Politics in the Federal District Courts*, 14.

# 10 Decision Making: The Special Case of Collegial Courts

Until now we have treated decision making by American judges at all levels as if it were essentially the product of identical influences—those from the legal and the democratic subcultures. To a substantial degree this is a valid approach to take. After all, jurists on multijudge appellate courts adhere to the same legal reasoning process as do their colleagues on the trial court bench; lower-court judges may be influenced in close cases by their political party affiliation just as are members of the appeals courts. But before an analysis of judicial decision making can be complete, we need to recognize one vital difference between trial courts on the one hand and the state and federal appellate courts on the other. The former render decisions that are largely the product of a single individual, whereas the latter are *collegial* courts, in which decision making is the product of group interaction. As one former trial judge, now a member of an appellate court, described it:

> The transition between a district judge and circuit judge is not an easy one, primarily because of, shall I say, the autocratic position occupied by the district court judge. He is the sole decider. He decides as he sees fit, and files the decision in a form as he sees fit. *A Court of Appeals decides by committee.* One of the first traumas I had was when opinions were sent back by the other judges asking me to add this sentence, change that, etc., to get concurrence. I admit at the beginning I resisted that. It was pride. I learned it was a joint project, but it was a very difficult thing. I see the same in others.[1] [Emphasis added.]

What are the extra ingredients that go into a decision made by the nine-member Supreme Court or by a three-judge state appellate panel? What is the essence of the dynamics of multijudge decision making that distinguishes it from a judgment made by a single jurist? We shall discuss several theoretical approaches that have attempted to get a handle on this interesting but slippery subject.

## Cue Theory

We have noted that as long as trial and appeals courts have jurisdiction over a case, the judges must render some type of decision on the merits; they have little discretion over the composition of their dockets. If the judges view a particular case as presenting a trivial question, they will not spend time agonizing over it, but they are still obliged to provide some kind of formal ruling on the substance of the matter. Not so with the Supreme Court. Recall from Chapter 5 that of the approximately 5,000 petitions presented to the Court each year, the justices agree to hear only a few hundred on the merits—and only about half of those carry with them full-blown written opinions. Since the passage of Public Law 100-352 in 1988, the Supreme Court has had complete control over its own docket— that is, the justices themselves decide which issues they want to tackle in a given term and which ones are not ripe for adjudication or must be summarily dismissed for "want of a substantial federal question." The importance of this is that what the Supreme Court decides *not* to rule on is often as significant as the cases it does summon forth for its scrutiny. (At the state level, as noted in the previous chapter, there is great variance in the amount of control that the supreme courts have over their dockets.[2])

Judicial scholars have sought to identify the reasons why some petitions are culled out for special attention and why the rest never receive those important four votes that are needed for the Supreme Court to grant certiorari and decide the case. A pioneering study of this question was conducted by a research team during the early 1960s.[3] Analysts began by examining the Court's official reasons for granting certiorari as set forth in Rule 17, which specifies that the Court might hear a case if (1) an appeals court has decided a point of local law in conflict with local decisions, (2) a court of appeals has departed from "the usual course of judicial proceedings," (3) a conflict is perceived between a lower-court decision and a Supreme Court precedent, (4) a conflict exists on a point of law among the various federal circuits, or (5) there exists a really important question on which the Court feels it must have the final word.

The research team tested these official reasons by comparing the cases for which certiorari was granted with those in which review was denied. To their surprise (or maybe not), the official reasons did not prove to be a very accurate or useful guide to the Court's decision making. For example, in over 50 percent of the cases that were selected for review, the Court's official reason for its actions was that the cases were "important"—a nebulous adjective at best. The researchers thought they could do better. They set out to identify certain key characteristics of those cases for which review was and was not granted. They hoped to develop some predictive statements that were more precise and reliable than Rule 17. The result was cue theory.

Cue theory is based on the assumption that the Supreme Court justices have neither the time nor the desire to wade through the myriad of pages in the thousands of petitions presented to them each year. Therefore, it is logical to assume that they must have developed some sort of shortcut to help them select the petitions that are interesting and important. The justices must, researchers hypothesized, look for cues in each petition—readily identifiable characteristics that trigger a positive response in the justices as they skim through the cumbersome assemblage of legal documents. After all, we ourselves have our own particular cue theories as we go about our daily lives. We wouldn't read through a four-page circular on a local store's white sale, for instance, if we already had an ample supply of bedding material. Just as we look for cues in sorting through the daily mail, so, too, do justices on the Supreme Court as they sort through the daily arrival of petitions for certiorari. At least this is what the research team reasoned.

The results of the team's hypotheses and investigations were encouraging. Of the several possible cues they tested for, three were found to contain substantial explanatory power. In order of importance they were (1) whether the U.S. government was a party to a case and was asking for Court review, (2) whether a civil rights or civil liberties issue was involved, and (3) whether there was dissension among the judges in the court that had previously heard the case (or disagreement between two or more courts and government agencies). If a case contained all three cues, there was an 80 percent chance that certiorari would be granted; if none were present, the chance dropped to a mere 7 percent. Clearly the researchers had developed a useful model to explain this one aspect of Supreme Court behavior.

During the past two decades judicial scholars have further tested, elaborated on, and revised cue theory. Some studies have found a relationship between the way the justices voted on a grant of certiorari and their eventual vote on the merits of the case at conference.[4] More recent studies have suggested that a fourth cue has considerable explanatory power—the ideological direction of the lower-court decision.[5] In comparing selected periods of the Warren Court (1967 and 1968 terms) and the Burger Court (1976 and 1977 terms) on certiorari voting, the analysts reached several conclusions. First, during the liberal Warren Court era, the justices were more likely to review economic cases that had been decided in a *conservative* manner by the lower court[6]—especially when the U.S. government was seeking Court review. Second, and conversely, the more conservative Burger Court tended to review *liberal* lower-court economic decisions. Third, the Burger Court was readier to scrutinize a civil libertarian position taken by a lower court than a lower-court decision limiting civil liberties.

Cue theory, then, is one predictor of High Court voting behavior. It is interesting to note the way the 1970s studies shed light on the 1960s research: The earlier team observed that the justices were likely to review cases involving civil rights or civil liberties issues; the later analysts found that the justices would most probably hear such cases when lower-court rulings had gone against the ideological grain of the Court's majority. One contemporary judicial scholar has summarized the certiorari behavior of the Court during the past several decades:

> Cues may change over time as political issues change throughout the country and as new justices come to the Court with their own ideas about public policy and law. During the 1950s, civil liberties were most important and made up a large part of the Court's total workload. In addition, during the 1950s and most of the 1960s, underdog appellants such as aliens, minorities, criminal defendants, laborers, and other have-nots were more successful in obtaining a hearing than during the 1970s, when the Supreme Court was shifting to more conservative policies under justices appointed by Republican President Richard Nixon. In recent years, upperdogs such as governments at all levels, businesses, and corporations have received more attention by the Supreme Court.[7]

In the remainder of the chapter we will examine several models of appellate court behavior that seek to explain how these collegial bodies make decisions once a case has been docketed. The models are small group analysis, attitude theory and bloc-formation analysis, and fact pattern analysis.

## Small-Group Analysis

As applied to the judiciary, most small-group research is based on the thesis that judges want to influence the judgments of their colleagues and to be on the winning side as often as possible. This school of thought assumes that judges' positions are not written in stone from the start but are susceptible to moderation or even to a 180-degree turn on occasion. More specifically, scholars believe that a good deal of interaction takes place among justices from the time a case is first discussed in conference to the moment the final decision is rendered in open court some weeks or months later. One researcher, in fact, has referred to the appellate judges' openness to change as "fluidity."[8]

It has been no secret that the way judges relate to one another affects their behavior on the court. Examination of the personal papers of members of the Supreme Court, interviews with appellate court jurists, and reminiscences of former law clerks all reveal the impact of group dynamics on voting behavior and on the content of written opinions.[9] Two characteristics in particular seem to carry weight as justices seek to influence their colleagues—personality and intellect. Judges who are considered to be warm, good-hearted, fair-minded, and so on seem able to put together winning coalitions and to hammer out compromises a bit more effectively than colleagues who have a reputation for condescension, self-righteousness, hostility, or vindictiveness.[10] As one researcher put it after interviewing supreme court justices in Louisiana, Pennsylvania, New Jersey, and Massachusetts:

> Generally, the judges believed it is important for court members to moderate their own personal idiosyncrasies in order to maintain as much harmony in the group as possible. Such things as arrogance, pride, sense of superiority, and loss of temper were condemned. . . . A pleasing personality . . . can be particularly important on collegial courts because the judges interact on a continuous basis: they operate as a small, permanent committee.[11]

This reflection on human nature should come as no surprise. A student who had served on his university's multimember student court gave us an illustration of this phenomenon, and though a student tribunal is certainly not a state or federal appellate court, we think the dynamics involved are similar:

> We had this guy on the court . . . who was one of these people that you just kind of naturally take to. I mean, he had a good sense of humor and was real decent and outgoing. I don't think he was that much of a "brain" or anything, but you always felt that he honestly wanted to do the right thing. Well, when we were split on some case—especially on matters of what punishment to hand down—and he suggested a way out, I think we all listened pretty carefully to what he thought was fair. He was just that sort of person.

The other personal attribute that is part of small-group dynamics is the knowledge and intellectual capacity of the individual judge.[12] A justice with a superior intellect or wide experience in a particular area of the law has a good deal more clout than a jurist who is seen as an intellectual lightweight. As one appeals court judge observed:

> Personality doesn't amount to so much as opinion-writing ability. Some judges are simply better than others. Some know more, think better. It would be strange if among nine men all had the same ability. Some simply have more respect than others. . . . That's bound to be so in any group. The first thing, is the judge particularly broad and experienced in the field? A couple of judges are acknowledged masters in admiralty. What they think carries more weight. I don't have much trouble being heard on criminal law or state government. I've been there. Ex-district judges on Courts of Appeals certainly carry more weight in discussion of trial procedures, instructions to juries, etc. Every judge is recognized for a particular proficiency obtained before or after his appointment. It saves enormous spadework and drudgery [to assign opinions accordingly]. No one could develop an expertise in all these fields.[13]

The techniques or strategies that justices use in their conscious (or even unconscious) efforts to maximize their impact on multijudge courts can be grouped into three general categories: persuasion on the merits, bargaining, and threat of sanctions. While the tactics overlap and are inherently interrelated, we shall take a look at their central focuses, which are in fact different.

## Persuasion on the Merits

This aspect of small-group dynamics takes us right back to the *legal subculture* discussed in Chapter 9. Quite simply, it means that because of their training and values, judges are open to persuasion based on sound legal reasoning bolstered by legal precedents. Unless judges have taken a hard-and-fast position from the start, most can be swayed by an articulate and well-reasoned argument from a colleague with a differing opinion.

One study of the Supreme Court concluded that the justices

> can be persuaded to change their minds about specific cases as well as about broad public policies, and intellectual persuasion can play an important role in such shifts. . . . Time and time again positions first taken at conference are changed as other Justices bring up new arguments. Perhaps most convincing in demonstrating the impact of intellectual factors are the numerous instances on record in which the Justice assigned the opinion of the Court has reported back to the conference that additional study had convinced him that he and the rest of the majority had been in error.[14]

For example, Justice Robert Jackson, hardly a wilting violet when it came to holding fast to a judicial point of view, once commented: "I myself have changed my opinion after reading the opinions of the other members of this Court. And I am as stubborn as most. But I sometimes wind up not voting the way I voted in conference because the reasons of the majority didn't satisfy me."[15]

Judges on state appellate courts appear to be just as willing to have their positions altered by arguments well seasoned by the spices of precedent and sound judicial reasoning. After interviews with supreme court justices in four states one scholar observed:

> When differences become evident, members of the court may attempt to persuade other judges to adopt their view by vigorously presenting their position or arguing the merits of their way of analyzing the case. Because of different amounts of influence exerted by the chief justice or by judges who have special personal status on the court, certain members of the court may be "persuaded" to abandon their own position and adopt the views of others.[16]

The persuasion-on-merits phenomenon can't be pushed too far, however. If the facts and legal arguments are straightforward enough, a justice may simply not be open to change. And judges who are deeply committed to a specific point of view or whose egos are sufficiently great will probably be impervious to legal arguments inconsistent with their own views. For instance, at the present time Justices Thurgood Marshall and William Brennan are profoundly and morally opposed to the principle of capital punishment and have often said so in their opinions. It is doubtful that any amount of legal reasoning or any calling up of "sacred precedents" could alter their belief that executions constitute "cruel and unusual punishment" by contemporary standards.

## Bargaining

*Bargaining* may sound like a strange word to use in talking about the personal interactions of judges on collegial courts. When students first hear the term, they often think of the vote-trading technique called *logrolling* that legislators sometimes use. For example, one lawmaker might say to another, "If you vote for a new federal dam in my district, I'll vote to build a couple of new post offices in yours." Is this what happens with judges, too? Is there evidence that they sometimes say to one another, "If you vote for me in this case, I'll decide with you in one of your 'pet cases' "? In fact, there is virtually *no* evidence for this in the judiciary. Bargaining does indeed take place, but it is more subtle and does not involve vote swapping. While some bargaining occurs in the give-and-take that goes on in conference, when the initial votes are taken, most is focused on the scope and contents of the majority (or even the dissenting) opinion.

To understand how the bargaining process works it is important to realize that usually much more is at stake in the outcome of a decision than merely whether party A or party B wins. Judges also have to discuss such questions as these: How broad should the decision be—that is, should we suggest in our written opinion that this case is unique, or should we open the gates and encourage other suits of this nature? Should we overturn what appears to be the obviously controlling precedent, or should we "distinguish around" it and let the precedent stand? Should we base our decision on constitutional grounds, or should we allow the victor to win on more technical and restrictive grounds? In other words, most decisions at the appellate level are not zero-sum games in which the winner automatically takes all; there are almost always important supplementary issues to be talked about or to be bargained for.

A landmark case of the 1970s provides a good example. In 1973 the Supreme Court handed down a joint decision on the matter of abortion.[17] To most citizens the only issue the Court had to decide was whether abortion was legal or not. While that may have been the bottom-line question, many other issues were in fact at stake, and the bargaining over them among the majority justices was intense.[18] What is human life and when does it begin? Should the decision rest on the Ninth Amendment or should it be based on the due process clause of the Fourteenth Amendment? Does a fetus have any constitutional rights? Is it a greater health risk to a woman to have an abortion or to deliver a child after carrying it to full term? Can a woman decide to have an abortion on her own or does a physician have to concur; if the latter, how many doctors need concur? And this by no means completes the list!

For the abortion case the justices spent over a year trying to hammer out a decision that would be acceptable to a majority. Draft opinions were sent around, altered, and changed again as the official opinion writer, Justice Harry Blackmun, tried to accommodate all views—or at least not to offend someone in the majority so strongly that he would join the dissenters. Woodward and Armstrong noted in *The Brethren* that the law clerks "in most chambers were surprised to see the Justices, particularly Blackmun, so openly brokering their decision like a group of legislators." [19] But the law clerks themselves were not immune to the bargaining process. In the Supreme Court's cafeteria, law library, and gymnasium the clerks asked one another whether "your Justice" could go along with this or that compromise or related that "my Justice" would never support an opinion containing such and such an offensive clause.

Bargaining of this nature is just as common on state collegial courts as it is at the national level. This statement by one state supreme court justice is quoted by a scholar who regards it as typical:

> You might say to another judge that if you take this line out, I'll go along with your opinion. You engage in a degree of compromise and if it doesn't hurt the point you're trying to make in an opinion, you ought to agree to take it out. . . . The men will write an opinion and circulate it. And then the other judges will write a letter or say at conference, can you change this or that, adjust the language here, etc. . . . Your object is to get a unanimous court. That's always best.[20]

With a significant portion of appellate court cases, then, bargaining is the name of the game—it is one way in which a group of jurists, in a unanimous or majority opinion, is able to present a united front. One classic study that focused on the Supreme Court has observed:

> For Justices, bargaining is a simple fact of life. Despite conflicting views on literary style, relevant precedents, procedural rules, and substantive policy, cases have to be settled and opinions written; and no opinion may carry the institutional label of the court unless five Justices agree to sign it. In the process of judicial decision-making, much bargaining may be tacit, but the pattern is still one of negotiation and accommodation to secure consensus. Thus how to bargain wisely—not necessarily sharply— is a prime consideration for a Justice who is anxious to see his policy adopted by the Court. A Justice must learn not only how to put pressure on his colleagues but how to gauge what amounts of pressure are sufficient to be "effective" and what amounts will overshoot the mark and alienate another judge. In many situations a Justice has to be willing to settle for less than he wants if he is to get anything at all. As Brandeis once remarked, the "great difficulty of all group action, of course, is when and what concession to make." [21]

Appellate judges do most of their face-to-face bargaining at the three-judge conferences and then iron out the details of the opinion later on using the telephone and short memos. As with Supreme Court decision making, a threat to dissent can often result in changes in the way the majority opinion is drafted.

> When a conservative minority sought to amend a middle-of-the-road compromise by which the 5th circuit achieved unanimity in the Mississippi school case, for example, a former legislator reportedly threatened to bolt to the left. "They came back into the fold in a hurry," a colleague remarked. "So you see, the judicial process is like legislation. All decisions are compromises." [22]

## Threat of Sanctions

Besides persuasion on the merits and bargaining, there is one other tactic that jurists use in their efforts to maximize their impact on the multimember appellate tribunals—the threat of sanctions. Basically there are three sanctions that a judge or justice can invoke against colleagues: the vote, the willingness to write a strong dissenting opinion, and the threat to "go public."

*The Judge's Vote.* The threat to take away one's vote from the majority, and thus dissent, may cause the majority to mollify its views. For example, back in 1889 Justice Horace Gray sent this subtle (or perhaps not so subtle) message to Justice Samuel Miller:

> After a careful reading of your opinion in *Shotwell v. Moore,* I am very sorry to be compelled to say that the first part of it . . . is so contrary to my conviction, that I fear, unless it can be a good deal tempered, I shall have to deliver a separate opinion on the lines of the enclosed memorandum.
>
> I am particularly troubled about this, because, if my scruples are not removed, and Justices Field, Bradley and Lamar adhere to their dissent, your opinion will represent only four judges, half of those who took part in the case. [23]

His back against the wall because of his narrow majority, Justice Miller was obliged to yield to his colleague's costly "scruples."

For the most part the potential effect of a threat to dissent from the majority depends on how small that majority is. Thus if the initial vote among a three-judge appellate panel were three-to-zero, the threat of one member to dissent would not be all that serious; there would still be a two-to-one majority. Conversely, if at a preliminary Supreme Court conference there were a five-to-four vote, the threat by one of those five to defect would be taken seriously indeed by the remaining four.

Sometimes, however, the impact of one's vote is not merely a function of how divided the court is. On occasion the perceived need for unanimity among the court may be so strong that *any* justice's threat to vote against the prevailing view may have a disproportionate effect. We know now, for example, that prior to the 1954 *Brown* decision, a majority on the Supreme Court opposed segregation in the schools. Chief Justice Warren and the other liberals believed, though, that a simple majority was not enough to confront the expected backlash if segregation were struck down; only a *unanimous* Court, they felt, could have any chance of seeing its will prevail throughout the nation. Therefore, the liberal majority bided its time during the early 1950s until the moment came when all nine judges were willing to take on the malignant giant of racial segregation.

A more recent example occurred when President Nixon declined to turn over the now famous tape recordings to the federal prosecutor. His refusal was challenged in the courts, and when the case reached the nation's highest tribunal, it became clear that only a unanimous court could effectively rebuke the chief executive and avert what was fast becoming a constitutional crisis. The colorful language of *The Brethren* tells the tale. When the eight justices (Justice Rehnquist had disqualified himself) met in conference to discuss the case, Justice

> Brennan saw the consensus immediately. The President did not have a single vote. Even more encouraging, there was reason to believe that the gaps among the justices could be bridged. A single opinion seemed within reach. That would be the greatest deterrent to a defiant President. Brennan decided to float again his suggestion of a single opinion, authored by, and signed by, all eight. Someone had to steer a middle ground between Powell and White—the emerging antagonists on the question of standards for Presidents and other citizens. The Court could erupt into a confusing mixture of opinions, concurrences and dissents. The Chief was not capable of preventing that, Brennan believed.
>
> Brennan spoke up. The Nixon challenge had to be met in the strongest way possible. An eight-signature opinion would do it. With the memos now in circulation, they could bang out an opinion in a week of concentrated effort. Each Justice might be given a section to work on, and they could convene in a few days to measure progress. Brennan reminded them of the impact of nine signatures on the Little Rock school opinion. It had been one of the Court's finest moments. The country would benefit from such a show of strength now.[24]

State judges, too, may well feel the need for unanimity in certain types of cases. For example, one New Jersey supreme court justice told a researcher: "We did have a case where we felt a unanimous opinion was necessary. No one felt strongly about a dissent, so no dissents were made. . . . A religious case, for example, needs a unanimous decision. Courts don't try to be divisive on this." [25]

Thus while the impact of the threat to abandon the majority is usually in direct proportion to the closeness of the vote, there are occasions when a majority will pay top dollar to keep any judge or justice from breaking ranks.

**The Willingness to Write a Strong Dissent.**   There are dissents and there are dissents. Appellate court jurists who intend to vote against the majority must decide whether to write a lengthy, assertive dissenting opinion or merely to dissent without opinion. For jurists who are not regarded by other justices—or by the public at large—as being prestigious or articulate, the threat to write a dissenting opinion may be taken with the proverbial grain of salt. If, however, potential dissenters are respected jurists with a reputation for a keen wit or for often being right in the long run, the situation is quite different. The other judges may be willing to alter their views to accommodate potential dissenters' positions or at least to dissuade them from attacking the majority position. As one court observer has noted:

> There are factors which push the majority Justices, especially the opinion writer, to accept accommodation. An eloquent, tightly-reasoned dissent can be an upsetting force. Stone's separate opinions during the thirties pointed up more sharply the folly of the conservative Justices than did any of the attacks on the Court by elected politicians. The majority may thus find it profitable to mute criticism from within the Court by giving in on some issues.[26]

Thus the second sanction—the threat to write a dissenting opinion— depends on the circumstances for its effectiveness. Sometimes it may be regarded as no more than a nuisance or the fruit of judicial egomania; on other occasions it may be viewed as likely to weaken the impact of the majority opinion.

With state courts the impact of a threat to author a strong dissent is smaller simply because dissents are more infrequent at that level. Consensus and unanimity are norms in most of the state appellate tribunals, whereas this is clearly not the case at the federal level. To be more specific, since the 1943 term at least 50 percent of Supreme Court decisions have produced dissents while the figures from the states reveal quite a different picture. Using data from the early to mid-1960s researchers have found that fewer than ten state supreme courts produced dissents in 20 percent or more of their cases, and only the high courts in Michigan, New York, and Pennsylvania produced dissents at or above the 40 percent mark.[27]

*The Threat to "Go Public."*    On rare occasions an appellate judge may use the ultimate weapon against colleagues—public exposure. Such strong medicine is usually administered only when a jurist believes a colleague (or a group of judges) has violated the basic rules of the game; the judge then threatens to hang out the dirty linen for all to see. For example, one appeals court judge told how, as a newcomer to the bench, he had threatened public exposure to force a senior colleague to withdraw an opinion filed without his consent, a possibility he had been warned against by another judge on the court: "It was my first sitting as a circuit judge," he recalled. "It was not a major case. But there was strong give and take!"[28]

In 1967, Judges John Danaher and Warren Burger (soon to be Chief Justice Burger) accused three of their appellate court colleagues of consciously attempting to foist on the Washington, D.C., Circuit a minority position on criminal procedures.[29] Ironically, some four years later it was Burger who was threatened with public exposure by a Supreme Court colleague who felt that Burger was trying to turn his minority status on a case into a majority position.

The incident occurred as follows. When the vote had been taken at conference on the abortion case, Chief Justice Burger was in the minority (the case was *Roe v. Wade*, considered jointly with *Doe v. Bolton*). According to Supreme Court practice, this would have meant that the senior member of the majority—in this case William O. Douglas—would have been assigned to speak for the Court. Ignoring Court protocol, Burger assigned the official opinion writing to his alter ego Harry Blackmun. This enraged Douglas. But the pot didn't really boil over until several months later when Burger lobbied from his minority status to have the case postponed until the next term. (Douglas wanted the decision to come down immediately.) These extracts from *The Brethren* capture something of the drama of the confrontation:

> This time Douglas threatened to play his ace. If the conference insisted on putting the cases over for reargument, he would dissent from such an order, and he would publish the full text of his dissent. Douglas reiterated the protest he had made in December about the Chief's assigning the case to Blackmun, Burger's response and his subsequent intransigence. . . . Douglas . . . continued: "When, however, the minority seeks to control the assignment, there is a destructive force at work in the Court. When a Chief Justice tries to bend the Court to his will by manipulating assignments, the integrity of the institution is imperiled."

Douglas's pen then became more acid:

> Borrowing a line from a speech he had given in September in Portland, Douglas then made it clear that, despite what he had said earlier, he did in fact view the Chief and Blackmun as Nixon's Minnesota Twins. "Russia once gave its Chief Justice two votes; but that was too strong even for the Russians." [30]

Douglas was ultimately prevailed upon to refrain from publishing this petulant opinion, but the illustration remains a classic example of the third sanction that one jurist can use against another—the threat to go public.

The threat to go public is probably a less potent weapon at the state level than it is with federal judges—particularly Supreme Court justices. This is because state appellate courts are generally much less visible to the general public except in the most unusual and controversial cases. Thus if a judge on a typical state appellate court threatened to go public and reveal to the populace some irregularity to which he or she had been subjected, the jurist might be told, "So, who cares?"

Despite the availability of several sanctions, it should be noted that they are usually invoked with varying degrees of hesitation—lest a judge or justice acquire a reputation for intransigence. For example, with regard to a justice's willingness to write a dissenting opinion, one perceptive scholar has noted:

> Although dissent is a cherished part of the common law tradition, a Justice who persistently refuses to accommodate his views to those of his colleagues may come to be regarded as an obstructionist. A Justice whose dissents become levers for legislative or administrative action reversing judicial policies may come to be regarded as disloyal to the bench.[31]

Or, putting it in more human terms, one appeals court judge observed that "you have to keep on living with each other. In the next case the situations may be reversed." [32]

## The Special Role of the U.S. Chief Justice, the U.S. Chief Judges, and State Supreme Court Chief Justices

As indicated in the previous chapters, the heads of the multijudge federal and state appellate tribunals have a number of special duties and responsibilities. At this point we shall examine their respective roles insofar as they constitute one more ingredient in the recipe for small-group interaction.

*The Chief Justice of the United States.*    The Constitution makes only passing reference to this official whose stature has come to loom so large in the eyes of the American people. Despite the constitutional slight, the chief justice can have considerable impact on the decision-making process. The key seems to be whether the chief justice possesses the capacity and the will to use the formal and informal powers that have accrued to the office during the past two centuries.

The chief justice's greatest potential for leadership is at the conference, where the cases are discussed and where the initial votes are taken among the justices. Because the chief has the primary responsibility for setting the agenda of the conference and traditionally is the first to offer an opinion about each case, the potential for influencing both the format and the tone of the deliberation is significant. As noted earlier, David J. Danelski has identified two types of roles for justices at conference: social leader and task leader. The social leader "attends to the emotional needs of his associates by affirming their values as individuals and as Court members, especially when their views are rejected by the majority. Ordinarily he is the best liked member of the Court. . . . In terms of personality, he is apt to be warm, receptive and reponsive." The task leader, on the other hand, is the intellectual force behind the conference deliberations, focusing on the actual decision and trying to keep the Court consistent with itself. Danelski describes how the two roles complement each other:

As presiding officer of the conference, the Chief Justice is in a favorable position to assert task and social ledership. His presentation of cases is an important task function. His control of the conference's process makes it easy for him to invite suggestions and opinions, seek compromises, and cut off debate which appears to be getting out of hand, all important social functions.[33]

One observer, commenting on the recent transition from the Burger to the Rehnquist Court, has noted these differences in leadership styles:

Differences are already apparent during oral arguments. Rehnquist is sharper, more thoughtful, more commanding and wittier than his predecessor in the center chair. And from the far right of the bench, Scalia almost bubbles over with energy and questions for counsel. No less revealing is that in the week before the start of the 1986-87 term on the first Monday in October, Rehnquist managed to get the justices to dispose of over 1,000 cases (granting 22 and denying or otherwise disposing of the rest). He did so in only two days, whereas it usually took Burger more than twice as long to get through about the same number.[34]

In the past the chief justice has also had a key role in setting up what is called the *discuss list*—that is, those special petitions selected out of the many to which the Court will give full consideration. The chief's law clerks obviously helped with this task, but the chief guided their judgment. Under the Burger and Rehnquist Courts the chief justice has played much less of a role in establishing the discuss list. At the present time a majority of the justices pool their law clerks and give a single clerk the authority to summarize a particular petition for all the justices who participate in the pool. However, the more liberal members of the Court (particularly Marshall and Brennan) refuse to participate in this practice—apparently because they mistrust the judgment of clerks serving under conservative justices. (Brennan examines each case himself when he has time, and Stevens has his clerks screen all petitions and write memos only on those they deem important enough for him to consider.) Whether the chief justice chooses to play a major or minor role in this process, the activity is important because it determines which cases the Court will consider as a group and which are to be summarily dismissed.

The final power of the chief justice is the assignment of opinions—that is, to designate who will write the official decision of the Court.[35] As noted earlier, this task falls to chief justices only if they are in the majority when the vote on a case is taken at conference; otherwise the most senior justice in the majority selects the opinion writer. The chief justices have the greatest control over an opinion when they assign it to themselves, and traditionally they have retained many important cases for that reason.[36] It will be recalled that in such cases as *Marbury v. Madison, Brown v. Board of Education,* and *United States v. Nixon,* the chief justice used his option to speak as the official voice of the Court.

Chiefs who choose not to write the opinion may assign it to that member of the majority whose views are closest to the dissenters', with the hope that some of the minority may subsequently switch their votes to the majority view.[37] Or, as has most often been the case in recent decades, chief justices will assign the opinion to an ideological alter ego so that the grounds for the decision will be favorable to their own.

When Warren Burger was chief justice, a new and somewhat unhappy wrinkle appeared in this overall process of opinion assignment. Using his option of being the last to vote on a case in conference, Burger occasionally sat back and waited to see how the vote was headed and then automatically joined the majority position—regardless of whether he had supported that position during the discussion of the case. This increased Burger's control over opinion assignment but at some real cost to the internal harmony within the Court. We get a flavor of this from the perspective of Justice Douglas:

> It took Douglas several moments to grasp the pattern of the assignments, and then he was flabbergasted. The Chief had assigned four cases in which Douglas was sure the Chief was not a member of the majority. These included the two abortion cases, which the Chief had assigned to Blackmun. He could barely control his rage as he ran down the list. Was there some mistake? He asked a clerk to check his notes from the conference. Douglas kept a docket book in which he recorded his tabulation of the votes. It was as he suspected. . . . "God, I miss Hugo," Douglas lamented to friends whenever Burger manipulated assignments. "Burger would never have dared pull that if Hugo were around." As senior Associate Justice, Black had helped keep the Chief within bounds. To Douglas's dismay, that role now fell almost exclusively to him.[38]

There is no evidence that Chief Justice Rehnquist has chosen to follow Burger's questionable activity in this regard.

Despite the considerable influence that a chief justice may have on the Court's small group, the crucial factor, as previously indicated, seems to be whether the chief has both the *capacity* and the *desire* to exert such potential authority. For example, the first great chief justice, John Marshall, possessed both these traits, and they helped fill the intellectual vacuum of the Court during the early 1800s:

> Marshall, like the majority of justices in the court's history, was an experienced politician. . . . He guided the court in a series of sweeping decisions . . . through force of personality and a talent for negotiation. Justice William Johnson, a Jefferson appointee, grumbled to his patron about Marshall's dominance. Wondering why Marshall invariably wrote the Court's opinions, Johnson reported to Jefferson that he had "found out the real cause. [William] Cushing was incompetent. [Samuel] Chase could not be got to think or write. [William] Paterson was a slow man and willingly declined trouble, and the other two judges [Marshall and Bushrod Washington] you know are commonly estimated as one judge." [39]

Although John Marshall had the skill and the desire to influence the Court, not all of his successors possessed these traits. For instance, the nation's chief justice between 1941 and 1946, Harlan Fiske Stone, had neither the talent nor the will for either task leadership or social leadership. As his biographer sadly wrote of him, "He was totally unprepared to cope with the petty bickering and personal conflict in which his court became engulfed." [40]

*The Chief Judges of the U.S. Appeals Courts.* As with the chief justice, the leadership potential of the administrative circuit heads is determined, in part, by their intellectual and negotiating skills and by their desire to put them to use. In reality, however, their potential effect on their respective circuits is probably less than the potential impact of the chief justice on the Supreme Court. First, since most appellate court decisions are made by three-judge panels on a rotating basis, the chief judge is not likely even to be a part of most cirucit decision making. Second, the circuits are more decentralized than the Supreme Court. Finally, the chief judge is not nearly so prominent a figure in the eyes of the public or of other government decision makers. Or, as one former chief judge said about the job: "The only advantage is that the title sounds more imposing if you are speaking in public or writing an article. Otherwise it's a pain in the ass." [41]

Much of a chief judge's work is administrative (such as docketing cases, keeping financial records, adjusting the caseloads), but it is also true that administration and policy making are not mutually exclusive endeavors. As the chief judge of the former U.S. Fifth Circuit once acknowledged: "So many times judicial problems slop over into administrative problems and vice versa" that the real questions are when and where this effect occurs. Commenting on the influence of the chief judges, one observer has said:

> As with strong presidents [or "as with strong chief justices," he might have added] . . . the spillover depends on the personality of the chief and the countervailing force of experienced colleagues. The impact of chief judges was most noticeable on freshmen and the composition of three-judge district courts. ("If all the judges are new, he'll pack a wallop out of proportion to one vote.") Southern judges made no bones about packing three-judge district courts in race relations cases. ([The liberal] "Tuttle was not about to set up a three-judge court with [segregationists like] Cameron and Cox on it; this occurs no more.") Of all administrative powers, plainly the most potent instruments of policy leadership involve the assignment of work.[42]

*The State Supreme Court Chief Justices.* To some extent the powers and leadership potential of state chief justices mirror those of the U.S. chief justice, but there are also significant differences, not only between the federal and state levels but also from one state to another. Recall that at the national level the chief justice is appointed by the president with the advice and consent of the Senate. In some states—Michigan, for example—the chief justice is chosen by fellow associate justices; in Texas and Ohio the chief justices are elected directly by the people.

The states also differ in regard to whether the chief justice has the most power in the assignment of opinions. There are only four states, including Hawaii, that follow very closely the opinion assignment practice of the U.S. Supreme Court. In more than a quarter of the states the chief justice assigns opinions in all cases, whether he or she is in the majority or not.[43] Well over half of the states use an automatic method of opinion assignment whereby a justice either draws cases by lot or, more often, receives them by rotation. In fewer than half of the twenty states that use the rotating system the assignments hold only if the justice to whom the case is assigned is in the majority.

On the effectiveness of the chief justice under the different opinion assignment methods, one scholar has concluded:

> A chief justice who is an extraordinary leader can make the court perform more effectively and efficiently by using selective opinion assignment. A court without an extraordinary leader may be better served by a rotational method of assignment. . . . Nondiscretionary methods best maintain social cohesion, but the chief justice's discretion in assigning opinions can best accomplish the efficient disposition of the workload.[44]

As with the U.S. chief justice, however, nothing inherent in the office guarantees that a chief justice will be an active and effective leader. Intellect, personality, political skills, and a fair degree of happenstance still churn and blend in mysterious ways to create chief justices whom court watchers term either "great" or "ineffectual." On the positive side there have been people such as Arthur Vanderbilt, who became chief justice of the New Jersey Supreme Court in 1948. As one scholar observed of him:

> Once installed as chief justice . . . he had to contend with a set of judges who had served under the old constitution and did not fully share either his vision or his aims. Nevertheless, Vanderbilt provided impetus and direction to the movement for judicial reform in the state, and, as chief justice, he secured the gains of the reform movement, gave the court stature, and ensured it the independence it needed to play a major role in the governance of the state. Despite the obvious differences, the comparison that springs to mind is with John Marshall, who—like Vanderbilt—assumed the leadership of a relatively moribund court and transformed it.[45]

Likewise one can point to Howell Heflin, chief justice of the Alabama Supreme Court, whose dynamic leadership and political skills during the 1970s brought about much needed judicial reforms in the state and effective leadership on the Court.[46]

On the negative side there are many examples of persons who came to the state high court bench with great potential but who lacked the ability or the political savvy (and perhaps the luck) to provide leadership in the wake of opposition or political lethargy. For instance, when Frank D. Celebrezze headed the Ohio Supreme Court during the early 1980s, he blatantly politicized the court until he was driven from office by the voters in the 1986 election. One observer summarized the unhappy period of his chief justiceship:

> Squabbles on the Celebrezze court were important because, owing to the Celebrezze agenda, the court was important. The irony of Celebrezze's stewardship is that as his court attained prominence, his actions, so visible on so many fronts, brought the court as an institution into disrepute. During [his term as chief justice] Ohioans perceived their court as a "circus." [47]

## Evidence of Small-Group Interaction

We have argued that small-group dynamics involve persuasion on the merits by one judge toward another, bargaining among the appellate jurists, and the threat of sanctions, such as a judge's vote, a willingness to write a strong dissent, and (at least for federal judges) the threat to go public. We have also contended that supreme court chief justices and chief judges of the appeals courts can potentially affect the decision making of their respective small judicial groups. The evidence we have cited for this so far has largely been anecdotal or subjective, but there are some more rigorous empirical data to back up our arguments.

One study compared U.S. Supreme Court justices' initial votes at conference with the final votes as they appeared in the published reports for the years 1946 to 1956.[48] Any change in the two sets of votes was attributed to small-group interaction. The findings tell us several things. First, there were vote changes in about 60 percent of all cases. Most of these changes occurred when a justice who had not participated in the first vote or who had been a dissenter opted to join the majority position. But when one considers all votes for all cases, the justices changed positions only 9 percent of the time. In such instances of vote change, the initial majority position lost out in only 14 percent of the cases. A study of conference and final votes surely underestimates the extent of small-group interaction, because there is plenty of such interaction prior to the initial conference vote. Many other empirical studies that deal with the federal appeals courts and with state supreme courts likewise suggest the importance of small-group dynamics as a factor in judicial decision making.[49]

Although it is unclear how many final outcomes are actually determined by small-group dynamics, we know that they are a major factor in the drawing up of the majority opinion and in setting forth its perimeters and corollaries. Scholars still lack a precise measure of the impact of small-group interaction, but it seems fair to say that it is considerable.

## Attitude Theory and Bloc-Formation Analysis

Many judicial scholars have been dissatisfied with small-group analysis, arguing that the fruits of such exploration are barely worth their efforts. While not denying that personal interactions make a difference in some cases and perhaps play a key role in a handful of decisions, they contend that the richest ore for explaining judicial behavior can be found in other mines. A decision-making model that claims greater explanatory power deals with the discovery of the justices' basic, judicially relevant attitudes and with the coalitions, or *blocs*, formed by jurists who share similar attitudes.[50] This approach rests on the assumption that judges—particularly appellate jurists—view cases primarily in terms of the broad political, socioeconomic issues they raise and that they generally respond to these issues in accordance with their own personal values and attitudes. The "official reasons" the justices give for their decisions (found in their published opinions) are regarded as "mere rationalizations." For example, let us suppose that Judge X strongly believes that the government should never tamper with freedom of the press. If a case comes before the court in which censorship is the central issue, then Judge X will go with his convictions and vote on the side of the news media. His written opinion may be full of impressive legal citations, quotations from eminent law reviews, or lofty discussions of the importance for democracy of a maximum of freedom of expression. But all this, the attitude scholars contend, is only a rationalization after the fact. The *real* reason for Judge X's vote was that he strongly dislikes the concept of government censorship.

The attitude theorists do not claim that their decision-making models explain everything, nor do they deny that judges must often decide cases *against* the grain of their personal values. For instance, a justice may be a strong environmentalist, but if a pro-environment petitioner has absolutely no standing to sue, it is not likely that the justice will yield to the tug of the heart. Nevertheless, supporters of the judicial attitude approach contend that it can explain a significant portion of judicial behavior and that it is well worth the research time and effort that such studies require.

Let us now examine some specific questions about this approach: Where do judicial attitudes originate? How does one learn about a judge's attitudes? What are some of the techniques that have been used to study attitudinal behavior and bloc formation? What have these techniques uncovered in terms of substance?

First, as noted in Chapters 8 and 9, appellate jurists acquire their relevant attitudes from the same sources that people in general do: from parents and friends, from educational institutions, from the media, from political activities, and so on. Thus, there is clearly an overlap between the attitude theorists and those who study judicial background characteristics. The difference is that the latter want to know *from where* the justices acquire their values, while the attitude theorists concentrate on measuring the effects of judges' values—regardless of their origin—on collegial decision making. The attitude scholars acknowledge that some beliefs change during the course of a jurist's tenure on the bench, but still they postulate "that attitudes are 'relatively enduring.' " [51]

Second, how can one compile a judge's attitudes in order to test for their manifestations in collegial court decisions? Unfortunately, judges have shown no willingness to answer the sort of in-depth questionnaires that might reveal judicially significant attitudes—particularly on matters that relate to issues that may come before them in court. Likewise judges are reluctant to give speeches, grant interviews, or write articles that bare their judicial souls. Judges consider such behavior inappropriate and many resist making it easy for reporters and social scientists to suggest a link between their personal values and the way they decide cases.

For the most part, scholars have turned to the contents of written opinions to categorize judges' primary values. Thus a justice who writes a strong opinion attacking government interference with the free operation of the marketplace is said to have a conservative economic attitude. This sort of approach has opened the researchers to the charge that they have created a tautology: A justice writes several conservative economic opinions; is classified as an economic conservative, and, lo and behold, aggregate analysis of his or her voting patterns reveals that the judge is a conservative on economic issues. Such theorists respond that this criticism is unfair because the patterns they have uncovered have proved to be consistent over time and susceptible to duplication by other researchers using similar methodologies. The next section will examine some of the research techniques that have been useful in measuring judicial attitudes and, in particular, the degree to which these attitudes cause likeminded judges to vote as blocs on similar cases.

### Content Analysis

One important method used by attitude theorists is *content analysis*— they search through hundreds of appellate court opinions for certain key words or phrases that indicate a particular judicial attitude.[52] For example, a judge whose opinions contain numerous references to "personal freedom" is probably going to be more of a civil libertarian than one whose published decisions are strewn with continual references to "law and order." Such an approach has been greatly enhanced by the advent of the computer; it has been possible to lay bare the attitudinal dimensions of scores of judges who jointly have rendered thousands of opinions.

## Bloc Analysis

The publication in 1948 of C. Herman Pritchett's *The Roosevelt Court: A Study of Judicial Votes and Values, 1937-1947* is regarded as the first attempt to study, in a rigorous, quantitative manner, voting blocs on the Supreme Court. Pritchett discovered two basic attitudinal coalitions on the Court: those who voted to sanction the liberal economic reforms of Roosevelt's New Deal and those who believed that such measures were unconstitutional. During the 1950s and beyond, the analysis of voting blocs based on similar attitudes became more sophisticated.[53] For example, researchers not only tested for the existence of a cohesive bloc on the Court, but they began to introduce such factors as an index of inter-agreement—that is, a mean agreement score of the justices in the bloc.

The dean of the attitude-bloc approach, Glendon Schubert, looked at the state of the art in 1974:

> Sociometric analysis of interagreement in voting behavior, which focused upon a pool of all the votes of all of the justices, in cases decided on the merits during a stipulated period, showed . . . that the Court characteristically divided into a liberal bloc and conservative bloc. But bloc analysis also showed that there were usually some justices who did not seem to affiliate with either bloc, and there seemed to be a considerable amount of inconsistent voting, even among the bloc members—inconsistent, that is, in the sense that in some decisions one or more justices would vote with members of the "opposing" bloc rather than with members of their own bloc. The latter findings were perplexing, and it was not until the introduction of more powerful research tools that they were understood. At first through linear cumulative scaling and subsequently through factor analysis and multidimensional scaling, studies of the voting behavior of Supreme Court justices have shown that there are three major attitudinal components of judicial liberalism and conservatism.

The three types of attitude dimensions developed by Schubert were political, social, and economic. The political liberal supports civil rights and liberties, while the conservative is more supportive of the law-and-order position. The social liberal upholds the egalitarian position on matters of voting, citizenship, and ethnic status; a conservative counterpart is more inclined to oppose equal access to the polity and the economic structure. Finally, the economic liberal is less of a defender of private property and vested interests than is a conservative colleague.[54]

The courts of appeals have also been subjected to bloc analysis during the past two decades, and there, too, researchers have been able to identify groups of judges with similar voting patterns on the same issue dimension.[55] Likewise state supreme courts have been subject to this type of analysis, with results similar to those for federal appellate tribunals. For instance, in an early classic study of the Michigan supreme court, Schubert demonstrated the existence of liberal and conservative blocs on a variety of issues such as workers' compensation cases and matters of contributory negligence in civil cases.[56] And more recent studies of the high court in Ohio have demonstrated the presence of ideologically based voting blocs.[57]

## Scaling

Almost simultaneously with the development of bloc analysis came the application of scaling techniques to the study of judicial behavior on collegial courts.[58] *Scaling* is founded on several basic assumptions. One is that there exists an underlying attitudinal continuum of beliefs about a given subject—for example, support for civil rights and liberties. In principle the stronger one's support for these freedoms, the higher one would fall on the scale. On a hypothetical 10-point scale a justice who was only moderately supportive of civil rights and liberties might be assigned a score of 3, whereas a justice who always voted on the libertarian side would be given a score of 10.

Scaling also assumes that there is a cutoff point somewhere along the scale for each justice—that is, the point at which the case stimuli will be so low that the justice will vote against rather than for the particular attitude dimension being studied. Judicial behavioralists like to use scaling because it permits them to predict how a judge or justice might vote (or would have voted) in any given case. For example, let us assume that Justice X can be assigned a 6 on a 10-point civil rights scale (with 1 representing total opposition to the cause and 10 indicating unqualified support for civil rights). Then let us suppose that a case comes up in which the stimuli to vote for the civil rights position will be only a 4. We would predict that the justice would *not* vote for the position because the stimuli to do so had not reached his threshold of 6. Scales are said to be accurate if their predictions are correct about 90 percent of the time, and to the delight of scholars most scales do meet this level of reliability.

Since 1946 two types of scales have worked particularly well in the analysis of nonunanimous Supreme Court decisions: the C scale (Schubert's scale for civil rights and liberties) and the E scale (Schubert's scale for matters in which an economic underdog is in litigation against a well-to-do opponent). Improving on his earlier analysis and techniques, Schubert developed what he called a "psychometric model." [59] In such a model justices hypothetically respond (in their votes) to various stimuli found in the cases. The key elements are (1) the nature of the stimulus and where it falls on the value continuum, and (2) the particular judge's attitude and where it appears on the value scale.

The use of the techniques of content analysis, bloc analysis, and scaling has greatly enhanced the capacity of judicial scholars to explain and predict the behavior of judges on collegial courts. One researcher, Harold Spaeth, has gained for himself a fair amount of popular acclaim for his accurate radio and newspaper predictions of pending Supreme Court decisions and votes. Using the very research techniques we have discussed here, he has scored hits on greater than 9 out of 10 predictions of judicial behavior.[60]

## Fact Pattern Analysis

There is another model for explaining the behavior of judges on collegial courts—*fact pattern analysis*. At first blush this approach seems to resemble that of the traditional legal subculture understanding of judicial decision making discussed in Chapter 9, because its central thesis is that the facts of a case are the primary determinants of how the case will be resolved. Recall that the legal subculture model contends that a judge will resolve an issue in favor of the side that is able to marshal the stronger set of factual evidence and legal precedents. While fact pattern scholars also believe that the facts of a case determine its outcome, they quickly part company with the traditional approach after that point.[61]

Several basic assumptions of the fact pattern approach set it apart from other models of judicial behavior. First, when fact pattern scholars refer to the "facts of a case," they have in mind quite a different set of items from the legal subculture adherents. "Facts" to these scholars include such elements as the gender of the litigants, whether an attorney in a criminal case is court appointed or privately retained, the social status of the parties, and whether the petitioner is a member of a racial minority. According to traditional scholars, such information is not supposed to affect the outcome of a case, but to the fact pattern theorists, cases are often won or lost because of just such extrajudicial variables. Let us look at an example.

One classic study using this approach focused on the voting behavior of Supreme Court justice Felix Frankfurter. The author found that Frankfurter was favorably disposed toward a petitioner in cases containing certain basic facts, or "signs," as the writer called them. The signs included the terms *confession-counsel*, meaning that the defendant's confession may not have been voluntary; *Negro*, indicating the minority status of the accused; and *state*, suggesting an insensitivity to correct criminal procedure. Referring to these signs, the study noted that there was

> a positive association between the presence of each and a favorable vote
> for civil liberties by Frankfurter in both years. Frankfurter's favorable
> vote was cast with the appearance of the 'Negro' sign in 13 of 15 cases;
> with the appearance of the 'state' sign 28 of 47 times; and with the

appearance of the 'confession-counsel' factor in 8 cases out of 9. These figures alone suggest that Frankfurter's willingness to draw negative inferences against a governmental unit in civil liberty cases might have been affected by the presence of these factors, with the presence of one or more of them improving the chances of a favorable vote.[62]

A second theoretical underpinning of fact pattern researchers is that they do not begin their analysis with any assumption

> regarding the existence or nonexistence of consistent patterns in the acceptance of facts or in decisions based on facts. Whether or not consistency does exist in a given area of adjudication is determined by the use of the methods. If consistent patterns cannot be identified, it must be concluded that judicial action in the given area of law cannot be understood in terms of the dependence of decisions on facts. If, on the other hand, consistent patterns are found, an important implication of the proposed methods is apparent. Should it be possible to predict only later cases from earlier cases, the underlying pattern of consistency could be explained in terms of stare decisis. But if earlier cases could be predicted from later ones, adherence to precedent would have to be explained in terms of an independent—although convergent—recognition and acceptance of similar standards of justice by different judges at different times. Thus not only the existence of consistent patterns but also the basis for their consistency can be evaluated.[63]

Finally, the fact pattern scholars believe that to explain judicial behavior they must learn how to weight each of the key facts of a case and also to learn how the facts combine to have the greatest (and the least) effect on any given judge. This is obviously a time-consuming and complicated procedure because the researcher is usually dealing with scores of possible facts and an enormous variety of possible weightings—combinations that literally run into the billions. Using sophisticated mathematical equations and the computer, fact pattern scholars have advanced into the unknown with considerable success. One of its key exponents explains how:

> Each case is represented by an equation, in which an index denoting the acceptance or rejection of a fact by an appellate court is set equal to the combination of appearances, nonappearances, and denials of the fact at the preceding stages. The weights of the fact at the various stages—in the sense of how persuasive its appearance at the respective stages is toward its acceptance by the appellate court—are the *unknowns* in the equations. As the equations are solved, the weights are determined. To be sure, the complex procedures which are required for the solutions of the equations again necessitate the use of a computer, especially because there is a separate system of equations for each fact. By using the weights in a case not previously encountered, one can predict for each fact an acceptance or rejection that would be consistent with the established pattern of past cases.[64]

Fact pattern analysis, like the other approaches to collegial court decision making, does not claim to explain the whole of judicial behavior. But like the other models discussed in this chapter, it has provided some key insights during the past several decades as to how and why appellate judges act as they do.[65]

## Summary

We began this chapter with the observation that decision making by judges on collegial, appellate courts is in some key ways different from the behavior of judges acting alone on trial benches. Because of these differences scholars have devised theories and research techniques to capture the special reality of decision making by jurists on federal and state multijudge appellate courts. We took a close look at the discretionary review process of the Supreme Court and noted that the issues it decides *not* to rule on are often as substantively important as those cases it selects for full review. In this context we discussed the importance of cue theory—the attempt by scholars to learn the characteristics of those few cases chosen from the many for Supreme Court consideration.

We then focused on three separate theoretical approaches to explain and predict the decision making of multijudge courts: small-group analysis, attitude theory and bloc-formation analysis, and fact pattern analysis. Each of these has its own working assumptions and research techniques used to glean the explanatory data. Although it is tempting to speculate on which of these several approaches provides the best insights into appellate court behavior, it is probably fairest to say that the jury of judicial scholars is still out.

## Notes

1. From an interview with an appeals court judge as quoted in J. Woodford Howard, Jr., *Courts of Appeals in the Federal Judicial System* (Princeton, N.J.: Princeton University Press, 1981), 135.
2. Alabama, for example, imposes a burdensome original jurisdiction on its supreme court, and Arizona requires its high court to hear appeals in a wide variety of cases. On the other hand, Florida has given its supreme court broad discretion in case selection. See G. Alan Tarr and Mary Cornelia Aldis Porter, *State Supreme Courts in State and Nation* (New Haven, Conn.: Yale University Press, 1988), 49.
3. Joseph Tanenhaus et al., "The Supreme Court's Certiorari Jurisdiction: Cue Theory," in *Judicial Decision-Making*, ed. Glendon Schubert (New York: Free Press, 1963), 111-132.
4. For example, see S. Sidney Ulmer, "The Decision to Grant Certiorari as an Indicator to Decision 'On the Merits,' " *Polity* 4 (1972): 429-447. Nevertheless, in a more recent study Ulmer found that despite the inordinate willingness of the High Court to hear cases brought by the U.S. government, such willingness did not translate into subsequent support for the government's position—at least in civil liberties cases. See S. Sidney Ulmer, "Governmental Litigants, Underdogs, and Civil Liberties in the Supreme Court: 1903-1968 Terms,"

*Journal of Politics* 47 (1985): 899-909.

5. For example, see Donald R. Songer, "Concern for Policy Outputs as a Cue for Supreme Court Decisions on Certiorari," *Journal of Politics* 41 (1979): 1185-1194, and S. Sidney Ulmer, "Selecting Cases for Supreme Court Review: An Underdog Model," *American Political Science Review* 72 (1978): 902-910.

6. Virginia C. Armstrong and Charles A. Johnson, "Certiorari Decisions by the Warren and Burger Courts: Is Cue Theory Time Bound?" *Polity* 15 (1982): 141-150.

7. Henry R. Glick, *Courts, Politics, and Justice*, 2d ed. (New York: McGraw-Hill, 1988), 232.

8. J. Woodford Howard, Jr., "On the Fluidity of Judicial Choice," *American Political Science Review* 62 (1968): 43-57.

9. For example, see Walter F. Murphy, *Elements of Judicial Strategy* (Chicago: University of Chicago Press, 1964); Bob Woodward and Scott Armstrong, *The Brethren: Inside the Supreme Court* (New York: Simon & Schuster, 1979); Howard, *Courts of Appeals in the Federal Judicial System;* Alpheus T. Mason, *Harlan Fiske Stone: Pillar of the Law* (New York: Viking, 1956).

10. In the parlance of judicial scholars, this is referred to as the *social leadership* function. See David J. Danelski, "The Influence of the Chief Justice in the Decisional Process," in *Courts, Judges, and Politics*, 3d ed., ed. Walter F. Murphy and C. Herman Pritchett (New York: Random House, 1979), 695-703. We will have more to say about Danelski's characterizations a little later in the chapter.

11. Henry Robert Glick, *Supreme Courts in State Politics* (New York: Basic Books, 1971), 59.

12. This is termed the *task leadership* function. See Danelski, "The Influence of the Chief Justice in the Decisional Process."

13. Howard, *Courts of Appeals in the Federal Judicial System*, 230-231.

14. Murphy, *Elements of Judicial Strategy*, 44.

15. As quoted in Murphy, *Elements of Judicial Strategy*, 44.

16. Glick, *Supreme Courts in State Politics*, 89.

17. *Roe v. Wade*, 410 U.S. 113 (1973), and *Doe v. Bolton*, 410 U.S. 179 (1973).

18. Woodward and Armstrong, *The Brethren*, chaps. entitled "1971 Term" and "1972 Term."

19. Ibid., 233.

20. Glick, *Supreme Courts in State Politics*, 66.

21. Murphy, *Elements of Judicial Strategy*, 57.

22. Howard, *Courts of Appeals in the Federal Judicial System*, 209.

23. As quoted in Charles Fairman, *Mr. Justice Miller and the Supreme Court, 1862-1890* (Cambridge, Mass.: Harvard University Press, 1939), 320.

24. Woodward and Armstrong, *The Brethren*, 309.

25. Henry Robert Glick and Kenneth N. Vines, *State Court Systems* (Englewood Cliffs, N.J.: Prentice-Hall, 1973), 79.

26. Murphy, *Elements of Judicial Strategy*, 63-64.

27. Henry R. Glick and George W. Pruet, Jr., "Dissent in State Supreme Courts: Patterns and Correlates of Conflict," in *Judicial Conflict and Consensus: Behavioral Studies of American Appellate Courts*, ed. Sheldon Goldman and Charles M. Lamb (Lexington: University Press of Kentucky, 1986), 200.

28. As quoted in Howard, *Courts of Appeals in the Federal Judicial System*, 209.

29. *Ross v. Sirica*, 380 F. 2d 557 (D.C. Cir. 1967).

30. Woodward and Armstrong, *The Brethren*, 187, 188.

31. Murphy, *Elements of Judicial Strategy*, 61.
32. As quoted in Howard, *Courts of Appeals in the Federal Judicial System*, 209.
33. Danelski, "The Influence of the Chief Justice in the Decisional Process," 696.
34. David M. O'Brien, "The Supreme Court: From Warren to Burger to Rehnquist," *PS* 20 (1987): 12.
35. For an excellent discussion of this subject, see David W. Rohde and Harold J. Spaeth, *Supreme Court Decision Making* (San Francisco: Freeman, 1976), chap. 8.
36. Elliot E. Slotnick, "The Chief Justice and Self-Assignment of Majority Opinions: A Research Note," *Western Political Quarterly* 31 (1978): 219-225.
37. However, some recent research has challenged the "conventional wisdom . . . that assignment of the majority opinion to the marginal member of the minimum winning original coalition might ensure its survival." In a study of the Warren Court the researchers found that "although the marginal justice is substantially advantaged in opinion assignment, coalition maintenance is not thereby enhanced." Saul Brenner and Harold J. Spaeth, "Majority Opinion Assignments and the Maintenance of the Original Coalition on the Warren Court," *American Journal of Political Science* 32 (1988): 72-81. Also, see Saul Brenner, "Reassigning the Majority Opinion on the United States Supreme Court," *Justice System Journal* 11 (1986): 186-195.
38. Woodward and Armstrong, *The Brethren*, 170-171.
39. Donald Dale Jackson, *Judges* (New York: Atheneum, 1974), 329.
40. As quoted in Danelski, "The Influence of the Chief Justice in the Decisional Process," 698. For a good recent discussion of the importance of Stone's leadership style as it affected future chief justiceships, see Thomas G. Walker et al., "On the Mysterious Demise of Consensual Norms in the United States Supreme Court," *Journal of Politics* 50 (1988): 361-389.
41. As quoted in Howard, *Courts of Appeals in the Federal Judicial System*, 228.
42. Howard, *Courts of Appeals in the Federal Judicial System*, 229. In a few instances the chief judges have been accused of "stacking" the three-judge panels, which are supposed to operate on a more or less random, rotational basis. For example, see *Armstrong v. Bd. of Educ. of Birmingham*, 323 F. 2d 333, 352-361 (5th Cir. 1963); 48 F.R.D. 141, 182 (1969). See also, Burton M. Atkins and William Zavoina, "Judicial Leadership on the Court of Appeals: A Probability Analysis of Panel Assignment in Race Relations Cases on the Fifth Circuit," *American Journal of Political Science* 18 (1974): 701-711.
43. Victor E. Flango et al., "Measuring Leadership through Opinion Assignments in Two State Supreme Courts," in Goldman and Lamb, eds., *Judicial Conflict and Consensus*, 217.
44. Ibid., 218-219.
45. Tarr and Porter, *State Supreme Courts in State and Nation*, 186.
46. Ibid., chap. 3.
47. Ibid., 148. For all the details, chap. 4.
48. Saul Brenner, "Fluidity on the United States Supreme Court: A Reexamination," *American Journal of Political Science* 24 (1980): 526-535.
49. For example, see Goldman and Lamb, *Judicial Conflict and Consensus*, pts. 2 and 3, and Glick, *Supreme Courts in State Politics*.
50. For a good discussion of the attitude approach to the study of judicial decision making, see Rohde and Spaeth, *Supreme Court Decision Making*, chap. 4, and Glendon Schubert, *The Judicial Mind Revisited* (New York: Oxford University Press, 1974). Also see James L. Gibson, "From Simplicity to Complexity:

The Development of Theory in the Study of Judicial Behavior," *Political Behavior* 5 (1983): 7-50.

51. Rohde and Spaeth, *Supreme Court Decision Making*, 75.

52. For example, see Glendon Schubert, "Jackson's Judicial Philosophy: An Exploration in Value Analysis," *American Political Science Review* 59 (1965): 940-963, and Werner F. Grunbaum, "A Quantitative Analysis of the 'Presidential Ballot' Case," *Journal of Politics* 34 (1972): 223-243.

53. For example, see Glendon Schubert, *Quantitative Analysis of Judicial Behavior* (New York: Free Press, 1959), and S. Sidney Ulmer, "The Analysis of Behavior Patterns in the United States Supreme Court," *Journal of Politics* 22 (1960): 629-653.

54. Glendon Schubert, *Judicial Policy Making* (Glenview, Ill.: Scott, Foresman, 1974), 160-161. For a good and more recent study of this phenomenon, see Craig R. Ducat and Robert L. Dudley, "Dimensions Underlying Economic Policymaking in the Early and Later Burger Courts," *Journal of Politics* 49 (1987): 521-539.

55. For example, see Sheldon Goldman, "Conflict on the U.S. Courts of Appeals 1965-1971: A Quantitative Analysis," *University of Cincinnati Law Review* 42 (1973): 635-658, and Charles M. Lamb, "Warren Burger and the Insanity Defense: Judicial Philosophy and Voting Behavior on a U.S. Court of Appeals," *American University Law Review* 24 (1974): 91-128.

56. Schubert, *Quantitative Analysis*, 129-141. For a more up to date analysis of the Michigan Court (as contrasted with the Pennsylvania Supreme Court), see Victor E. Flango et al., "Measuring Leadership through Opinion Assignment in Two State Supreme Courts," in Goldman and Lamb, eds., *Judicial Conflict and Consensus*, 215-239.

57. For a discussion of these studies, see Tarr and Porter, *State Supreme Courts in State and Nation*, chap. 4.

58. For a good discussion of scaling and its application to judicial studies, see Joseph Tanenhaus, "The Cumulative Scaling of Judicial Decisions," *Harvard Law Review* 79 (1966): 1583-1594.

59. Schubert, *The Judicial Mind Revisited*.

60. "Computer Helps Predict Court Rulings," *New York Times*, August 15, 1971, 1:75, and "Court Handicappers: Computer Predictions of Supreme Court Decisions," *Newsweek*, August 12, 1974, 53.

61. A recent study combined fact pattern analysis with a study of judges' background attributes. The researcher found that such a "combination . . . is more successful at explaining judicial voting in equal protection cases than either set of variables alone. This difference is particularly notable with respect to background variables. These traits alone allowed 63 per cent for the votes to be classified correctly, compared with 73 per cent of case variables and 80 per cent for a combination of the two sets of variables." Jilda M. Aliotta, "Combining Judges' Attributes and Case Characteristics: An Alternative Approach to Explaining Supreme Court Decisionmaking," *Judicature* 71 (1988): 277-281. Also see Jeffrey A. Segal, "Supreme Court Justices as Human Decision Makers: An Individual-Level Analysis of the Search and Seizure Cases," *Journal of Politics* 48 (1986): 938-955.

62. S. Sidney Ulmer, "The Discriminant Function and a Theoretical Context for Its Use in Estimating the Votes of Judges," in *Frontiers of Judicial Research*, ed. Joel B. Grossman and Joseph Tanenhaus (New York: Wiley, 1969), 365.

63. Fred Kort, "Quantitative Analysis of Fact-Patterns in Cases and Their Impact

on Judicial Decisions," in *American Court Systems*, ed. Sheldon Goldman and Austin Sarat (San Francisco: Freeman, 1978), 334.

64. Ibid., 332.

65. For other examples of fact pattern studies, see S. Sidney Ulmer, "Supreme Court Behavior in Racial Exclusion Cases: 1935-1960," *American Political Science Review* 56 (1962): 325-330; Stuart S. Nagel, *The Legal Process from a Behavioral Perspective* (Homewood, Ill.: Dorsey Press, 1969), chaps. 10-13; and Reed C. Lawlor, "Personal Stare Decisis," *Southern California Law Review* 41 (1967): 73-118.

# 11　Implementation and Impact of Judicial Policies

In the two previous chapters we have focused on decision making by judges. In this chapter we extend the discussion to examine what happens *after* a decision is reached. Decisions made by judges are not self-executing, and a wide variety of individuals—other judges, public officials, even private citizens—may be called upon to implement or carry out a court's decisions. As we study the implementation process we will look at the various actors involved, their reactions to judicial policies, and the methods by which they may respond to a court's decision.

Depending upon the nature of the court's decision, the judicial policy may have a very narrow or a very broad impact. A suit for damages incurred in an automobile accident would directly affect only the persons involved, and perhaps their immediate families. On the other hand, the famous *Gideon v. Wainwright* decision has directly affected literally millions of people in one way or another.[1] In *Gideon* the Supreme Court held that states must provide an attorney for indigent defendants in felony trials. Scores of people—defendants, judges, lawyers, taxpayers—have felt the effects of that judicial policy. As we discuss the implementation process, then, we will also look at the impact judicial policy making has had on society.

As noted above, a wide range of public officials, and even private citizens, may play a role in implementing a judicial policy. Lower-court judges, however, are so frequently involved in enforcing a higher court's decision that they deserve especially careful attention. Therefore, we begin our analysis of the implementation process with the lower-court judges.

## The Impact of Upper-Court Decisions on Lower Courts

As we noted in Chapter 2, Americans often view the appellate courts, notably the U.S. Supreme Court, as most likely to be involved in policy making. The trial courts, on the other hand, are frequently seen as norm enforcers rather than policy makers. Given this traditional view, the picture that often emerges is one in which the Supreme Court makes a decision which is then implemented by a lower court. In short, some envision a judicial bureaucracy with a hierarchy of courts much like superiors and subordinates.[2] Recent studies, however, have cast doubt on the bureaucracy theory, arguing instead that "most of the work of the lower courts seems less dependent on the Supreme Court than ... bureaucracy [theory] would indicate."[3] In other words, we now realize that lower-court judges have a great deal of independence from the appellate courts and may be viewed as "independent actors ... who will not follow the lead of higher courts unless conditions are favorable for their doing so."[4]

For example, it is well known that not all federal district judges immediately enforced the Supreme Court's public school desegregation decision.[5] Instead, some judges allowed school districts to engage in a variety of tactics ranging from evasion to postponement of the Supreme Court mandate.[6]

## Lower-Court Discretion

Why do the lower-court judges have so much discretion when it comes to implementing a higher court's policy? In part, the answer may be found in the structure of our judicial system. You will recall from our discussions in Chapters 2 and 3 that the judiciary has always been characterized by independence, decentralization, and individualism. Federal judges, for example, are protected by life tenure and traditionally have been able to run their courts as they see fit. Disciplinary measures are not at all common, and federal judges have historically had little fear of impeachment. To retain their positions, the state trial court judges do not have to worry about the appellate courts in their system, either. They simply have to keep the electorate satisfied. In short, lower-court judges have a good deal of freedom to make their own decisions and to respond to upper-court rulings in their own way.

The discretion exercised by a lower-court judge may also be a product of the higher court's decision itself. Let us look at a couple of examples. Following the famous school desegregation decision in 1954, the Supreme Court heard further arguments on the best way to implement its new policy. In 1955 it handed down its decision in *Brown v. Board of Education of Topeka II*.[7] In that case the Court was faced with two major questions: (1) How soon were the public schools to start desegregating and (2) how much time should they be given to complete the process? Federal district judges given the task of enforcing the High Court's ruling were told that the public schools were to make a prompt and reasonable start and then proceed with all deliberate speed to bring about desegregation. What constitutes a prompt and reasonable start? How rapidly must a school district proceed in order to be moving with all deliberate speed? Since the Supreme Court justices did not provide specific answers to these questions, many lower-court judges were faced with school districts that continued to drag their feet while at the same time claiming they were acting within the High Court's guidelines.

A second example concerns the Supreme Court's decision in the 1962 reapportionment case, *Baker v. Carr.*[8] In that case the Court held that allegations of malapportioned state legislative districts in Tennessee presented a justiciable rather than a political question; that is, apportionment cases could properly be litigated in the courts. The case was remanded (sent back down) to the federal court for the middle district of Tennessee in Nashville for implementation. Justice Brennan's opinion for the Court concluded with the statement, "The cause is remanded for further proceedings consistent with this opinion." No guidelines were provided for the federal district judge, who was not told how rapidly to proceed nor what methods to use. Justice Clark, in a concurring opinion, pointed out that the Court "fails to give the District any guidance whatever." [9]

It is obvious, then, that federal district judges implementing either of the policies described above could exercise a wide degree of latitude and still legitimately say that they were in compliance with the Supreme Court's mandate. While not all High Court decisions allow such discretion, a good number of them do. Opinions that are vague, ambiguous, or simply poorly written are almost certain to encounter problems during the implementation process.

A court's decision may be unclear for several reasons. Sometimes the issue or subject matter may be so complex that it is difficult to fashion a clear policy. In obscenity cases, for instance, the Supreme Court has had little difficulty in deciding that pornographic material is not entitled to constitutional protection. Defining obscenity has proven to be another story. Phrases such as "prurient interest," "patently offensive," "contemporary community standards," and "without redeeming social value" became commonplace in obscenity opinions. Obviously, these terms leave a good deal of room for subjective interpretation. It is little wonder that a Supreme Court justice admitted that he could not define obscenity but added that "I know it when I see it." [10]

Policies established by collegial courts are often ambiguous because the majority opinion is written to accommodate several judges. At times such opinions may read more like committee reports than forceful, decisive statements. Another situation that often occurs in a collegial setting is that the majority opinion is accompanied by several concurring opinions. When this happens, lower-court judges are left without a clear-cut precedent to follow. The death penalty cases serve as an example. In 1972 the Supreme Court struck down the death penalty in several states, but for a variety of reasons. Some justices opposed the death penalty per se, on the ground that it constituted cruel and unusual punishment in violation of the Eighth

Amendment to the Constitution. Others voted to strike down the state laws because they were applied in a discriminatory manner.[11] The uncertainty created by the 1972 decision affected not only lower-court judges but also state legislatures. There was a rash of widely divergent death penalty statutes passed by the states as well as a considerable amount of new litigation.

A lower-court judge's discretion in the implementation process may also be affected by the manner in which a higher court's policy is communicated. Quite obviously, the first step in implementing a judicial policy is actually to learn of the new appellate court ruling. Although we probably assume that lower-court judges automatically are made aware of a higher court's decision, such is not always the case. Certainly the court from which a case has been appealed will be informed of the decision. In our example above, for instance, the federal district court for the middle district of Tennessee was told of the Supreme Court's decision in *Baker v. Carr* because its earlier decision was reversed, and the case was remanded to it for further action. However, systematic, formal efforts are not made to inform other courts of the decision or to see that lower-court judges have access to a copy of the opinion. Instead, the decisions that contain the new judicial policy are simply made available to the public in printed form, and judges are expected to read them if they have the time and inclination.

Although opinions of the Supreme Court, lower federal courts, and state appellate courts are available in a large number of courthouse, law school, and university libraries, that does not guarantee that they will be read and understood. The problem is especially acute for judges in rural areas. One study reported that copies of the *United States Reports*, which contain Supreme Court decisions, are available in only three cities in the entire state of Wyoming.[12] Further complicating things is the fact that many lower-level state judges, such as justices of the peace and juvenile court judges, are nonlawyers who have little interest or skill in reading complex judicial decisions.[13] Finally, even those judges who have an interest in higher-court decisions and the ability to understand them do not have adequate time to keep abreast of all the new opinions.

Given the problems described above, how do judges become aware of upper-court decisions? One way is through lawyers presenting cases in the lower courts. It is generally assumed that the opposing attorneys will present relevant precedents in their arguments before the judge. As we noted in Chapter 3, those judges who are fortunate enough to have law clerks may also rely upon them to search out recent decisions from higher courts.

Thus some higher-court policies are not quickly and strictly enforced simply because lower-court judges are not aware of them. Even those which they are aware of may not be as clear as a lower-court judge might like. Either reason contributes to the discretion exercised by lower-court judges placed in the position of having to implement judicial policies.

## Interpretation by Lower Courts

A recent study notes that "important policy announcements almost always require interpretation by someone other than the policy maker." [14] This is certainly true in the case of judicial policies established by appellate courts. Thus the first exercise of a lower-court judge's discretion may be to interpret what the higher court's decision actually means.

Consider for a moment an example from a famous Supreme Court decision concerning what types of speech are protected by the Constitution. In a 1919 case the Court announced that "the question in every case is whether the words used are used in such circumstances and are of such a nature as to create a clear and present danger that they will bring about the substantive evils that Congress has a right to prevent." [15] With that statement the Court announced what is known as the "clear-and-present-danger" doctrine. Although it may seem simple in the abstract to say that a person's right to speak is protected unless the words create a "clear and present danger," lower-court judges do not decide cases in the abstract. They must fit higher-court policy decisions to the concrete facts of an actual case. Place yourself in the position of a lower-court judge deciding a case shortly after the announcement of the clear-and-present-danger policy. Assume that you were presiding over the trial of an individual who, in the course of a speech to a group of onlookers on a busy street corner in a large city, advocated violent overthrow of the U.S. government. You might well have had to answer one or more of the following questions in your own mind as you tried to interpret the clear-and-present-danger doctrine: (1) How well defined must the danger be in order for it to be clear? (2) How imminent must the danger be in order for it to be present? (3) Is the danger in question one the government has a right to prevent? (4) Did the speech actually bring about any danger? (5) At what point is the government allowed to intervene or stop the speech? As you can see, interpreting what is meant by the clear-and-present-danger policy is no simple task. In fact, modern courts grapple with the free speech question just as did the courts in 1919.

The manner in which a lower-court judge interprets a policy established by an upper court depends upon many factors. We have already noted that many policies are simply not clearly stated. Thus reasonable people may disagree over the proper interpretation. Even policy pronouncements that do not suffer from ambiguity, however, are sometimes interpreted differently by different judges.

A judge's own personal policy preferences will also have an effect upon the interpretation he or she gives to an upper-court policy. We saw in

Chapters 8, 9, and 10 that judges come to the courts with their own unique background characteristics. Some are Republican, others are Democrats; one judge may be liberal, another conservative. They come from different regions of the country. Some have been prosecutors; others have been primarily defense lawyers or corporate lawyers. In short, their backgrounds may influence their own particular policy preferences. Thus the lower-court judges, given their wide latitude anyway, may read their own ideas into an upper-court policy. The result is that a policy may be enthusiastically embraced by some judges yet totally rejected by others.

## Strategies Employed by Lower Courts

We have seen that appellate court policies are open to different interpretations; so we now turn our attention to the actual strategies employed by the implementing judges. Those who favor and accept a higher court's policy will naturally try to enforce it and perhaps even expand upon it. On the other hand, a judge who does not like an upper court's policy decision may well implement it sparingly or only under duress.

We first examine the strategies that may be employed by a judge who basically disagrees with a policy established by an upper court. One rarely used strategy is defiance, whereby a judge simply does not apply the higher court's policy in a case before a lower court. A recent study of judicial implementation offers this example:

> Desegregation brought out considerable trial court defiance; in one extreme case, a Birmingham, Alabama, municipal judge not only refused to follow Supreme Court decisions desegregating municipal facilities but also declared the Fourteenth Amendment unconstitutional.[16]

Such outright defiance is highly unusual, since there are other strategies that are not quite so extreme. For example, a study of the libel decisions of the U.S. courts of appeals between 1964 and 1974 did not find a single case of noncompliance with Supreme Court mandates.[17] Another study, focusing on compliance with the Supreme Court's *Miranda* decision, found only one instance of noncompliance among 120 cases decided by the courts of appeals in 1968.[18]

Another strategy often employed by judges not favorably inclined toward an upper-court policy is simply to avoid having to apply the policy. Sometimes a case may be disposed of on technical or procedural grounds so that the judge does not have to rule on the actual merits of the case. It may be determined, for example, that the plaintiff does not have standing to sue or that the case has become moot because the issue was resolved before the trial commenced. Lower-court judges sometimes avoid accepting a policy by declaring a portion of the upper-court decision to be "dicta." *Dicta* refers to the part of the opinion that does not contribute to the central logic of the decision. It may be useful as guidance but is not seen as binding. Obviously, what constitutes dicta is open to varying interpretations.

Yet another strategy often employed by judges who are in basic disagreement with a judicial policy is to apply it as narrowly as possible. One method of accomplishing this is for the lower-court judge to rule that a precedent is not controlling because there are factual differences between the higher-court case and the case before the lower courts. In other words, because the two cases may be distinguished, the precedent does not have to be followed. Let's look at an example.

In its *Miranda* decision the Supreme Court held that suspects taken into custody must be advised of their constitutional rights and that any confession made by a suspect who has not been so advised is invalid. A leading judicial scholar notes that some judges saw *custody* as the key word, and he provides several examples of situations in which *Miranda* was distinguished and therefore not applied:

1. Detention and interrogation at the Mexican border leading to a seizure of heroin and cocaine held not custodial.
2. A request for proof of ownership of a car on the street held not custodial.
3. Questioning of an erratic driver at roadside, with lack of *Miranda* warnings, did not void a conviction, although the policeman did intend to arrest, because he had not told driver he was free to go.
4. Questioning of the wife of a stabbing victim at the station house, when the interrogation had not focused on her, held noncustodial.[19]

State court judges faced with interpreting or implementing civil liberties policies often rely on what is termed "new judicial federalism."[20] This idea originated in the early 1970s, primarily in response to Warren Burger's appointment as chief justice of the U.S. Supreme Court. Many civil libertarians, fearful that the new Burger Court would erode or overturn major Warren Court decisions, began to look to state bills of rights as alternative bases for their court claims. The Burger Court in fact encouraged a return to state constitutions by pointing out that the states could offer greater protection under their own bills of rights than was available under the federal Bill of Rights.

In the beginning, state civil liberties suits focused most frequently on the rights of defendants, and only the supreme courts of California and New Jersey showed much interest in new judicial federalism. Initially, courts used this approach to circumvent specific Burger Court decisions. By the late 1980s, however, a national campaign to revive state civil liberties law was underway. Since 1970 there have been more than 300 decisions in which the state courts "have either afforded greater protection to rights under their state constitutions than was granted by the Supreme Court or have based their decisions upholding rights claims solely on state constitutional grounds."[21]

A recent study of state court activity involving new judicial federalism says that state courts have been most active in the areas of criminal justice and freedom of speech and press. The author also notes that state judges, unlike U.S. Supreme Court justices, are not constrained by considerations of federalism. Therefore, they may use their own state constitutions and go beyond federal court rulings that "underprotect" civil liberties.[22]

Not all lower-court judges are opposed to a policy announced by a higher court. Some judges, as we have noted earlier, have risked social ostracism and various kinds of harassment in order to implement policies they believed in but that were not popular in their communities.[23]

A judge who is in basic agreement with an upper-court policy is likely to give that policy as broad an application as possible. In fact, the precedent might be expanded to apply to other areas. Let's look at one instance of judges expanding a precedent.

In *Griswold v. Connecticut* the Supreme Court held that a Connecticut statute forbidding the use of birth control devices was unconstitutional because it infringed upon a married couple's constitutional right to privacy.[24] In other words, the Court said that a decision whether to use birth control devices was a personal one to be made without interference from the state. Five years later a three-judge federal district court expanded the Griswold precedent to justify its finding that the Texas abortion statute was unconstitutional.[25] The court ruled that the law infringed upon the right of privacy of an unmarried woman to decide, at least during the first trimester of pregnancy, whether to obtain an abortion. Thus the lower court actually went further than the Supreme Court in striking down state involvement in such matters.

## Influences on Lower-Court Judges

It should be quite evident by now that lower courts are not slaves of the upper courts when it comes to implementing judicial policies but instead have a high degree of independence and discretion. At times the lower courts must decide cases for which there are no precise standards from the upper courts. Whenever this occurs, lower-court judges must turn elsewhere for guidance in deciding a case before them.

A recent study notes that lower-court judges in such a position "may take their cues on how to decide a particular case from a wide variety of factors including their party affiliation, their ideology, or their regional norms."[26] Several analyses, for example, point out that differences between Democratic and Republican lower-court judges are especially pronounced when Supreme Court rulings are ambiguous, when there is a transition from one Supreme Court period to another, or when the issue area is so new and controversial that more definite standards have not yet been formulated.[27]

Regional norms have also been mentioned prominently in the literature as having an influence on lower-court judges when they interpret and apply upper-court decisions.[28] One study found, for example, that "federal judges tend to be more vigilant in enforcing national desegregation standards in remote areas than when similar issues arise within the judge's immediate work/residence locale." In other words, the prevailing local norms may mean that "when faced with desegregating his own community a judge may be more concerned with public reaction than when dealing with an outlying area."[29]

To this point we have examined only one actor in the implementation process—the lower-court judge. It is now time to turn our attention to others in the political system who influence the way judicial policies are implemented. We begin our discussion with Congress because it is the body that most often registers and mirrors public reactions to major federal judicial policies.[30]

## Congressional Influences on the Implementation Process

Once a federal judicial decision is made, Congress can offer a variety of responses. It may aid the implementation of a decision or hinder it. In addition, it can alter a court's interpretation of the law. Finally, Congress can mount an attack on individual judges. Naturally, the actions of individual members of Congress will be influenced by their partisan and ideological leanings.

In the course of deciding cases, the courts are often called upon to interpret federal statutes. On occasion the judicial interpretation may differ from what a majority in Congress intended. When that situation occurs, the statute can simply be changed in new legislation that in effect overrules the court's initial interpretation. A good example of this occurred in March 1988, when Congress effectively overruled the Supreme Court's decision in *Grove City College v. Bell*.[31] At issue in the case was the scope of Title IX of the 1972 Education Act Amendments, which forbids sex discrimination in education programs. In the *Grove City* case, which involved a small Pennsylvania college, the Court ruled that only the specific "program or activity" receiving federal aid was covered by Title IX. Under that interpretation only Grove City College's financial aid office was affected by the law. Many in Congress interpreted Title IX to mean that the entire college was subject to the act's prohibitions.

In order to overturn the Court's decision and restore the interpretation favored by many legislators, a bill known as the Civil Rights Restoration Act was passed by Congress. The bill was vetoed by President Reagan. However, on March 22, 1988, the House and Senate mustered the necessary two-thirds vote to override the president's veto. In this way Congress established its view that if one part of an entity receives federal funds, the entire entity is covered by Title IX of the Education Act.[32] Still, the vast majority of the federal judiciary's statutory decisions are not touched by Congress. A study focusing on the Supreme Court's labor and antitrust decisions in the 1950-1972 period found that only 27 of the 222 decisions were the objects of reversal attempts in Congress, and that only 9 of those attempts were successful.[33]

Besides ruling on statutes, the federal courts interpret the Constitution. There are two methods Congress can use to reverse or alter the effects of a constitutional interpretation it does not like. First, Congress can respond with another statute. After the Supreme Court struck down government prohibitions on abortion, Congress passed the Hyde Amendment and other laws restricting the use of federal funds for elective and therapeutic abortions. The Court, in later cases, indicated that the congressional action was constitutionally permissible.[34]

Second, a constitutional decision can be overturned directly by an amendment to the U.S. Constitution. Although many such amendments have been introduced over the years, it is not easy to obtain the necessary two-thirds vote in each house of Congress to propose the amendment and then achieve ratification by three-fourths of the states. In fact, only four Supreme Court decisions in the entire history of the country have been overturned by constitutional amendments. The Eleventh Amendment overturned *Chrisholm v. Georgia* (dealing with suits against a state in federal court); the Thirteenth Amendment overturned *Scott v. Sandford* (dealing with the legality of slavery); the Sixteenth Amendment overturned *Pollock v. Farmer's Loan and Trust Co.* (pertaining to the constitutionality of the income tax); and the Twenty-sixth Amendment overturned *Oregon v. Mitchell* (giving eighteen-year-olds the right to vote in state elections).

Congressional attacks on the federal courts in general and on certain judges in particular are another method of responding to judicial decisions. Sometimes these attacks are in the form of verbal denouncements that allow a member of Congress to let off steam over a decision or series of decisions. For example, a member of the House once expressed his disapproval of the Supreme Court by declaring that it was "a greater threat to this Union than the entire confines of Soviet Russia."[35]

Federal judges may be impeached and removed from office by Congress. Although the congressional bark may be worse than its bite in the use of this weapon, it is still a part of its overall arsenal, and the impeachments of three federal judges in recent years serve as a reminder of that fact.

Finally, the confirmation process offers a chance for an attack on the courts. As a new federal judicial appointee goes through hearings in the Senate, individual senators sometimes use the opportunity to denounce individual judges or specific decisions. Without doubt, the most observed hearings in history involved President Reagan's nomination of Judge Robert Bork (of the D.C. Circuit Court of Appeals) to a position as an associate justice of the Supreme Court. A number of senators on the Judiciary Committee took Judge Bork to task for opinions he had written in specific cases, his writings while he served as a law professor at Yale University, and his views on several controversial Supreme Court decisions (notably *Roe v. Wade*).[36]

It should be noted, however, that Congress and the federal courts are not natural adversaries even though it occasionally may appear that way. Retaliations against the federal judiciary are fairly rare, and often the two branches work in harmony toward similar policy goals. For example, Congress played a key role in implementing the Supreme Court's school desegregation policy by enacting the Civil Rights Act of 1964, which empowered the Justice Department to initiate suits against school districts. Title VI of the act also provided a potent weapon in the desegregation struggle by threatening the denial of federal funds to schools guilty of segregation. The Department of Health, Education, and Welfare was given the authority to compile desegregation guidelines as a basis for determining whether districts were complying with the law. That department met its responsibilities under the law by assigning personnel to visit the school districts. They investigated conditions in the district to see whether discrimination existed and, if they found that it did, they tried to negotiate plans to bring about desegregation. If such a plan could not be negotiated, an administrative process culminating in loss of federal educational funds was commenced. In 1965 Congress further solidified its support for a policy of desegregated public schools by passing the Elementary and Secondary Education Act. This act gave the federal government a much larger role in financing public education and thus made the threat to cut off federal funds a most serious problem for many segregated school districts.[37] Such support from Congress was significant because it has been noted that the chances of compliance with a policy are increased when there is unity between branches of government.[38]

A recent study lends support to the notion that passage of the 1964 Civil Rights Act was an important step in the implementation of a policy of racial equality. The authors examined minority discrimination cases heard by federal district courts during the ten-year period 1960-1969 and found that the cases decided in 1965-1969 (after passage of the 1964 Civil Rights Act) were significantly more liberal than those decided in 1960-1964.[39]

## Executive Branch Influences on the Implementation Process

At times the president may be called upon directly to implement a judicial decision. Such an example occurred in the famous Nixon tapes case, which arose during the investigation into the coverup of the break-in at the Democratic party headquarters in the Watergate Hotel.[40] As the investigation unfolded, it became apparent that the coverup led directly to high government officials working close to the president. It was also revealed during a Senate committee investigation into the matter that President Nixon had installed an automatic taping system in the Oval Office. Leon Jaworski, who had been appointed special prosecutor to investigate the Watergate affair, subpoenaed certain tapes that he felt might provide evidence needed in his prosecutions of high-ranking officials. President Nixon refused voluntarily to turn over the tapes on grounds of executive privilege and the need for confidentiality. The Supreme Court's decision—which, ironically, was announced on the day that the Judiciary Committee in the House of Representatives began holding hearings on whether to impeach Nixon—instructed the president to surrender the subpoenaed tapes to Judge John J. Sirica, who was handling the trials of the government officials. President Nixon did, of course, comply with the High Court's directive and thus implemented a decision that led to his downfall. Within two weeks he resigned from the presidency, in August 1974.

Even when not directly involved in the enforcement of a judicial policy, the president may still be able to influence its impact. Because of the stature of the position and the visibility that accompanies it, a president simply by words and actions may encourage support for, or resistance to, a new judicial policy. For instance, it has been argued that President Eisenhower's lack of enthusiasm for the *Brown v. Board of Education* decision and "his unwillingness to condemn southern resistance in more than a pro forma fashion encouraged Arkansas Governor Orval Faubus to block integration of Little Rock Central High School in 1957." [41] As a consequence, Eisenhower was later forced to send federal troops to Little Rock to enforce the district court's integration order. Sending in troops of course made President Eisenhower's participation in the implementation process more direct.

A president can propose legislation aimed at retaliating against the courts. President Franklin D. Roosevelt, for instance, urged Congress to increase the size of the Supreme Court so he could "pack" it with justices who supported New Deal legislation. President Reagan adopted this tactic in another way. He was a consistently strong supporter of constitutional amendments to overturn the Supreme Court's school prayer and abortion decisions.

The appointment power also gives the president an opportunity to influence federal judicial policies. Although the White House shares the power to appoint federal judges with the Senate, evidence points to the fact that the president dominates the process at the Supreme Court and courts of appeals levels. As we noted in Chapter 8, on the other hand, senatorial courtesy is a major consideration in the appointment of federal district judges.

During his campaign for the presidency in 1968, Richard Nixon made the Supreme Court an issue by criticizing the Warren Court for its liberal decisions and activist approach. He promised that, if elected, he would appoint "strict constructionists" to the Supreme Court and lower federal courts. In his first year in office Nixon appointed Warren Burger as chief justice and Harry Blackmun as an associate justice. Two years later Nixon was able to appoint another pair of justices—Lewis Powell and William Rehnquist.

How successful was Nixon in accomplishing his goal of altering the policy direction of the Supreme Court? One student of the transition from the Warren Court to the Burger Court says:

> The Burger Court, even before it consolidated its position and reversed precedents directly, showed through both doctrine and results considerable withdrawal from and undercutting of Warren Court policies affecting the entire range of civil liberties problems but particularly noticeable in the criminal procedure and free speech areas.[42]

Thus President Nixon was generally able to accomplish his goal for the Supreme Court. Also, the uncertainty and ambiguity in Supreme Court precedents brought about by the transition from the Warren Court to the Burger Court left the lower federal courts with more discretion. A study of the federal district courts, for example, says:

> With the advent of the Burger Court, the trial court jurists could no longer count on the Supreme Court for as clear and unambiguous legal guidelines as they had received from the Warren Court's more stable majority. With the decline of the fact-law congruence after 1968 the trial court judges became more free to take their decision-making cues from personal-partisan values rather than from guidelines set forth by the High Court. Consequently, the level of partisan voting increased markedly.[43]

Presidents have long realized that lower federal judges are important in the judicial policy-making process. For this reason, as we noted in Chapter 8, many chief executives have shown an interest in appointing lower court judges who share their basic ideologies and values.[44] A study of the opinions of federal district judges appointed by Presidents Wilson through Ford confirms that "to a noticeable and substantively significant degree, the appointing president does have an ideological impact on the output of the trial court judiciary."[45] Another study focused on support for criminal defendants in decisions handed down by the federal district appointees of Presidents Nixon, Johnson, and Kennedy. The authors noted that presidential influence is shaped by several legal and extralegal factors, some beyond White House control. Still, they concluded that "the value basis of presidential appointment is reflected in the subsequent policy choices of district court appointees."[46]

The most careful screening of lower-court nominees in recent times, however, has been carried out by the Reagan administration.[47] The Reagan team established the Office of Legal Policy to screen potential judicial nominees for ideological compatibility with the president. Furthermore, recent studies of the voting patterns of lower federal judges show that the Reagan appointees differ significantly from those placed on the bench by Jimmy Carter or other recent presidents of either party.[48]

A president can also influence judicial policy making through the activities of the Justice Department, a part of the executive branch that we discussed briefly in Chapter 4. The attorney general and staff subordinates can emphasize specific issues according to the overall policy goals of the president. Recall, for example, that the 1964 Civil Rights Act authorized the Justice Department to file school desegregation suits. This allowed the executive branch to become more actively involved in implementing the policy goal of racial equality. The other side of the coin, however, is the fact that the Justice Department may, at its discretion, deemphasize specific policies by not pursuing them vigorously in the courts. The Nixon administration was accused of applying the brakes to the momentum that had developed in the effort to desegregate southern public schools.[49]

Another official discussed in Chapter 4 who is in a position to influence judicial policy making is the solicitor general. Historically, this official has been seen as having dual responsibility, to both the judicial and executive branches. Because of the solicitor general's close relationship with the Supreme Court this official is sometimes referred to as the "tenth justice."[50] In other words, the solicitor general is often seen as a counsellor who advises the Court about the meaning of federal statutes and the Constitution. As we noted earlier, the solicitor general also determines which of the cases involving the federal government as a party will be appealed to the Supreme Court. Furthermore, he or she may file an *amicus curiae* brief urging the Court to grant or deny another litigant's certiorari petition or supporting or opposing a particular policy being urged upon the High Court. The solicitor general thus reacts to the policy decisions of the Supreme Court.

In performing these functions the solicitor general traditionally "avoids a conflict between his duty to the executive branch and his respect for Congress or his deference to the judiciary through a higher loyalty to the law." [51] Recently, however, the Reagan administration was accused of trying to use the solicitor general's office to "campaign for the Administration's agenda in the Supreme Court." [52]

Many judicial decisions are actually implemented by the various departments, agencies, bureaus, and commissions that abound in the executive branch. In one instance, a Supreme Court decision called upon the U.S. Air Force to play the major implementation role. That case was *Frontiero v. Richardson*.[53] The *Frontiero* case called into question congressional statutes that provided benefits for married male members of the Air Force but did not provide similar benefits for married female members. Under the laws, a married Air Force serviceman who lived off the base was entitled to an allowance for living quarters regardless of whether his wife was employed or how much she earned. Married female members of the Air Force, on the other hand, were not entitled to such an allowance unless their husbands were physically or mentally incapable of self-support and dependent on their wives for more than half their support. Lieutenant Sharron Frontiero challenged the policy on the ground that it constituted sexual discrimination in violation of the Fifth Amendment. Her suit was filed in a federal district court in Alabama on December 23, 1970. It was not until April 5, 1972, that the three-judge district court announced its decision upholding the Air Force policy. Lieutenant Frontiero appealed to the Supreme Court, which overturned the lower-court decision on May 14, 1973. The Air Force was then required to implement a policy it had fought for nearly three years.

## Other Implementors

To this point we have concentrated primarily upon lower-court judges, Congress, the president, and others in the executive branch as interpreters and implementors of judicial policies. There are, of course, many other actors involved in the implementation process.[54]

While our focus thus far has been primarily on various federal officials, it should be noted that implementation of judicial policies is often performed by state officials as well. Many of the Supreme Court's criminal due process decisions, such as *Gideon v. Wainwright* and *Miranda v. Arizona*, have been enforced by state court judges and other state officials. State and local police officers, for instance, have played a major role in implementing the *Miranda* requirement that criminal suspects must be advised of their rights. The *Gideon* ruling that an attorney must be provided at state expense for indigent defendants in felony trials has been implemented by public defenders, local bar associations, and individual court-appointed lawyers.

State legislators and executives are also frequently drawn into the implementation process, quite often as unwilling participants. A judge who determines that a wrong has been committed may use the power to issue an equitable decree as a way of remedying the wrong. The range of remedies available is broad since cases vary in the issues they raise and the types of relief sought. Among the more common affirmative remedy options from which a judge may choose are process remedies, performance standards, and specified remedial actions.[55] *Process remedies* involve providing for such things as advisory committees, citizen participation, educational programs, evaluation committees, dispute resolution procedures, and special masters; the remedies do not specify a particular form of action. *Performance standards* call for specific remedies—a certain number of housing units or schools or a certain level of staffing in a prison or mental health facility; the specific means of attaining these goals are left to the discretion of the officials named in the suit. Examples of *specified remedial actions* are school busing, altered school attendance zones, and changes in the size and condition of prison cells or hospital rooms. This type of remedy provides the defendant with no flexibility concerning the specific remedy or the means of attaining it.

Implementation of these remedial decrees often falls, at least partially, to the state legislatures. An order calling for a certain number of prison cells or a certain number of guards in the prison system might require new state expenditures, which the legislature would have to fund. Similarly, an order to construct more modern mental health facilities or provide more modern equipment would mean an increase in state expenditures. Governors would also naturally be involved in carrying out these types of remedial decrees since they typically are heavily involved in state budgeting procedures. Also, they may sign or veto laws. Some even have an item veto power, which permits them to veto certain budget items while approving others.

Sometimes judges appoint certain individuals to assist in carrying out the remedial decree. Special masters are usually given some decision-making authority. Court-appointed monitors are also used in some situations, but they do not relieve the judge of decision-making responsibilities. Instead, the monitor is an information gatherer who reports on the defendant's progress in complying with the remedial decree. In some circumstances a judge may name someone as a receiver. This person is employed when there is a failure to implement orders or because barriers of one kind or another block progress in providing a remedy. A good example occurred in the 1970s when the fights within Alabama's mental health agencies and facilities made it virtually impossible to obtain the action Judge Frank Johnson wanted. Finally, Judge Johnson ordered the governor to take over as receiver and empowered him to disregard normal organizational barriers.[56]

While space does not permit us to discuss every state and local public official in the implementation process, one group of individuals has been so deeply involved in implementing judicial policies that we feel compelled to deal with them here, if only briefly. These implementors are the thousands of men and women who constitute school boards throughout the country.

Two major policy areas stand out as having embroiled school board members in considerable controversy as they faced the inevitable task of trying to carry out Supreme Court policy. First, when the High Court ruled in 1954 that segregation has no place in the public schools, it was school boards and school superintendents, along with federal district judges, who bore the brunt of implementing that decision.[57] Their role in this process has affected the lives of millions of schoolchildren, parents, and taxpayers all over America.

The second area that has involved school boards is the Supreme Court's policies on religion in the public schools. In *Engel v. Vitale* the Court held unconstitutional a New York requirement that a state-written prayer be recited daily in the public schools.[58] Some school districts responded to the decision by requiring instead the recitation of a Bible verse or the Lord's Prayer. Their reasoning was that since the state did not write the Lord's Prayer or the Bible, they were not violating the Court's policy. A year later the Supreme Court struck down these new practices, pointing out that the constitutional violation lay in endorsing the religious activity and did not depend on whether the state had written the prayer.[59] Some school districts continued to evade the spirit, if not the letter, of the High Court's policy by requiring a period of silent meditation during which students could pray if they wished. The Alabama silent meditation law was declared void by the Supreme Court June 4, 1985, because students were instructed that they could use the time for prayer. This action was said to unconstitutionally endorse religion as a "favored practice." The Court indicated, however, that "moment of silence" laws not endorsing prayer would pass constitutional muster.[60]

Both of these policy areas involve basically private citizens—school board officials—in implementing controversial, emotion-charged policies that they may neither clearly understand nor agree with. The lack of understanding of the Supreme Court's school prayer decisions, for example, led some school districts to take no action at all, while other school boards placed a ban on all religious activities.[61]

## The Impact of Judicial Policies

Thus far, we have focused primarily on the implementation of judicial policies by various government officials. This is entirely appropriate, since court decisions are often specifically directed at other public policy makers. However, as a recent study of the Supreme Court tells us, "the ultimate importance of the Court's decisions rests primarily on their impact outside government, on American society as a whole." [62] We will explore briefly a few policies that have had significant effects on "society as a whole": the courts' role in developing a policy of racial equality, legislative reapportionment, criminal due process, and abortion.

### Racial Equality

Not long ago, one team of judicial impact scholars said:

> Perhaps the judiciary's biggest impact on modern America came in the *Brown* decision, which initiated the drive for racial equality. However, it took the active participation of Congress and the president to sustain this effort and ensure substantial implementation of such policies. The state of race relations in America might be quite different if the courts had ignored the issue, but it also might be different if Congress and the president had not joined the effort.[63]

Quite clearly, the United States could not have achieved as much as it has in the quest for racial equality had Congress and the president stayed out of the picture. However, as the statement correctly points out, it was the courts that initiated the pursuit for a national policy of racial equality with its ruling in *Brown*. Thus one of the most important ways the federal judiciary can influence policy is to place issues on the national political agenda.

In the beginning, the court decisions were often vague, leading to evasion of the new policy. The Supreme Court justices and many lower federal judges were persistent in decisions following *Brown* and in this way kept the policy of racial equality on the national political agenda; their persistence paid off with passage of the 1964 Civil Rights Act, ten years after *Brown*. That act, which had the strong support of Presidents Kennedy and Johnson, squarely placed Congress and the president on record as being supportive of racial equality in America.

One other aspect of the federal judiciary's importance in the policy-making process is illustrated by *Brown* and the cases that followed it. Although the courts stood virtually alone in the quest for racial equality for several years, their decisions did not go unnoticed. It is argued that "the psychological impact of the decision far exceeded its immediate legal consequences. *Brown* stood as a symbol to blacks and whites alike that racial equality now had an institutional champion at the highest level."

Spurred on by this knowledge, civil rights activists engaged in sit-ins, freedom marches, freedom rides, demonstrations, and other types of protests. Such actions "stirred up so much attention and emotion that the other branches of government could no longer avoid a major policymaking role." [64]

While no one would argue that the United States has achieved complete racial equality, some gains have been made. The federal courts are not totally responsible for those gains, of course, but they have played a major role in their achievement.

## Reapportionment

Prior to the involvement of the federal judiciary in the drawing of legislative districts, malapportionment was widespread throughout the states. The problem of malapportionment, which occurs when legislative districts with different populations have the same number of legislators, had become especially acute by the early 1960s because multitudes of people had, for many years, been moving from rural areas to urban areas. Failure of the state legislatures to take these population shifts into account meant that rural areas with small populations were able to elect many more legislators than the heavily populated urban areas.

In 1962, in the famous *Baker v. Carr* decision, the Supreme Court ruled that malapportionment presented a judicial question. The remedy eventually called for by the Supreme Court was reapportionment. However, as we noted early in this chapter, the case was remanded to the federal district court with no clear guidelines as to how the High Court's decision was to be implemented.

The Supreme Court, as it frequently does, developed more specific guidelines for the lower federal courts in subsequent cases.[65] In these follow-up decisions the Court instituted the "one-person, one-vote" principle for districts pertaining to both houses of a state legislature and for congressional districts. The one-person, one-vote ideal is achieved, of course, by creating districts that are as nearly equal in population as possible. With considerable effort on the part of federal district judges, the state legislatures were eventually brought into compliance with the one-person, one-vote principle. Today, census updates dictate that state legislatures go through the reapportionment process periodically.

In one sense, then, the policy goal of the federal courts was realized. Changes in the makeup of state legislatures and the U.S. House of Representatives occurred. Furthermore, urban and suburban areas gained strength at the expense of rural areas in the legislative bodies.

In another way, however, the courts' reapportionment policy has not had the effect some expected. Many believed that state expenditures for such things as aid to the cities, public education, public welfare, and urb?

renewal would increase considerably. Examined from this perspective, we must conclude that the impact of reapportionment on the states has been rather modest.[66]

## Criminal Due Process

Judicial policy making in this area is most closely associated with the Warren Court period. Speaking of this era, a former solicitor general said, "Never has there been such a thorough-going reform of criminal procedure within so short a time." [67] The Warren Court decisions were aimed primarily at changing the procedures followed by the states in dealing with criminal defendants. By the time Warren left the Supreme Court, new policies had been established to deal with a wide range of activities. Although a complete list of the Court's decisions is too lengthy to discuss here, among the more far reaching were *Mapp v. Ohio, Gideon v. Wainwright*, and *Miranda v. Arizona*.[68]

The *Mapp* decision extended the exclusionary rule, which had applied to the national government for a number of years, to the states. This rule simply required state courts to exclude from trials evidence that had been illegally seized by the police. Although some police departments, especially in major urban areas, have tried to establish specific guidelines for their officers to follow in obtaining evidence, such efforts have not been universal. Because of variations in police practices and differing lower-court interpretations of what constitutes a valid search and seizure, implementation of *Mapp* has not been consistent throughout the country.

Perhaps even more important in reducing the originally perceived impact of *Mapp* has been the lack of solid support for the exclusionary rule among the Supreme Court justices. The decision was not a unanimous one to begin with, and over the years some of the justices, notably former chief justice Warren Burger, have been openly critical of the exclusionary rule. Furthermore, Burger Court decisions broadened the scope of legal searches, thus limiting the applicability of the rule. As we saw earlier in this chapter, ambiguity and the absence of clear guidelines from the High Court increase the discretion of lower-court judges who are asked to implement a policy.

The *Gideon v. Wainwright* decision held that indigent defendants must be provided attorneys when they go to trial in a felony case in the state courts. Many states routinely provided attorneys in such trials even before the Court's decision. The other states began to comply in a variety of ways. Public defender programs were established in many regions. In other areas local bar associations cooperated with judges to implement some method of complying with the Supreme Court's new policy.

The impact of *Gideon* is clearer and more consistent than that of *Mapp*. One reason, no doubt, is the fact that many states had already implemented the policy called for by *Gideon*. In other words, it was simply more widely accepted than the policy established by *Mapp*. The policy announced in *Gideon* was also more sharply defined than the one in *Mapp*. Although the Court did not specify whether a public defender or a court-appointed lawyer must be provided, it is still quite clear that the indigent defendant must have the help of an attorney. It should also be noted that the Burger Court did not retreat from the Warren Court's policy of providing an attorney for indigent defendants as it did in the search and seizure area addressed by *Mapp*. All these factors add up to a more recognizable impact for the policy announced in *Gideon*.

In *Miranda v. Arizona* the Supreme Court went a step further and ruled that police officers must advise suspects taken into custody of their constitutional rights, one of which is to have an attorney present during questioning. Suspects must also be advised that they have a right to remain silent and that any statement they make may be used in court; that if they cannot afford an attorney, one will be provided at state expense; and that they have the right to stop answering questions at any time. These requirements are so clearly stated that police departments have actually copied them down on cards for officers to carry in their shirt pockets. Then, when suspects are taken into custody, the police officers simply remove the card and read the suspects their rights.

If we measure compliance simply in terms of whether police officers read the *Miranda* rights to persons they arrest, we would have to say that there has been a high level of compliance with the Supreme Court policy. Some researchers, however, have questioned the impact of *Miranda* because of the method by which suspects may be advised of their rights. It is one thing to simply read to a person from a card, while it is quite another to explain what is meant by the High Court's requirements and then try to make the suspect understand them. Looked at in this manner, the impact of the policy announced in *Miranda* is not quite as clear.

The Burger Court did not show an inclination to lend its solid support to the Warren Court's *Miranda* policy. Although *Miranda* has not been overruled, its impact has been limited somewhat. In the *Harris v. New York* case, for example, the Burger Court ruled that statements made by an individual who had not been given the *Miranda* warning could be used to challenge the credibility of his testimony at trial.[69]

In sum, we would emphasize that the impact of the Supreme Court's criminal justice policies has been rather mixed. The reason for this assessment must be attributed to several factors. In some instances vagueness or ambiguity is a problem. In other cases it may be less than solid support for the policy among justices or eroding support as one Court replaces another. All these variables translate into greater discretion for the implementors.

## Abortion

In *Roe v. Wade* the Supreme Court ruled (1) that a woman has an absolute right to an abortion during the first trimester of pregnancy; (2) that a state may regulate the abortion procedure during the second trimester in order to protect the mother's health; and (3) that during the third trimester the state may regulate or even prohibit abortions, except where the life or health of the mother is endangered.[70]

The reaction to this decision was immediate, and primarily negative.[71] It came in the form of letters to individual justices, public speeches, the introduction of resolutions in Congress, and the advocacy of "right to life" amendments in Congress. As might be expected given the controversial nature of the Court's decision, hospitals did not wholeheartedly offer to support the decision by changing their abortion policies. In fact, one study, using a national sample of hospitals, found that less than one-half changed their abortion policies following the Supreme Court's decision in *Roe*.[72]

Response to the Court's abortion policy was not short-lived. It has not only continued but has moved into new areas. State legislatures have enacted numerous laws aimed at regulating abortion in one way or another, some of which have passed constitutional muster, others of which have not. Interest groups representing both sides of the issue are active participants in elections. The 1984 presidential election saw the two major party platforms take opposing stands on the abortion issue. The Democratic platform expressed support for *Roe v. Wade*, while the Republicans called for a constitutional amendment to protect the right to life of unborn children. This pattern was repeated in the 1988 presidential election. Democratic candidate Michael Dukakis expressed support for *Roe v. Wade*. Republican George Bush, on the other hand, supports abortions only in cases of rape or incest or when the mother's life is endangered.

Although the abortion controversy now exists in many political arenas, Congress continues to be a hotbed of activity. Unable to secure passage of a constitutional amendment to overturn the Court's abortion decision, antiabortion forces have used another approach. For several years they successfully obtained amendments to appropriations bills preventing the expenditure of federal funds for elective abortions. In 1980 the Supreme Court, in a five-to-four vote, upheld the constitutionality of such a prohibition.[73]

With its July 3, 1989, decision in *Webster v. Reproductive Health Services*, the Supreme Court reignited the controversy over abortion, which has smoldered for sixteen years. Although *Roe v. Wade* was not overturned, the Court, in a five-to-four vote, upheld several provisions of a Missouri law aimed at making abortions more difficult to obtain. Most significant perhaps was the majority's ruling that states may require doctors to determine whether a fetus at twenty weeks old is viable (capable of surviving outside the womb). The Court also indicated that abortion would get further attention in its next term. Slated for attention are cases from Illinois, Ohio, and Minnesota. More changes in abortion policy may be forthcoming.

## Conclusions

There is no doubt that some judicial policies have a greater impact on society than others. Because many reasons for this situation have been offered throughout this chapter, an extended discussion of them is not needed here. Instead, we simply want to offer some concluding thoughts about the ability of courts to effectuate changes in society.

Quite clearly, the judiciary plays a greater role in developing the nation's policies than the constitutional framers envisioned. Yet the courts are not as powerful as the rhetoric of some politicians would have us believe. The judiciary is but one of three coequal branches of the government and is subject to the checks and balances that may be exercised by Congress, the president, or others. The legal and democratic subcultures that have been discussed throughout the book also serve to limit the courts' policy-making powers.

Within this complex framework of competing political and social demands and expectations, however, there *is* a policy-making role for the courts. Because the other two branches of government are sometimes not receptive to the demands of certain segments of society, the only alternative for those individuals or groups is to turn to the courts. Civil rights organizations, for example, made no real headway until they found the Supreme Court to be a supportive forum for their school desegregation efforts. They were then able to use the *Brown* and other decisions as a springboard to attack a variety of areas of discrimination. Thus a champion at a high government level may offer hope to individuals and interest groups.

As civil rights groups attained some success in the federal courts, others were encouraged to employ litigation as a strategy. For example, several scholars tell us that women's rights supporters followed a pattern established by minority groups when they began taking their grievances to the courts.[74] In this manner, what began as a more narrow pursuit for racial equality was broadened to a quest for equality for other disadvantaged groups in society.

Clearly, then, the courts can announce policy decisions that attract national attention and perhaps stress the fact that other policy makers have failed to act. In this way the judiciary may invite the other branches to exercise their policy-making powers. Follow-up decisions indicate the judiciary's determination to pursue a particular policy and help keep alive the invitation for other policy makers to join in the endeavor.

All things considered, the courts seem best equipped to develop and implement narrow policies that are less controversial in nature. The policy established in the *Gideon* case provides a good example. The decision that indigent defendants in state criminal trials must be provided with an attorney did not meet any strong outcries of protest. Furthermore, it was a policy that primarily required the support of judges and lawyers; action by Congress and the president was not really necessary. A policy of equality for all segments of society, on the other hand, is so broad and controversy-laden that it must move beyond the judiciary. As it does so, the courts become simply one part, albeit an important part, of the policy-making process.

## *Summary*

We began this chapter by pointing out that judicial decisions are not self-executing. The courts depend upon a variety of individuals, both inside and outside the judicial branch, to carry out their rulings.

Lower-court judges are prominent in the implementation process. Our discussion of their role in carrying out decisions of higher courts emphasized the discretion they exercise. Factors that account for the flexibility that rests with the lower-court judge include the decentralization of the judicial system, ambiguity or vagueness in higher-court rulings, and poor intercourt communication. The chapter examined, as well, the strategies that balking lower-court judges may employ in resisting appellate court decisions they dislike.

Congress and the president may also be involved in the implementation process. Each of these two branches can react either positively or negatively to a court decision. The wide range of influences the president and Congress exert in enforcing a judicial decision were described in some detail.

It was also noted that some policies call upon state officials to take part in the implementation process. State court judges, for example, played the major role in enforcing the Warren Court's criminal due process decisions. Local school boards have also been called upon to carry out Supreme Court policies.

The chapter concluded with a discussion of the impact on society of several important federal court policies. Explanations were offered as to why some policies have a more obvious impact on society than others; most important, perhaps, is that if a ruling—like the Supreme Court's original decision on abortion—faces opposition, Congress and other implementors are likely to drag their feet. A final section of the chapter offered some concluding thoughts on the role of courts in bringing about changes in society. It noted that the judiciary can act as a kind of beacon for traditionally underrepresented groups seeking to achieve their goals.

# Notes

1. *Gideon v. Wainwright*, 372 U.S. 335 (1963).
2. For a good description of the bureaucratic theory, see Walter F. Murphy, "Chief Justice Taft and the Lower Court Bureaucracy: A Study in Judicial Administration," *Journal of Politics* 24 (1962): 453-476.
3. Richard J. Richardson and Kenneth N. Vines, *The Politics of Federal Courts* (Boston: Little, Brown, 1970), 144.
4. Lawrence Baum, "Implementation of Judicial Decisions: An Organizational Analysis," *American Politics Quarterly* 4 (1976): 91.
5. The desegregation policy was announced in *Brown v. Board of Education of Topeka*, 347 U.S. 483 (1954). For a study of the lower federal courts involved in implementing *Brown*, see Jack W. Peltason, *Fifty-Eight Lonely Men* (New York: Harcourt, Brace & World, 1961).
6. For an excellent account of the school desegregation struggle in Georgia, see Harrell R. Rodgers, Jr., and Charles S. Bullock III, *Coercion to Compliance* (Lexington, Mass.: Lexington Books, 1976).
7. *Brown v. Board of Education of Topeka II*, 349 U.S. 294 (1955).
8. *Baker v. Carr*, 369 U.S. 186 (1962).
9. Ibid., 237, 251.
10. The statement was made by Justice Potter Stewart in *Jacobellis v. Ohio*, 378 U.S. 184 (1964).
11. *Furman v. Georgia*, 408 U.S. 238 (1972). A good account of the various views held by the justices, as well as the behind-the-scenes events leading to the final decision, may be found in Bob Woodward and Scott Armstrong, *The Brethren: Inside the Supreme Court* (New York: Simon & Schuster, 1979), 205-220.
12. See Stephen L. Wasby, "The Communication of the Supreme Court's Criminal Procedure Decisions," *Villanova Law Review* 18 (1973): 1090.
13. For a good discussion of this point with pertinent examples, see Charles A. Johnson and Bradley C. Canon, *Judicial Policies: Implementation and Impact* (Washington, D.C.: CQ Press, 1984), 55-56.
14. Ibid., 29.
15. *Schenck v. United States*, 249 U.S. 47 (1919).
16. Johnson and Canon, *Judicial Policies*, 40.
17. See John Gruhl, "The Supreme Court's Impact on the Law of Libel: Compliance by Lower Federal Courts," *Western Political Quarterly* 33 (1980): 517.
18. See Donald R. Songer, "The Impact of the Supreme Court on Outcomes in the U.S. Courts of Appeals: A Comparison of Four Issue Areas" (Paper delivered at the annual meeting of the Southern Political Science Association, Birmingham, Alabama, November 1983), 6. The *Miranda* decision is *Miranda v. Arizona*, 384 U.S. 436 (1966).
19. Stephen L. Wasby, *The Impact of the United States Supreme Court: Some Perspectives* (Homewood, Ill.: Dorsey Press, 1970), 158.
20. See G. Alan Tarr, "Civil Liberties under State Constitutions," *The Political Science Teacher* 1 (Fall 1988): 8-9.
21. Ibid., 8.
22. Ibid.
23. See Peltason, *Fifty-Eight Lonely Men*, and Richardson and Vines, *The Politics of Federal Courts*, 98-99.
24. *Griswold v. Connecticut*, 381 U.S. 479 (1965).

25. *Roe v. Wade*, 314 F. Supp. 1217 (1970).
26. Ronald Stidham and Robert A. Carp, "U.S. Trial Court Reactions to Changes in Civil Rights and Civil Liberties Policies," *Southeastern Political Review* 12 (1984): 7.
27. See, for example, Kathleen L. Barber, "Partisan Values in the Lower Courts: Reapportionment in Ohio and Michigan," *Case Western Reserve Law Review* 20 (1969): 406-407; Robert A. Carp and C. K. Rowland, *Policymaking and Politics in the Federal District Courts* (Knoxville: University of Tennessee Press, 1983), chap. 2; C. K. Rowland and Robert A. Carp, "A Longitudinal Study of Party Effects on Federal District Court Policy Propensities," *American Journal of Political Science* 24 (1980): 301; and Ronald Stidham, Robert A. Carp, and C. K. Rowland, "Women's Rights before the Federal District Courts, 1971-1977," *American Politics Quarterly* 11 (1983): 214.
28. See, for example, Peltason, *Fifty-Eight Lonely Men;* Kenneth N. Vines, "Federal District Judges and Race Relations Cases in the South," *Journal of Politics* 26 (1964): 338-357; Richardson and Vines, *The Politics of Federal Courts*, 93-100; and Micheal W. Giles and Thomas G. Walker, "Judicial Policy-Making and Southern School Segregation," *Journal of Politics* 37 (1975): 917-936.
29. Giles and Walker, "Judicial Policy-Making and Southern School Segregation," 931.
30. For a good study of the relationship between Congress and the Supreme Court, see John R. Schmidhauser and Larry L. Berg, *The Supreme Court and Congress: Conflict and Interaction, 1945-1968* (New York: Free Press, 1972).
31. 465 U.S. 555 (1984).
32. See *Congressional Quarterly Weekly Report*, March 12, 1988, 677; and March 26, 1988, 774, for accounts of the hearings.
33. Beth M. Henschen, "Statutory Interpretations of the Supreme Court: Congressional Response," *American Politics Quarterly* 11 (1983): 441-458.
34. See *Maher v. Roe*, 432 U.S. 464 (1977), and *Harris v. McRae*, 448 U.S. 297 (1980).
35. Quoted in Lawrence Baum, *The Supreme Court*, 2d ed. (Washington, D.C.: CQ Press, 1985), 217.
36. See *Congressional Quarterly Weekly Report*, September 12, 1987, 2159-2177; September 26, 1987, 2301-2304, 2329-2338; and October 3, 1987, 2366-2369, 2416.
37. See James E. Anderson, David W. Brady, and Charles S. Bullock III, *Public Policy and Politics in America* (North Scituate, Mass.: Duxbury Press, 1978), 291-292; and Charles S. Bullock III, "Equal Education Opportunity," in *Implementation of Civil Rights Policy*, ed. Charles S. Bullock III and Charles M. Lamb (Monterey, Calif.: Brooks/Cole, 1984), 57-58.
38. See Wasby, *The Impact of the United States Supreme Court*, 256.
39. See Stidham and Carp, "U.S. Trial Court Reactions to Changes in Civil Rights and Civil Liberties Policies," 13-14. A liberal opinion was defined as one that favored the minority litigant or supported the demise of racial, social, and political discrimination.
40. *United States v. Nixon*, 418 U.S. 683 (1974).
41. Johnson and Canon, *Judicial Policies*, 160.
42. Stephen L. Wasby, *The Supreme Court in the Federal Judicial System* (New York: Holt, Rinehart & Winston, 1978), 10.
43. Carp and Rowland, *Policymaking and Politics in the Federal District Courts*, 43.

44. For a discussion of this point, see Ronald Stidham, Robert A. Carp, and C. K. Rowland, "Patterns of Presidential Influence on the Federal District Courts: An Analysis of the Appointment Process," *Presidential Studies Quarterly* 14 (1984): 548-560.
45. Ibid., 554.
46. See C. K. Rowland, Robert A. Carp, and Ronald Stidham, "Judges' Policy Choices and the Value Basis of Judicial Appointments: A Comparison of Support for Criminal Defendants among Nixon, Johnson, and Kennedy Appointees to the Federal District Courts," *Journal of Politics* 46 (1984): 898.
47. See Sheldon Goldman, "Reagan's Second Term Judicial Appointments: The Battle at Midway," *Judicature* 70 (1987): 324-339.
48. See Ronald Stidham and Robert A. Carp, "Judges, Presidents, and Policy Choices: Exploring the Linkage," *Social Science Quarterly* 68 (June 1987): 395-404; and C. K. Rowland, Donald R. Songer, and Robert A. Carp, "Presidential Effects on Criminal Justice Policy in the Lower Federal Courts: The Reagan Judges," *Law and Society Review* 22 (1988): 191-200.
49. See Rodgers and Bullock, *Coercion to Compliance*, 20. Also see Leon E. Panetta and Peter Gall, *Bring Us Together: The Nixon Team and the Civil Rights Retreat* (Philadelphia: Lippincott, 1971).
50. See Lincoln Caplan, "Annals of Law: The Tenth Justice," pt. 1, *The New Yorker*, August 10, 1987, 32. Also see Lincoln Caplan, *The Tenth Justice: The Solicitor General and the Rule of Law* (New York: Knopf, 1988).
51. Caplan, "Annals of Law: The Tenth Justice," 37.
52. Ibid., 47. Also see Lincoln Caplan, "Annals of Law: The Tenth Justice," pt. 2, *The New Yorker*, August 17, 1987, 30-62; and Caplan, *The Tenth Justice: The Solicitor General and the Rule of Law*.
53. *Frontiero v. Richardson*, 411 U.S. 677 (1973).
54. A recent study, for example, analyzes judicial implementation and impact from the standpoint of the roles of four populations: an interpreting population, an implementing population, a consumer population, and a secondary population. See Johnson and Canon, *Judicial Policies*.
55. Our discussion of the use of equitable powers to provide remedial decrees is drawn from Phillip J. Cooper, *Hard Judicial Choices* (New York: Oxford University Press, 1988), 12-14, 342, 348-349.
56. Ibid., 348-349.
57. See Rodgers and Bullock, *Coercion to Compliance*, and Giles and Walker, "Judicial Policy-Making and Southern School Segregation."
58. *Engel v. Vitale*, 370 U.S. 421 (1962).
59. See *Abington School District v. Schempp*, 374 U.S. 203 (1963).
60. *Wallace v. Jaffree*, 472 U.S. (1985).
61. For good studies of the responses of school boards to the Court's school prayer decisions, see Kenneth Dolbeare and Phillip Hammond, *The School Prayer Decisions: From Court Policy to Local Practice* (Chicago: University of Chicago Press, 1971); William Muir, *Prayer in the Public Schools: Law and Attitude Change* (Chicago: University of Chicago Press, 1967); Richard Johnson, *The Dynamics of Compliance* (Evanston, Ill.: Northwestern University Press, 1967); and Robert Birkby, "The Supreme Court and the Bible Belt: Tennessee Reaction to the *Schempp* Decision," *Midwest Journal of Political Science* 10 (1966): 304-319.
62. Baum, *The Supreme Court*, 226.
63. Johnson and Canon, *Judicial Policies*, 269.
64. Ibid., 257, 258.

**354  Judicial Process in America**

65. See *Gray v. Sanders*, 372 U.S. 368 (1963); *Wesberry v. Sanders*, 376 U.S. 1 (1964); and *Reynolds v. Sims*, 377 U.S. 533 (1964).

66. See Roger A. Hanson and Robert E. Crew, Jr., "The Policy Impact of Reapportionment," *Law and Society Review* 8 (1973): 69-94; Eric Uslaner, "Comparative State Policy Formation, Interparty Competition and Malapportionment," *Journal of Politics* 40 (1978): 409-432; and Douglas G. Feig, "Expenditures in American States: The Impact of Court-Ordered Reapportionment," *American Politics Quarterly* 6 (1978): 309-324.

67. Archibald Cox, *The Warren Court* (Cambridge, Mass.: Harvard University Press, 1968), 74.

68. *Mapp v. Ohio*, 367 U.S. 643 (1961); *Gideon v. Wainwright*, 372 U.S. 335 (1963); and *Miranda v. Arizona*, 384 U.S. 436 (1966).

69. *Harris v. New York*, 401 U.S. 222 (1971).

70. *Roe v. Wade*, 410 U.S. 113 (1973).

71. For a good case study of the impact of *Roe v. Wade*, including reactions to the decision, see Johnson and Cannon, *Judicial Policies*, 4-14. Our discussion draws heavily on this study.

72. See Jon R. Bond and Charles A. Johnson, "Implementing a Permissive Policy: Hospital Abortion Services after *Roe v. Wade*," *American Journal of Political Science* 26 (1982): 1-24.

73. See *Harris v. McRae*, 448 U.S. 297 (1980).

74. See Richard C. Cortner, "Strategies and Tactics of Litigants in Constitutional Cases," *Journal of Public Law* 17 (1968): 287-307; Jo Freeman, *The Politics of Women's Liberation* (New York: David McKay, 1975); Leslie Friedman Goldstein, "Sex and the Burger Court: Recent Judicial Policy Making toward Women," in *Race, Sex and Policy Problems*, ed. Marian Lief Palley and Michael B. Preston (Lexington, Mass.: Lexington Books, 1979), 103-113; and Karen O'Connor, *Women's Organizations' Use of the Courts* (Lexington, Mass.: Heath, 1980).

# 12 Policy Making by American Judges: An Attempt at Synthesis

"An education," the saying goes, "is what you have left after you've forgotten what you've learned." This text has presented you with many facts, theories, statistics, and examples about the federal and state court systems. But as time goes on and the myriad of facts and illustrations are largely forgotten, what *education* ought you to have about the operation and policy making of American courts? It is the purpose of this chapter to pull out of the previous eleven chapters certain key ideas and significant themes that we would like you to remember long after most factual tidbits have faded from memory.

By this time it is surely clear that the decisions of federal and state judges and justices affect all our lives. Whether it be the norm enforcement rulings or the broader policy-making decisions, the output of federal and state courts permeates the warp and woof of the body politic in the United States. No one can have a full and accurate understanding of the American political system without being cognizant of the work of the men and women who wear the black robe. As we look at the matter of decision making by the judiciary, two basic questions are worthy of consideration. First, what are the conditions that cause judges to engage in policy making and to do so boldly? Second, does the literature give any clues as to the substantive direction of this policy making—that is, will it be conservative or liberal, supportive of or antagonistic toward the status quo? In seeking answers to these two basic questions, we have synthesized four sets of variables that shed some light in this realm: (1) the nature of the case or issue presented to the court, (2) the values and orientations of the judges, (3) the nature of the judicial decision-making process, and (4) extraneous variables that serve to implement and sustain judicial decisions.

## The Nature of the Case or Issue

One critical variable that clearly affects the degree to which (and sometimes the direction in which) American jurists influence our lives rests with the type of dispute or controversy that might serve as grist for the judicial mills. If it is the sort of issue that judges can resolve with room for significant maneuver, the impact of the case on public policy may be impressive. Conversely, if American jurists are forbidden to enter a certain decision-making realm or may enter with only limited options, the policy impact will be nil. There are several aspects of this general proposition, as we shall indicate.

## Jurisdiction

In Chapter 5 we outlined the jurisdiction of the three levels of the federal and state judiciaries. A knowledge of this is important in and of itself, but it takes on a second meaning in the context of this discussion—namely, that judges may not make policy in subject areas over which they have no legal authority. The controversy between the United States and the Soviet Union over the deployment of nuclear weapons in space is of great significance to the American people—and indeed our very lives may be dependent on its successful resolution—but judges will not affect this matter because they have no jurisdiction over war-and-peace disputes between the United States and its adversaries. Conversely, the courts will have considerable policy impact over matters of racial segregation and disputes over reapportionment because such disputes fall squarely within the legal jurisdiction of the U.S. judiciary.

While the courts do have some leeway in determining whether or not they have jurisdiction over a particular subject matter, for the most part jurisdictional boundaries are set forth in the U.S. and state constitutions and by acts of Congress and the state legislatures. In this same context a legislative body's power to create and restrict the courts' jurisdiction can often affect greatly the *direction* of judicial decision making. For example, Congress, by virtue of the Voting Rights Act, has granted citizens the right to sue local governments in federal courts if those governments alter the contours of electoral districts so as to dilute significantly the voting strength of minorities. By giving courts jurisdiction in this area and by telling judges in effect how to decide the cases (by establishing the decision-making goals), Congress has obviously had a major impact on judicial policy making. Likewise, the current threat by some members of Congress to remove certain matters from federal court jurisdiction, such as the power to use busing as a tool of desegregation, has policy-making potential of equal magnitude.

## Judicial Self-Restraint

The nature-of-the-case variable is also related to whether a controversy falls into one of those forbidden realms into which the "good judge" ought not to set foot. One judge might well like to sink his judicial teeth into a particular matter that is crying for adjudication, but if the litigant has not yet exhausted all legal or administrative remedies, the jurist will have to stay his hand. Another judge might well like to overturn a particular presidential action because she thinks it "smacks of fascism," but if no specific portion of the Constitution has been violated, she will have to express her displeasure in the voting booth—not in the courtroom. As we have indicated, the various maxims of judicial self-restraint may come from a variety of sources, including the Constitution, tradition, and acts of Congress and state legislatures; some have been imposed by the judges themselves. But whatever their source, they serve to channel the potential areas of judicial policy making. Judges would have little success in attempting to adjudicate matters that would soon bring reversal, censure, or organized opposition from those who are in a position to "correct" a judge who has strayed from the accepted pathway of judicial behavior.

## Norm Enforcement Versus Policy Making

Throughout this book we have discussed judicial behavior as being that of both norm enforcement and significant policy making. Most cases, as we have noted, fall into the former category—particularly for the lower judiciary. That is, for the majority of cases, judges routinely cite the applicable precedents, yield to the side with the weightiest evidence, and apply the statutes that clearly control the given fact situation; discretion is at a minimum. For these routine cases judges are not so much making policy as they are applying and enforcing *existing* norms and policy. In addition to norm enforcement, however, judges are presented with cases in which their room to maneuver—that is, their potential to make policy—is much greater. Such opportunities exist at all levels of the judiciary, but appellate judges and justices probably have more options for significant policy making than do their colleagues on the trial court bench. We would also recall that since the late 1930s, it has been Bill of Rights issues rather than labor and economic questions that have provided judges with the greatest opportunities for significant policy making.

In exploring this subject, we identified several situations (or case characteristics) that greatly enhance the judge's capacity to make policy rather than merely to enforce existing policy. One such opportunity occurs when the legal evidence is contradictory or equally strong on both sides. That is, it is not uncommon for judges to preside over a case for which the facts and evidence are about equally compelling or for which there are about an equal number of precedents that would sustain a finding for either party. Being pulled in several directions at once may not be an entirely comfortable position, but it does allow the jurists freer rein to strike out on their own than if prevailing facts and law impelled them toward one position.

Likewise, judicial policy making can flower when jurists are asked to resolve new types of controversies for which statutory law and past judicial precedents are virtually absent. For example, when the federal courts were asked whether artificially created life forms could be patented, there was no way they could avoid making policy. (Even the refusal to decide is a decision, as the existentialists have long argued.) Thus some cases by their very nature invite judicial policy making, while others carry with them no such invitation. Of course, judges differ in their perceptions of whether or not there is an opportunity in a given case for creative, innovative decision making. To some extent such differences are a function of the judges themselves—a point we shall address momentarily. But our contention here is that whether a case is of the garden-variety norm enforcement genre or whether it invites major judicial policy making depends to a large degree on the nature of the controversy itself.

### Summary

In considering whether and in what direction judges' decisions will significantly affect our lives, we can say this: the nature of the case itself is a vital component in this line of inquiry. Judges can make policy only in those areas over which the U.S. and state constitutions and the legislative branches have granted them jurisdiction and only in a manner consistent with the norms of judicial self-restraint. Also, if the controversies presented to the judges provide them with some room to maneuver—such as many current civil rights and liberties issues do—there will likely be more policy making than if the cases were tightly circumscribed by clearly controlling precedents and law.

## The Values and Orientations of the Judges

A second set of variables to be considered if we want to know about judicial policy making and about the direction it will take involve the judges themselves. What are their background characteristics? How were they appointed (or elected) and by whom? What are their judicial role conceptions? By learning something about the values and orientations of the men and women who are tapped for judicial service, we are better able to explain and predict what they will do on the bench. (Also recall from Chapters 4, 6, and 7 that the attitudes and values of other actors in the judicial process—for example, police officers, prosecutors, and the solicitor general—likewise affect the content and direction of their important duties.)

We have looked at judicial background characteristics in a variety of contexts in this book. Here we shall examine several that have particular relevance vis-à-vis judicial policy making and its direction.

### Judges as a Socioeconomic Elite

In Chapter 8 we made much of the fact that America's jurists come from a very narrow segment of social and economic strata. To an overwhelming degree they are offspring of upper- and upper-middle-class parents and come from families with a tradition of political, and often judicial, service. They are the men and women to whom our system has been good, who fit in, who have "made it." The mavericks, malcontents, and ideological extremists are discreetly weeded out by the judicial recruitment process.

What does all this suggest about judicial policy making and its direction? Given the striking similarity of the jurists and the backgrounds from which they come, their overall policy making is generally going to be within fairly modest, conventional, and ideologically moderate boundaries. While many judges have a commitment to reform and will use their policy making opportunities to this end, still it is to adjust and enhance a way of life that they basically believe in. Seldom bitten is the hand of the socioeconomic system that feeds them. Although an occasional maverick may slip in or develop within the judicial ranks, most judges are basically conservative in that they hold dear the traditional institutions and rules of the game that have brought success to them and their families. While America's elite has its fair share of both liberals and conservatives, it does not contain many who would use their discretionary opportunities to alter radically the basic social and political system.

## Judges as Representatives of Their Political Parties

While the nature of the judicial recruitment process gives virtually all U.S. judges a similar and fairly conventional cast, there are differences. The prior political party affiliation of jurists does alter the way they exercise their policy-making discretion when the circumstances of a case give them room to maneuver. As we have noted, judges and justices who come from the ranks of the Democratic party have been somewhat more liberal than their colleagues from Republican ranks. This has meant, for one thing, that Democrats on the bench are more likely to favor government regulation of the economy—particularly when such regulation appears to benefit the underdog or the worker in disputes with management. In criminal justice matters, Democratic jurists are more disposed toward the motions made by defendants. Finally, in questions involving civil rights and liberties, the Democrat on the bench tends to establish policies that favor a broadening position.

In this same context we stress the important policy link between the partisan choice made by voters in a presidential election, the judges whom the chief executive appoints, and the subsequent policy decisions of these jurists. When voters make a policy choice in electing a conservative or a liberal to the presidency, they also have a discernible impact upon the judiciary as well. Despite the many participants in the judicial selection process and the variety of forces that would thwart policy-oriented presidents (and governors) from getting "their kind of people" on the bench, it is still fair to say that to an impressive degree chief executives tend to get the type of men and women they want in the judiciary.

In a speech made just prior to the 1984 presidential election, conservative Supreme Court justice William Rehnquist discussed this phenomenon with unusual candor. Although he was speaking primarily about the Supreme Court, his remarks pertain to the entire U.S. judiciary. There is "no reason in the world," said Rehnquist, why President Reagan should not attempt to "pack" the federal courts. The institution has been constructed in such a way that the public will, in the person of the president, have something to say about the membership of the Court and thereby indirectly about its decisions. Thus, Rehnquist felt, presidents may seek to appoint people who are sympathetic to their political and philosophical principles. After calling new judicial appointments "indirect infusions of the popular will," Rehnquist added that it "should come as no surprise" that presidents attempt to pack the courts with people of similar policy values, but "like murder suspects in a detective novel, they must have motive and opportunity." [1]

## Judges as Manifestations of "Localism"

Another aspect of the values and orientations of the judges themselves has an impact upon their policy-making process: the attributes and mores that the judges carry with them from the region in which they grew up or in which they hold court. For both trial and appellate jurists we have documented a wide variety of geographic variations in the way they view the world and react to its demands. On a regional basis, for example, we noted that on many policy issues northern jurists have been more liberal than their colleagues in the South. Not only does judicial policy making vary from one region of the land to another, but studies reveal that each of the circuits tends to be unique in the way its appellate and trial court judges administer the law and make decisions. The presence of significant state-by-state differences in U.S. trial judge behavior is further evidence that judges bring with them to the bench certain local values and orientations that subsequently affect their policy-making patterns. Finally, we showed that judges in larger cities (particularly in the South) tend to be somewhat more liberal than their colleagues in smaller towns and in rural districts. This evidence, too, bespeaks the impact of localism on the decision-making values of the jurists.

## Judges' Conceptions of Their Judicial Roles

In our discussion of this phenomenon we noted three basic ways in which judges conceive of their roles vis-à-vis the policy-making process. At one end of the spectrum are the "law makers," who take a rather broad view of the judicial role. These jurists, often referred to as "activists" or "innovators," contend that they can and sometimes must make significant public policy when they render many of their decisions. At the other end of the spectrum are the "law interpreters," who take a very narrow view of the judicial function. Sometimes called "strict constructionists," they believe that norm enforcement rather than policy making is the only proper role of the judge. In between are the "pragmatists," or "realists," who contend that judging is primarily a matter of enforcing norms but that on occasion they can and must formulate new judicial policy.

Understanding the role conception that a judge brings to the bench (or develops on the bench) will not tell us much about the substantive direction of his or her policy making: it is possible to be a conservative activist just as well as a liberal activist. One can go out on a judicial limb and give the benefit of the doubt to the economic giant or to the underdog, to the criminal defendant claiming police brutality or to the police officer urging renewed emphasis on law and order. But a knowledge of the judges' role conceptions will tell us a good deal about whether they are more inclined to defer to the norms and policies set by others or to strike out occasionally and make policy on their own.

### Summary

In attempting to learn about policy making by judges and its substantive direction, we have set forth a second factor that helps channel our thinking—namely, the values and orientations that the judges bring with them to the bench. Here we have suggested four items that are particularly relevant in this regard: (1) that America's judges come from the establishment's elite, a fact that serves to discourage radical policy making; (2) that judges' policy making is reflective of their partisan orientations and that of the executive who nominated them; (3) that policy decisions manifest the local values and attitudes that judges possess when they first put on the black robe; and (4) that judges will engage in more policy making if they bring to the bench a belief that it is right and proper for judges to act in this manner.

## The Nature of the Judicial Decision-Making Process

Knowing how judges think and reason, how they are influenced in their decision-making process, provides us with a good clue about policy making by U.S. judges. While this factor is inexorably intertwined with the first two we have outlined here, it is distinct enough to warrant a separate discussion. The account in Chapter 9 of the legal subculture examined the nature of the legal reasoning process that is at the very heart of the system of jurisprudence in America. We noted that this is essentially a three-step process described by the doctrine of precedent as follows: (1) similarity is seen between cases, (2) the rule of law inherent in the first case is announced, and (3) the rule of law is made applicable to the second case. Adherence to past precedents, to the doctrine of *stare decisis*, is also part and parcel of the legal reasoning process. Skillfully shaping and crafting the wisdom of the past, as found in previous court rulings, and applying it to contemporary problems is what this time-honored process is all about.

Decision making on collegial courts contains some dimensions not inherent in the behavior of trial judges sitting alone. In Chapter 10 we examined several approaches that judicial scholars have used to get a theoretical handle on the way appellate court judges and justices think and act. One of these is small-group dynamics, an approach that sees the output of the appellate judiciary as strongly influenced by three general phenomena: persuasion on the merits, bargaining, and the threat of sanctions.

The first of these, persuasion, lies at the heart of small-group dynamics. It means quite simply that because of their training and values, judges are receptive to arguments based on sound legal reasoning, often spiced with relevant legal precedents. Both hard and anecdotal evidence exists to indicate that judicial policies are indeed influenced in the refining furnace of the judicial conference room.

Bargaining, too, molds the content and direction of judicial policy outputs. The compromises that are made among jurists—during the decision-making conference and while an opinion is being drafted—to satisfy the majority judges are almost always the product of bargaining. It's not that judges say to one another: "If you vote for my favorite judicial policy position, I'll vote for yours." Rather, a justice might phrase a "bargaining offer" more like this—say, in a case dealing with the right of students to appeal adverse disciplinary rulings from a state university to the federal courts: "I don't agree with your opinion as it now stands permitting students to appeal *all* adverse disciplinary decisions to the local federal district court. That's just too liberal for me, and I don't approve of interfering in university affairs to that degree. However, I could go along with a majority opinion that permitted appeals in *really serious* disciplinary matters that might result in the permanent suspension of a student." The first justice must then decide how badly the colleague's vote is needed—badly enough to water down the opinion to include only cases dealing with permanent suspension rather than all cases, as in the original opinion? Such is the grist for the bargaining mill that spews forth judicial policies.

The sanctions that we discussed include a variety of items in the genteel arsenal of judicial weaponry. A judge's threat to take a vote away from the majority and dissent may cause the majority judges to alter the content of a policy decision. A judge's willingness to write a strong, biting dissent is another sanction that occasionally causes a unity-conscious majority to consider policy changes in an opinion. The threat to go public is a third tactic that judges use in collegial courts to alter the policy course of other jurists. Public exposure of an objectionable internal court practice or stance is probably the least pleasant of the sanctions. Finally, we noted that chief justices of the U.S. and state supreme courts and their counterparts at the appellate and trial court levels all have singular opportunities to guide and shape the policy decisions of the courts. The stature and options that are part of their unique leadership positions provide them an opportunity for crafting court policy if they have the desire and innate ability to make the most of it.

Besides small-group dynamics we also looked at an approach to appellate court decision making known as attitude and bloc formation analysis. This school of thought sees judges as possessing a stable set of attitudes that guide their policy choices. Such attitudes exist on dimensions like civil rights and liberties, social issues (matters of voting and ethnic status), and economic questions dealing with the equal distribution of wealth. Justices with similar attitudes on these several dimensions tend to vote in a similar manner on cases and thus form into voting blocs. Scholars have used the techniques of content analysis of opinions (to find and measure attitudes), scaling, and bloc analysis to test this theory. Their research has borne some impressive fruit because it has been possible to demonstrate that members of the appellate judiciary do decide cases in accordance with consistent underlying value dimensions and that voting blocs do form and behave according to predictable patterns.

Fact pattern analysis competes effectively with the small-group approach and with attitude and bloc analysis to account for appellate judge behavior. As we have seen in Chapter 10 the fact pattern approach would explain the individual behavior of appellate court judges in terms of their response to key facts inherent in the cases. Unlike traditional scholars, who postulate that judges respond only to the *legal* facts of a case, the fact pattern school argues that the jurists are alert to a wide variety of extrajudicial factors, such as the race and gender of a defendant, or whether a petitioner's attorney was court-appointed or privately retained. This approach does not assume the existence (or nonexistence) of consistent patterns in the acceptance of facts or in decisions based on facts. Finally, the fact pattern scholars have used sophisticated mathematical equations to weight the key facts they have identified and have learned the various fact combinations that have the maximum (and minimum) effect on each justice.

What does this third general factor—the nature of the judicial decision-making process—tell us about judicial policy making and its substantive direction? We would offer two observations about this. First, most policy making by judges is likely to be slow and incremental. Indeed, this is exactly what one would expect from a reasoning process that relies so heavily on respecting past precedents and that places such emphasis on stability and continuity. The decision-making process of American judges does not lend itself to radical and abrupt departures from past precedents and behavior. Yet change does occur and new policies are made. But legal history suggests that American jurists have often "reformed to preserve," and that is a principle often associated with conservatism.

Second, an understanding of the judicial thought process and of the small-group dynamics of collegial courts does not in itself tell us anything about the substantive direction of a court's policy making. However, knowing which judges and justices are masters at persuasion, bargaining, and the use of sanctions does give us some insight into explaining and predicting the content of judicial policy decisions. If on a given court it is the conservatives who have developed a mastery of these tactics, then the bettor would do well to wager a few dollars on more conservative judicial decisions; vice versa if it is the liberals who have perfected their interactive skills.

## The Impact of Extraneous Influences

At this point there should be little doubt that the making and implementation of judicial policy decisions are influenced by a variety of actors and forces quite outside the courtroom. It is not just judges and law clerks, leather-bound casebooks, and arguments by silk-tongued lawyers that go into the shaping and carrying out of judicial decisions. Into the calculus must also go such unwieldy variables as these: the values and ability of the executive, the will of Congress or the legislature, the temper of public opinion, the strength and ideological orientation of key interest groups, and the attitudes and good will of those called on to implement judicial decisions in the "real world."

The executive input into the making and implementation of key judicial decisions is considerable. Selected as a policy choice of the citizenry in the past election, the chief executive has the opportunity to fill the courts with men and women who share the basic political and judicial philosophies of the administration. Once on the court, judges may be encouraged or discouraged in their policy making by the words and deeds emanating from the White House or the governor's mansion. For instance, the willingness of Presidents Eisenhower and Kennedy to use federal troops to help enforce judicial integration orders must have encouraged subsequent policy decisions in this realm; conversely, the public statements of Presidents Nixon and Reagan about judges having gone too far in tampering with our local schools must have caused many federal judges to think at least twice before issuing new school integration orders. The overall role of the chief executive in implementing judicial policy decisions was examined more systematically in Chapter 11.

Congress, too, has its impact on the creation and nurturing of judicial policy decisions just as the legislature does at the state level. In its power to establish most of the original and appellate jurisdiction of the federal judiciary, it has the capacity to determine the subject-matter arenas where judicial policy battles are fought. In its capacity to establish the number of courts and the financial support they will have, Congress can show its approval or displeasure at the third branch of government. By accepting or rejecting presidential nominees to the courts, the Senate helps to determine who the judicial decision makers will be and hence the value orientations of these jurists. Finally, the implementation of many key judicial policy decisions is absolutely dependent on legislation that Congress must pass to make the ruling a meaningful reality for those affected by it. Had not Congress passed several key bills to implement the courts' desegregation orders (discussed in Chapter 11), integration of the public schools would be little more than a nice idea for those whom the rulings were intended to benefit.

Public opinion also has a role to play in this policy-making process—not an outrageous prospect for a nation that calls itself a democracy. In rendering key policy decisions, judges can hardly be oblivious to the mood and values of the citizenry of which they themselves are a part. And indeed in many policy areas (such as obscenity, desegregation, and legislative apportionment) judges have actually been ordered by the Supreme Court to take the local political and social climate into consideration as they tender their rulings. In the implementation of court decisions, the support or opposition of the public is often a key variable in determining whether or not the judge's orders are carried out in the spirit as well as the letter of the law.

Interest-group activity is another thread in the tapestry of judicial policy making. Such organizations often provide the president (or a state governor) with the names of individuals whom they support for judicial office, and they lobby against those whose judicial values they consider suspect. They often provide the vehicle for key judicial decisions by instigating legislation, by sponsoring test cases, and by giving legal and financial aid to those litigants whose cases they favor. At the implementing stage we have seen (in Chapter 11) how they can thwart or help carry out more effectively judicial decisions.

The final group of extraneous forces are those individuals and organizations who are expected to implement the judicial policy decision on a day-by-day basis out on the street: the police officer who is asked to be *sure* that the accused understand their legal rights; the physician who must certify that a requested abortion is *really* in the mental health interests of the pregnant woman; the personnel officer at a state institution who could readily find some technicality for refusing to hire a minority applicant; or the censor on the town's movie review board who is told that nudity and obscenity are not synonymous but who doesn't want to believe it. It is the values, motivations, and actions of individuals such as these that we must consider if we are to understand fully the judicial policy-making process. Their good-faith support of a judicial policy decision is vital to making it work; their indifference or opposition will cause the judge's ruling to die aborning.

It was our intention in this chapter to get some grip on the slippery handle of policy making by American judges. While many more questions have been raised than answered, perhaps we know a little better now at least where to search for some answers. If we want to learn the conditions that allow for bold policy making and if we want some clue as to the direction that policy making will take, here is where we must focus our attention: on the nature of the case or controversy that can properly be brought into court; on the values and orientations of the jurists who preside over these courts; on the precise nature of the decision-making process of American judges; and, finally, on a variety of extraneous individuals and groups whose values filter into the American judicial process from beginning to end.

## Note

1. "Rehnquist Says It's OK for a President to Pack High Court," *Houston Chronicle*, October 19, 1984, 1:3.

# Selected Bibliography

## Books

Abadinsky, Howard. *Law and Justice*. Chicago: Nelson-Hall 1988.

Abraham, Henry J. *The Judicial Process*. 4th ed. New York: Oxford University Press, 1980.

Ball, Howard. *Courts and Politics: The Federal Judicial System*. Englewood Cliffs, N.J.: Prentice-Hall, 1980.

Bass, Jack. *Unlikely Heroes*. New York: Simon & Schuster, 1981.

Baum, Lawrence. *The Supreme Court*. 3d ed. Washington, D.C.: CQ Press, 1988.

Berkson, Larry C., and Susan B. Carbon. *The United States Circuit Judge Nominating Commission: Its Members, Procedures and Candidates*. Chicago: American Judicature Society, 1980.

Berkson, Larry C., Steven W. Hays, and Susan J. Carbon, eds. *Managing the State Courts*. St. Paul, Minn.: West, 1977.

Birkby, Robert H. *The Court and Public Policy*. Washington, D.C.: CQ Press, 1983.

Cannon, Mark W., and David M. O'Brien. *Views from the Bench*. Chatham, N.J.: Chatham House, 1985.

Caplan, Lincoln. *The Tenth Justice: The Solicitor General and the Rule of Law*. New York: Knopf, 1988.

Carp, Robert A., and C. K. Rowland. *Policymaking and Politics in the Federal District Courts*. Knoxville: University of Tennessee Press, 1983.

Chase, Harold W. *Federal Judges: The Appointing Process*. Minneapolis: University of Minnesota Press, 1972.

Cooper, Phillip J. *Hard Judicial Choices*. New York: Oxford University Press, 1988.

Dolbeare, Kenneth, and Phillip Hammond. *The School Prayer Decisions: From Court Policy to Local Practice*. Chicago: University of Chicago Press, 1971.

Early, Stephen T., Jr. *Constitutional Courts of the United States*. Totowa, N.J.: Littlefield, Adams, 1977.

Eisenstein, James. *Counsel for the United States: U.S. Attorneys in the Political and Legal Systems*. Baltimore: Johns Hopkins University Press, 1978.

Epstein, Lee. *Conservatives in Court*. Knoxville: University of Tennessee Press, 1985.

Fish, Peter G. *The Politics of Federal Judicial Administration*. Princeton, N.J.: Princeton University Press, 1973.

Frank, Jerome. *Courts on Trial: Myth and Reality in American Justice*. Princeton, N.J.: Princeton University Press, 1950.

Frank, John P. *Marble Palace*. New York: Knopf, 1968.

Frankfurter, Felix, and James M. Landis. *The Business of the Supreme Court.* New York: Macmillan, 1928.

Friedenthal, Jack H., Mary Kay Kane, and Arthur R. Miller. *Civil Procedure.* St. Paul, Minn.: West, 1985.

Friedman, Lawrence M. *American Law.* New York: Norton, 1984.

_____. *History of American Law.* 2d ed. New York: Simon & Schuster, 1985.

Friesen, Earnest C., Jr., Edward C. Gallas, and Nesta M. Gallas. *Managing the Courts.* Indianapolis: Bobbs-Merrill, 1971.

Glick, Henry R. *Courts, Politics, and Justice.* 2d ed. New York: McGraw-Hill, 1988.

_____. *Supreme Courts in State Politics.* New York: Basic Books, 1971.

Goldman, Sheldon. *Constitutional Law and Supreme Court Decision-Making.* New York: Harper & Row, 1982.

Goldman, Sheldon, and Thomas P. Jahnige. *The Federal Courts as a Political System.* 3d ed. New York: Harper & Row, 1985.

Goldman, Sheldon, and Charles M. Lamb, eds. *Judicial Conflict and Consensus: Behavioral Studies of American Appellate Courts.* Lexington: University Press of Kentucky, 1986.

Goldman, Sheldon, and Austin Sarat. *American Court Systems: Readings in Judicial Process and Behavior.* 2d ed. New York: Longman, 1989.

Goulden, Joseph C. *The Benchwarmers: The Private World of the Powerful Federal Judges.* New York: Weybright & Talley, 1974.

Grossman, Joel B. *Lawyers and Judges: The ABA and the Politics of Judicial Selection.* New York: Wiley, 1965.

Grossman, Joel B., and Joseph Tanenhaus. *Frontiers of Judicial Research.* New York: Wiley, 1969.

Henderson, Dwight F. *Courts for a New Nation.* Washington, D.C.: Public Affairs Press, 1971.

Hepperle, Winifred L., and Laura Crites, eds. *Women in the Courts.* Williamsburg, Va.: National Center for State Courts, 1978.

Howard, J. Woodford, Jr. *Courts of Appeals in the Federal Judicial System.* Princeton, N.J.: Princeton University Press, 1981.

Jackson, Donald Dale. *Judges.* New York: Atheneum, 1974.

Jacob, Herbert. *Justice in America.* 4th ed. Boston: Little, Brown, 1984.

Johnson, Charles A., and Bradley C. Canon. *Judicial Policies: Implementation and Impact.* Washington, D.C.: CQ Press, 1984.

Johnson, Richard. *The Dynamics of Compliance.* Evanston, Ill.: Northwestern University Press, 1967.

Kalven, Harry, Jr., and Hans Zeisel. *The American Jury.* Boston: Little, Brown, 1966.

Kitchin, William. *Federal District Judges.* Baltimore: Collage Press, 1978.

Klein, Mitchell S. G. *Law, Courts, and Policy.* Englewood Cliffs, N.J.: Prentice-Hall, 1984.

Levi, Edward H. *An Introduction to Legal Reasoning.* Chicago: University of Chicago Press, 1948.

Levin, Martin A. *Urban Politics and the Criminal Courts.* Chicago: University of Chicago Press, 1977.

Lieberman, Jethro K. *The Litigious Society.* New York: Basic Books, 1983.

Mason, Alpheus T. *Harlan Fiske Stone: Pillar of the Law.* New York: Viking Press, 1956.

McLauchlan, William P. *Federal Court Caseloads.* New York: Praeger, 1984.

Milner, Neal. *The Court and Local Law Enforcement.* Beverly Hills, Calif.: Sage, 1971.

Muir, William. *Prayer in the Public Schools: Law and Attitude Change.* Chicago: University of Chicago Press, 1967.

Murphy, Walter F. *Elements of Judicial Strategy.* Chicago: University of Chicago Press, 1964.

Murphy, Walter F., and C. Herman Pritchett, eds. *Courts, Judges, and Politics.* 3d ed. New York: Random House, 1979.

Nagel, Stuart S. *The Legal Process from a Behavioral Perspective.* Homewood, Ill.: Dorsey Press, 1969.

Neubauer, David W. *America's Courts & the Criminal Justice System.* 2d ed. Monterey, Calif.: Brooks/Cole, 1984.

Oakley, John Bilyeu, and Robert S. Thompson. *Law Clerks and the Judicial Process.* Berkeley: University of California Press, 1980.

O'Connor, Karen. *Women's Organizations' Use of the Courts.* Lexington, Mass.: Heath, 1980.

Partridge, Anthony, and Allan Lind. *A Reevaluation of the Civil Appeals Management Plan.* Washington, D.C.: Federal Judicial Center, 1983.

Peltason, Jack W. *Fifty-Eight Lonely Men.* New York: Harcourt, Brace & World, 1961.

Porter, Mary Cornelia, and G. Alan Tarr. *State Supreme Courts: Policymakers in the Federal System.* Westport, Conn.: Greenwood, 1982.

Pritchett, C. Herman. *The Roosevelt Court: A Study of Judicial Votes and Values, 1937-1947.* New York: Macmillan, 1948.

Richardson, Richard J., and Kenneth N. Vines. *The Politics of Federal Courts.* Boston: Little, Brown, 1970.

Rodell, Fred. *Nine Men.* New York: Random House, 1955.

Rodgers, Harrell R., Jr., and Charles S. Bullock III. *Coercion to Compliance.* Lexington, Mass.: Heath, 1976.

Rohde, David W., and Harold J. Spaeth. *Supreme Court Decision Making.* San Francisco: Freeman, 1976.

Ryan, John Paul, et al. *American Trial Judges: Their Work Styles and Performance.* New York: Free Press, 1980.

Schantz, William T. *The American Legal Environment.* St. Paul Minn.: West, 1976.

Schmidhauser, John R. *Judges and Justices: The Federal Appellate Judiciary.* Boston: Little, Brown, 1979.

———. *The Supreme Court: Its Politics, Personalities, and Procedures.* New York: Holt, Rinehart & Winston, 1960.

Schubert, Glendon. *Judicial Behavior: A Reader in Theory and Research.* Chicago: Rand McNally, 1964.

———. *The Judicial Mind Revisited.* New York: Oxford University Press, 1974.

———. *Judicial Policy Making.* Glenview, Ill.: Scott, Foresman, 1974.

———. *Quantitative Analysis of Judicial Behavior.* New York: Free Press, 1959.

Schubert, Glendon, ed. *Judicial Decision-Making.* New York: Free Press, 1963.

Seron, Carroll. *The Roles of Magistrates: Nine Case Studies.* Washington, D.C.: Federal Judicial Center, 1985.

———. *The Roles of Magistrates in Federal District Courts.* Washington, D.C.: Federal Judicial Center, 1983.

Simon, James F. *In His Own Image.* New York: McKay, 1973.

Smigel, Erwin O. *The Wall Street Lawyer: Professional Organization Man.*

Glencoe, Ill.: Free Press, 1964.
Steamer, Robert J. *Chief Justice: Leadership and the Supreme Court.* Columbia: University of South Carolina Press, 1986.
Stumpf, Harry P. *American Judicial Politics.* San Diego: Harcourt Brace Jovanovich, 1988.
Tarr, G. Alan, and Mary Cornelia Aldis Porter. *State Supreme Courts in State and Nation.* New Haven, Conn.: Yale University Press, 1988.
Vago, Steven. *Law and Society.* Englewood Cliffs, N.J.: Prentice-Hall, 1981.
Vetter, Harold J., and Leonard Territo. *Crime and Justice in America.* St. Paul, Minn.: West, 1984.
Wasby, Stephen L. *The Impact of the United States Supreme Court: Some Perspectives.* Homewood, Ill.: Dorsey Press, 1970.
Watson, Richard A., and Rondal G. Downing. *The Politics of the Bench and the Bar.* New York: Wiley, 1969.
Wheeler, Russell R., and Charles Nihan. *Administering the Federal Judicial Circuits: A Study of Chief Judges' Approaches and Procedures.* Washington, D.C.: Federal Judicial Center, 1982.
Wheeler, Russell R., and Howard R. Whitcomb, eds. *Judicial Administration: Text and Readings.* Englewood Cliffs, N.J.: Prentice-Hall, 1977.
Williston, Samuel. *Life and Law.* Boston: Little, Brown, 1940.
Wirt, Frederick M. *Politics of Southern Equality: Law and Social Change in a Mississippi County.* Chicago: Aldine, 1970.
Woodward, Bob, and Scott Armstrong. *The Brethren: Inside the Supreme Court.* New York: Simon & Schuster, 1979.
Wright, Charles Alan. *Handbook of the Law of Federal Courts.* 2d ed. St. Paul, Minn.: West, 1970.

## Articles

Adamany, David W. "Legitimacy, Realigning Elections, and the Supreme Court." *Wisconsin Law Review* (1973): 790-846.
_____. "The Party Variable in Judges' Voting: Conceptual Notes and a Case Study." *American Political Science Review* 63 (1969): 57-74.
Alfini, James J. "Alternative Dispute Resolution and the Courts: An Introduction." *Judicature* 69 (1986): 252-253, 314.
Aliotta, Jilda M. "Combining Judges' Attributes and Case Characteristics: An Alternative Approach to Explaining Supreme Court Decisionmaking." *Judicature* 71 (1988): 277-281.
Armstrong Virginia C., and Charles A. Johnson. "Certiorari Decisions by the Warren and Burger Courts: Is Cue Theory Time Bound?" *Polity* 15 (1982): 141-150.
Ashman, Allan, and Pat Chapin. "Is the Bell Tolling for Nonlawyer Judges?" *Judicature* 59 (1976): 417-421.
Atkins, Burton M., and William Zovoina. "Judicial Leadership on the Court of Appeals: A Probability Analysis of Panel Assignment on Race Relations Cases on the Fifth Circuit." *American Journal of Political Science* 18 (1974): 701-711.
Baar, Carl. "Federal Judicial Administration: Political Strategies and Organizational Change," pp. 97-109 in *Judicial Administration: Text and Readings.* Ed. Russell R. Wheeler and Howard R. Whitcomb. Englewood Cliffs, N.J.: Prentice-Hall, 1977.
Barnum, David G. "The Supreme Court and Public Opinion: Judicial Decision

Making in the Post-New Deal Period." *Journal of Politics* 47 (1985): 652-666.

Baum, Lawrence. "Implementation of Judicial Decisions: An Organizational Analysis." *American Politics Quarterly* 4 (1976): 86-114.

———. "Policy Goals in Judicial Gatekeeping: A Proximity Model of Discretionary Jurisdiction." *American Journal of Political Science* 21 (1977): 13-35.

Bermant, Gordon, and Russell R. Wheeler. "From within the System: Educational and Research Programs at the Federal Judicial Center," pp. 102-145 in *Reforming the Law*. Ed. Gary B. Melton. New York: Guilford, 1987.

Birkby, Robert. "The Supreme Court and the Bible Belt: Tennessee Reaction to the *Schempp* Decision." *Midwest Journal of Political Science* 10 (1966): 304-319.

Bond, Jon R. "The Politics of Court Structure: The Addition of New Federal Judges, 1949-1978." *Law and Policy Quarterly* (1980): 181-188.

Bond, Jon R., and Charles A. Johnson. "Implementing a Permissive Policy: Hospital Abortion Services after *Roe v. Wade*." *American Journal of Political Science* 26 (1982): 1-24.

Brenner, Saul. "Fluidity on the United States Supreme Court: A Reexamination." *American Journal of Political Science* 24 (1980): 526-535.

———. "Reassigning the Majority Opinion on the United States Supreme Court." *Justice System Journal* 11 (1986): 186-195.

Brenner, Saul, and Harold J. Spaeth. "Majority Opinion Assignments and the Maintenance of the Original Coalition on the Warren Court." *American Journal of Political Science* 32 (1988): 72-81.

Broach, Glen T., et al. "State Political Culture and Sentence Severity in Federal District Courts." *Criminology* 16 (1978): 373-382.

Burbank, Stephen B. "Politics and Progress in Implementing the Federal Judicial Discipline Act." *Judicature* 71 (1987): 13-28.

Canon, Bradley C. "Characteristics and Career Patterns of State Supreme Court Justices." *State Government* 45 (1972): 34-41.

———. "The Impact of Formal Selection Process on the Characteristics of Judges— Reconsidered." *Law and Society Review* 6 (1972): 575-593.

Canon, Bradley C., and S. Sidney Ulmer. "The Supreme Court and Critical Elections: A Dissent." *American Political Science Review* 70 (1976): 1215-1218.

Carbon, Susan. "Women in the Judiciary." *Judicature* 65 (1982): 285.

Carp, Robert A. "The Behavior of Grand Juries: Acquiescence or Justice?" *Social Science Quarterly* 55 (1975): 853-870.

Carp, Robert, and Russell Wheeler. "Sink or Swim: The Socialization of a Federal District Judge." *Journal of Public Law* 21 (1972): 359-393.

Casper, Jonathan D. "The Supreme Court and National Policy Making." *American Political Science Review* 70 (1976): 50-63.

Cook, Beverly Blair. "Public Opinion and Federal Judicial Policy." *American Journal of Political Science* 21 (1977): 567-600.

Cooley, John W. "Arbitration vs. Mediation—Explaining the Differences." *Judicature* 69 (1986): 263-269.

Curran, Barbara A. "American Lawyers in the 1980s: A Profession in Transition." *Law and Society Review* 20 (1986): 19-52.

Dahl, Robert A. "Decision-Making in a Democracy: The Supreme Court as a National Policy-Maker." *Journal of Public Law* 6 (1957): 279-295.

Daniels, Stephen. "A Tangled Tale: Studying State Supreme Courts." *Law and Society Review* 22 (1988): 833-863.

Dolbeare, Kenneth M. "The Federal District Courts and Urban Public Policy: An Exploratory Study (1960-1967)," pp. 373-404 in *Frontiers of Judicial Research*.

Ed. Joel B. Grossman and Joseph Tanenhaus. New York: Wiley, 1969.

Dubois, Philip L. "The Illusion of Judicial Consensus Revisited: Partisan Conflict on an Intermediate State Court of Appeals," *American Journal of Political Science* 32 (1988): 946-967.

Ducat, Craig R., and Robert L. Dudley. "Dimensions Underlying Economic Policymaking in the Early and Later Burger Courts." *Journal of Politics* 49 (1987): 521-539.

Edelman, Peter. "Institutionalizing Dispute Resolution Alternatives." *Justice System Journal* 9 (1984): 134-150.

Feeley, Malcolm M. "Another Look at the 'Party Variable' in Judicial Decision-Making: An Analysis of the Michigan Supreme Court." *Polity* 4 (1971): 91-104.

Feig, Douglas G. "Expenditures in American States: The Impact of Court-Ordered Reapportionment." *American Politics Quarterly* 6 (1978): 309-324.

Fitzpatrick, Collins T. "Misconduct and Disability of Federal Judges: The Unreported Informal Responses." *Judicature* 71 (1988): 282-283.

Flanders, Steven, and Jerry Goldman. "Screening Practices and the Use of Para-Judicial Personnel in a U.S. Court of Appeals," pp. 241-258 in *Judicial Administration: Text and Readings*. Ed. Russell R. Wheeler and Howard R. Whitcomb. Englewood Cliffs, N.J.: Prentice-Hall, 1977.

Funston, Richard. "The Supreme Court and Critical Elections." *American Political Science Review* 69 (1975): 795-811.

Gibson, James L. "From Simplicity to Complexity: The Development of Theory in the Study of Judicial Behavior." *Political Behavior* 5 (1983): 7-50.

Glick, Henry R., and Craig F. Emmert. "Selection Systems and Judicial Characteristics." *Judicature* 70 (1987): 228-235.

Glick, Henry, and Craig Emmert. "Stability and Change: Characteristics of Contemporary State Supreme Court Judges." *Judicature* 70 (1986): 107-112.

Goldman, Sheldon. "Conflict on the U.S. Courts of Appeals, 1965-1971: A Quantitative Analysis." *University of Cincinnati Law Review* 42 (1973): 635-658.

_____. "Reagan's Judicial Appointments at Mid-Term: Shaping the Bench in His Own Image." *Judicature* 66 (1983): 335-347.

_____. "Reagan's Second Term Judicial Appointments: The Battle at Midway." *Judicature* 70 (1987): 324-339.

_____. "Should There Be Affirmative Action for the Judiciary?" *Judicature* 62 (1979): 488-496.

_____. "Voting Behavior on the United States Courts of Appeals, 1961-1964." *American Political Science Review* 60 (1966): 370-385.

_____. "Voting Behavior on the United States Courts of Appeals, Revisited." *American Political Science Review* 69 (1975): 491-506.

Gottschall, Jon. "Carter's Judicial Appointments: The Influence of Affirmative Action and Merit Selection on Voting on the U.S. Courts of Appeals." *Judicature* 67 (1983): 165-173.

Gruhl, John. "The Supreme Court's Impact on the Law of Libel: Compliance by Lower Federal Courts." *Western Political Quarterly* 33 (1980): 502-519.

Grunbaum, Werner F. "A Quantitative Analysis of the 'Presidential Ballot' Case." *Journal of Politics* 34 (1972): 223-243.

Hall, Melinda Gann. "Small Group Influences in the United States Supreme Court." *Justice System Journal* 12 (1987): 359-369.

Handberg, Roger, and Harold F. Hill, Jr. "Court Curbing, Court Reversals, and Judicial Review: The Supreme Court Versus Congress." *Law and Society Review*

14 (1980): 309-322.

Hanson, Roger A., and Robert E. Crew, Jr. "The Policy Impact of Reapportionment." *Law and Society Review* 8 (1973): 69-94.

Henschen, Beth M. "Statutory Interpretations of the Supreme Court: Congressional Response." *American Politics Quarterly* 11 (1983): 441-458.

Holland, Kenneth M. "The Federal Rules of Civil Procedure." *Law and Policy Quarterly* 3 (1981): 209-224.

Howard, J. Woodford, Jr. "On the Fluidity of Judicial Choice." *American Political Science Review* 62 (1968): 43-57.

Jacob, Herbert. "The Effect of Institutional Differences in the Recruitment Process: The Case of State Judges." *Journal of Public Law* 13 (1964): 104-119.

Johnson, Charles A. "Judicial Decisions and Organizational Change: A Theory." *Administration and Society* 11 (1979): 27-51.

Kort, Fred. "Quantitative Analysis of Fact-Patterns in Cases and Their Impact on Judicial Decisions," pp. 330-334 in *American Court Systems*. Ed. Sheldon Goldman and Austin Sarat. San Francisco: Freeman, 1978.

Kuklinski, James H., and John E. Stanga. "Political Participation and Government Responsiveness: The Behavior of California Superior Courts." *American Political Science Review* 73 (1979): 1090-1099.

Lamb, Charles M. "Warren Burger and the Insanity Defense: Judicial Philosophy and Voting Behavior on a U.S. Court of Appeals." *American University Law Review* 24 (1974): 91-128.

Lawlor, Reed C. "Personal Stare Decisis." *Southern California Law Review* 41 (1967): 73-118.

Miller, Richard E., and Austin Sarat. "Grievances, Claims and Disputes: Assessing the Adversary Culture." *Law and Society Review* 15 (1980-1981): 525-566.

Murphy, Walter F. "Chief Justice Taft and the Lower Court Bureaucracy: A Study in Judicial Administration." *Journal of Politics* 24 (1962): 453-476.

Neiser, Eric. "The New Federal Discipline Act: Some Questions Congress Didn't Answer." *Judicature* 65 (1981): 142-160.

Newland, Chester A. "Press Coverage of the United States Supreme Court." *Western Political Quarterly* 17 (1964): 15-36.

Puro, Steven. "United States Magistrates: A New Federal Judicial Officer." *Justice System Journal* 2 (1976): 141-156.

Rohde, David W. "Policy Goals, Strategic Choice and Majority Opinion Assignments in the United States Supreme Court." *Midwest Journal of Political Science* 16 (1972): 652-682.

Rowland, C. K., and Robert A. Carp. "A Longitudinal Study of Party Effects on Federal District Court Policy Propensities." *American Journal of Political Science* 24 (1980): 291-305.

Rowland, C. K., Robert A. Carp, and Ronald Stidham. "Judges' Policy Choices and the Value Basis of Judicial Appointments: A Comparison of Support for Criminal Defendants among Nixon, Johnson, and Kennedy Appointees to the Federal District Courts." *Journal of Politics* 46 (1984): 886-902.

Rowland, C. K., Donald R. Songer, and Robert A. Carp. "Presidential Effects on Criminal Justice Policy in the Lower Federal Courts: The Reagan Judges." *Law and Society Review* 22 (1988): 191-200.

Schmidhauser, John R. "Judicial Behavior and the Sectional Crisis of 1837-1860." *Journal of Politics* 23 (1961): 615-640.

———. "The Justices of the Supreme Court: A Collective Portrait." *Midwest Journal of Political Science* 3 (1959): 1-57.

Schubert, Glendon. "Jackson's Judicial Philosophy: An Exploration in Value Analysis." *American Political Science Review* 59 (1965): 940-963.

Segal, Jeffrey A. "Supreme Court Justices as Human Decision Makers: An Individual-Level Analysis of the Search and Seizure Cases." *Journal of Politics* 48 (1986): 938-955.

Slotnick, Elliot E. "The Changing Role of the Senate Judiciary Committee in Judicial Selection." *Judicature* 62 (1979): 502-510.

_____. "The Chief Justice and Self-Assignment of Majority Opinions." *Western Political Quarterly* 31 (1978): 219-225.

_____. "Federal Appellate Judge Selection: Recruitment Changes and Unanswered Questions." *Justice System Journal* 6 (1981): 283-305.

_____. "Judicial Selection Systems and Nominations Outcomes: Does the Process Make a Difference?" *American Politics Quarterly* 12 (1984): 222-240.

_____. "The Paths to the Federal Bench: Gender, Race and Judicial Recruitment Variation." *Judicature* 67 (1984): 371-388.

_____. "Reforms in Judicial Selection: Will They Affect the Senate's Role? pt. 2." *Judicature* 64 (1980): 114-131.

_____. "Review Essay on Judicial Recruitment." *Justice System Journal* 13 (1988): 109-124.

_____. "Who Speaks for the Court? Majority Opinion Assignment from Taft to Burger." *American Journal of Political Science* 23 (1979): 60-77.

Songer, Donald R. "Concern for Policy Outputs as a Cue for Supreme Court Decisions on Certiorari." *Journal of Politics* 41 (1979): 1185-1194.

Stidham, Ronald, and Robert A. Carp. "Judges, Presidents, and Policy Choices: Exploring the Linkage." *Social Science Quarterly* 68 (1987): 395-404.

_____. "Trial Courts' Responses to Supreme Court Policy Changes: Three Case Studies." *Law and Policy Quarterly* 4 (1982): 215-235.

_____. "U.S. Trial Court Reactions to Changes in Civil Rights and Civil Liberties Policies." *Southeastern Political Review* 10 (1984): 3-27.

Stidham, Ronald, Robert A. Carp, and C. K. Rowland. "Patterns of Presidential Influence on the Federal District Courts: An Analysis of the Appointment Process." *Presidential Studies Quarterly* 14 (1984): 548-560.

_____. "Women's Rights Before the Federal District Courts, 1971-1977." *American Politics Quarterly* 11 (1983): 205-218.

Tanenhaus, Joseph. "The Cumulative Scaling of Judicial Decisions." *Harvard Law Review* 79 (1966): 1583-1594.

Tanenhaus, Joseph, et al. "The Supreme Court's Certiorari Jurisdiction: Cue Theory," pp. 111-132 in *Judicial Decision-Making*. Ed. Glendon Schubert. New York: Free Press, 1963.

Tate, C. Neal. "Personal Attribute Models of the Voting Behavior of U.S. Supreme Court Justices: Liberalism in Civil Liberties and Economic Decisions, 1946-1978." *American Political Science Review* 75 (1981): 355-367.

Ulmer, S. Sidney. "The Analysis of Behavior Patterns in the United States Supreme Court." *Journal of Politics* 22 (1960): 629-653.

_____. "Are Background Models Time-Bound?" *American Political Science Review* 80 (1986): 957-967.

_____. "The Decision to Grant Certiorari as an Indicator to Decision 'on the Merits.'" *Polity* 4 (1972): 429-447.

_____. "The Discriminant Function and a Theoretical Context for Its Use in Estimating the Votes of Judges," pp. 335-369 in *Frontiers of Judicial Research*.

Ed. Joel B. Grossman and Joseph Tanenhaus. New York: Wiley, 1969.

————. "Governmental Litigants, Underdogs, and Civil Liberties in the Supreme Court: 1903-1968 Terms." *Journal of Politics* 47 (1985): 899-909.

————. "The Political Party Variable in the Michigan Supreme Court." *Journal of Public Law* 11 (1962): 352-362.

————. "Selecting Cases for Supreme Court Review: An Underdog Model." *American Political Science Review* 72 (1978): 902-910.

————. "Supreme Court Behavior in Racial Exclusion Cases: 1935-1960." *American Political Science Review* 56 (1962): 325-330.

————. "Toward a Theory of Sub-Group Formation in the United States Supreme Court." *Journal of Politics* 27 (1965): 133-152.

Walker, Thomas, et al. "On the Mysterious Demise of Consensual Norms in the United States Supreme Court." *Journal of Politics* 50 (1988): 361-389.

Wasby, Stephen L. "The Communication of the Supreme Court's Criminal Procedure Decisions." *Villanova Law Review* 18 (1973): 1086-1118.

## Government Publications

*The Third Branch.* Washington, D.C.: Administrative Office of the United States Courts and the Federal Judicial Center. Monthly.

# Index

ABA. *See* American Bar Association
Abadinsky, Howard, 106-107, 199, 200
*Abington School District v. Schempp,* 353
Abortion
  decisions of courts, 44-45, 303-304, 308, 334, 336, 339, 348-349
  protests, 11, 348
Abraham, Henry J., 58, 132, 252, 253, 292
*Actus reus,* 142
Adamany, David W., 47, 57, 293
Adams, John, 22-23, 31, 40, 86
Administrative law, 5
Administrative Office Act of 1939, 64, 70
Administrative Office of the U.S. Courts, 39, 64-66
Advisory opinions
  of judges, 21-22, 121
  of state attorneys general, 96
*Alberts v. California,* 296
Alfini, James J., 200
Aliotta, Jilda M., 324
Alternative dispute resolution, 193-198
American Bar Association (ABA)
  philosophical orientation, 220
  in selection of judges, 205, 216, 220-221, 232
American Civil Liberties Union (ACLU), 104-105
American Jewish Congress, 104
American Revolution, 9
*Amicus curiae* briefs, 102, 104-105, 277, 340-341
Anarchists, 6-7
Anderson, James E., 352
Anticipatory socialization. *See* Social-ization of judges
Appellate court decisions, implementa-tion of
  communication of, 330-331

examples, 48-49, 280-281, 327-350
  influenced by Congress, 26, 283-285, 335-338
  influenced by lower courts, 26, 280-281, 327-335, 341, 345
  influenced by the president, 26, 283-285, 338-341
Appellate jurisdiction
  of state appeals courts, 50-52, 54, 117-118, 172-173
  of state supreme courts, 50-52, 54-55, 117-118, 298
  of U.S. appeals courts, 31-36, 112-113, 125, 172-173
  of U.S. Supreme Court, 27, 45, 113-117, 121, 125, 298
Appointments, judicial
  ideologically based, 19-20, 23, 219, 229-240, 338-340, 359-360
  recess, 217
Arbitration, 196-197
Armstrong, Scott, 83, 253, 322, 323, 351
Armstrong, Virginia C., 322
*Armstrong v. Board of Education of Birmingham,* 323
Arnold, Thurman, 145
Arraignment, 152
Arrests
  and discretion of police officers, 144-148, 346-347
  types of, 144-145
Articles of Confederation, 17-18
Ashman, Allan, 58
Assigned defense counsel, 97. *See also* Public defenders
Assistant U.S. attorneys, 92-93. *See also* U.S. attorneys
Atkins, Burton M., 323
Attitude theory and bloc-formation analysis, 315-319, 363
Attorneys
  contributions to state judicial cam-

Media
communication of court decisions,
31, 282-283, 319
influence on judicial selection and
judges, 232, 240, 280, 316
Mediation, 195-196
Mennonite Central Committee, 104
*Mens rea*, 142, 143
Merit selection of state judges, 60, 226,
227-228
Mexican-American Legal Defense and
Education Fund, 101
Miller, Arthur R., 82, 200
Miller, Richard E., 199
Miller, Samuel F., 305
*Miller v. California*, 295, 296
Minitrials, 198
Minton, Sherman, 236
*Miranda v. Arizona*, 56, 149, 173, 174,
175, 332, 333, 341-342, 346-347, 354
Misdemeanor (definition of), 136
Missouri Plan, 227-228
Mitchell, John, 221
Mize, Sidney, 260-261
Monitors, 342
*Moore v. U.S.*, 175
Moral Majority, 219
Moran, Tom, 175
Motion for directed verdict, 191
Motion to dismiss, 188
Motion to make more definite, 188
Motion to quash, 187
Motion to strike, 187-188
Muir, William, 353
Murphy, Frank, 242
Murphy, Walter F., 251, 252, 292, 322,
323, 351
*Muskrat v. United States*, 133

NAACP. *See* National Association for
the Advancement of Colored People
NAACP Legal Defense Fund, 101, 103
Nader, Ralph, 101
Nagel, Stuart S., 325
National Association for the Advance-
ment of Colored People (NAACP), 37,
101, 102
National Center for State Courts, 117-
118
National Committee for Amish Reli-
gious Freedom, 103

National Council of Churches of Christ
in the United States, 104
National Jewish Commission on Law
and Public Affairs, 104
*National Labor Relations Board v.
Jones and Laughlin Steel Corp.*, 56,
296
National Organization for Women, 101,
219
*Nectow v. City of Cambridge*, 199
Nelson, Jack, 252
Neubauer, David W., 58, 174
New Deal programs and court decisions, 24, 64, 233, 235, 317
New judges bills and presidential influence on courts, 231
New Judges Seminars, 67, 68, 243
New judicial federalism, 333-334
Nihan, Charles, 82
Nixon Richard M.
and the ABA, 220-221
appointment of Warren Burger, 25,
216
appointment strategy, 101, 232
courts of appeals appointments, 205-
207, 233, 234, 240
criticism of Warren Court, 25, 339
district court appointments, 202, 205,
233-234, 238, 240, 266, 340
liberalism of district court appointees, 237
rejection of Supreme Court nominees, 211, 222
school desegregation, 364-365
southern strategy, 272
Supreme Court appointments, 25,
211, 300
and tapes case, 306, 338
No-fault divorce, 182-183
*Nolle prosequi*, 154
*Nolo contendere*, 152
Nonpartisan election of state judges,
226-227
Norm enforcement by courts, 25-27,
35-38, 42-44, 287-290, 327-328, 357-
358
*Northern Pipeline Construction Co. v.
Marathon Pipe Line Company*, 57

Oakley, John Bilyeu, 83
O'Brien, David M., 83, 323

# PRESS

A Division of Congressional Quarterly Inc.

Designed as a primary text for courses in judicial process and behavior, *Judicial Process in America* provides a lucid, comprehensive study of the complex environment in which the American judiciary functions. In this examination of federal, state, civil, and criminal courts, the authors contend that judges' decisions today play a powerful role in shaping public policy and that the courts themselves are strongly influenced by other institutions and forces. The text offers a thorough, balanced look at the procedural and human variables that affect the judicial process. Carp and Stidham draw on observations from historians, psychologists, court administrators, and journalists to complement the core research of political scientists and legal scholars.

*Judicial Process in America* assesses major changes and trends in the courts, including the behavior of individual judges versus those in a collegial setting, the impact of the Reagan era on the judiciary, and possible influences on President Bush's court appointments. This blend of traditional scholarship with tenets of modern behaviorism gives students a solid understanding of the factors that guide judges to decisions affecting our daily lives.

Robert A. Carp is associate dean at the University of Houston. He is coauthor of *Policymaking and Politics in the Federal District Courts* (1983) and, with Ronald Stidham, of *The Federal Courts* (CQ Press, 1985). He has published numerous articles on the judicial process and judicial behavior in both political science and law journals.

Ronald Stidham is an associate professor of political science at Lamar University. The federal district courts are his major research interest; his articles have appeared in the *Journal of Politics* and *American Politics Quarterly*.

ISBN 0-87187-485-7